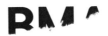

Color Atlas of Oral Diseases

Diagnosis and Treatment

Fourth Edition

George Laskaris, MD, DDS, PhD
Associate Professor of Oral Medicine
Medical School
University of Athens
Athens, Greece
Former Consultant of Oral Medicine
Department of Dermatology
"A. Sygros" Hospital
Athens, Greece
Visiting Professor
University of London
London, England

1003 illustrations

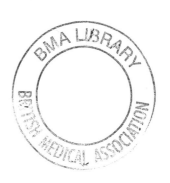
Thieme
Stuttgart • New York • Delhi • Rio de Janeiro

Library of Congress Cataloging-in-Publication Data

Names: Laskaris, George, author.
Title: Color atlas of oral diseases : diagnosis and treatment / George Laskaris.
Description: Fourth edition. | Stuttgart ; New York : Thieme, [2017] | Includes bibliographical references and index. |
Identifiers: LCCN 2017018592 (print) | LCCN 2017019890 (ebook) | ISBN 9783131647542 (ebook) | ISBN 9783137170044 (hardcover) |
Subjects: | MESH: Mouth Diseases | Atlases
Classification: LCC RC815 (ebook) | LCC RC815 (print) | NLM WU 17 | DDC 617.5/2200222--dc23
LC record available at https://lccn.loc.gov/2017018592

© 2017 Georg Thieme Verlag KG,

Thieme Publishers Stuttgart
Rüdigerstrasse 14, 70469 Stuttgart, Germany
+49 [0]711 8931 421, http://www.thieme.de

Thieme Publishers New York
333 Seventh Avenue, New York, NY 10001 USA
+1 800 782 3488, http://www.thieme.com

Thieme Publishers Delhi
A-12, Second Floor, Sector-2, Noida-201301
Uttar Pradesh, India
+91 120 45 566 00, customerservice@thieme.in

Thieme Publishers Rio, Thieme Publicações Ltda.
Edifício Rodolpho de Paoli, 25º andar
Av. Nilo Peçanha, 50 - Sala 2508
Rio de Janeiro 20020-906 Brasil
+55 21 3172 2297 / +55 21 3172 1896

Cover design: Thieme Publishing Group
Typesetting by DiTech Process Solutions Pvt. Ltd., India

Printed in India by Replika Press Pvt. Ltd.   5 4 3 2 1

ISBN 978-3-13-717004-4

Also available as an e-book:
eISBN 978-3-13-164754-2

Important Note: Medicine is an ever-changing science undergoing continual development. Research and clinical experience are continually expanding our knowledge, in particular our knowledge of proper treatment and drug therapy. Insofar as this book mentions any dosage or application, readers may rest assured that the authors, editors, and publishers have made every effort to ensure that such references are in accordance with **the state of knowledge at the time of production of the book.**

Nevertheless, this does not involve, imply, or express any guarantee or responsibility on the part of the publishers with respect of any dosage instructions and forms of application stated in the book. **Every user is requested to examine carefully** the manufacturer's leaflets accompanying each drug and to check, if necessary in consultation with a physician or specialist, whether the dosage schedules mentioned therein or the contraindications stated by the manufacturer differ from the statements made in the present book. Such examination is particularly important with drugs that are either rarely used or have been newly released on the market. Every dosage schedule or every form of application used is entirely at the user's risk and responsibility. The authors and publishers request every user to report to the publishers any discrepancies or inaccuracies noticed.

Some of the product names, patents, and registered designs referred to in this book are in fact registered trademarks or proprietary names, even though specific reference to this fact is not always made in the text. Therefore, the appearance of a name without a designation as proprietary is not to be construed as a representation by the publisher that it is in the public domain.

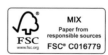

*This book is dedicated to my sweetest son **Christos G. Laskaris**, whose memory continues to inspire and give me the strength to create, love, and offer.*

*To my wife **Vivi**, constant and unique partner to any step along the family, social, and scientific way.*

*To my daughters, **Christina** and **Marina,** as a small indication of reward for their love.*

Nikon Medical Camera

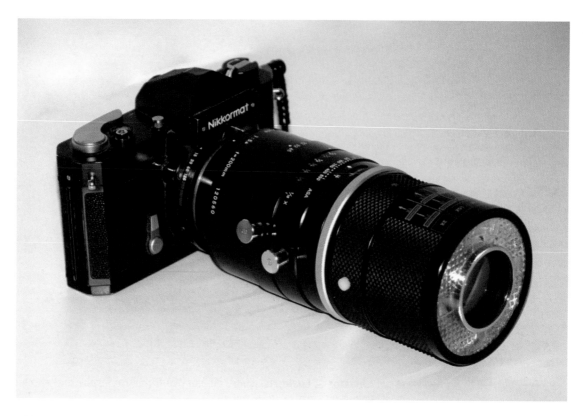

This camera has been an irreplaceable technological instrument, which, for 43 years, has helped me impress in color photographs, accurately, a great variety of oral and skin diseases in thousands of patients.

Contents

35. Reactive Tumors 536

36. Nonneoplastic Lesions of the Salivary Glands 542

37. Potentially Malignant Disorders 554

38. Potentially Malignant Disorders 562

39. Malignant Neoplasms 568

Foreword

It is a pleasure and privilege for me to write the foreword to the new English edition of Professor Laskaris' *Color Atlas of Oral Diseases*. This work reflects the vast experience and expertise that Professor Laskaris has gained in clinical practice and research during his professional life spanning over 40 years.

Since the publication of the first edition of the atlas, there have continued to be immense social and medical changes across the globe that have led to a substantial increase in the number of individuals with diseases that require intervention by specialists in oral medicine. For example, HIV disease led to many affected persons developing a wide range of oral disorders, including oral hairy leukoplakia and Kaposi's sarcoma that oral specialists had never encountered previously, and while now becoming less frequent (in view of the widening availability of antiretroviral therapy), they are also now recognized as complications of iatrogenic immunosuppression. Life expectancy has continued to improve, and with this there are many more patients than in the past developing the oral consequences of immunologically mediated disease, oral and other malignancy, and paraneoplastic disease. Similarly, as early life health care improves, so the number of children and adults with complex genetically based orofacial disease increases, while at the same time the widening availability of novel agents of systemic disease (e.g., disease-modifying biologicals, other immunotherapies, and antiretrovirals among others) has led to an increase in the frequency and spectrum of disorders of the oral mucosa and salivary glands.

All of these, and many other, changes in oral disease and the need for appropriate treatment are reflected in the contents of Professor Laskaris' book. This is not merely an atlas providing excellent clinical examples of common (as well as uncommon, rare, and very rare!) diseases, but a book that provides synopses that are of significant benefit to both the nonspecialist and specialist to safely and effectively manage patients with diseases that can greatly lessen their quality of life. Professor Laskaris is to be commended on his discipline of securing such high-quality images of diseases and industry in writing such an informative and practically useful text.

This is an important and essential book for the practice of oral medicine across the globe.

Professor Stephen Porter, MD, PhD, FDSRCS (Eng)
Institute Director and Professor of Oral Medicine
UCL Eastman Dental Institute
London, UK

Preface

Oral medicine is a demanding clinical specialty. Beyond possessing adequate theoretical knowledge, the oral physician (stomatologist) must be a keen and diligent observer and an astute clinician with extensive outpatient and inpatient experience. The visual approach is the most powerful tool at the disposal of the oral physician. Acquisition of the skill to "see" lesions in a particular way requires extensive and intensive clinical training and is rewarded with a high degree of diagnostic accuracy. To this effect, I felt that the format of juxtaposition of text and pictures is ideal and was chosen for the presentation of the subject matter of this text.

Twenty-nine years have elapsed since the first edition and 3 years since the third edition of this book were published in Greek, and the impact was beyond the wildest expectation.

The three English editions that followed were embraced by the international community and had an impressive track record. The numerous favorable comments by international leaders in the field of oral medicine and reviews in the most prestigious specialty journals, where the reviewers ranked this book among the standard texts forming the canon of the specialty, are cherished rewards to the author.

The tally so far is three editions in Greek, four editions in English, translations into seven more languages, and Greek and international prizes. This fourth English edition contains the distillation of my experience and service at the Medical School, University of Athens, Department of Dermatology, "A. Sygros" Hospital and other major hospitals of the city as well as in my private practice.

This new edition has been entirely rewritten and adapted to contemporary publishing and scientific demands.

Numerous changes and additions have been made. Ten new chapters, enriched with many new clinical entities, have been added. The pictorial material has been renewed and enriched at a level of over 90% with high-standard color pictures from the 130,000 pictures and slides comprising my personal collection.

The structure of the text has changed. In the beginning of the book, rules for the diagnostic and therapeutic approach to the patient with oral disease have been codified. For every disease entity, the basic characteristics (key points) and the differential diagnosis are presented in boxes. The clinical description is precise, followed by clear, representative pictures. The histopathologic findings and the rest of the laboratory tests are then presented, followed by the therapeutic strategies in detail. At the end of the book, there is an appendix with tables of differential diagnosis of oral lesions classified according to morphology and color, and with tables presenting the performance of biopsy and interpretation of the histopathologic findings. These changes will provide the reader with a concise, comprehensive, and reliable book. Furthermore, students of medicine and dentistry can acquire basic and up-to-date knowledge, which, in combination with the rich pictorial material, provides an excellent introduction to clinical oral medicine. Finally, I hope that the book will be a useful diagnostic and therapeutic tool in the medical practice of oral medicine specialists, dentists, otorhinolaryngologists, dermatologists, pediatricians, and internists.

George Laskaris, MD, DDS, PhD

Acknowledgments

Creating a scientific book requires discipline and is a lonely journey during which you come closer to people who will contribute in their own different ways. Therefore, I would like to thank the following individuals.

First of all, I wish to acknowledge the important contribution of **Dr. Annie Argyriades Porter**, specialist in special care dentistry, for her initial excellent translation of the Greek text to English. There is no doubt that without her help it would have been difficult for me to complete this book.

My special thanks also go to **Dr. Stephen Porter**, Professor of Oral Medicine, University of London, for the final editing and the foreword of the book.

To **Dr. Christos Kittas,** Professor of Pathology, Medical School, University of Athens, I owe special recognition for over 40 years of scientific collaboration and the useful suggestions in the pathology part of this book.

Many thanks to **Dr. Eleana Stoufi, Dr. Marina Doukas,** and **Dr. Eleni Georgakopoulos,** my collaborators in oral medicine, for their constant help during this project.

Finally, my thanks go to the staff of Thieme Publishers for the excellent professional commitment they have shown.

The following figures were sourced from the collection of the colleagues listed below and who I thank greatly.

Dr. G. Goumenos for figs. 11.4, 11.26; Prof. A. Katsabas for fig. 30.17; Prof. I. Iatrou for fig. 42.7; Prof. A. Katsarou for figs. 25.18, 25.19, 25.20; Dr. A. Panagiotopoulos for fig. 28.9; Prof. N. Papadogeorgakis for fig. 39.57; Dr. Ahsan A. (India) for figs. 2.5, 30.9, 43.4; Prof. Almeida O. (Brazil) for figs. 19.19, 19.20; Profs. Blozis G. and Neiders M. (USA) for figs. 25.91, 25.92; Dr. Ribeiro (Brazil) for fig. 20.4; Prof. Carozzo M. (England) for fig. 25.45; Dr. Delgando-Azanero W. (Peru) for figs. 18.25, 20.6; Dr. Glick M. (USA) for fig. 17.33; Drs. Romero de Leon and Aguirre A. (USA) for fig. 20.5; Prof. Scully C. (England) for figs. 25.93, 27.27, 31.8; Prof. Shklar G. (USA) for figs. 5.10, 5.11, 31.9.

Introduction to Oral Medicine

Diagnostic and Therapeutic Approach

This brief introduction offers codified information that a practicing oral physician (stomatologist) must implement in order to successfully overcome diagnostic and therapeutic dilemmas. Oral medicine is an important subspecialty of general internal medicine. A specialist in oral diseases is required to possess a certain level of clinical and laboratory expertise in medicine and dentistry along with clinical experience. These will allow the practitioner to negotiate with diagnostic and therapeutic challenges successfully.

The training framework of the specialist in oral medicine includes internal medicine, dermatology, otorhinolaryngology, pediatrics, clinical pharmacology, therapeutics, histopathology, and others.

The mouth and the structures within the oral cavity offer significant clinical advantages: (1) It is a cavity readily accessible for inspection and palpation, (2) it is easy to be biopsied, (3) it is repeatedly examined because dental and gingival problems are common, thereby necessitating repeated visits to the dentist, and (4) it is readily accessible for self-examination. On the other hand, the oral cavity also offers many diagnostic difficulties due to the following factors: (1) A plethora of local and systemic diseases with morphologically similar lesions manifest in the mouth, and (2) local factors, such as saliva, dentures, foodstuffs, and the mechanical action of the teeth themselves may alter the appearance of the elementary lesion. The clinical diagnostic methodology follows fundamental principles that we must adhere to in order to arrive at a correct diagnosis. These principles are summarized in **Table I.1**. Laboratory tests follow the clinical evaluation. The laboratory is an aid and not a substitute for sound clinical methodology. Clinicians should be familiar with laboratory errors and the disorientation that they may cause in the diagnostic process. Thus, it is a basic principle of practice that laboratory results are always evaluated by the clinician in relation to the clinical presentation of the disease.

A correct decision for therapy is based on a correct diagnosis. The rules and parameters that must be followed in implementing appropriate therapy are summarized in **Table I.1**. In cases of therapeutic failure, provided all the rules and guidelines have been followed, the clinician must revise the diagnostic hypothesis and investigate other alternatives.

The reader of this book is encouraged to study the cited bibliography at the end of this Introduction for additional information on oral medicine, pathology, dermatology, internal medicine, immunology, and therapeutics that were used by the author in this book as basic, classic reference material.

Table I.1 Diagnostic and therapeutic approach

I. Diagnosis

- Complete history and physical examination
- Evaluation of oral lesions
- Examination and evaluation of skin and mucosal lesions elsewhere in the body
- Evaluation of symptoms and signs in other systems
- Intake of medications prior to the beginning of the disease
- Grouping of disease entities according to clinical criteria
- Reevaluation of symptoms and signs in cases where the diagnosis is doubtful
- Consultation with the family physician if necessary
- Performance of biopsy on the basis of clinical indications
- Histopathologic examination by an experienced pathologist
- Evaluation of pathology report by the clinician, in relation to the symptoms and signs of the patient
- Repeat biopsy if in doubt
- Further laboratory evaluation if clinically indicated
- Is the diagnosis correct
- Reevaluation of the patient after initiation of therapy

II. Differential diagnosis

- Initiation of symptoms and signs
- Duration (acute–subacute–chronic course)
- General symptoms (fever, pain, malaise, anorexia, weight loss, arthralgias)
- Lesion morphology (macules, papules, blisters, bullae, pustules, plaques, nodules)
- Color of the lesions (white, red, black, brown, yellow)
- Location (tongue, buccal mucosa, palate, floor of the mouth, gingiva, lips)
- Coexisting skin lesions, mucosal lesions
- Biopsy and histopathologic examination
- Laboratory work-up (microbiology, immunology, hematology, imaging studies, molecular studies)

III. Therapy

- Choice of the right medication
- Administration of the medication in the right form (pills, injections, ointments)
- Exact dosage and dosage schedule
- Consideration of clinical pharmacology issues, such as interaction between the administered drug and other medications that the patient is taking
- Extreme care concerning contraindications for the drug that we intend to administer
- Side effects due to our therapy
- Adherence to the therapeutic program
- Evaluation of the therapeutic result 2–4 days after initiation of therapy
- In case of therapeutic failure, reevaluation of the diagnostic hypothesis
- It is a general principle that correct therapy presupposes correct diagnosis

Textbooks—Basic References

Bolognia JL, Jorizzo JL, Rapini RP. Dermatology. 2nd ed. Philadelphia, PA: Saunders; 2012

Bradley P, Guntinas-Lichius O. Salivary Gland Disorders and Diseases: Diagnosis and Management. Stuttgart, Germany: Thieme Verlag; 2011

Chan LS. Blistering Skin Diseases. London, UK: Manson Publishing; 2009

Fletcher CDM. Diagnostic Histopathologic of Tumors. 4th ed. Philadelphia, PA: Elsevier; 2013

Goldsmith LA, Katz SI, Gilchrest BA, et al. Dermatology in General Medicine. 8th ed. New York, NY: McGraw-Hill; 2012

Greer JP, Arber D, Glader B, et al. Wintrobe's Clinical Hematology. 13th ed. Philadelphia, PA: Lippincott Williams and Wilkins; 2013

James JD, Berger TG, Elston DM. Andrew's Diseases of the Skin: Clinical Dermatology. 12th ed. Philadelphia, PA: Elsevier; 2015

Kumar P, Clark M. Clinical Medicine. 8th ed. Philadelphia, PA: W.B.Saunders; 2012

Laskaris G, Scully C. Periodontal Manifestations of Local and Systemic Diseases. Berlin, Germany: Springer; 2003

Laskaris G. Clinical Stomatology (in Greek). Athens, GR: Listas Publications; 2012

Laskaris G. Color Atlas of Oral Diseases. 3rd ed. Stuttgart, Germany: Thieme Verlag; 2003

Laskaris G. Oral Diseases in Children and Adolescents. Stuttgart, Germany: Thieme Verlag; 2000

Laskaris G. Treatment of Oral Diseases. Stuttgart, Germany: Thieme Verlag; 2005

Neville BW, Damm DD, Allen CM, Chi AC. Oral and Maxillofacial Pathology. 4th ed. St. Louis, Missouri: Elsevier; 2015

Papadakis MA, McPhee SJ. Current Medical Diagnosis and Treatment. New York, NY: McGraw-Hill; 2016

Spitz JL. Genodermatoses: A Clinical Guide to Genetic Skin Disorders. 2nd ed. Philadelphia, PA: Lippincott Williams and Wilkins; 2004

Walker BR, College NB, Ralston SH, Penman IPN. Davidson's Principles and Practice of Medicine. 22nd ed. Philadelphia, PA: Churchill Livingstone; 2014

1 Normal Mucosal Variants

Leukoedema

Key points
- Common normal variation of the oral mucosa.
- It is more frequent in black-skinned people than in whites.
- Leukoedema usually occurs on the buccal mucosa, frequently bilaterally and rarely on the lateral border of the tongue and the mucosal surface of the lips.
- The diagnosis is based on the clinical features.

Introduction

Leukoedema is a common normal oral mucosal variant due to increased thickness of the epithelium and intracellular edema of the spinous layer cells. A similar clinical pattern may be seen at the mucosa of the larynx and the vagina. It occurs more frequently in black-skinned people, with a prevalence ranging between 70 and 90%. In contrast, the prevalence rate in whites is much less.

Clinical features

As a rule, leukoedema occurs bilaterally and involves most often the buccal mucosa and rarely the lateral border of the tongue (**Figs. 1.1**, **1.2**). Clinically, the oral mucosa presents as opalescent or grayish-white with slight wrinkling, which characteristically disappears if the mucosa is distended, by pulling or stretching the cheek. Leukoedema has a normal consistency on palpation.

The disorder is usually discovered as an incidental finding by the patient or during a routine oral examination by the dentist. The diagnosis is based exclusively on the clinical features.

Differential diagnosis
- Chronic biting
- Pseudomembranous candidiasis
- Lichen planus
- Leukoplakia
- Cinnamon contact stomatitis
- White sponge nevus
- Hereditary benign intraepithelial dyskeratosis

Pathology

It is not necessary. On histologic examination, leukoedema demonstrates thickness of the epithelium, increased parakeratosis, and acanthosis with broad and elongated rete ridges. Characteristically, the cells of the spinous layer are large with small pyknotic nuclei due to marked intracellular edema.

Treatment

No treatment is necessary.

Racial Pigmentation

Key points
- Physiologic findings due to increased melanin production.
- The pigmentation is more common in black-skinned people and in dark-skinned whites.
- The gingiva and the buccal mucosa are the most frequently affected areas.
- The disorder is asymptomatic and benign.

Introduction

Melanin is a normal skin and oral mucosal pigment produced by melanocytes. Increased melanin deposition in the oral mucosa may occur in various diseases. Dark discoloration may often be a normal finding in black- and dark-skinned people.

Clinical features

In healthy people there may be clinically asymptomatic black or brown areas of varying size and distribution in the oral mucosa, usually on the gingiva, buccal mucosa, palate and less often on the tongue, floor of the mouth, and the lips (**Fig. 1.3**). The pigmentation is more prominent in areas of pressure or friction and becomes more intense with aging. A biopsy may be justified if the clinical features are atypical, causing a diagnostic dilemma.

Differential diagnosis
- Smoking-associated melanosis
- Pigmentation due to drugs
- Freckles
- Lentigo simplex
- Lentigo maligna
- Pigmented nevi
- Melanoma
- Addison's disease
- Peutz-Jeghers syndrome
- Albright's syndrome
- Amalgam tattoo

Pathology

Histologically, increased melanin production is observed while the number of melanocytes is normal. The overlying epithelium is normal.

Treatment

No treatment is required.

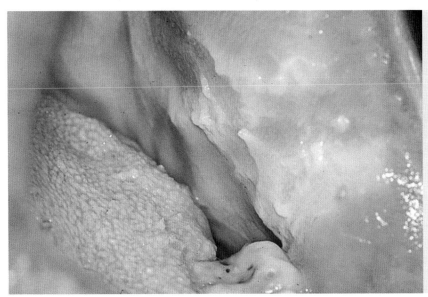

Fig. 1.1 Leukoedema of the buccal mucosa.

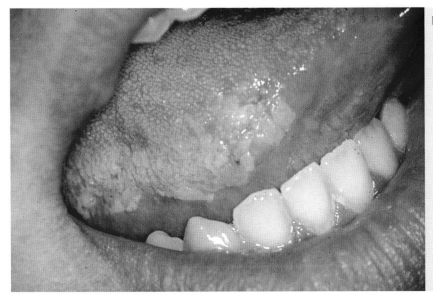

Fig. 1.2 Leukoedema of the tongue.

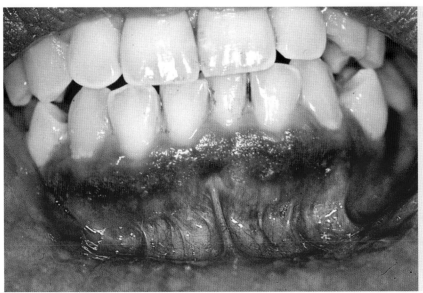

Fig. 1.3 Normal pigmentation of the gingiva.

Linea Alba

Key points

- Linea alba is a common alteration of the buccal mucosa, and is usually bilateral.
- It is located on the buccal mucosa at the level of the occlusal line, usually behind the premolars.
- Mechanical pressure or irritation from the buccal surface of the teeth is the etiologic factor.

Introduction

Linea alba is a relatively common linear elevation of the buccal mucosa, extending from the corner of the mouth to the third molar, at the occlusal line. It is more prominent along the premolar and molar teeth. Usually, it is associated with mechanical irritation or sucking from the buccal surfaces of the teeth. The change is more prominent around occlusal defects.

Clinical features

Clinically, linea alba presents as unilateral or usually bilateral linear elevation of normal or slightly whitish color and normal consistency on palpation (**Fig. 1.4**). Occasionally, it may be scalloped and characteristically it appears on the buccal mucosa along the occlusal level. Linea alba varies in prominence and can be more frequent in obese people. The diagnosis is based exclusively on the clinical features.

Differential diagnosis

- Chronic biting
- Leukoplakia
- Candidiasis
- Cinnamon contact stomatitis
- Leukoedema

Pathology

It is not needed. On histologic examination, the epithelium is normal with slight hyperorthokeratosis and intracellular edema of the spinous cells.

Treatment

No treatment is required.

Fordyce's Granules

Key points

- Fordyce's granules represent a normal anatomical variation characterized by collection of sebaceous glands in the oral mucosa.
- They occur in approximately 70 to 80% of the population.
- The upper lip, commissures, buccal mucosa, and retromolar area are most frequently affected.
- The diagnosis is based on the clinical features.

Introduction

Fordyce's granules are ectopic sebaceous glands in the oral mucosa which are functionally inactive. A similar pattern may be seen on the genital mucosa. They are a frequent oral finding that occurs in approximately 70 to 80% of population, in both sexes. With aging, the granules may become more prominent as a result of moving toward the mucosal surface.

Clinical features

Clinically, Fordyce's granules appear as multiple small, slightly raised whitish-yellow, well-circumscribed spots that rarely coalesce to form plaques (**Figs. 1.5**, **1.6**). They most often occur in the mucosal surface of the upper lip, commissures, buccal mucosa adjacent to the molars, and the retromolar region, in a symmetrical bilateral pattern. The majority of the patients have multiple lesions while some may have only a few. Characteristically, the granules become more evident when the mucosa is stretched. They are asymptomatic and the diagnosis is usually made during a routine oral examination or incidentally by the patients.

Differential diagnosis

- Lichen planus
- Candidiasis
- Leukoplakia

Pathology

It is not necessary. On histologic examination, multiple, well-formed, ectopic sebaceous glands, without hair follicles, can be seen in the superficial part of the connective tissue.

Treatment

No treatment is required as Fordyce's granules represent a normal anatomical variation of the oral mucosa.

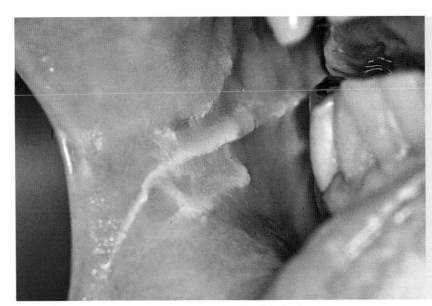

Fig. 1.4 Linea alba.

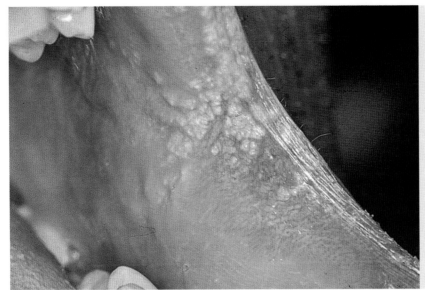

Fig. 1.5 Fordyce's granules in the buccal mucosa.

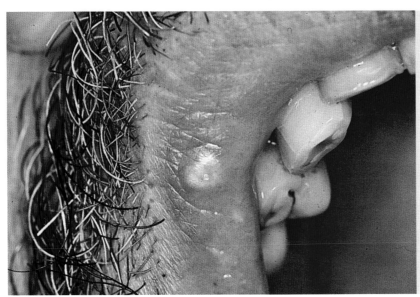

Fig. 1.6 Sizeable Fordyce's granule of the upper lip.

2 Developmental Defects

Orofacial Clefts

The fetal development of the face and the oral cavity is a marvelous multilateral and complicated procedure which results in the formation of the most exceptional part of the human body, the face. Every derangement of the formation and the completion of the tissues can cause disorders in the facial region, the facial clefts.

Types of facial clefts
- Cleft lip
- Cleft palate
- Cleft maxilla/mandible
- Bifid uvula
- Medium upper lip cleft
- Oblique facial cleft

Causes of cleft formation
- Genetic
- Environmental
- Smoking during pregnancy
- Alcohol abuse during pregnancy
- Medication during pregnancy
- Malnutrition and vitamin deficiency

Cleft Lip

Key points
- The most common cleft.
- It can be solitary or part of a syndrome.
- Often coexists with palatal cleft.
- It causes esthetic defect.

Introduction

Cleft lip is a derangement of the development which mainly involves the upper lip and very rarely the lower lip. It can present as a solitary disorder or as part of a genetic syndrome.

Clinical features

A unilateral or more rarely bilateral deficit on the lip with higher frequency on the left side is observed (**Fig. 2.1**). It occurs more often in males than females. It is usually combined with palatal or maxillary cleft. It has been estimated that the incidence of cleft lip is 1 per 9,000 births and in combination with palatal malformation it is 1 per 1,000 births. Usually, the defect is unilateral and it causes esthetic and functional deficit.

Treatment

Plastic reconstructive surgery.

Cleft Palate

Key points
- A common cleft.
- In several cases it coexists with maxillary and lip cleft.
- Many times it is part of genetic syndromes.
- It causes functional defects.

Introduction

The cleft palate is a developmental derangement caused by the failure to fuse the two embryonic palatal processes. The cleft palate often coexists with maxillary and lip cleft. The incidence of cleft palate alone varies from 0.29 to 0.56 per 1,000 births.

Clinical features

The deficit is located on the hard palate alone or on both hard and soft palates (**Figs. 2.2, 2.3**). In major cases functional and psychological problems may occur. Bifid uvula represents a minor expression of the cleft palate and may be seen alone or in combination with more severe malformations (**Fig. 2.4**).

Treatment

Early surgical treatment is recommended. The role of the orthodontist and the prosthodontist is pivotal for the functional restoration of the deficit.

Oblique Facial Cleft

Key points
- A rare form of cleft.
- It extends from the upper lip to the ocular orbit.
- The disorder causes major esthetic and functional defects.
- Often combined with palatal and labial cleft.

Introduction

Oblique facial cleft is a sporadic, exceedingly rare form of cleft. The incidence is 1 case per 1,300 facial clefts. The disorder is nearly always associated with cleft lip and palate. Occasionally it is incompatible with life.

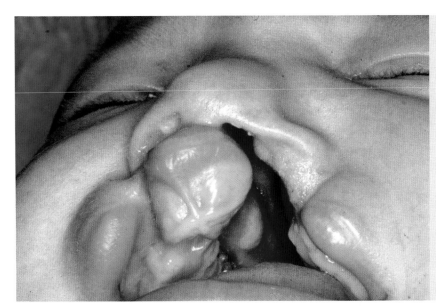

Fig. 2.1 Cleft lip and palate.

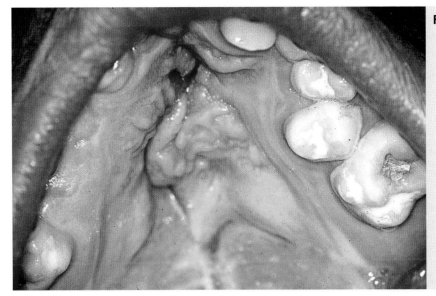

Fig. 2.2 Cleft palate.

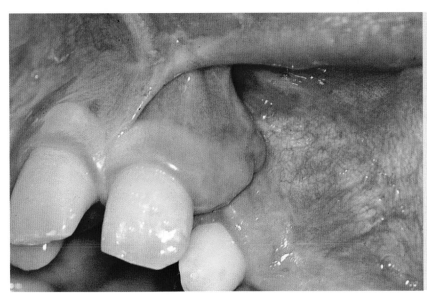

Fig. 2.3 Cleft maxilla.

Clinical features

Oblique facial cleft may extend through the upper lip to the nose to involve the eye (oro-ocular type) (**Fig. 2.5**). In 20 to 30% of the cases it is bilateral. It may coexist with other developmental malformations such as facial asymmetry, ocular and nasal abnormalities.

Treatment

Plastic reconstructive surgery.

Oral Hair

Key points

- Hair and hair follicles are extremely rare on the oral mucosa.
- Few cases have been reported, all in whites.
- Oral hair may offer an explanation of oral keratoacanthoma.

Introduction

Original hair and hair follicles are a very unusual phenomenon within the oral tissues. Only seven cases have been reported in the literature by 2015. All the reported cases have been registered in whites. There is no satisfactory explanation for the occurrence of oral hair although a developmental anomaly is the most possible cause.

Clinical features

Clinically, oral hair presents as a single, asymptomatic black hair of 0.3 to 3.5 cm in length, usually surrounded by a whitish mucosa (**Fig. 2.6**). Occasionally, the lesion may cause minor problems during kissing. The presence of oral hair may result in psychological problems and the patients can be quite anxious to solve the problem. The tongue, gingival and buccal mucosa are the most frequently affected sites. The presence of oral hair and follicles may offer an explanation for the rare occurrence of keratoacanthoma intraorally. The diagnosis of oral hair is based on the clinical features, but it can be confirmed by a biopsy.

Differential diagnosis

- Skin graft with hair
- Implantation of hair to the oral mucosa following an accident

Pathology

On histologic examination, hair follicles in the lamina propria are observed, associated with several sebaceous glands.

Treatment

Conservative surgical excision is the treatment of choice.

Congenital Lip Pits

Key points

- A rare developmental malformation.
- Occasionally, it may be associated with cleft lip and/or cleft palate.
- It usually occurs on the lower lip.
- The diagnosis is based on the clinical features.

Introduction

Congenital lip pits are relatively rare developmental invaginations that occur exclusively on the lower lip. They originate from persistent lateral sulci, on the embryonic mandibular arch. The malformation may occur alone or in combination with commissural pits, cleft lip, and/or cleft palate. Congenital lip pits are frequently inherited as an autosomal dominant trait.

Clinical features

Clinically, congenital lip pits present as bilateral, asymptomatic, and symmetric depressions in the middle of the vermilion border of the lower lip (**Fig. 2.7**). A small amount of mucous may accumulate at the deep aspect of the pit which is blind and may vary in size from 0.2 to 1 cm. The lip may be enlarged and swollen, but the defect is not associated with pain. The diagnosis is based on the clinical features and the history.

Differential diagnosis

- Mechanical trauma
- Surgical deformity
- van der Woude syndrome
- Other rare syndromes

Pathology

It is not usually required. On histologic examination, a sulcus lined by normal epithelium may be seen. A mild chronic inflammation by plasma cells and leukocytes is a common finding. In addition, minor salivary glands may communicate with the pits.

Treatment

Treatment of choice is reconstructive surgical repair of the irregularity for aesthetic purposes.

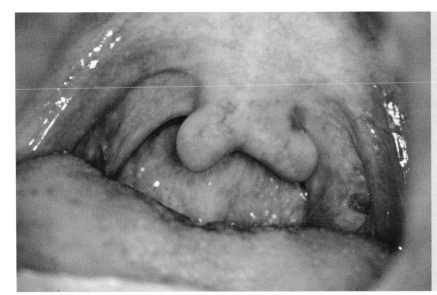

Fig. 2.4 Bifid uvula.

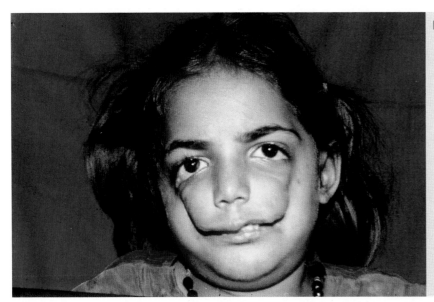

Fig. 2.5 Oblique facial cleft.

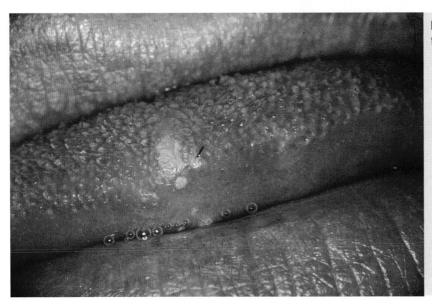

Fig. 2.6 Black hair with accessories on the tip of the tongue.

Commissural Lip Pits

Key points
- A relatively common developmental invagination that characteristically occurs at the corners of the mouth.
- Very rarely, the disorder may be associated with other orofacial defects.
- The diagnosis is based on the clinical features.

Introduction

Commissural lip pits are a developmental invagination due to failure of normal fusion of the embryonal mandibular and maxillary processes. Occasionally, an autosomal dominant trait has been recorded. They appear to be more common in adult men and are not obvious during childhood. Usually, the disorder is not associated with other orofacial defects.

Clinical features

Clinically, commissural lip pits usually present as bilateral small blind asymptomatic fistulas 1 to 3 mm in depth. Characteristically, the pits develop at the corner of the vermilion border of the lips (**Fig. 2.8**). Occasionally, small amount of mucous may accumulate at the deep aspect of the pits which becomes evident after squeezing its base. The diagnosis is based exclusively on the clinical features.

Differential diagnosis
- Mechanical trauma
- Surgical deformity

Pathology

It is not required. On histologic examination a small invagination lined by normal epithelium is the common feature. Usually, ducts from minor salivary glands may drain into the invaginated epithelium.

Treatment

No treatment is required. In rare cases where the pits may cause mild topical problems, reconstructive surgery is recommended.

Ankyloglossia

Key points
- A developmental malformation of the tongue.
- Ankyloglossia may occasionally cause speech defects or gingival recession, which may lead to periodontal disease.
- The diagnosis is based on clinical criteria and is frequently incidental.

Introduction

Ankyloglossia or tongue-tie is a rare developmental malformation characterized by a short and thick lingual frenum leading to limitation of tongue movement. Most often the anomaly is the result of fusion and attachment of the lingual frenum to the floor of the mouth or the alveolar mucosa. In other cases the short lingual frenum stems from the tip of the tongue.

Clinical features

Clinically, the lingual frenum is short and usually thick and inelastic (**Fig. 2.9**). Occasionally, it can be thin and short, extending from the floor of the mouth or the alveolar mucosa to the tip of the tongue. In severe cases the tongue is tied down with limited movement. In such cases it may lead to speech difficulties. However, in the majority of the cases the functional problems are minor or absent. Short and thick frenum of the lips may also occur (**Fig. 2.10**). The diagnosis is based on the clinical features.

Pathology

It is not required.

Treatment

In most cases treatment is not required. In severe cases, with speech and swallowing problems, frenectomy (surgical clipping of the lingual frenum) will correct the problems.

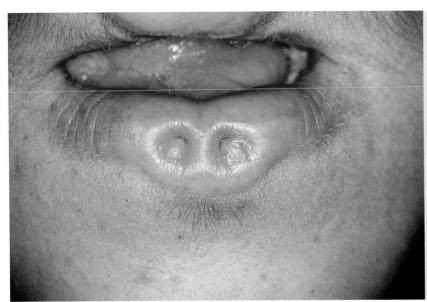

Fig. 2.7 Congenital lip pits.

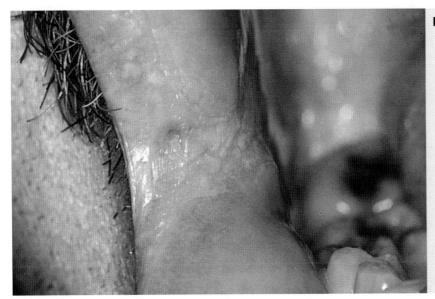

Fig. 2.8 Congenital commissural pits.

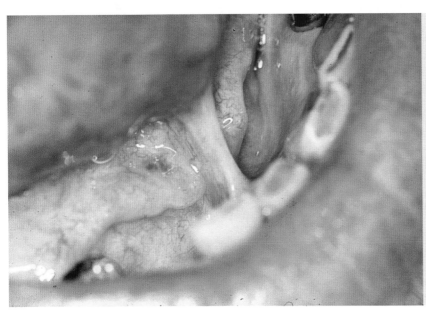

Fig. 2.9 Ankyloglossia.

Bifid Tongue

Key points
- A rare developmental malformation.
- It may be in complete or incomplete form.
- The lesion is usually asymptomatic.

Introduction

Bifid tongue is a rare developmental anomaly that may appear in *complete* or *incomplete* form. It may develop as an isolated defect, coexist with the oro-facial-digital syndrome or occur as a complication of tongue piercing.

Clinical features

Clinically, the incomplete form of bifid tongue manifests as a deep furrow along the midline of the dorsum of the tongue or as a double ending of the tip of the tongue (**Figs. 2.11, 2.12**). The complete form is very rare and appears as two separate parts of the anterior portion of the tongue, each of them controlled independently. The malformation is usually asymptomatic. The diagnosis is based on the clinical features.

Differential diagnosis
- Trauma of the tongue
- Surgical complication
- Lingual piercing complication
- Oro-facial-digital syndrome

Pathology

It is not required.

Treatment

The incomplete form usually requires no therapy. The complete form requires reconstructive surgical reconstruction.

Double Lip

Key points
- A rare oral malformation that usually affects the upper lip.
- Double lip may be congenital or acquired.
- It is more evident during smiling.

Introduction

Double lip is a rare oral malformation that affects more often the upper lip and less often the lower lip or both. The disorder is usually *congenital*, but it can also be *acquired*. The acquired form can occur as a result of trauma, surgical complication, radiation, and repeated sucking of the lip by the patient. Frequently, double lip is a part of Ascher's syndrome.

Clinical features

Clinically, double lip is characterized by an asymptomatic protruding horizontal fold on the mucosal surface of the lip (**Fig. 2.13**). The abnormality becomes prominent during speech or smiling, while when the lip is at rest the disorder is usually invisible. In a case of double lip, the clinician should bear in mind Ascher's syndrome with the classical clinical triad: blepharochalasis, nontoxic thyroid goiter, and congenital double lip. The diagnosis of double lip is based exclusively on the clinical features.

Differential diagnosis
- Ascher's syndrome
- Repeated mechanical trauma
- Surgical complication
- Radiation of the orofacial area

Pathology

It is not required.

Treatment

It is usually not required. In severe cases, surgical correction may be attempted for aesthetic reasons only.

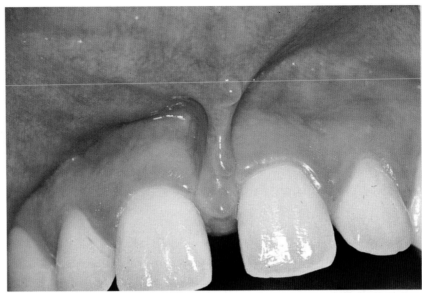

Fig. 2.10 Short bridle of the upper lip.

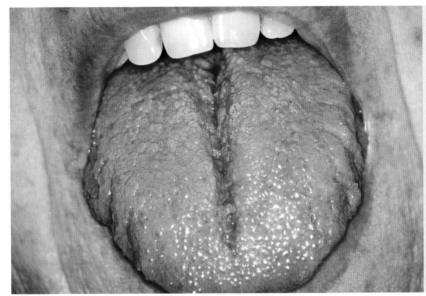

Fig. 2.11 Deep central fissure on the middle of the tongue.

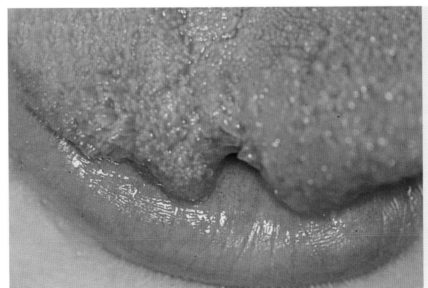

Fig. 2.12 Bifid tongue.

Torus Palatinus

Key points
- A relatively common bony exostosis.
- Characteristically, it occurs along the midline of the vault of the hard palate.
- The disorder is usually asymptomatic and the diagnosis is usually made incidentally during routine oral examination.
- The diagnosis is based on the clinical features.

Introduction

Torus palatinus is a bony exostosis that occurs along the midline of the hard palate. The etiology and pathogenesis remain uncertain. However, it is thought that genetic and environmental influences (multifactorial etiology) participate in the development of the lesion. The prevalence of torus palatinus varies from 20 to 30% or less with a female-to-male ratio of 2:1.

Clinical features

Clinically, torus palatinus appears as a sessile, asymptomatic, bony hard mass that develops during normal growth along the middle of the hard palate and is covered by thin normal mucosa. However, occasionally the mucosa may become ulcerated and painful if traumatized (**Fig. 2.14**). Recently, cases have been recorded with mucosal ulcerations and osteonecrosis of torus palatinus in patients who received bisphosphonates and RANKL inhibitor (denosumab). The size of the mass usually varies from 1 to 3 cm in diameter. There are several clinical forms of torus palatinus: the *nodular, lobular, spindled, flat,* and *completely irregular.* The lesion usually appears during the second or third decade of life. Because of its slow asymptomatic growth, it is usually an incidental finding during routine dental examination. The diagnosis is based on the clinical features.

Differential diagnosis
- Osteoma
- Gardner's syndrome
- Osteosarcoma

Pathology

It is usually not required. On histologic examination, a normal mass of lamellar cortical bone is recorded. The dental and occlusal radiographs are usually normal. However, large lesions may present as diffuse radiopaque lesions.

Treatment

Usually, no treatment is needed. However, surgical excision is necessary in edentulous patients if a full or partial denture is required and possibly in cases of osteonecrosis after bisphosphonates or denosumab therapy.

Torus Mandibularis

Key points
- A relatively common bony exostosis.
- It occurs along the lingual aspect of the mandible in the premolar area.
- Torus mandibularis usually develops bilaterally.
- The exostosis is usually asymptomatic and the diagnosis is based on the clinical features.

Introduction

Torus mandibularis is a relatively common bony exostosis that characteristically appears along the lingual aspect of the mandible superior to the mylohyoid ridge at the premolar area. In over 80 to 90% of the cases the lesions are bilateral. They may rarely be associated with torus palatinus. The prevalence ranges between 6 and 40%, affecting both sexes almost equally.

Clinical features

Clinically, torus mandibularis presents as slow-growing, asymptomatic, hard bony modules that may be single or multiple, three to five in number (**Fig. 2.15**). The size varies from 0.5 to several centimeters. Usually, the patients are not aware of the lesion unless secondary erosion or ulcer develops after mechanical trauma. Tori mandibulares usually reach their final size by the end of the third decade of life. The diagnosis is based on the clinical features.

Differential diagnosis
- Osteoma
- Gardner's syndrome
- Chronic dental abscess
- Osteosarcoma

Pathology

It is not usually required. On histologic examination, a mass of dense lamellar cortical bone is seen. Occlusal radiograph usually shows a dense radiopacity at the area of exostosis.

Treatment

It is usually not required. In severe cases surgical correction is needed particularly if a full or partial denture has to be constructed.

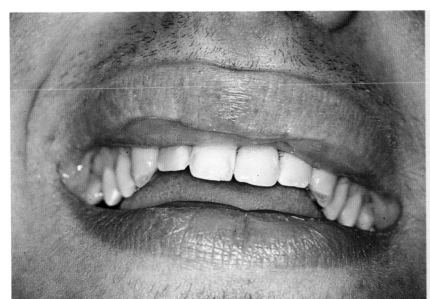

Fig. 2.13 Double lip.

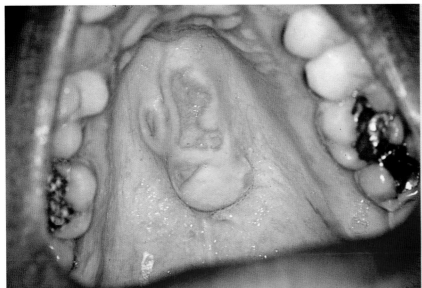

Fig. 2.14 Torus palatinus on the center of the hard palate superficially ulcerated.

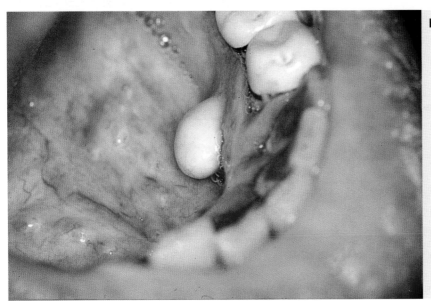

Fig. 2.15 Torus mandibularis.

Multiple Exostoses

Key points
- A relatively rare type of bony exostoses.
- They occur on the buccal aspect of the maxilla and the mandible, usually bilateral.
- Their occurrence is related to increasing age.
- Rarely multiple exostoses may be concurrent with torus palatinus and/or torus mandibularis.

Introduction

Multiple exostoses occur as multiple bony hard masses along the buccal aspect of the alveolar ridges of the jaws. The lesions usually develop bilaterally and are more common in the maxilla than the mandible. They occur less frequently than torus palatinus and torus mandibularis, and may rarely coexist with them. Occasionally, a single exostosis may be seen in the tuberosity area of the maxilla. The etiology of multiple exostoses involves interplay of multifactorial genetic and environmental factors.

Clinical features

Clinically, multiple exostoses present as multiple, asymptomatic, nodular bony elevations along the buccal aspect of the alveolar bone of the jaws, covered by normal mucosa (**Fig. 2.16**). However, occasionally ulceration may develop on the overlying mucosa, following mechanical trauma, leading to pain. The diagnosis is based on the clinical features.

Differential diagnosis
- Multiple osteomas
- Gardner's syndrome
- Paget's disease of bone
- Fibrous dysplasia

Pathology

It is not usually required. On histologic examination, a mass of normal dense lamellar cortical bone is seen.

Treatment

No treatment is required. Problems may be encountered during full or partial denture fitting. In such cases surgical recontouring can be performed.

Fibrous Developmental Malformation

Key points
- A rare developmental malformation of fibrous proliferation.
- It usually occurs in the maxillary tuberosity region and less frequently in the retromolar region of the mandible.
- The lesions usually occur bilateral in a symmetrical pattern.

Introduction

Fibrous developmental malformation is a rare fibrous overgrowth of unknown etiology. The lesions most frequently begin during childhood or puberty and may exhibit rapid or insidious growth. Usually, after the third decade of life the lesions remain stable.

Clinical features

Clinically, fibrous developmental malformations appear as a painless fibrous overgrowth that classically develops bilaterally, in a symmetrical pattern in the maxillary tuberosity region and rarely in the retromolar region of the mandible (**Figs. 2.17, 2.18**). The surface of lesion is smooth and is covered by normal mucosa with pale color. It is firm on palpation. The fibrous mass is firmly attached to the underlying bone, but on occasion may be movable. The lesion is asymptomatic and benign. Its size may extend to several centimeters and occasionally may even touch each other causing problems in speech, mastication, and swallowing. The diagnosis is based on the clinical criteria and a biopsy is rarely necessary.

Differential diagnosis
- Fibroma
- Hereditary gingival fibromatosis
- Neurofibroma
- Oral focal mucinosis

Pathology

Microscopic examination of fibrous developmental malformation shows large amount of dense collagen with few spindle-shaped cells and mild, chronic, scattered inflammation, mainly of plasma cells and lymphocytes. The covering epithelium is thin with flat rete ridges.

Treatment

Conservative surgical excision is the treatment of choice.

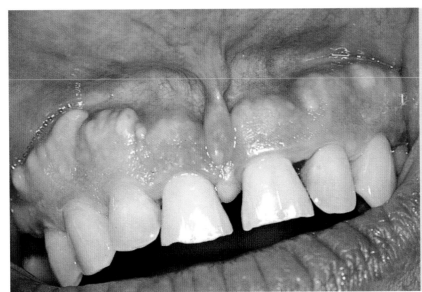

Fig. 2.16 Multiple exostoses of the maxilla.

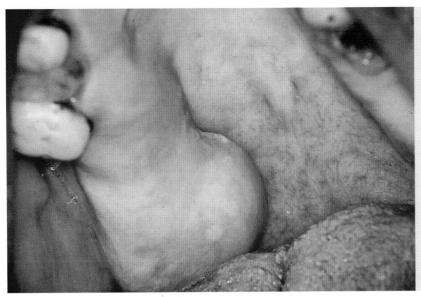

Fig. 2.17 Fibrous developmental hyperplasia of the maxillary tuberosities on the right.

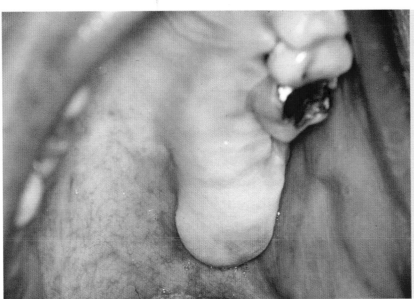

Fig. 2.18 Fibrous developmental hyperplasia of the maxillary tuberosities on the left.

Masseter Hypertrophy

Key points

- A relatively rare disorder that may be congenital or acquired.
- The congenital form may be part of several syndromes associated with hemifacial hypertrophy.
- The masseter hypertrophy is usually acquired and is unilateral.

Introduction

Masseter hypertrophy is a relatively rare disorder which is usually caused by increased muscle function, bruxism, or habitual overuse of the masseters during mastication. Anabolic steroids may also be responsible for masseter hypertrophy. In most cases the condition is unilateral due to the continued use of one side of the jaws during mastication.

Clinical features

Clinically, masseter hypertrophy appears as an asymptomatic swelling over the ascending ramus of the mandible, which characteristically becomes more prominent and firm when the patient clenches the teeth (**Fig. 2.19**). In most cases the diagnosis is based on clinical criteria.

Differential diagnosis

- Tonic-clonic spasm of masseter
- Hemifacial hypertrophy
- Syndromes associated with hemihypertrophy
- Sjogren's syndrome
- Mikulicz's syndrome
- Heerfordt's syndrome
- Muscular benign or malignant tumors
- Cellulitis

Laboratory tests

Usually, laboratory tests are not required. Electromyogram and computed tomography may be useful. Biopsy is performed only in rare cases when a diagnostic problem arises.

Treatment

No treatment is necessary. Education of the patient to use the opposite side of the jaws during mastication can be helpful. Botulinum toxin may be of use.

Hemifacial Atrophy

Key points

- A rare disorder characterized by progressive unilateral atrophy of the facial tissues.
- The cause remains unknown.
- Most cases are sporadic, but few hereditary cases have been described.
- Unilateral tongue and lip atrophy and occlusal problems are the most common oral manifestations.

Introduction

Hemifacial atrophy is a rare developmental disorder characterized by unilateral atrophy of the face. It may occasionally affect other parts of the same side of the body. The cause of the disorder remains unknown. In most cases hemifacial atrophy is sporadic. However, familial cases have been recorded leading to a possible hereditary pattern. The lesions begin during childhood and become more prominent during puberty and remain stable thereafter. Girls are most frequently affected than boys in a ratio of 3:2.

Clinical features

Clinically, the affected side appears atrophic and the skin is wrinkled and shriveled and is frequently associated with hyperpigmentation (**Fig. 2.20**). The lipocytes of the affected side disappear first, followed by skin, muscle, cartilage, and bone hypoplasia. The oral manifestations include unilateral tongue, lip, and major salivary glands atrophy (**Fig. 2.21**). Developing teeth may show deficient root development and delayed eruption, leading usually to occlusal problems. The lips and nose are deviated toward the affected site. Hemifacial atrophy may occur in association with epilepsy, trigeminal neuralgia, enophthalmos, alopecia, and sweat gland disorders (*Bomberg's syndrome*). The diagnosis is mainly based on the clinical features.

Differential diagnosis

- Hemifacial hypertrophy
- Unilateral masseter hypertrophy
- Facial lipodystrophy
- Bell's palsy with facial muscles paralysis
- Scleroderma, localized form

Pathology

Histologic examination shows atrophy of epidermis with mild perivascular infiltration mainly by lymphocytes.

Treatment

Surgical reconstruction may be of benefit when the lesion becomes stable. In addition, orthodontic therapy for occlusal problems is suggested.

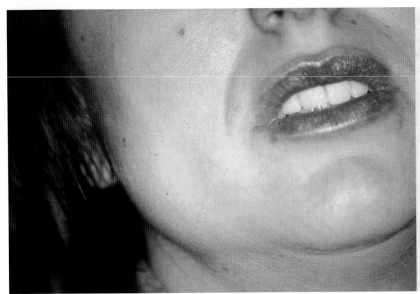

Fig. 2.19 Hypertrophy of the right masseter.

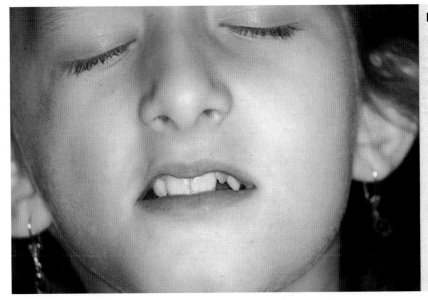

Fig. 2.20 Right hemifacial atrophy.

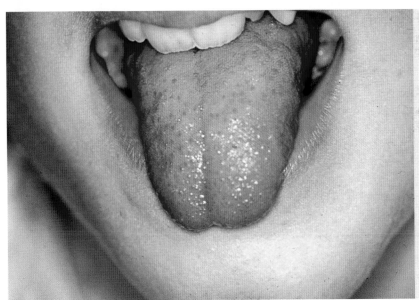

Fig. 2.21 Atrophy of the right side of the tongue.

3 Mechanical Injuries

Traumatic Ulcer

Key points

- It is the most common ulcer of the mouth.
- A close relationship between an ulcerogenic factor (mechanical damage) and the ulcer is necessary for the diagnosis.
- Self-limiting process that heals within 5 to 8 days following removal of the etiologic factor.
- Clinically may mimic oral squamous cell carcinoma.
- Frequently occurs on the tongue, buccal mucosa, lips, and gingiva.

Introduction

Traumatic ulcerations are the most common oral lesions. Acute or chronic injury to the oral mucosa may lead to an ulcer. There are several causes of traumatic ulcers; the most common causes are a sharp or broken tooth, rough fillings, sharp parts of full or partial dentures, sharp foodstuff and other foreign bodies, biting of the mucosa, mistake during use of dental instruments, and overzealous toothbrushing. Some of the causes are clinically obvious while others are difficult to be established.

Clinical features

Traumatic ulcers may occur anywhere in the mouth, but most commonly develop on the lateral borders of the tongue (**Figs. 3.1, 3.2**), buccal mucosa, gingiva, lips, and labial sulcus (**Figs. 3.3, 3.4**). The clinical presentation is variable, but usually traumatic ulcers appear as solitary, painful lesions with a smooth red or white-yellow surface and thin erythematous or even whitish halo due to hyperkeratosis. They are usually soft to palpation and heal spontaneously without scarring within 6 to 10 days after removal of the cause. The size of the ulcer may vary from a few millimeters to several centimeters in diameter and depends on the intensity, duration, and type of the trauma as well as any superimposed infection. Occasionally, when the cause is sustained and intense, the ulcer's surface may become irregular with vegetations, the border raised, and the base indurated, due to scar formation and chronic inflammation. In these cases the traumatic ulcer may clinically mimic oral squamous cell carcinoma.

Complaints, such as pain, bleeding, and burning sensation, vary from mild to severe depending on the depth and location of the ulcer. The diagnosis is mainly based on the history and the clinical features. However, if an ulcer persists over 10 days, it must be biopsied to rule out cancer.

Differential diagnosis

- Squamous cell carcinoma
- Salivary gland adenocarcinomas
- Eosinophilic ulcer
- Riga-Fede ulceration
- Aphthous ulcer
- Tuberculosis
- Chancre
- Wegener's granulomatosis
- Chemical burn
- Thermal burn
- Non-Hodgkin's lymphoma
- Necrotizing sialadenometaplasia
- Ulcer due to Epstein-Barr virus in immunosuppressed patients

Pathology

Usually, it is not needed. On histologic examination, traumatic ulcer exhibits loss of the epithelium. The surface is covered by a fibrinopurulent network containing mainly neutrophils. The floor of the ulcer consists of granulation tissue intermixed with lymphocytes, neutrophils, histiocytes, plasma cells, and eosinophils.

Treatment

The best choice is to remove or correct the causative factor. This usually leads to rapid healing of the ulcer. Topical corticosteroid ointments in Orabase or gel improve the symptoms and help healing. Systemic oral corticosteroids in low dose and for a short period of time, e.g., prednisolone 10 to 20 mg/d for 4 to 6 days, can be used successfully for chronic and painful traumatic ulcers. Oxygenating mouthwashes may also be helpful.

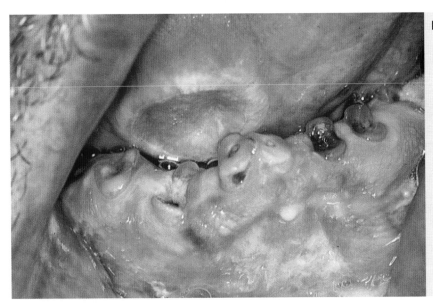

Fig. 3.1 Traumatic ulcer of the tongue.

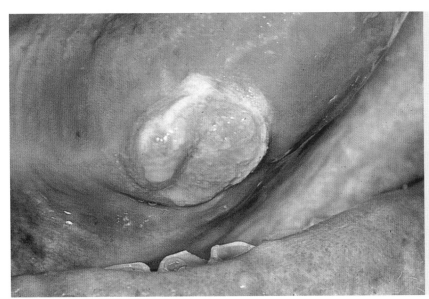

Fig. 3.2 Traumatic ulcer of the tongue.

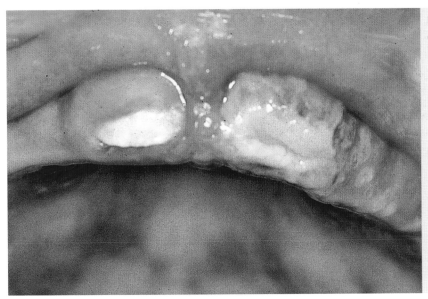

Fig. 3.3 Traumatic ulcer of the upper gingiva.

Riga-Fede Ulceration

Key points

- It occurs exclusively in infants usually between 1 and 12 months of age.
- Repeated mechanical trauma of the tongue by the natal incisors of the mandible during breast feeding is the cause.
- It is located on the anterior ventral surface of the tongue and lingual frenum.
- Riga-Fede ulceration is a variation of traumatic granuloma.
- The diagnosis is based on the history and the clinical features.

Introduction

Riga-Fede ulceration is a form of traumatic granuloma which characteristically develops on the anterior ventral surface of the tongue and the lingual frenum. The ulceration classically occurs during infancy and is closely related with the natal front teeth of infants.

Clinical features

Clinically, Riga-Fede ulceration appears as a painful ulcer usually with vegetating granulomatous surface which is covered by whitish-yellow pseudomembrane (**Fig. 3.5**). Its size varies from 1 to 2 cm in diameter. Characteristically, the lesion is located on the ventral aspect of the tongue, beneath the tip, and is developed in close relationship with the natal incisors. The diagnosis is made on clinical criteria.

Differential diagnosis

- Traumatic ulcer
- Eosinophilic granuloma
- Pyogenic granuloma
- Factitial trauma

Pathology

On histologic examination, Riga-Fede ulceration shows a base of granulation tissue and mixed inflammatory infiltrate predominantly by histiocytes, eosinophils, lymphocytes, and many dilated capillaries. The surface of the ulcer is covered by fibrin intermixed with inflammatory cells.

Treatment

It is suggested to cover the natal incisors with a cellulose film or oral base and to discontinue nursing. Surgical correction is suggested only in severe and persistent cases.

Traumatic Bulla

Key points

- A relatively common phenomenon in the oral cavity.
- It is due to a sharp mechanical injury of the oral mucosa.
- Traumatic bulla appears suddenly, is usually single, and characteristically hemorrhagic.
- There are not similar lesions on the other mucosae and the skin.
- The lesion usually recedes automatically soon (1–3 days).

Introduction

Acute traumatic injury of the oral mucosa, usually caused by biting or prosthetic appliances, may form abrupt subepithelial hemorrhages that sometimes detach the epithelium at the basement membrane level forming a hemorrhagic bulla.

Clinical features

Clinically, the lesion appears as a bulla containing blood (**Fig. 3.6**). The bulla is tense, well defined with a size of few millimeters to 1 cm. It usually occurs as a single lesion, but more may occur. The lesion is asymptomatic and usually disappears within 1 to 3 days without treatment.

The buccal mucosa is the site of predilection; however, rarely it may be seen in other oral sites. The diagnosis is usually made on clinical criteria.

Differential diagnosis

- Angina bullosa hemorrhagica
- Epidermolysis bullosa acquisita
- Mucous membrane pemphigoid
- Bullous pemphigoid
- Pemphigus
- Linear immunoglobulin A (IgA) disease
- Pemphigoid gestationis
- Lichen planus, bullous type

Pathology

On histologic examination, a subepithelial bulla formation containing blood is observed. The epithelium is normal without acantholysis. Direct and indirect immunofluorescences are negative.

Treatment

No treatment is required.

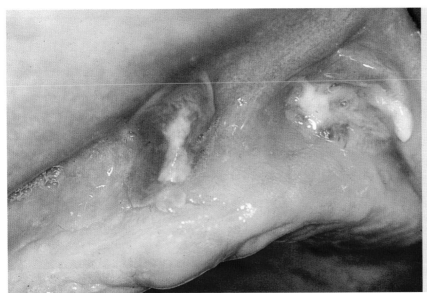

Fig. 3.4 Two traumatic ulcers of the upper labioalveolar sulcus.

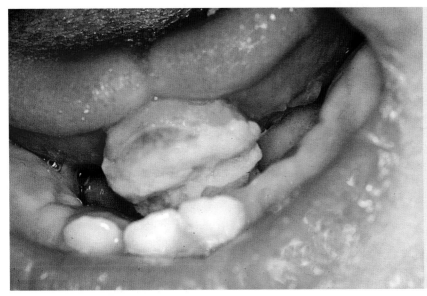

Fig. 3.5 Riga-Fede ulcer on the frenum and the ventral surface of the tongue.

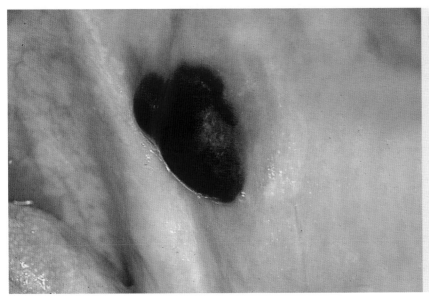

Fig. 3.6 Traumatic hemorrhagic bulla of the buccal mucosa.

Traumatic Hematoma

Key points

- It appears suddenly, after a mechanical injury.
- The overlying oral mucosa is usually intact.
- The color of the lesion is deep red.
- The lesion disappears usually in 8 to 10 days without treatment.

Introduction

Traumatic hematoma of the oral mucosa occurs under the influence of mild or severe mechanical forces that provoke vessel breakage, hemorrhage, and entrapment of blood within the oral tissues, depending on the size, petechiae, purpura, ecchymosis, and hematoma. The most common cause is biting of the oral mucosa by the patient or careless use of dental and surgical instruments.

Clinical features

Clinically, traumatic hematoma appears as an irregular, painless or with mild pain, mass with a deep red hue. The hematoma is usually slightly elevated and is associated with edema. The size may vary from 2 cm to several centimeters. The tongue, buccal mucosa, and the lips are the most common affected sites (**Figs. 3.7, 3.8**). Patients under anticoagulant therapy may be at risk of developing hematomas. The diagnosis is based on the history and the clinical features.

Differential diagnosis

- Hematoma due to anticoagulant therapy
- Thrombocytopenia
- Thrombasthenia
- Hemangiomas
- Vascular malformations

Pathology

It is not required.

Treatment

Usually, no treatment is required as the lesion resolves spontaneously. However, with large hematomas, high doses of ascorbic acid, e.g., 2 to 3 g/d for about 1 week, may reduce the time to resolution. Surgical intervention may be useful in rare cases.

Chronic Biting

Key points

- A relatively common habit particularly with anxiety and other psychological problems.
- The buccal mucosa, the lateral border of the tongue, and the labial mucosa are most frequently involved.
- The lesions are innocent without risk of malignancy.

Introduction

Chronic biting of the oral mucosa or maceration of the oral mucosa can be a chronic habit with a psychological background. The patients repeatedly bite the oral mucosa, pull it between the teeth, and tear the superficial epithelial layers.

Clinical features

Clinically, chronic biting appears as a localized or diffused irregular whitish lesion of small furrows, with desquamation of the affected epithelium. Infrequently, superficial erosions of the epithelium and petechiae may occur (**Figs. 3.9, 3.10**). Usually, the lesions are bilateral although unilateral lesions may be seen.

The buccal mucosa, at the level of occlusal plane, is the site of predilection, followed by the lateral borders of the tongue and the labial mucosa.

Differential diagnosis

- Leukoedema
- Fordyce's granules
- Cinnamon contact stomatitis
- Candidiasis
- Hairy leukoplakia
- Lichen planus
- Leukoplakia
- White sponge nevus
- Chemical burn

Pathology

It is not required. On histologic examination, epithelial hyperplasia with detached parts of the epithelium colonized by bacteria and hyphae of candida are common findings.

Treatment

Usually, no treatment is required. However, patients should be made aware of the habit and suggestions to stop it are necessary.

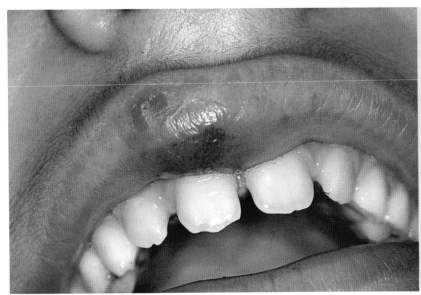

Fig. 3.7 Traumatic hematoma of the upper lip.

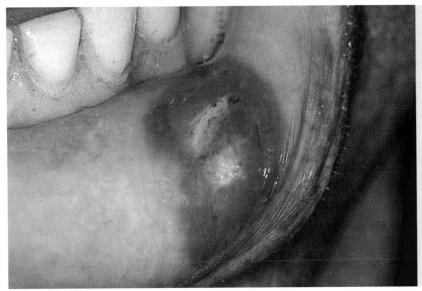

Fig. 3.8 Traumatic hematoma of the lower lip.

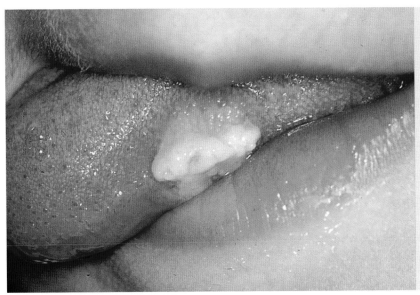

Fig. 3.9 Localized chronic biting of the lateral border of the tongue.

Trauma from Toothbrush

Key points
- Toothbrushing-induced trauma most commonly occurs on the gingiva.
- The canine and premolars' region on the buccal aspect are most frequently affected.
- It is due to the overzealous brushing of the teeth.
- The diagnosis is based on the history and the clinical features.

Introduction

Toothbrushing-induced lesions, either frictional keratosis or erosions, may be observed on the gingiva and the alveolar mucosa. These lesions may occur during aggressive toothbrushing, with a hard brush. Erosions more frequently occur as an acute event. In contrast, frictional keratosis is the result of a chronic irritation.

Clinical features

Clinically, toothbrushing erosions appear as small, oval, round, or band-like superficial epithelial loss that is covered by a whitish pseudomembrane (**Fig. 3.11**). These lesions cause usually mild subjective complains and heal rapidly in 3 to 4 days after stopping the brushing. The attached gingiva and the interdental papillae are more frequently affected. The diagnosis is based on the history and the clinical features.

Differential diagnosis
- Secondary herpetic lesions
- Aphthous ulcers
- Traumatic lesions from other causes
- Thermal burn
- Mucous membrane pemphigoid
- Pemphigus

Pathology

It is not required.

Treatment

The lesion is self-healing in 3 to 4 days.

Factitious Trauma

Key points
- It occurs usually in patients with serious emotional problems or mental impairment.
- The trauma is usually inflicted by tooth biting, fingernails, or by the use of a sharp object.
- The most common clinical feature is small-to-large ulceration.
- The diagnosis is based on the clinical criteria.

Introduction

Patients with mental impairment or those with serious emotional problems may have self-inflicted oral trauma and ulcerations. The trauma and ulceration is usually inflicted by tooth biting, fingernails, or by the use of a sharp object. The lesions are more commonly observed in children and adolescents.

Clinical features

Clinically, factitious trauma usually appears as a mild or severe ulceration few or several centimeters in diameter (**Fig. 3.12**). The lesions are painful and are frequently located on the tongue, lips, and gingiva. Similar lesions may be observed on the skin either alone or in association with oral lesions (**Fig. 3.13**). The diagnosis depends on strong clinical suspicion and the history, although many patients deny that they are responsible for lesions.

Differential diagnosis
- Ulcerations from mechanical injuries, thermal or electrical burn
- Aphthous ulcer
- Malignant ulceration
- Tuberculosis
- Syphilis
- Eosinophilic ulcer

Pathology

It is not required. However, when a diagnostic dilemma exists, a biopsy and histologic examination is necessary to rule out other diseases. An ulcer is seen microscopically. The surface is covered by fibrinopurulent network containing inflammatory cells. The floor of the ulcer consists of granulation tissue intermixed with neutrophils, lymphocytes, histiocytes, plasma cells, and eosinophils.

Treatment

Local measures, such as corticosteroid paste in Orabase, antibacterial mouthwashes, and psychiatric support are the suggested measures.

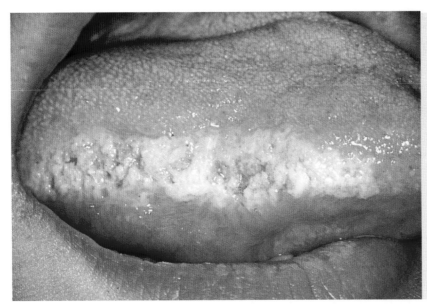

Fig. 3.10 Extensive chronic biting of the lateral border of the tongue.

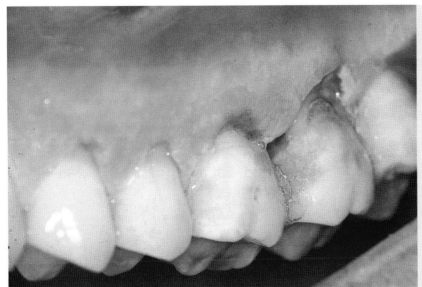

Fig. 3.11 Toothbrush trauma of the upper gingiva.

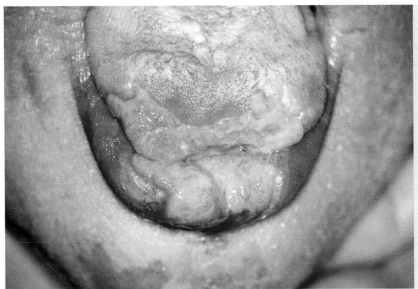

Fig. 3.12 Extensive factitious ulceration of the tongue and the lower lip of a patient with severe psychological upset.

Oral Trauma from Sexual Practices (Fellatio and Cunnilingus)

Key points
- Orogenital contact is a common sexual practice.
- The most common oral lesions related to this practice are *fellatio* and *cunnilingus*.
- Sucking, negative pressure, and mechanical irritation from the teeth are the cause of the lesions.
- The diagnosis is made on the history and the clinical features.

Introduction

Orogenital sexual practices are common in both heterosexual and homosexual couples. Apart from sexually transmitted diseases, oral lesions may occur due to negative pressure or mechanical irritation applied during orogenital sex. The two most common oral lesions are *fellatio* and *cunnilingus*.

Clinical features

Clinically, the lesions due to fellatio appear as asymptomatic petechiae, erythema, and ecchymoses at the junction of the hard and soft palates or the uvula (**Fig. 3.14**). These lesions are the result of submucosal hemorrhage due to negative pressure. They disappear spontaneously in 5 to 8 days. However, it may recur with repetition of this sexual practice. The oral lesion due to cunnilingus appears as a small nonspecific erosion or ulceration covered by a whitish pseudomembrane usually surrounded by erythema. Characteristically, the lesion develops at the lingual frenum (**Fig. 3.15**). As the tongue moves forward to back the taut, lingua frenum is rubbed over the rough incisal edges of the mandibular incisors. The diagnosis of both lesions from fellatio and cunnilingus is based on the history and the clinical features.

Differential diagnosis
- Thermal burn
- Erythematous candidiasis
- Infectious mononucleosis
- Petechiae and purpura due to coughing or vomiting
- Traumatic erosion or ulcer
- Chancre
- Aphthous ulceration
- Secondary herpetic lesions
- Thrombocytopenic purpura
- Aplastic anemia
- Leukemia

Pathology

It is not required.

Treatment

Usually, no treatment is required as the lesions resolve spontaneously in 5 to 8 days.

Cotton Roll Trauma

Key points
- It is a form of traumatic lesion.
- Cotton rolls are applied in dental practice for moisture control.
- Erythema or/and superficial atypical erosion may be seen.
- The common use of the rubber dam has reduced this form of lesion.

Introduction

Cotton roll trauma or cotton roll stomatitis may occur after placing cotton rolls in the mouth to keep the dental surfaces dry. In such cases, excessive drying of the mucosal surfaces may result in erosions during a rough removal of the cotton roll, which adheres to the mucosa. The wide use of the rubber dam in the dental practice in recent decades has reduced this iatrogenic event.

Clinical features

Clinically, cotton roll trauma appears as a painful erosion, usually covered with a whitish pseudomembrane and an erythematous base (**Fig. 3.16**). The lesion disappears without any treatment in 4 to 6 days. The diagnosis is made exclusively on the history and the clinical features.

Differential diagnosis
- Traumatic erosions due to other causes
- Thermal burn
- Aphthous ulcers
- Secondary herpes simplex

Pathology

It is not required.

Treatment

No treatment is necessary as the lesions heal spontaneously in 4 to 6 days.

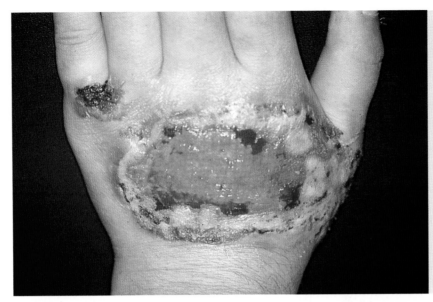

Fig. 3.13 Factitia, large ulcer on the dorsum of the hand of the patient of Fig. 3.12

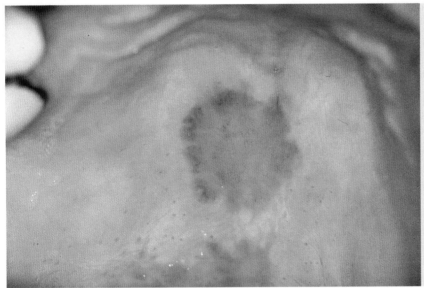

Fig. 3.14 Fellatio, erythema of the palate.

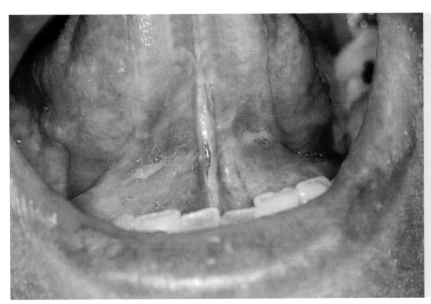

Fig. 3.15 Cunnilingus, erosions on the frenum of the tongue.

Denture Stomatitis

Key points

- Denture stomatitis is a common disorder in people who wear dentures for long periods of time.
- Etiologic factors are irritation from ill-fitting dentures and poor denture hygiene.
- It is usually confined to the maxilla.
- Denture stomatitis is usually asymptomatic.

Introduction

Denture stomatitis is a common disorder in people who wear dentures continuously for long periods of time. The prevalence varies between 30 and 70%. Usually, the lesion is confined to the maxilla and only rarely occurs on the mandibular-mucosal surface. Several etiologic factors have been incriminated; the most important factors are continuous irritation from ill-fitting dentures, food debris, *Candida albicans*, and bacterial accumulation under the denture surface. Rarely, allergic reaction of the mucosa to the acrylic base of the denture may play a role.

Clinical features

Clinically, the mucosa beneath the denture is edematous and erythematous with or without whitish spots that represent accumulation of food remnants or/and hyphae of *C. albicans* (**Fig. 3.17**). The mucosal surface may be smooth or granular or nodular. Most patients are asymptomatic, but some complain of a burning sensation, irritation, or mild pain. The lesions are benign and may be localized or generalized.

Differential diagnosis

- Papillary palatal hyperplasia
- Allergic contact stomatitis due to acrylic monomer
- Erythematous candidiasis

Pathology

Usually, it is not necessary. The skin punch test to acrylic resin is usually negative while the cytologic smear for *Candida* is of limited value. On histologic examination, the epithelium is hyperplastic. The mucosa is irregular with multiple papillary projections with or without hyphae presentation.

Treatment

Improvement of denture fit, oral hygiene, and antifungal drugs systematically, e.g., fluconazole 100 mg/d or itraconazole caps 100 mg/d for 6 to 7 days, are the first-line therapy. In cases with extensive papillary hyperplasia, the lesions must be removed by electrosurgery or CO_2 laser and a new denture should be constructed.

Papillary Palatal Hyperplasia

Key points

- Papillary palatal hyperplasia is a variety of denture stomatitis.
- It may also occur in edentulous people.
- Mechanical irritation by food or mouth breathing with a high palatal vault is the causative factor in edentulous people.
- Classically, it is localized at the midline of the anterior part of the palate.

Introduction

Although papillary palatal hyperplasia is a clinical form of denture stomatitis, on rare occasions the disorder may develop in edentulous people usually with high-arched palate. In such cases the lesions are usually localized and rarely generalized. The causative factor is primarily mechanical irritation by food stuffs or mouth breathing and secondarily infection by *C. albicans*.

Clinical features

Clinically, papillary palatal hyperplasia appears as multiple coalescing, small edematous, and reddish capillary projection that usually measures 1 to 2 mm or more in diameter (**Fig. 3.18**). The lesions are usually asymptomatic, confluent, and may occupy part or rarely all of the hard palate, giving it a cauliflower-like pattern. As the lesions are asymptomatic, they may be accidentally discovered by the patients or during a routine mouth examination by the dentist. Some patients become anxious, fearing cancer. However, the disorder is benign and should not be a cause for alarm.

Differential diagnosis

- Denture stomatitis
- Hyperplastic candidiasis
- Acanthosis nigricans
- Tuberous sclerosis
- Focal dermal hypoplasia syndrome
- Neurofibromatosis type 1
- Darier's disease

Pathology

It is not necessary. On histologic examination, inflammatory papillary hyperplasia with multiple papillary projections of the mucosa is present. Pseudoepithelial hyperplasia may also be seen. Inflammatory infiltrations by lymphocytes, plasma cells, and neutrophils are common findings.

Treatment

Excision of the severe lesion by electrosurgery or CO_2 laser is the treatment of choice.

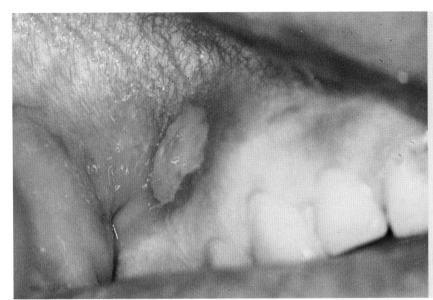

Fig. 3.16 Erosion on the alveolabial sulcus caused by cotton roll.

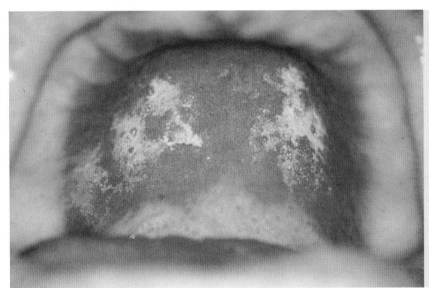

Fig. 3.17 Denture stomatitis, erythema, and edema of the palate with *Candida albicans* infection.

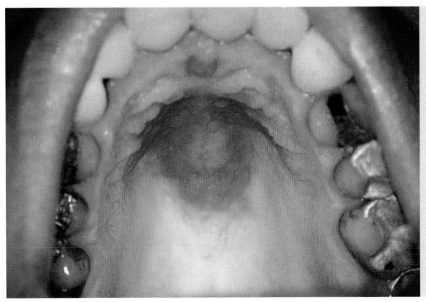

Fig. 3.18 Papillary palatal hyperplasia.

33

Hyperplasia due to Negative Pressure

Key points
- Commonly occurs on the hard palate.
- The cause is a vacuum at the center of the basal plate of the upper denture.
- It is an innocent lesion.

Introduction

In patients wearing upper denture, usually a mucosal elevation may appear at the center of the hard palate. The lesion occurs if a relief vacuum exists at the center of the basal plate of the upper denture and is the result of the negative pressure that develops.

Clinical features

Clinically, the mucosa may be slightly elevated and appears red with a smooth or papillary surface at the center of the hard palate (**Fig. 3.19**). The mucosal hyperplasia usually has a heart shape or is rounded. A similar lesion may develop on the upper lip if a wide middle space between central incisors exists (**Fig. 3.20**). The lesion is asymptomatic and innocent and the diagnosis is made on the clinical features.

Differential diagnosis
- Denture stomatitis
- Papillary palatal hyperplasia
- Fibroma
- Fibroepithelial polyp

Pathology

It is not required.

Treatment

No treatment is necessary. Only in the case of new denture construction the lesion may be removed by electrosurgery.

Atrophy of Alveolar Ridge

Key points
- The area most frequently affected is the anterior process of the maxilla.
- It appears only in edentulous patients.
- The atrophy appears as flabby ridges and folds.
- The disorder may cause problems in the retention of the denture.

Introduction

Atrophy of the alveolar ridge may be the result of excessive occlusal trauma due to a poor fitting denture and inflammation. This may cause resorption of the alveolar ridge. However, cases without any obvious factors may arise. The anterior part of the maxilla is more frequently affected, but the mandible may also be affected.

Clinical features

Clinically, the alveolus becomes flabby and dark red in color than the adjacent normal mucosa and may occasionally be associated with a denture fibrous hyperplasia (**Fig. 3.21**). The flabby ridge is movable with firm consistency. The lesion occurs more frequently in women than in men. The diagnosis is made on the clinical features.

Differential diagnosis
- Bone loss
- Fibrous hyperplasia from denture
- Osteoporosis

Pathology

It is not required.

Treatment

Usually, no treatment is necessary. In severe cases, bone grafting and surgical reconstruction is recommended.

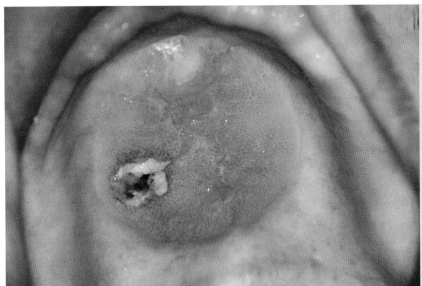

Fig. 3.19 Hyperplasia and ulceration of the palatal mucosa caused by negative pressure from the denture.

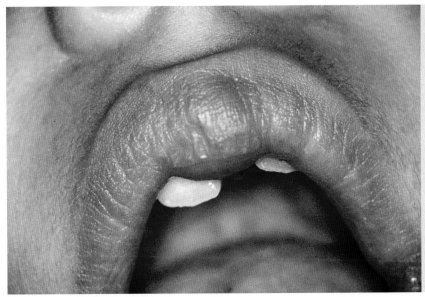

Fig. 3.20 Hyperplasia of the upper lip by negative pressure caused by the wide interdental space between the central incisors.

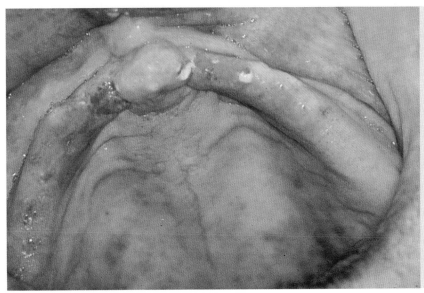

Fig. 3.21 Atrophy of the maxillary alveolar ridge.

Mucosal Necrosis due to Injection

Key points
- Local anesthetic injection may occasionally be followed by mucosal necrosis.
- Local ischemia is usually the cause.
- The hard palate is the site of predilection.
- The necrotic ulcer is usually a self-healing lesion.

Introduction

Mucosal necrosis of the hard palate may occur after palatal injection with a local anesthetic containing epinephrine. Rapid injection of the solution results in local ischemia, which may be followed by tissue necrosis. The hard palate is particularly sensitive to these lesions due to local pressure, because of the firm adherence of mucosa to the bone and the absence of loose connective tissue.

Clinical features

Clinically, palatal necrosis appears as a well-circumscribed deep ulcer, exactly at the site of injection (**Fig. 3.22**). The size varies from few millimeters to 1 cm or more in diameter. The ulcer develops 3 to 6 days after the procedure and frequently heals spontaneously within 2 weeks. Rarely, bone necrosis may occur. The diagnosis is made on the history and the clinical features.

Differential diagnosis
- Necrotizing sialometaplasia
- Traumatic ulcer
- Bisphosphonate-associated necrosis
- Denosumab-associated necrosis
- Salivary gland adenocarcinomas
- Squamous cell carcinoma

Pathology

Usually, it is not required. A biopsy is recommended only if a diagnostic dilemma exists to rule out malignancy.

Treatment

No therapy is necessary. Mouthwashes with oxygen-releasing substrates for 10 to 15 days are recommended.

Eosinophilic Ulceration

Key points
- A self-limiting benign inflammatory lesion unrelated to eosinophilic granuloma of Langerhans cell histiocytosis.
- Trauma is considered to be the causative factor.
- The tongue is the site of predilection.
- A sudden-onset painful ulcer is the main clinical feature.
- The diagnosis is based on the histologic examination.

Introduction

Eosinophilic ulceration or traumatic eosinophilic granuloma is a benign self-limiting inflammatory lesion unrelated to eosinophilic granuloma of Langerhans cell histiocytosis. The exact etiology remains obscure, although a traumatic background has been suggested. It has been proposed that some cases of eosinophilic ulceration are probably T-cell mediated which react with CD30. If the lesion represents a lymphoproliferative disorder or a low-grade non-Hodgkin's lymphoma, molecular studies are essential for clarity.

Clinical features

Clinically, eosinophilic ulceration appears as sudden-onset painful ulcer with an irregular surface, covered with a whitish-yellow membrane, and raised inflammatory and indurated border (**Figs. 3.23, 3.24**). Usually, the ulcer is single but multiple lesions may occur. The tongue is the site of predilection (> 74%), followed by the lips, buccal mucosa, and rarely the gingiva. Men are more frequently affected than women (ratio 5:1) with mean age of 57-59 years. The sudden onset and the pain is a cause of concern for the patient. The diagnosis is based on biopsy and histopathologic examination.

Differential diagnosis
- Traumatic ulcer
- Riga-Fede ulceration
- Histiocytic granuloma
- Major aphthous ulcer
- Wegener's granulomatosis
- Non-Hodgkin's lymphoma
- Malignant granuloma
- Leukemia
- Tuberculosis
- Syphilitic ulcer (chancre)
- Squamous cell carcinoma
- Necrotizing sialoadenometaplasia
- Epstein-Barr ulceration in immunosuppressed patients

Pathology

Histopathologic examination is important to establish the diagnosis. Microscopically, a deep ulcer that is covered by a fibrin intermixed with neutrophils and eosinophils is the common feature. The base of the ulcer consists of granulation tissue with inflammatory infiltration by lymphocytes, histiocytes, plasma cells, neutrophils, and numerous eosinophils. However, in some cases these cells may exhibit pleomorphism and mitotic activity. Large atypical CD30+ T cells, occasionally monoclonal, can be seen. In such cases further immunohistochemical or molecular studies, e.g., by polymerase chain reaction (PCR), should be performed to diagnose a low-grade non-Hodgkin's lymphoma.

Treatment

The lesion is usually self-limiting and heals over several weeks or months. Spontaneous healing after a biopsy may also occur. However, the healing time can be shortened by systemic treatment with corticosteroids. Prednisone 20 to 30 mg/d or betamethasone 2 to 3 mg/d for 1 week and then tapering the dose and stopping it in approximately 1 to 2 weeks is often the treatment of choice as the ulcer heals quickly (~ 8–12 days).

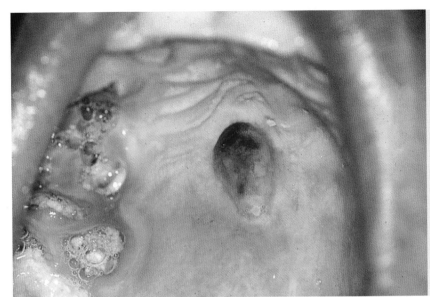

Fig. 3.22 Necrosis of the palate due to injection.

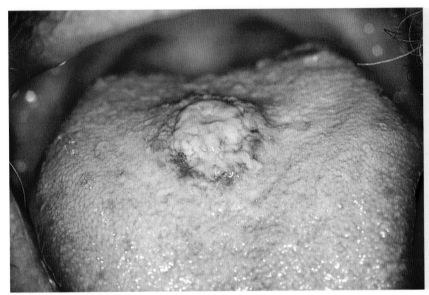

Fig. 3.23 Eosinophilic ulcer of the dorsum of the tongue, early stage.

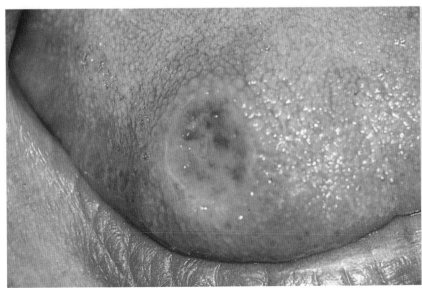

Fig. 3.24 Eosinophilic ulcer on the tongue, late stage.

4 Chemical Burns

Aspirin Burn

Key points

- It is one of the most common chemical injuries of the oral mucosa.
- It is usually caused when patients with toothache apply an aspirin tablet topically on the oral mucosa.
- The lesion heals spontaneously within 4 to 6 days.

Introduction

Careless or inappropriate use of a large number of caustic chemical agents and drugs in dental practice may cause oral lesions. In addition, accidental ingestion of household chemicals such as kitchen, toilet and metal cleansers, or even agricultural drugs may cause mild or severe damage of the oral mucosa. Some of these agents may be introduced into the mouth by the patient in an attempt to resolve oral problems and others by the dentist. The wide use of the rubber dam has reduced the frequency of such lesions. The severity of the lesion depends on the type of chemical utilized, its concentration, and the time of contact with the oral tissues. Aspirin is a very popular drug to relieve dental pain, systemically. However, some patients apply aspirin tablets repeatedly and directly to the painful tooth and the adjacent tissues for long periods. In such cases, the drug dissolves locally causing necrosis of the oral mucosa.

Clinical features

Clinically, aspirin burn initially presents as an irregular whitish and wrinkled mucosal area (**Fig. 4.1**). Later, the necrotic epithelium desquamates exposing an underlying painful erosion. The nonkeratinized movable mucosa is more sensitive than the keratinized one. The lesion heals within 4 to 6 days after stopping the agent. The diagnosis is based on the history and the clinical features.

Differential diagnosis

- Other chemical burns
- Thermal burns
- Traumatic lesions
- Candidiasis
- Cinnamon contact stomatitis
- Chronic biting
- Leukoplakia
- Lichen planus
- Secondary herpetic lesions

Pathology

It is not required. Histologic examination of chemical burns, including aspirin burn, is characterized by coagulative necrosis of the epithelium while the underlying connective tissue is infiltrated by acute inflammatory cells. Similar histologic features are usually found in almost all the forms of oral chemical burns.

Treatment

Usually, no treatment is necessary as the lesion heals spontaneously within 4 to 6 days. In severe persistent lesions, oral corticosteroids, in low doses for a short time, e.g., prednisone 10 to 15 mg/d for 3 to 5 days, improve the symptoms dramatically. Topically, oxygen-releasing mouthwashes are also helpful in severe cases.

Alcohol and Iodine Burn

Key points

- Repeated application of concentrated alcohol or iodine solution may result in mucosal damage.
- Lesions may be painful or painless depending on the severity of damage.
- The lesion heals spontaneously within 2 to 4 days.
- The diagnosis is based on the history and the clinical features.

Introduction

Concentrated alcohol in the form of absolute alcohol or spirits with high alcohol content are used occasionally by patients as a local anesthetic for mouth pain or as antiseptic. For the same purpose concentrated alcoholic iodine solutions may also be used. Repeated application of both chemicals may result in a mild-to-severe burn depending on the duration of the contact as well as the concentration and the quantity of the solutions.

Clinical features

Clinically, the affected mucosa is whitish or reddish, wrinkled, and tender (**Figs. 4.2, 4.3**). Superficial erosions in more severe cases may occur. The lesion usually heals spontaneously within 2 to 4 days. The diagnosis is based on the history and the clinical features.

Differential diagnosis

- Other chemical burns
- Thermal burns
- Traumatic lesions
- Chronic biting
- Cinnamon contact stomatitis
- Candidiasis
- Leukoplakia

Pathology

It is not required.

Treatment

Usually, no treatment is necessary as the lesion heals spontaneously in 2 to 4 days. Topically, oxygen-releasing mouthwashes may be used for a week's time.

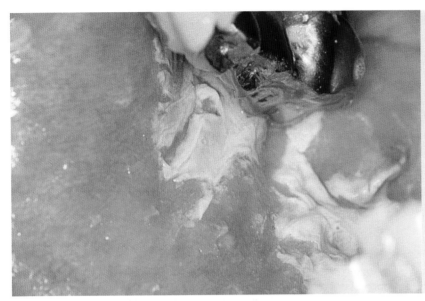

Fig. 4.1 Chemical burn of the buccal mucosa due to acetylsalicylic acid (aspirin).

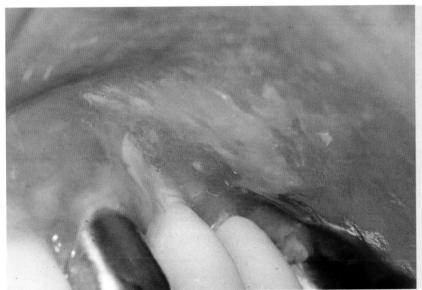

Fig. 4.2 Chemical burn of the labioalveolar sulcus caused by local application of iodine.

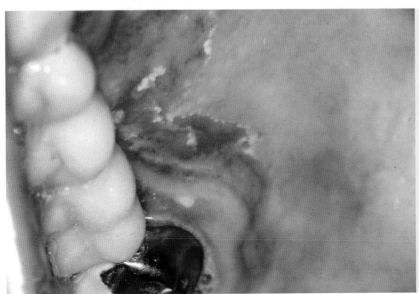

Fig. 4.3 Chemical burn of the palate caused by local application of Tsicoudia (alcohol-containing drink).

Trichloroacetic Acid Burn

Key points
- Trichloroacetic acid was used frequently in the past and rarely in the last decades, as a caustic agent for dental surgery.
- It is an extremely caustic agent that may cause a severe chemical burn.
- A white necrotic ulcer/erosion is the main clinical feature.
- The lesion heals spontaneously in 1 to 2 weeks.
- The diagnosis is based on the history and the clinical features.

Introduction

Trichloroacetic acid was often used in the past for cautery of the gingiva, for hemostasis, and to destroy granulation tissue. It is a highly caustic agent and improper use may result in serious chemical burn. Recently, the rarity of application of the agent and use of the rubber dam has reduced the frequency of this form of burn.

Clinical features

Clinically, trichloroacetic acid burn characteristically appears as a white and wrinkled surface due to tissue necrosis (**Figs. 4.4, 4.5**). Removal of the necrotic epithelium reveals severe inflammation and superficial painful erosion of the oral mucosa. The severity of the epithelial damage depends on the concentration of the agent and the duration of contact. The lesion usually heals spontaneously in 6 to 8 days. The diagnosis is based on the history and the clinical features.

Differential diagnosis
- Chemical burns due to other agents
- Thermal burns
- Physical trauma
- Leukoplakia
- Lichen planus
- Cinnamon contact stomatitis

Pathology

It is not required. Histologically, it is almost the same pattern as the aspirin burn.

Treatment

Usually, no treatment is necessary as the lesion heals spontaneously in 6 to 8 days. However, in severe and extensive lesions administration of oral corticosteroids in low dose for a short time, e.g., prednisone 10 to 15 mg/d for 3 to 5 days, causes rapid resolution.

Eugenol Burn

Key points
- Eugenol has a wide use in the dental practice.
- Mild chemical epithelial damage can arise after topical use of this agent.
- Itching and burning sensation associated with erythema and occasionally superficial mucosal erosion are the common features.
- The lesions usually heal spontaneously, after withdrawal of the agent, in 3 to 5 days.
- The diagnosis is based on the history and the clinical features.

Introduction

Eugenol is an agent that has been widely used in dentistry for many reasons such as an antiseptic, part of a gingivectomy pack, dry socket treatment, or local pulp anesthetic. The noxious potential of the drug is limited, but on occasion may cause a mucosal burn. Rarely, eugenol may also cause allergic contact stomatitis or even allergic contact dermatitis to the dentist.

Clinical features

Clinically, eugenol burn presents as a white-brownish surface with an underlying inflammation and superficial erosion (**Fig. 4.6**). Itching and burning sensation are the common symptoms. The lesion is self-healing in 3 to 5 days. The diagnosis is based on the history and the clinical features.

Differential diagnosis
- Other chemical burns
- Thermal burns
- Candidiasis
- Lichenoid amalgam reaction
- Cinnamon contact stomatitis

Pathology

It is not required.

Treatment

Usually, no treatment is necessary as the lesion heals spontaneously in 3 to 5 days.

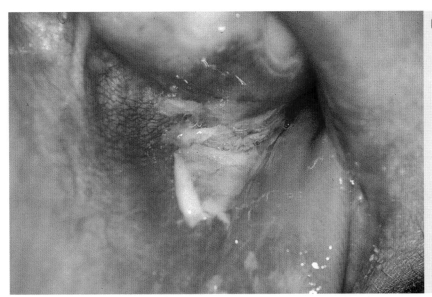

Fig. 4.4 Trichloroacetic acid burn.

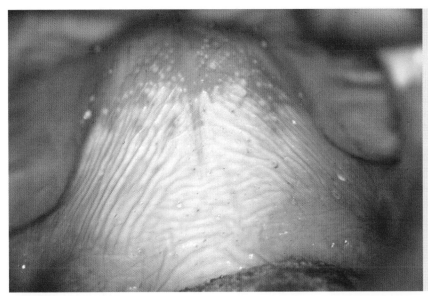

Fig. 4.5 Chemical burn of the palate caused by inept use of trichloroacetic acid.

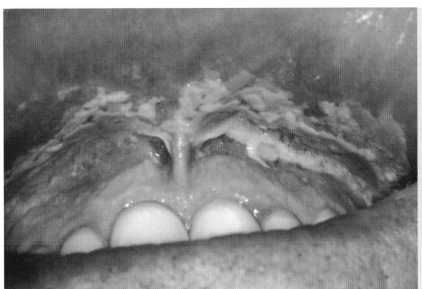

Fig. 4.6 Chemical burn of the upper labioalveolar sulcus caused by eugenol.

Hydrogen Peroxide Burn

Key points

- It was widely used in the past as a mouthwash medication for the prevention of periodontal disease.
- It is also commonly used as a bleaching agent.
- A high concentration of the solution usually is associated with mucosal damage where the offending agent contacts the mucosa.
- Epithelial necrosis and erosion are the common features.
- Removal of the causative agent is curative.

Introduction

Hydrogen peroxide has over the last two decades become the most frequently used tooth bleaching agent. It is used either as an in-office technique by the dentist at high concentration or applied at low concentration by the patient at home. Careless use and contact with the oral mucosa usually causes an epithelial damage.

Clinical features

Clinically, hydrogen peroxide epithelial damage presents as an erythematous area with a superficial erosion covered by a whitish necrotic fibrinopurulent membrane (**Fig. 4.7**). The lesion is self-healing in 3 to 6 days, depending on the severity. The diagnosis is based on the history and the clinical features.

Differential diagnosis

- Other chemical burns
- Thermal burns
- Bullous diseases
- Drug reaction
- Cinnamon contact stomatitis
- Desquamative gingivitis

Pathology

It is not required.

Treatment

Usually, no treatment is necessary as the lesions heal spontaneously in 3 to 6 days.

Phenol Burn

Key points

- Phenol has rarely been used in modern dentistry.
- Careless application may cause tissue necrosis.
- The severity of damage depends on the duration of contact and the concentration of the agent.
- The diagnosis is based on the history and the clinical features.

Introduction

Phenol is used in dentistry as an antiseptic agent and for local cautery. In modern dentistry its use is very rare. It is an extremely caustic chemical agent, and careless local application may cause severe mucosal damage, mainly depending on the concentration of the material and the duration of contact.

Clinical features

Clinically, phenol burn appears as a whitish mucosal surface that soon desquamates exposing a painful erosion or ulceration that heals slowly (**Fig. 4.8**). Rarely, superficial bone necrosis may occur. The diagnosis is based on the history and the clinical features.

Differential diagnosis

- Other chemical burns
- Thermal burns
- Traumatic erosion or ulcer

Pathology

It is not required.

Treatment

Usually, no treatment is necessary as the lesion heals spontaneously within 4 to 8 days. In severe persistent cases oral corticosteroids in low doses for a short time, e.g., prednisone 10 to 15 mg/d for 3 to 5 days, improve the symptoms and shorten the time of healing.

Sodium Perborate Burn

Key points

- The use of the agent has reduced in dentistry.
- It may occasionally produce local irritation or superficial erosion.
- The diagnosis is based on the history and the clinical features.

Introduction

Sodium perborate has been used in the past as an antiseptic and hemostatic mouthwash. With repeated use, it may cause a mild burn on the oral mucosa.

Clinical features

Clinically, the lesion appears as an erythematous surface or rarely as a superficial erosion covered by a whitish membrane, usually associated with mild pain (**Fig. 4.9**). The lesion heals spontaneously within 3 to 6 days. The diagnosis is made on clinical criteria.

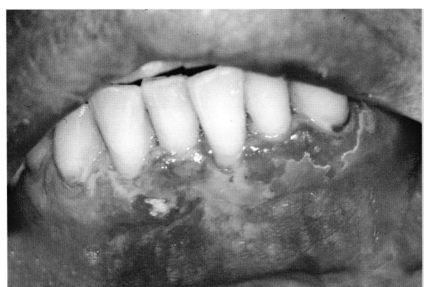

Fig. 4.7 Chemical burn caused by hydrogen peroxide.

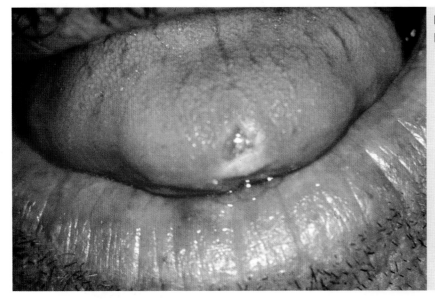

Fig. 4.8 Chemical burn caused by phenol.

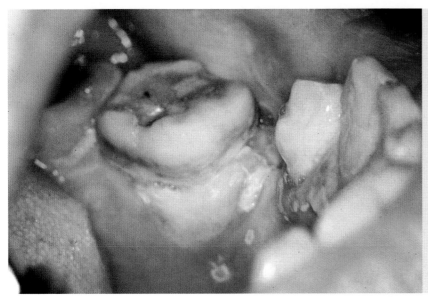

Fig. 4.9 Chemical burn of the gingiva caused by sodium perborate.

Differential diagnosis

- Other chemical burns
- Thermal burns
- Traumatic lesion
- Candidiasis
- Leukoplakia
- Cinnamon contact stomatitis
- Lichen planus

Pathology

It is not required.

Treatment

Usually, no treatment is necessary as the lesions heal spontaneously within 3 to 6 days.

Silver Nitrate Burn

Key points

- It is rare nowadays as the use of the agent has been reduced.
- Whitish or brown or mixed lesions may develop occasionally with ulceration.
- Lesions usually are located where the silver nitrate contacts the mucosa.
- The lesions heal spontaneously.

Introduction

Silver nitrate was used in the past by dentists and otolaryngologists for chemical cautery or as a sterilizing agent for various oral lesions, e.g., aphthous ulcers, small benign tumors, or gingival hemorrhage. However, the extent of mucosal damage can be severe. Silver nitrate is now rarely used in dentistry.

Clinical features

Clinically, at the site of application of the agent a painful mucosal damage occurs with a brownish or whitish surface erosion or ulceration (**Fig. 4.10**). The lesions heal within 4 to 8 days. The diagnosis is based on the history and the clinical features.

Differential diagnosis

- Other chemical burns
- Thermal burns
- Traumatic lesion

Pathology

It is not required.

Treatment

Usually, no treatment is necessary as the lesions heal spontaneously within about a week.

Sodium Hypochlorite Burn

Key points

- Earlier, it was considered as a relatively common accident during dental work.
- Painful erythema and erosion are the main features.
- The diagnosis is made on clinical criteria.
- Use of rubber dam reduces the possibility of this event.

Introduction

Sodium hypochlorite is widely used as endodontic material for mechanical irrigation of root canals and as a mild antiseptic. In contact with the oral soft tissues it may cause mild mucosal damage.

Clinical features

Clinically, the affected mucosa is erythematous and painful, with superficial erosions covered by a whitish-yellowish necrotic membrane (**Fig. 4.11**). The lesion usually resolves spontaneously without scarring within 4 to 6 days. The use of rubber dam provides protection from this iatrogenic lesion. The diagnosis is based on the history and the clinical features.

Differential diagnosis

- Other chemical burns
- Thermal burns
- Traumatic lesions

Pathology

It is not required.

Treatment

Usually, no treatment is necessary as the lesion heals spontaneously within 4 to 6 days.

Paraformaldehyde Burn

Key points

- It was used in the past for pulp mummification.
- Gingival, oral mucosal, and bone damage have been documented.
- Paraformaldehyde is not typically used any longer.

Introduction

Paraformaldehyde was often used in the past for pulp mummification in patients undergoing root canal therapy. It is an extremely caustic chemical agent and in contact with the oral mucosa and the bone may cause severe soft and hard tissue necrosis.

Clinical features

Clinically, soft tissue damage presents as a painful ulceration covered by a yellowish or brownish fibrinopurulent pseudomembrane surrounded by severe inflammation (**Fig. 4.12**).

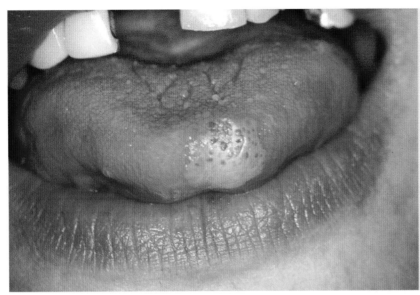

Fig. 4.10 Chemical burn of the tip of the tongue caused by silver nitrate.

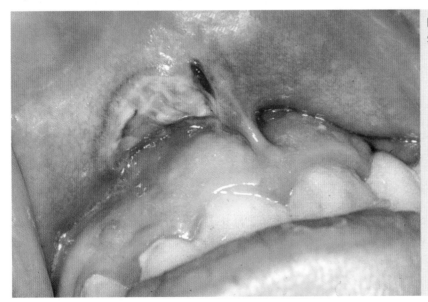

Fig. 4.11 Chemical burn caused by sodium hypochlorite.

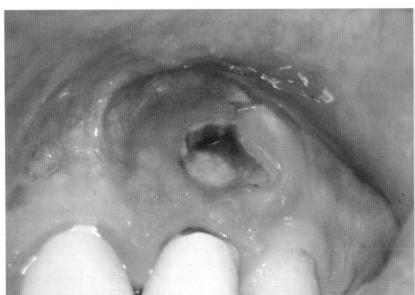

Fig. 4.12 Chemical burn caused by local application of paraformaldehyde resulting in a deep ulcer.

Bone necrosis may also occur as a consequence of leakage of the agent from the pulp chamber into the surrounding hard tissues. Paraformaldehyde is not used in modern dentistry. The diagnosis is made on the history and the clinical features.

Differential diagnosis

- Other chemical burns
- Traumatic ulcer
- Osteomyelitis
- Medication-related osteonecrosis

Pathology

It is not required.

Treatment

The lesions usually heal within 1 to 2 weeks after discontinuation of the agent. However, in severe persistent cases local oxygen-releasing mouthwashes or systemic antibiotics systemically in 4 to 6 days may be useful.

Acrylic Resin Burn

Key points

- This is the result of the use of acrylic resins for temporary oral prostheses.
- Inflammation of the oral mucosa with or without erosions is the main feature.
- It is the result of chemical and thermal damage.
- The diagnosis is based on the history and the clinical features.

Introduction

Autopolymerizing acrylic resins are occasionally used in dental practice for the construction of temporary prostheses. This may cause a local burn either due to heat from polymerization or chemical damage by any excess of monomer.

Clinical features

Clinically, the oral mucosa is diffuse red with or without superficial erosions (**Fig. 4.13**). A burning sensation or mild pain is the common symptom. The extent of the reaction depends on the duration of contact with the prosthesis. The lesion is not an allergic reaction. The diagnosis is based on the history and the clinical features.

Differential diagnosis

- Allergic stomatitis due to acrylic resin
- Other chemical burns
- Thermal burns
- Erythematous candidiasis

Pathology

It is not required.

Treatment

Usually, no treatment is necessary as the lesions resolve spontaneously in 4 to 6 days following removal of the prosthesis. However, in severe and extensive cases oral corticosteroids in low doses for a short time, e.g., prednisone 10 to 15 mg/d for 3 to 4 days, lessen the symptoms dramatically.

Chlorine Compound Burn

Key points

- This is a rare event.
- The severity of tissue damage depends on the concentration of the agent and the duration of contact.
- The diagnosis is based on the history and the clinical features.

Introduction

Accidental contact of chlorine compounds with the oral mucosa may cause a chemical burn and mucosal necrosis. Chlorine compounds in various concentrations are used as housecleaning material, hence their accidental (or deliberate) ingestion is the cause.

Clinical features

Clinically, a whitish painful erosion or ulceration of the oral mucosa is observed, covered by a necrotic membrane (**Fig. 4.14**). The lower lip, the tongue, and the floor of the mouth are most frequently affected. The diagnosis is based on the history and the clinical features.

Differential diagnosis

- Other chemical burns
- Thermal burns
- Traumatic ulcer

Pathology

It is not required.

Treatment

Usually, no treatment is necessary as the lesions heal spontaneously within 4 to 6 days. However, with persistent deep ulceration, corticosteroids in low doses for a short time, e.g., prednisone 10 to 15 mg/d for 4 to 6 days, improve the symptoms and shorten the healing time.

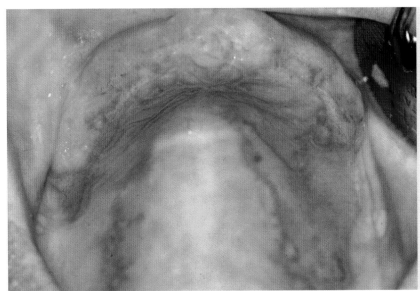

Fig. 4.13 Chemical and thermal burn of the palate caused by acrylic resin.

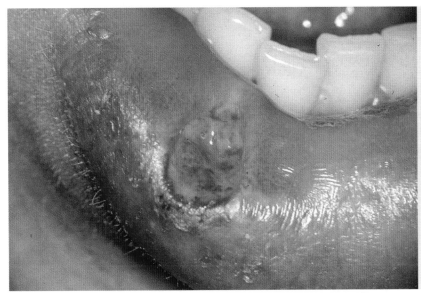

Fig. 4.14 Chemical burn of the lower lip caused by chlorine compound.

Agricultural Chemical Agents Burn

Key points

- It usually reflects accidental ingestion.
- The severity of the oral mucosal damage and the systemic reaction depends on the nature and concentration of the agent and its duration of contact.
- Occasionally, such an incident may be life threatening.
- The diagnosis is based on the history.

Introduction

A wide range of chemical agents are used in agriculture. Accidental contact of agricultural compounds with the oral mucosa may cause chemical burns in addition to systemic complications. These accidents are found most likely in rural areas.

Clinical features

The severity and extent of oral mucosal damage depend on the nature, concentration, and quantity of the compound and the duration of its contact with the oral tissues. Clinically, oral lesions present in a variety of ways, ranging from edema, redness to painful extensive erosions or ulcers covered with whitish or brownish necrotic epithelial debris (**Fig. 4.15**). The duration of oral lesions varies from 1 to 2 weeks. The diagnosis is based on the history and the clinical features.

Differential diagnosis

- Other chemical burns
- Thermal burns
- Erythema multiforme

Pathology

It is not required.

Treatment

This depends on the severity of the lesion and the nature of the particular agent. Severe cases with systemic symptoms warrant urgent hospitalization. In less severe cases without systemic complications the oral lesions should be managed by local anesthetics and antiseptic mouthwashes in association with systemic corticosteroids, e.g., prednisone 10 to 20 mg/d for 4 to 6 days.

Sanguinaria-Associated Oral Leukoplakia

Key points

- This is a unique form of leukoplakia due to the use of toothpastes or mouthwashes containing the herbal alkaloid sanguinaria.
- This type of leukoplakia is usually located on the maxillary mucobuccal fold, the alveolar mucosa, or the attached gingiva of the maxilla.
- Clinically, it appears as a homogeneous white plaque.
- A biopsy and histologic examination are necessary.

Introduction

Sanguinaria-associated leukoplakia is a unique form of leukoplakia that is attributed to long-term use of a mouthwash or toothpaste containing the herbal alkaloid sanguinaria. The use of such products was popular in the past to prevent periodontal disease. In recent years sanguinaria has been withdrawn from dental use.

Clinical features

Clinically, the lesion presents as an asymptomatic white homogeneous plaque that does not detach from the oral mucosa. Characteristically, the great majority of the lesions are located in the anterior maxillary mucobuccal fold or the alveolar mucosa or the attached gingiva (**Fig. 4.16**). The white plaque usually does not disappear even after the patient stops using the sanguinaria-containing products. Malignant transformation of the lesion is uncertain. The diagnosis is based on the history, clinical features, and the histologic examination.

Differential diagnosis

- Other forms of leukoplakia
- Lichen planus
- Candidiasis
- Chemical burn
- Cinnamon contact stomatitis
- Epithelial peeling

Pathology

A biopsy and histologic examination are important. The affected epithelium exhibits hyperorthokeratosis and hyperparakeratosis. Mild-to-moderate epithelial dysplasia may also be present.

Treatment

Surgical excision of the lesion is the treatment of choice. Use of products containing sanguinaria should be stopped.

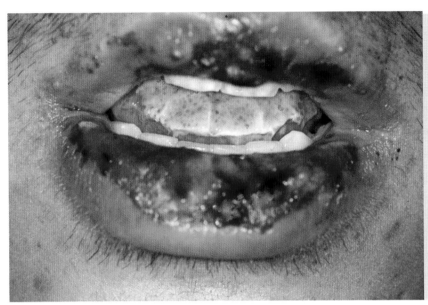

Fig. 4.15 Heavy chemical burn of the lips and the tongue caused by an agricultural agent.

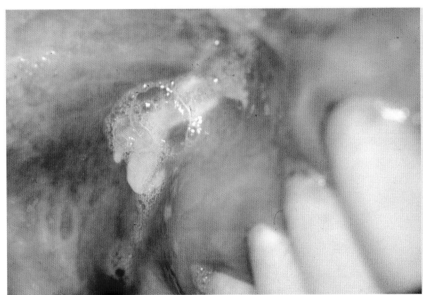

Fig. 4.16 Sanguinaria-associated leukoplakia on the upper alveobuccal sulcus.

Epithelial Peeling

Key points

- A superficial desquamation of the oral mucosa.
- White lesions that can be easily detached from the oral mucosa are the clinical features.
- The lesions are asymptomatic and harmless.
- The diagnosis is based on the clinical features.

Introduction

Epithelial peeling or epitheliolysis is a superficial desquamation of the oral mucosa that is usually caused by the direct irritating effect of toothpastes that contain high amounts of pyrophosphate or sodium lauryl sulfate (SLS) (**Figs. 4.17, 4.18**). However, the same phenomenon may be associated with several mouthwashes. It is not an allergic reaction.

Clinical features

Clinically, epithelial peeling presents as a superficial, asymptomatic white membrane that can be easily lifted from the oral mucosa. The lesion may be localized or generalized. The buccal mucosa and the mucobuccal folds are more commonly affected. The lesions usually disappear when patients stop using the causative toothpaste or mouthwash. The diagnosis is based on the history and the clinical features.

Differential diagnosis

- Chemical burns
- Thermal burns
- Chronic biting
- Leukoedema
- Candidiasis
- Cinnamon contact stomatitis

Pathology

It is not required.

Treatment

No treatment is necessary other than cessation of the causative agent.

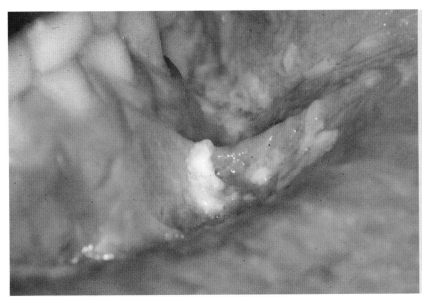

Fig. 4.17 Epithelial peeling.

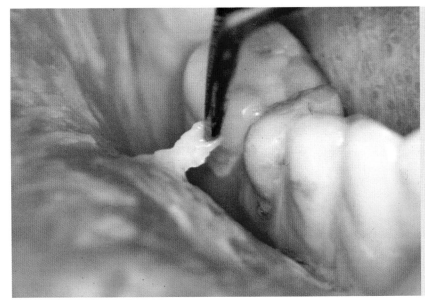

Fig. 4.18 Epithelial peeling.

5 Thermal and Electricity Lesions

Nicotinic Stomatitis

Key points
- This develops in response to heat rather than the chemicals in tobacco smoke.
- The palatal lesions are primarily due to pipe and less commonly due to cigar or cigarette smoking.
- The palatal mucosa assumes a grayish-white color associated with multiple nodules with red dots in the center.
- The lesion is not premalignant.

Introduction

Nicotinic stomatitis or smoker's palate is a thermal chemical reaction of the palatal mucosa that occurs most commonly in pipe smokers and rarely in cigarette or cigar smokers or even in nonsmokers who very often consume hot drinks. The disorder is not premalignant.

Clinical features

Clinically, nicotinic stomatitis is characterized by redness of the palatal mucosa, which later assumes a grayish-white color and multinodular formation due to keratinization of the epithelium (**Fig. 5.1**). A characteristic finding is the multiple red dots, 1 to 5 mm in diameter, in the center of the nodules, which represent the inflamed orifices of the secretory ducts of the minor salivary glands. In heavy smokers, fissures, furrows, and elevations may occur forming an irregular wrinkled surface (**Fig. 5.2**). The changes are more prominent toward the middle of the posterior hard palate. The prognosis of nicotinic stomatitis is good as it is not a potentially malignant disorder. However, it should not be confused with lesions associated with reversed smoking, which have serious consequences and high risk of malignant transformation. The diagnosis of nicotine stomatitis is made on the history and the clinical features while a biopsy only rarely may be necessary.

Differential diagnosis
- Reverse smoker's palate
- Leukoplakia
- Thermal burn
- Chemical burn
- Darier's disease

Pathology

Histologically, nicotinic stomatitis is characterized by hyperkeratosis, parakeratosis, and acanthosis of the palatal epithelium associated with mild chronic inflammation of the minor salivary glands and the subepithelial connective tissue. Epithelial dysplasia is rarely seen.

Treatment

The treatment is cessation of smoking. The palate returns to normal, usually within 2 to 4 weeks after smoking ceases.

Palatal Erosions due to Smoking

Key points
- It may occur in heavy smokers consuming more than 60 cigarettes a day.
- It is a severe thermal burn with erosions of the palatal mucosa.
- The lesions usually disappear after cessation of smoking.

Introduction

In heavy smokers, people consuming more than 60 cigarettes a day, palatal erosions may occur. The lesions are due to continuous high temperature in the oral cavity.

Clinical features

Clinically, the lesions appear as diffuse erythema on the palatal mucosa associated with painful erosions (**Fig. 5.3**). Thickening of the epithelium and white lesions as in nicotine stomatitis may also occur. The diagnosis is mainly based on the history and the clinical features and rarely a biopsy is needed to rule out epithelial dysplasia or malignancy.

Differential diagnosis
- Other forms of thermal burn
- Traumatic erosions
- Chemical burns
- Erythematous candidiasis
- Erythroplakia
- Lupus erythematosus
- Lichen planus

Pathology

On histologic examination, necrosis of the epithelium may be present associated with parakeratosis and acanthosis at the periphery of the erosion. The underlying connective tissue presents a mixture of acute and chronic inflammatory reaction.

Treatment

Cessation of smoking usually provokes retreating of the lesion within 2 to 4 weeks.

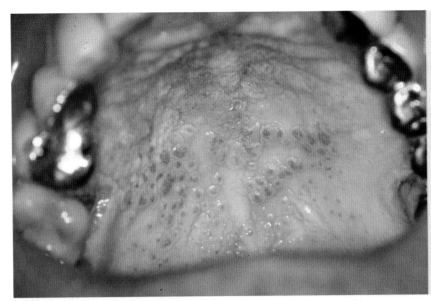

Fig. 5.1 Typical nicotine stomatitis.

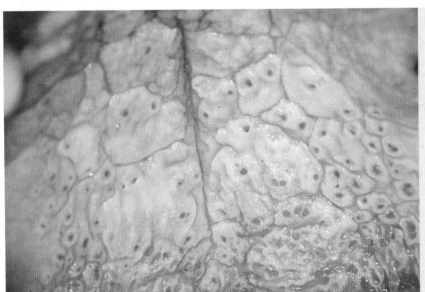

Fig. 5.2 Heavy nicotine stomatitis.

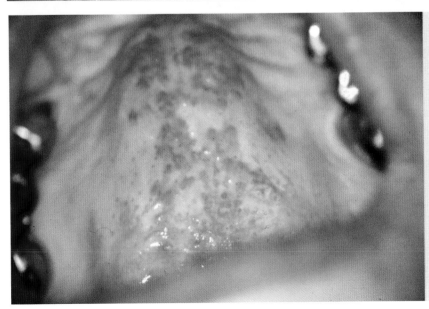

Fig. 5.3 Erythema and erosions of the palate due to heavy smoking.

Cigarette Smoker's Lip Lesions

Key points

- The lesions usually develop on the mucosal surface of the lower lip.
- Heavy smokers of nonfiltered cigarettes are more frequently affected.
- If smoking is stopped, the lip lesions may completely resolve.
- The lesions are not premalignant.

Introduction

Cigarette smoker's lip lesions arise commonly in heavy smokers of nonfiltered cigarettes (> 40 cigarettes daily) who hold them between the lips for a long time until short cigarette butts remain. The lesions are due to high temperature which develops during smoking in the area.

Clinical features

Characteristically, the lesions appear on the mucosal surface of the lower lip corresponding to the site at which the cigarette is held. Clinically, the lesions appear as flat or slightly elevated asymptomatic whitish wide lines intermixed with red striations (**Fig. 5.4**). The lesions are not premalignant. The diagnosis is based on the history and the clinical features.

Differential diagnosis

- Chronic biting
- Chemical burn
- Lichen planus
- Leukoplakia
- Discoid lupus erythematosus
- Candidiasis
- Cinnamon contact stomatitis

Pathology

Usually, it is not necessary. On histologic examination, hyperplasia of the epithelium and hyperorthokeratosis, parakeratosis, and acanthosis are common findings. A mild subepithelial inflammatory infiltrate may be seen.

Treatment

The lesions usually disappear after smoking cessation in 1 to 2 months.

Smoker's Melanosis

Key points

- Oral pigmentation is increased in heavy smokers.
- About 20 to 30% of tobacco users display smoker's melanosis.
- The anterior facial (i.e., labial) gingival are more frequently affected.
- Cessation of smoking results in gradual retreating of pigmentation within 2 to 3 years.

Introduction

Smoker's melanosis is a benign focal pigmentation of the oral mucosa more commonly encountered in women usually after the third decade of life. About 20 to 30% of heavy smokers exhibit areas of increased melanin pigmentation. The disorder is due to increased melanin production as a result of oral melanocyte stimulation mainly by nicotine and benzopyrene and probably due to the prolonged elevated temperature in the mouth.

Clinical features

Clinically, the pigmentation usually presents as asymptomatic multiple brown-pigmented macules or plaques localized mainly at the attached labial anterior gingiva and the interdental papillae of the mandible (**Figs. 5.5, 5.6**). The buccal mucosa, tongue, palate, and lips are less commonly affected. The areas of pigmentation increase during the first 2 years of smoking and are related to the number of cigarettes consumed per day. The diagnosis is usually based on the history and the clinical features and only rarely a biopsy is needed.

Differential diagnosis

- Racial pigmentation
- Traumatic pigmentation
- Drug-induced pigmentation
- Amalgam tattoo
- Pigmented nevi
- Lentigo simplex
- Freckles
- Malignant melanoma
- Endocrine disturbances
- Addison's disease
- Peutz-Jeghers syndrome
- Albright's syndrome
- von Recklinghausen's disease
- Hemochromatosis

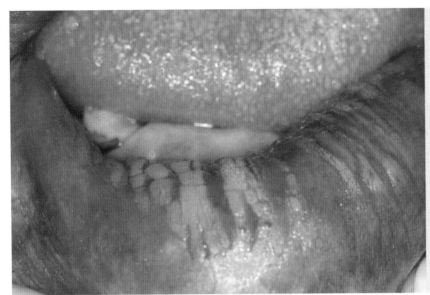

Fig. 5.4 White lines of the lower lip due to heavy smoking.

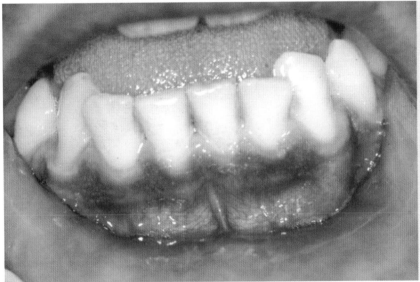

Fig. 5.5 Gingival melanosis due to smoking.

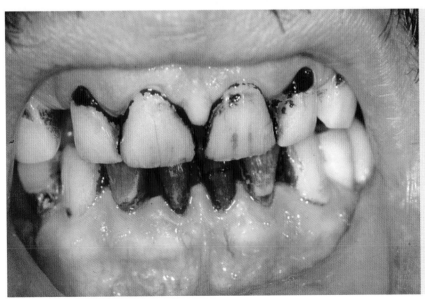

Fig. 5.6 Intense melanotic pigmentation of the teeth due to heavy smoking.

Pathology

Histologically, smoker's melanosis is characterized by increased melanin granules in the basal cell layer of the oral epithelium. Incontinent melanin is usually seen within the connective tissue and in melanophages of the lamina propria.

Treatment

Usually, no treatment is required. The pigmentation can gradually diminish after smoking cessation and may disappear after several months or years.

Thermal Burn

Key points

- This is a relatively common lesion on the oral mucosa.
- Very hot foods such as pizzas, melted cheese, beverages, or metal objects are the most common causes.
- The severity and extent of the lesion depends on the temperature of the responsible food or material.
- Erythema and erosions are the common clinical features.

Introduction

Thermal burn of the oral mucosa is caused by direct contact with very hot foods (pizzas, melted cheese), beverages, or hot metal objects. It is a relatively common incident which may produce mild or severe epithelial damage.

Clinical features

Clinically, the oral mucosa is red, and may undergo epithelial desquamation leaving small or extensive painful erosions (**Figs. 5.7, 5.8**). Vesicles may also develop. The palate, lips, tongue, and the floor of the mouth are most frequently affected. The diagnosis is based on the history and the clinical features. The patients usually remember the causative incident.

Differential diagnosis

- Chemical burns
- Traumatic erosions
- Herpes simplex
- Drug-induced stomatitis
- Cinnamon contact stomatitis
- Vesiculobullous diseases
- Fellatio
- Cunnilingus

Pathology

It is not required. Histologic examination reveals no specific epithelial necrosis with mild or severe inflammatory reaction.

Treatment

Mild lesions usually resolve within a week without treatment. Cold chamomile mouthwashes are helpful. In severe cases systemic corticosteroid in low dose for a short time, e.g., prednisone 10 mg/d for 3 to 4 days, dramatically improves the symptoms.

Electrical Burn

Key points

- Most electrical burns of the mouth occur in children younger than 6 years.
- The inappropriate use of a faulty electrical device or biting an electrical wire are the most usual causes.
- Two forms of electrical burns exist: the *contact* and *arc*.
- The lips, commissures, and perioral skin are the most frequently affected sites.
- Serious long-term functional and aesthetic consequences may occur.
- The diagnosis is based on the history and the clinical features.

Introduction

Electrical burns of the mouth are the most common electrical injuries in children younger than 6 years and may cause significant deformity. The majority of these burns occur when the child is sucking on the female end of a live extension cord or at the junction of an extension cord or when the child sucks or chews on exposed electrical wires. Less frequently, electrical burn may be a sign of child abuse. The most common electrical burns of the mouth are *arc* type, in which the saliva acts as a conducting medium and an electrical arc flows between the electrical source and the oral cavity, in such cases 2,500 to 3,000°C temperature can be generated.

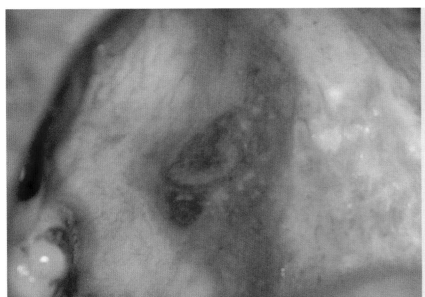

Fig. 5.7 Thermal burn of the palate caused by pizza.

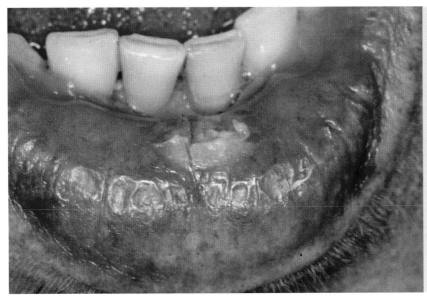

Fig. 5.8 Thermal burn of the lower lip caused by hot coffee.

Clinical features

Clinically, electrical burns of the oral cavity present as painful grayish-white, edematous lesions without bleeding (**Fig. 5.9**). Progressively, the affected area becomes brownish, necrotic, and finally sloughs, leaving a deep ulcerated area that may hemorrhage (**Figs. 5.10, 5.11**). The commissures, the lips, and perioral area are most frequently involved. The adjacent teeth may become nonvital. Drooling of food and saliva commonly occurs as a result of destruction of the sensory innervation of the lips. Scarring and microstomia are the most common long-term complications. The diagnosis is based on the history and the clinical features.

Differential diagnosis

- Traumatic injuries
- Severe thermal burn
- Noma

Pathology

It is not required.

Treatment

A multidisciplinary approach by oral medicine, oral and maxillofacial surgery, reconstructive surgery, and pediatric dentistry is important for the management of oral electrical burns. Treatment may be conservative and supportive. Surgical reconstruction may be necessary in severe cases.

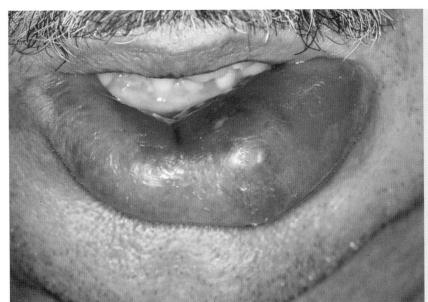

Fig. 5.9 Electrical burn of the lower lip.

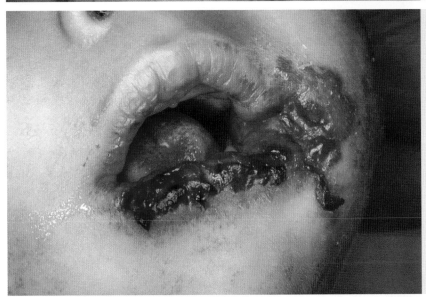

Fig. 5.10 Heavy electrical burn of the lower lip.

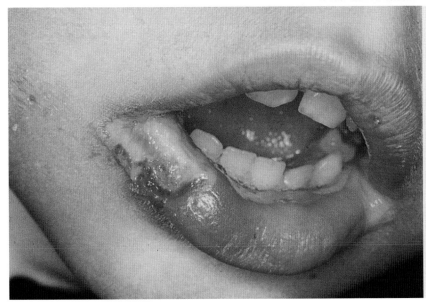

Fig. 5.11 Electrical burn of the lower lip.

6 Metal and Other Deposits

Amalgam Tattoo

Key points

- Amalgam tattoo is the most common form of pigmented exogenous materials that may be implanted within the oral mucosa.
- The lesions may be small or extensive.
- The gingiva, alveolar mucosa, floor of the mouth, and buccal mucosa are the sites most commonly involved.
- The differential diagnosis includes several other pigmented lesions including malignant melanoma.
- The diagnosis is based on the clinical features, radiographic findings, and histopathology.

Introduction

Amalgam tattoo is the most common exogenous oral implantation material causing pigmentation of the oral mucosa. Amalgam deposition into the oral mucosa may occur in several ways. It may develop as a result of continuous contact between an amalgam restoration and the gingiva or from embedding of amalgam fragments in the oral tissues during restoration of a tooth or surgical operation of the adjacent tissues. In addition, during tooth extraction, fragments of amalgam restorations often leave residues of the metal that may then be embedded within the adjacent soft tissues. Amalgam from endodontic retrofill procedures may also be a source of the tattoo. The use of the rubber dam has decreased much of the risk of amalgam tattoo.

Clinical features

Clinically, amalgam tattoo appears as a well-defined bluish or black, usually flat, irregular discoloration of varying size (**Figs. 6.1, 6.2**). The lesions may be solitary or multiple, are asymptomatic, and are usually found accidentally by the patient or during routine oral examination. The gingiva, alveolar mucosa, floor of the mouth, and buccal mucosa are more frequently affected. The diagnosis is based on the clinical features, radiographic findings, and biopsy results.

Differential diagnosis

- Pigmented nevi
- Ephelides
- Lentigo simplex
- Melanoacanthoma
- Lentigo maligna
- Malignant melanoma
- Silver and graphite implantation
- Cosmetic tattooing

Pathology

Histologic examination reveals numerous dark fragments of amalgam within the connective tissue usually surrounded by inflammatory infiltration, mainly by lymphocytes, histiocytes, and plasma cells. Occasionally, metallic fragments are visible radiographically as radiopaque material varying in size from one to several millimeters.

Treatment

Usually, no treatment is necessary if the clinical features are sufficient for diagnosis or the metallic fragments are evident radiographically. Conservative surgical excision is the treatment of choice along with histologic examination of the specimen, to rule out any other benign or malignant melanocytic lesion.

Silver and Graphite Deposits

Key points

- Silver and graphite implantation is rare on the oral mucosa.
- The gingiva, alveolar mucosa, and hard palate are more frequently affected.
- They present as gray or black discolorations and can cause diagnostic dilemmas.
- The diagnosis is usually based on the history and the clinical features.

Introduction

Silver and graphite deposits are a rare phenomenon in the oral mucosa. Silver discoloration may be the result of migration and deposition in the oral soft tissues after an endodontic procedure where silver cones were used for the packing of the root canals. Graphite discolorations are usually the result of a repeated self-traumatic implantation of pencil tip material by the patient, usually a child.

Clinical features

Clinically, both lesions present as a brownish-black or gray-brown asymptomatic macule or small plaque. Characteristically, silver discoloration usually appears near the apex of a tooth, several months after the endodontic treatment (**Fig. 6.3**). Graphite discoloration usually occurs on the gingiva, palate, and buccal mucosa (**Fig. 6.4**). The diagnosis is usually based on the history and the clinical features.

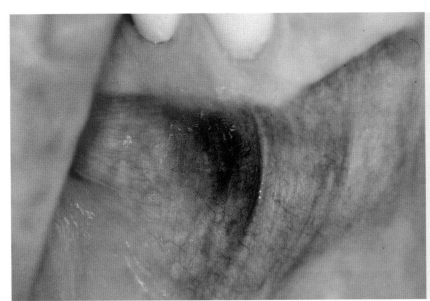

Fig. 6.1 Amalgam tattoo on the lower buccal sulcus.

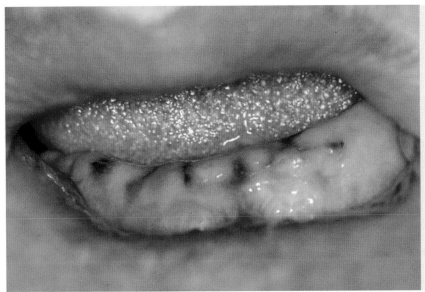

Fig. 6.2 Multiple foci of amalgam tattoo on the mucosa of an edentulous mandible.

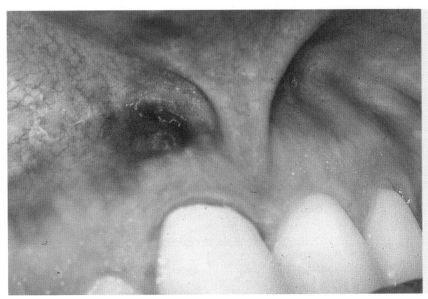

Fig. 6.3 Melanotic silver deposit.

Differential diagnosis

- Amalgam tattoo
- Pigmented nevi
- Ephelides
- Lentigo simplex
- Melanoacanthoma
- Malignant melanoma

Pathology

Usually, it is not required. Histologic examination reveals similar pattern as in amalgam tattoo.

Treatment

Usually, no treatment is required. Conservative surgical excision is the treatment of choice usually for cosmetic reasons or if there is a diagnostic dilemma.

Bismuth Deposition

Key points

- Systemic chronic bismuth compounds exposure may result in skin and mucosal discoloration.
- Bismuth oral mucosal discoloration is a rare phenomenon nowadays.
- A bluish line along the marginal gingiva is the characteristic pattern.

Introduction

Systemic bismuth compounds were formerly used for treatment of syphilis and a few other skin diseases. In addition, it is also used as a surgical pack. However, in recent years antibiotics and other medications have replaced bismuth compounds for those purposes. Oral discolorations due to bismuth are now rarely encountered except in patients where occupational exposure occurred or those who have been treated for syphilis in the preantibiotic era.

Clinical features

Clinically, bismuth deposition forms a characteristic bluish-gray line along the marginal gingiva and papillae (**Fig. 6.5**). Less frequently, bismuth may be deposited in other parts of the oral mucosa causing discoloration, mainly at the border of an ulcer, areas of inflammation, or the filiform and fungiform papillae. Burning mouth sensation, increased salivation, and rarely, ulceration may occur. Poor oral hygiene is a predisposing factor for the oral lesions. The diagnosis is based on the history and the clinical features.

Differential diagnosis

- Lead deposition
- Silver deposition
- Drug-related discoloration
- Addison's disease
- Normal pigmentation
- Amalgam tattoo

Pathology

It is not required.

Treatment

Discontinuation of further exposure to the bismuth is suggested. The oral discoloration does not need any treatment.

Lead Deposition

Key points

- Oral manifestation from injection or exposure of lead is a rare phenomenon.
- Gingival lead line, oral ulceration, and bluish-gray spots are the most common oral lesions.
- Chronic exposure to lead may cause symptoms and signs from several organs.
- The diagnosis is based on the history and clinical features.

Introduction

Lead poisoning may occur in different ways, most commonly in people working in the metal processing industry and in battery making factories. Another source of lead is food and drinks which come from lead-contaminated soil or water. In addition, another source of lead poisoning is lead-based paints.

Clinical features

Chronic lead intoxication may result in severe systemic symptoms and signs from the kidneys, bone marrow, bones, joints, nervous system, and gastrointestinal tract. Fatigue, headache, weakness, irritability, abdominal pain, and musculoskeletal pain are the common symptoms. Oral manifestation may also occur. Clinically, in the mouth a characteristic bluish-black line is observed along the marginal gingiva which is called lead line (**Fig. 6.6**). It is a lead sulfide precipitate resulting from the reaction of bacterial hydrogen sulfide and lead. Less frequently, nonspecific ulceration and bluish-gray spots may be observed on the tongue and buccal mucosa. Excessive salivation, metallic taste, aggressive periodontal disease, and tremor of the tongue may also occur. The diagnosis is based on the history and the clinical features.

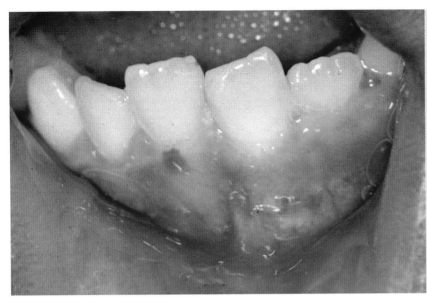

Fig. 6.4 Graphite fragments in the gingival crevice of the right central incisor.

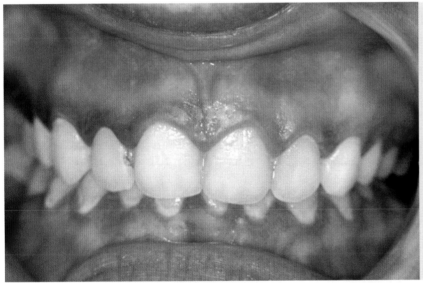

Fig. 6.5 Blue-black linear bismuth deposition on the gingiva—"bismuth line."

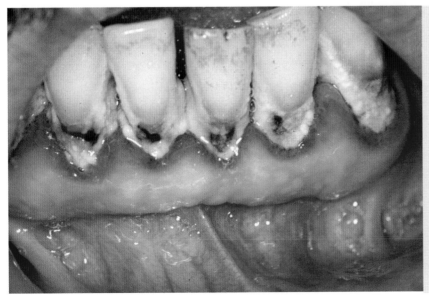

Fig. 6.6 Blue-black lead deposition on the marginal gingiva—"lead line."

Differential diagnosis
- Bismuth deposition
- Other heavy metal deposition
- Amalgam tattoo

Pathology

Histologic examination is not required for the oral lesions. Measurement of lead levels in the blood may be useful for diagnosis.

Treatment

Discontinuation of exposure to lead, supportive care, and administration of chelating agents such as 2,3-dimercaptosuccinic acid (DMSA) and 2,3-dimercaptopropane-1-sulfonate (DMPS) or D-penicillamine are the medications of choice in cases of severe lead poisoning.

Materia Alba of the Oral Mucosa

Key points
- Materia alba is usually found at the dentogingival margins.
- Materia alba of the oral mucosa is a relatively rare phenomenon.
- It presents as a whitish surface which is characteristically easily detached with mild pressure.
- The diagnosis is based on clinical criteria.

Introduction

Materia alba is the result of bacteria, dead epithelial cells, and food debris accumulation. It is commonly found at the dentogingival margins of people with poor oral hygiene and can be a factor for gingival disease. Materia alba may also be seen along the attached gingiva and alveolar mucosa of the sulci, or the oral mucosa of patients who are unable to brush and clean their gingiva and the mucosa because of painful oral diseases or neurologic dysfunction.

Clinical features

Clinically, materia alba of the oral mucosa appears as a whitish or white-gray soft plaque which is characteristically easily detached after slight pressure by a wooden spatula, leaving a reddish surface (**Fig. 6.7**). The diagnosis is based exclusively on the clinical features.

Differential diagnosis
- Candidiasis
- Chemical burn
- Cinnamon contact stomatitis
- Leukoplakia

Pathology

It is not required.

Treatment

No treatment is required other than measures to improve oral hygiene.

Phleboliths

Key points
- Small phleboliths are relatively rare in the mouth of older people.
- They are asymptomatic with blackish color.
- The diagnosis is usually made incidentally during routine oral examination.

Introduction

Phleboliths are calcified thrombi that occur in veins. The thrombi are formed by slowing of the peripheral blood flow which then becomes secondarily organized and mineralized. Such calcified thrombi constitute the core of the phlebolith. The phenomenon is usually common in elderly people and is also a characteristic feature of cavernous hemangiomas.

Clinical features

Clinically, oral phleboliths appear as relatively hard, painless, black or bluish swellings of the oral soft tissues usually associated with vascular malformations (**Figs. 6.8, 6.9**). The size varies from few millimeters to several centimeters. The diagnosis is usually based on the clinical features.

Differential diagnosis
- Vascular malformations
- Hemangioma
- Other soft tissue tumors
- Salivary gland calculi
- Calcified lymph nodes

Pathology

It is usually not required. Histologic and radiographic examination, angiography, and computed tomography may be used in some cases.

Treatment

Usually, no treatment is required. Surgical excision is suggested for aesthetic reasons or if there is diagnostic dilemma.

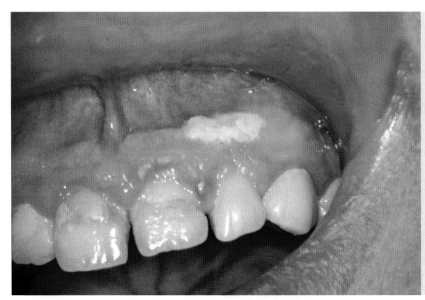

Fig. 6.7 Materia alba deposition on the alveolar mucosa of the maxilla.

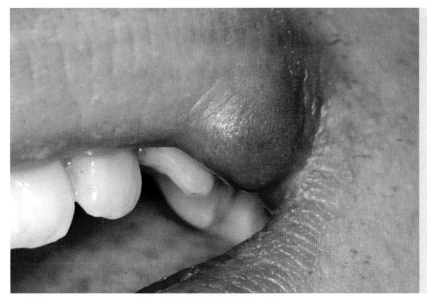

Fig. 6.8 Big phlebolith of the upper lip.

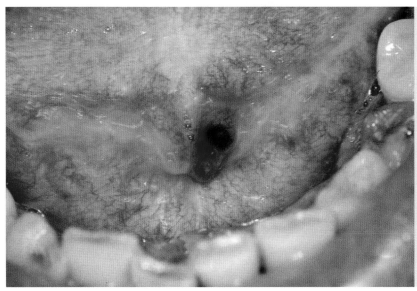

Fig. 6.9 Small phlebolith on the floor of the mouth.

7 Foreign Materials

Various Foreign Bodies

Key points

- Foreign body impaction in the mouth is a relatively common phenomenon.
- It may be the result of an accident, hard foodstuff, or dental and medical procedures in the oral cavity.
- The signs and symptoms vary and are usually associated with pain.
- The diagnosis is made on clinical criteria.

Introduction

Implantation of foreign bodies and materials in the oral soft tissues is a relatively common phenomenon. It may be the result of an accident, of chewing hard and sharp foodstuff, or following surgical and other dental or medical procedures. The most common types of foreign bodies include fish and animal bones, glass fragments, synthetic materials, sand particles, buttons, oral piercings, local medication, and others.

Clinical features

The clinical presentation varies depending on the kind of the foreign body implanted, its size, the way it has entered the oral tissues, the amount that is present in the tissues, and the location in the mouth. The most common features are a nonspecific painful ulcer associated with intense inflammation or hard growths with or without inflammation (**Figs. 7.1–7.4**). Discoloration of the surrounding tissues may occur, depending on the color and the size of the foreign body. Occasionally, metallic or plastic rings and firmly impacted bodies such as buttons in the mouth of children may cause diagnostic problems (**Figs. 7.5, 7.6**). Repeated intralesional injections of triamcinolone acetonide may also lead to the formation of hard nodules due to salt deposition. The diagnosis of foreign bodies in the mouth is based on the history and the clinical features. However, occasionally a biopsy is necessary for definite diagnosis.

Differential diagnosis

- Traumatic lesions
- Metallic deposits
- Benign and malignant tumors

Pathology

Examination of biopsy specimens of the affected area reveals the presence of foreign body (metal, bone, etc.) usually surrounded by dense inflammatory infiltration by lymphocytes, plasma cells, histiocytes, eosinophils, and multinucleated giant cells. Radiographic examination can be useful to identify the type of the foreign body.

Treatment

Conservative surgical excision is the treatment of choice or just a simple removal of the foreign material if it is possible.

Skin Grafts

Key points

- Skin grafts are often used to cover oral mucosal deficits following extensive oral surgery.
- The color of the skin graft may be whitish or grayish-white or even black due to melanin production.
- Hair and hair follicles may be observed in the graft.
- The diagnosis is made on clinical criteria.

Introduction

Skin grafts are often used in the oral cavity to cover mucosal deficits after extensive surgery for malignant or benign tumors' removal or reconstructive surgery reconstruction for other pathologic conditions.

Clinical features

Clinically, skin grafts present as an asymptomatic, whitish or grayish-white surface (**Fig. 7.7**). Occasionally, the color of the skin graft is black, due to melanin overproduction by the graft melanocytes. The size of the surface depends on the size of the graft. The border may be smooth or irregular. Hair and hair follicles may be observed in the graft (**Fig. 7.8**). The buccal mucosa, tongue, palate, lips, and alveolar mucosa are the areas where most skin grafts are placed. The diagnosis is based exclusively on the history and the clinical features.

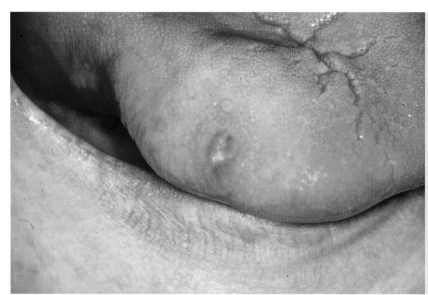

Fig. 7.1 Foreign body in the tongue—thorn from a plant.

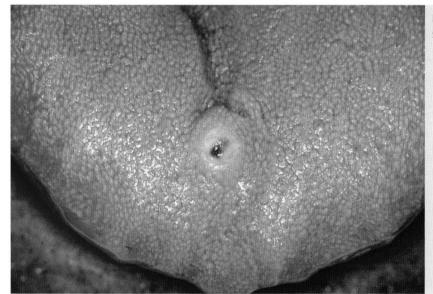

Fig. 7.2 Foreign body in the tongue—sand granule.

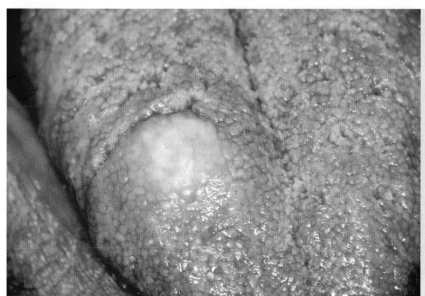

Fig. 7.3 Foreign body in the tongue—thorn from a plant.

Differential diagnosis

- Mucosal grafts
- Traumatic scar
- Leukoplakia
- Melanoma

Pathology

It is not required.

Treatment

None required.

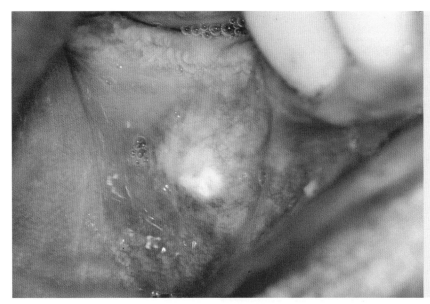

Fig. 7.4 Salt deposition in the tongue caused by repeated intralesional injection of triamcinolone acetonide.

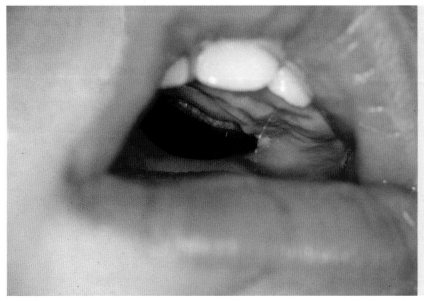

Fig. 7.5 Black button on the palate of a child.

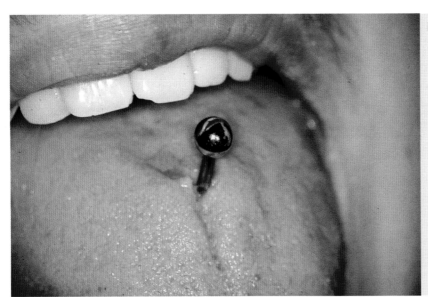

Fig. 7.6 Piercing on the tongue.

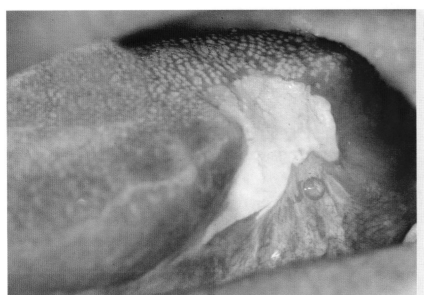

Fig. 7.7 Skin graft on the lateral border of the tongue.

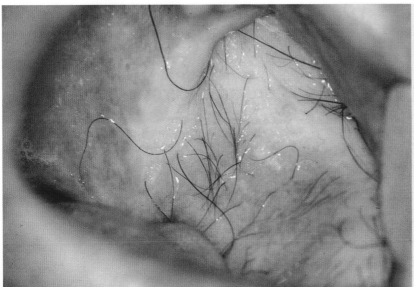

Fig. 7.8 Skin graft with hair on the buccal mucosa.

8 Oral Complications of Radiation and Chemotherapy

Mucositis due to Radiation Therapy

Key points

- Radiation therapy is an important tool in the armamentarium against oral cancer.
- Oral complications can be a frequent and clinically significant events during or after radiation treatment.
- The complications may be caused by the treatment itself (directly) or by side effects of the radiation (indirectly) and may be acute (early) or chronic (late).
- The most common oral complications due to radiation are mucositis, osteonecrosis of the jaws, salivary gland dysfunction, taste changes, pain, tooth decay, periodontal disease, fibrosis of the mucous membrane, and infections.
- Management of the oral complications includes preventive measures during and after the radiation therapy.

Introduction

Radiation therapy has an important place in the treatment of oral and other head and neck cancers. The most common form of radiation used is ionizing radiation delivered by an external source, or radioactive implants, e.g., iridium, gold, radium, cobalt. Radiation beyond its therapeutic levels may also cause changes or damage of the tissues, particularly those with a high cellular turnover, such as those of the oral mucosa, salivary glands, and bone. Oral mucositis is the culmination of a series of biologically complex and interactive events that can affect all oral mucosal surfaces.

Clinical features

The oral mucosal side effects of radiation mainly depend on the dose and duration of the treatment and perhaps the preventive oral care measures before the initiation of the cancer treatment. Oral mucositis is the most common oral complication during and after radiation therapy. It may be classified as acute (early) or chronic (late). Acute mucositis, usually occurs at the end of the first week of therapy and clinically presents as diffuse erythema and edema associated with a burning sensation or pain (**Fig. 8.1**). During the second week, the erythema becomes more severe and painful erosions or ulceration may develop, which are covered by a whitish-yellow necrotic membrane (**Figs. 8.2–8.4**).

Oral mucositis due to radiation therapy primarily affects almost all the mucosal surfaces within the direct radiation field. Malaise, dry mouth, burning sensation, loss of taste, pain during mastication, speech, and swallowing are common symptoms. Oral infections (by viruses, bacteria, or fungi), dental decay, jaw bone necrosis, gingivitis and periodontitis, atrophy and fibrosis of the oral mucosa, mucosal pigmentation, and dermatitis associated with atrophy (**Fig. 8.5**) are common complications. The lesions usually last 6 to 10 weeks, depending on the length of the treatment and the dose of radiation administered. The diagnosis is based on the history and the clinical features.

Differential diagnosis

- Mucositis following stem cell transplant
- Mucositis due to chemotherapy
- Bisphosphonates-related oral complications
- Monoclonal antibodies oral complications
- Drug reactions
- Allergic contact stomatitis
- Erythema multiforme
- Erosive lichen planus
- Pemphigus
- Mucous membrane pemphigoid
- Leukemia

Pathology

Usually, it is not required. Occasionally, the initial erythematous phase is followed by a breakdown of the oral mucosa resulting in the formation of ulcerative lesions. The ulcers are covered by a pseudomembrane composed of dead cells and fibrin, sometimes colonized by bacteria.

Treatment

Prevention of the oral complications includes a healthy diet, high level of oral hygiene, dental and periodontal care, and cessation of smoking and alcohol, before the initiation of radiation therapy. Treatment of oral mucositis during and after the radiation therapy includes cleaning the mouth, relieving any pain, promoting the healing of ulceration if possible, and managing any infections. It can be classified into *local* and *systemic*. The local treatment includes topical anesthetics, e.g., viscous lidocaine, topical corticosteroids, and tacrolimus, 0.15% benzydamine oral rinse, mouthwashes with granulocyte-macrophage colony-stimulating factor (GM-CSF) or oxygen-releasing mouthwashes, and saliva substitutes. Systemic corticosteroids in low doses, e.g., prednisone 15 to 20 mg/d for 2 to 3 weeks, in combination with high doses of B-complex vitamins can lead to relief in the signs and symptoms dramatically. Oral zinc sulfate supplementation may also be helpful.

Osteoradionecrosis

Key points

- Jaw bone osteonecrosis is a chronic (late) and possibly the most serious complication of radiation therapy for head and neck cancer.
- The etiology is linked mostly to radiation-induced hypoxic, hypocellular, hypovascular tissue and defective wound healing rather than infection.
- The mandible is more frequently affected than the maxilla and dentate patients are at higher risk than edentulous patients.
- Conservative surgical excision of bone sequestra and antibiotics are the treatments of choice.

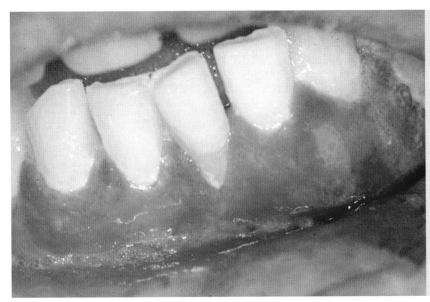

Fig. 8.1 Radiation-induced mucositis, severe erythema of the gingiva, and the alveolar ridge.

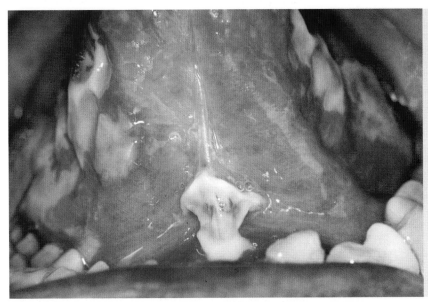

Fig. 8.2 Radiation-induced mucositis, lesions on the tongue.

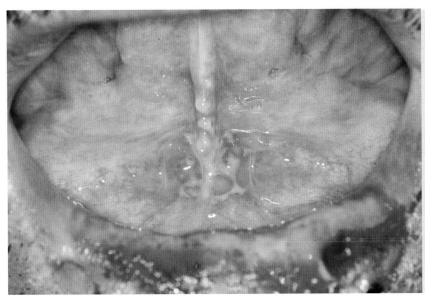

Fig. 8.3 Radiation-induced mucositis, lesions on the tongue, the floor of the mouth, and the lip.

Introduction

Osteoradionecrosis of the jaws is a serious complication of radiation therapy. It may occur in cases of high-dose radiation, especially if inadequate measures have been taken to reduce the radiation dosage delivered to the bone. The risk of osteoradionecrosis increases after topical trauma to the jaw or surgery during or after radiation. Osteoradionecrosis is the result of damage of small blood vessels or destruction within the jaws and damage of bone cell function. Although several instances of osteonecrosis develop secondary to local trauma, a minority of instances appear to occur spontaneously.

Clinical features

Clinically, jaw bone osteonecrosis presents as a painful or painless bone necrosis and bone exposure that may become a secondary infection and leads to the development of sequestration and rarely of a sinus tract or fistula (**Figs. 8.6, 8.7**). Extensive osteonecrosis may be associated with anesthesia or paresthesia. There is a higher incidence of osteonecrosis in the mandible than the maxilla due to the lower vascular network and the presence of more cortical bone in the mandible. The risk of this complication is increased in dentate patients especially if teeth, within the radiation field, are extracted after the radiation therapy. Osteonecrosis is usually a late complication of radiotherapy occurring within 2 to 6 months or even longer. Dental extractions or surgical procedures involving bone must be avoided during radiation therapy. The diagnosis is based on the medical history and the clinical features.

Differential diagnosis
- Bisphosphonate-induced osteonecrosis
- Monoclonal antibodies–induced osteonecrosis (e.g., denosumab)
- Bacterial osteomyelitis
- Osteosarcoma
- Chondrosarcoma

Pathology

Usually, it is not necessary. However, radiology, a biopsy, and microbial examination may be needed in some cases. Histologically, fragments of nonviable bone tissue with empty osteocyte lacunae are seen within vascularized fibrous tissue of bone marrow.

Treatment

Preventive care can make bone loss less severe. Before radiotherapy, all unrestorable, abscessed, or periodontally involved teeth should be extracted, dental treatment should be performed to the ones that can be restored, oral infection foci should be eliminated, and high levels of oral hygiene should be implemented. In severe cases of osteonecrosis, healing may occur after conservative therapy consisting of conservative local debridement, antibiotics, and efforts to keep teeth and gingiva healthy. In more severe cases, healing may be delayed for several months. In such cases more aggressive surgical debridement and hyperbaric oxygen use is suggested. The use of stem cells (induced pluripotent stem cells [IPS] or stimulus-triggered acquisition of pluripotency [STAP]) may be the future therapy.

Histologically, within vascularized fibrous tissue of marrow spaces fragments of nonviable bone tissue with empty osteocyte lacunae are seen.

Other Side Effects of Radiation

Key points
- Several other oral complications may be associated with head and neck radiation.
- The most common side effects are hyposalivation, mouth sores, infections, tooth decay, periodontal disease, taste disturbances, and mouth and jaw stiffness (trismus).
- Prevention of these complications includes high level of oral hygiene, a healthy diet, and dental and periodontal care.

Hyposalivation is a common complication of radiotherapy, particularly if the major salivary glands are included in the fields of radiation. Reduction in salivary flow may occur depending on the dose of radiation received. However, irreparable damage often occurs when the total dose is greater than 50 Gy and the salivary glands are in the field of radiation. Affected patients have difficulty speaking, chewing, and swallowing which ultimately lessens their quality of life.

In addition, patients are more susceptible to dental caries, periodontal disease, and bacterial, viral, and fungal infections. Trismus may develop as a late complication and can cause difficulties in mouth opening and mastication. Taste alteration affects patients usually from the third or fourth week of radiotherapy and may last for several months. It occurs in approximately 60 to 70% of all cases.

Atrophy of the oral mucosa and hyperpigmentation in the field of radiation may also occur.

Mucositis from Chemotherapy

Key points
- Chemotherapy causes neutropenia, neutrophil dysfunction, and impaired inflammatory response, which may delay tissue healing and lead to damage of the oral and periodontal tissues.
- Oral mucositis is the principal manifestation of acute oral toxicity related to chemotherapy and develops in 40 to 50% of patients.
- Chemotherapy-induced mucositis depends on patient's age, degree of oral toxicity of the chemotherapeutic agent, the dose and the number of chemotherapeutic agents used, and any preexisting oral conditions.
- Oral mucositis related to chemotherapy and oral mucositis due to radiation are similar in their clinical features.
- Upon completion of chemotherapy, oral mucositis gradually resolves within 3 to 4 weeks.
- Less commonly, xerostomia, oral infections, gingival bleeding, and alteration in taste may occur.
- The prevalence of oral complications from chemotherapy varies from 20 to 70%.

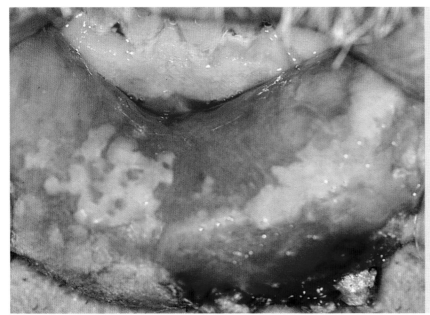

Fig. 8.4 Radiation-induced mucositis, lesions on the lower lip.

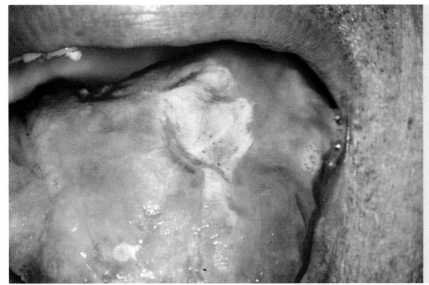

Fig. 8.5 Radiation-induced mucositis, late-stage lesions with atrophy of the mucosa, and pigmentation.

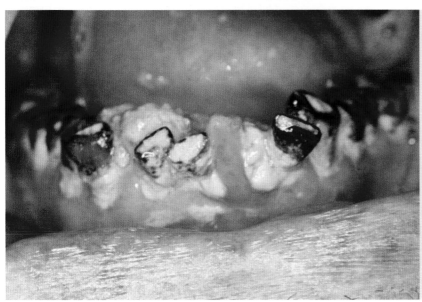

Fig. 8.6 Osteoradionecrosis of the mandible with dental damage, bone fistula, and sequestra.

Introduction

Chemotherapy is another weapon against several types of malignancies of the oral cavity, the head and neck region, and other organs. Chemotherapy can be used to treat extensive cancers that have spread too far to be treated by surgery or radiation alone. The drugs that are most commonly used for the treatment of cancer include cisplatin, 5-fluorouracil, carboplatin, paclitaxel, docetaxel, methotrexate, bleomycin, and others. Besides the targeted action of these agents against the neoplastic cells, there are side effects against normal cells and tissues, particularly those with higher mitotic index. Chemotherapy-induced oral mucositis depends on the patient's age, the degree of oral toxicity of the chemotherapeutic agent used, poor oral hygiene, and gender. The oral mucosa of younger patients has a higher mitotic index that increases their susceptibility to mucositis. They have, however, higher amounts of epithelial-related growth factors that favor a more rapid recovery. Myelosuppression caused by these agents and an inability to defend against local factors often exacerbate the oral lesions. Additional factors such as smoking, alcohol, xerostomia, and periodontal disease are high-risk parameters for developing oral mucositis. Oral mucositis affects an average of 40 to 60% of patients receiving cytotoxic chemotherapy.

Clinical features

Oral complications related to chemotherapy are classified as *acute* and *late*. Etiologically, they may be *direct*, where cytotoxicity is directed against the epithelial cells or *indirect*, where lesions are the result of oral infections (*Candida*, viruses, bacteria) and hemorrhage due to bone marrow suppression. Acute complications are mucositis, saliva changes, taste alterations, bleeding, and infections. Late complications are xerostomia and mucosal atrophy. Oral mucositis is the principal manifestation related to chemotherapy. It usually develops within 2 to 3 weeks of starting chemotherapy. Clinically, the oral mucosa appears red, edematous, usually with multiple painful erosions or ulcerations covered by white-yellowish pseudomembrane (**Figs. 8.8–8.10**). The patients complain about a burning sensation, dry mouth, taste changes, and gingival bleeding. Candidiasis, herpetic and bacterial infections may occur, particularly in patients with hematopoietic cell

transplantation, leukemias, and those receiving high-doses of chemotherapeutic agents. Oral lesions are more common on the nonkeratinized mucosa (tongue, buccal mucosa, floor of the mouth, soft palate). Oral mucositis from chemotherapy gradually resolves within 3 to 6 weeks. The diagnosis is based on medical history and clinical features.

Differential diagnosis

- Oral mucositis due to radiation
- Drug-induced oral lesions
- Erythema multiforme
- Herpetic stomatitis
- Graft-versus-host disease

Pathology

It is not required. Histologically, the lesions are nearly similar to those seen in mucositis due to radiation.

Treatment

Several agents have been used to manage oral mucositis caused by chemotherapy. The goal of therapy is to minimize the pain, improve the oral function, and reduce the secondary infections. Topical application of lidocaine and benzocaine, the use of mouthwashes with diphenhydramine, benzydamine hydrochloride, or ketoprofen lysine salt 1.6% have beneficial palliative effects. Local use of oxygen-releasing mouthwashes helps to remove degenerated tissue debris. Systemic administration of low doses of corticosteroids such as prednisolone tablets 20 to 30 mg/d for 1 week followed by tapering and cessation in 2 weeks of time promotes healing of the lesions, particularly if simultaneously vitamin B complex is administered in high doses. Recently, palifermin has been used for the treatment of oral mucositis. The oncologist in charge is responsible for the treatment of oral infections, if they develop. It is important that any treatment of oral lesions has to be performed in cooperation with the oncologists.

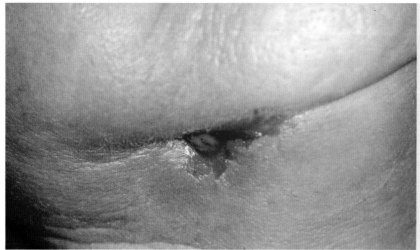

Fig. 8.7 Osteoradionecrosis, skin fistula.

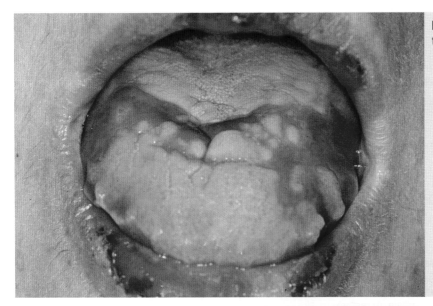

Fig. 8.8 Extensive erosions of the tongue caused by chemotherapy.

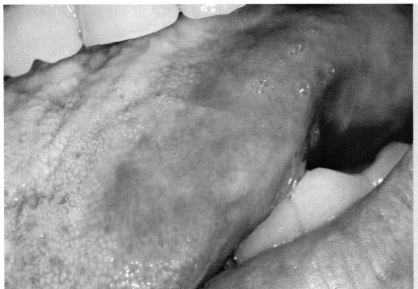

Fig. 8.9 Localized erosion on the lateral border of the tongue caused by chemotherapy.

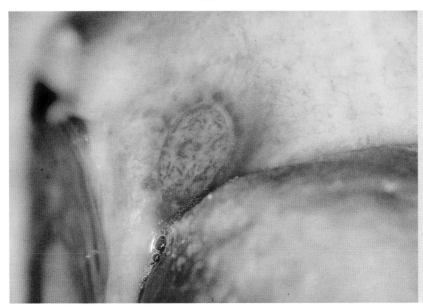

Fig. 8.10 Ulceration of the soft palate caused by chemotherapy.

9 Contact Allergic Reactions

Amalgam Contact Stomatitis

Key points
- Most commonly mercury and rarely other trace metals contained in amalgam are implicated in such hypersensitivity reactions.
- The mucosal reaction can be acute or chronic.
- Lichenoid reaction of the oral mucosa due to amalgam is relatively common.
- Oral allergic reactions are less common compared with the skin.

Introduction

Continuous contact of the oral mucosa with amalgam restorations (usually oxidized) may lead to hypersensitivity or toxic reactions, usually due to mercury and rarely due to other trace metals (zinc, copper, silver, and tin). The hypersensitivity reaction can be acute, manifesting within 24 hours following contact with the amalgam, and is rare or chronic, caused by hypersensitivity or by toxic action on the oral mucosa from the minerals and is more common.

Clinical features

Clinically, erythema is observed with irregular white areas or striae. Occasionally, erosions may occur accompanied by pain and a burning sensation particularly to certain foods (**Figs. 9.1–9.3**). As the lesions are clinically and histologically similar to lichen planus, this reaction is described by the term "lichenoid reaction." Characteristically, the lesions develop exactly at the sites of contact of the oral mucosa with the amalgam restorations and most commonly affect the buccal mucosa and the lateral surface of the tongue at the premolar/molar area. Another characteristic is the complete healing of the lesions when the amalgam restorations are replaced with other materials. The diagnosis is usually based on the history and the clinical features.

Differential diagnosis
- Lichen planus
- Discoid lupus erythematosus
- Drug-induced lesions
- Cinnamon contact stomatitis
- Leukoplakia
- Chronic biting

Pathology

Histopathologic examination reveals hyperkeratosis of the epithelium or atrophy. Hydropic degeneration of the basal layer and dense band-like chronic inflammatory infiltration on the superficial lamina propria, mainly by lymphocytes and plasma cells are usually present. A perivascular infiltrate composed primarily of lymphocytes and plasma cells is frequently observed. The histologic picture is similar with that of lichen planus. Cutaneous patch testing may be helpful.

Treatment

Polishing of old amalgam restorations or replacement with other materials is recommended. In very serious hypersensitivity cases systemic steroids in low dose can be helpful (10–20 mg of prednisolone for a week followed by a 2-week taper).

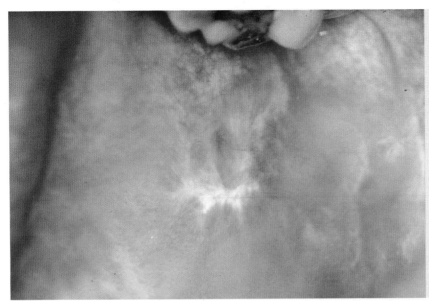

Fig. 9.1 Lichenoid reaction of the buccal mucosa caused by contact with an amalgam restoration.

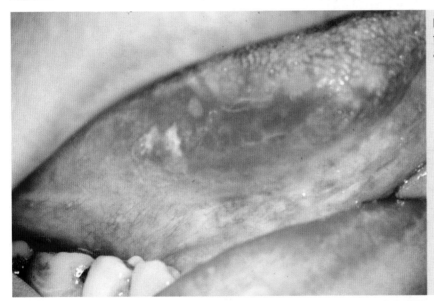

Fig. 9.2 Erosion and white areas of the tongue caused by contact with amalgam restorations.

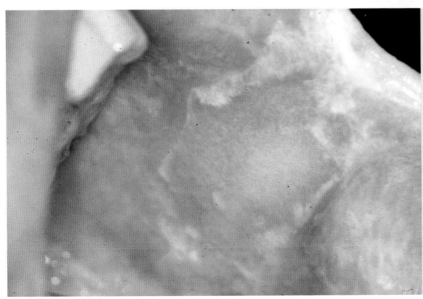

Fig. 9.3 Prominent lichenoid reaction of the buccal mucosa caused by contact with amalgam restorations.

Allergic Contact Stomatitis

Key points

- It is relatively rare, despite the fact that the oral mucosa is exposed to a multitude of antigens.
- It can develop within hours (acute) or days (chronic) when exposed to an allergen.
- The most common symptoms and signs include a burning sensation, erythema, edema, vesicles, and erosions.
- Removal of the offending agent should be curative.

Introduction

Contact allergic reactions of the oral mucosa are relatively rare compared with the skin, despite the fact that the oral mucosa is exposed to a multitude of antigens. The most important reasons are the presence of saliva which does not allow prolonged period of contact with the antigens, the limited epithelial keratinization that makes it difficult for antigens to bind, and the reduced presence of antigen-recognizing cells (T lymphocytes, Langerhans cells). The allergens mostly implicated can be found in foods and drinks, chewing gum, sweets, toothpastes, mouthwashes and medications used in dentistry, restorative dental materials, etc.

Clinical features

Clinically, a burning sensation or even pain, associated with erythema, and edema are the most frequent symptoms and signs. Rarely vesicles and erosions are noticed (**Figs. 9.4, 9.5**). The presence of oral symptoms and signs can be *acute* or *chronic*. Diagnosis is based on the history and the clinical features. Quite often diagnosis can be challenging, especially in the chronic type, as it is difficult to determine the responsible antigen.

Differential diagnosis

- Specific allergic stomatitis
- Drug-induced lesions
- Plasma cell stomatitis

Pathology

Histopathologic examination is not pathognomonic. Cutaneous patch testing can be helpful as it might confirm a suspected allergen.

Treatment

Avoidance of any suspected allergen and good oral hygiene are recommended. In severe cases systemic steroids in low dose can be helpful (10–20 mg of prednisolone for a week followed by a 2–3 weeks taper).

Dental Resin Contact Stomatitis

Key points

- A rare allergic reaction of the oral mucosa.
- Acrylic monomer is believed to be responsible.
- There is a close clinical correlation between the acrylic material and the reaction.

Introduction

Contact stomatitis of the oral mucosa due to the acrylic used in dentures is rare. The residual acrylic monomer, due to inadequate polymerization, is usually responsible. However, it has also been suggested that traces of other allergenic substances or microbial elements that are absorbed within the denture base may lead to acrylic antigenic action.

Clinical features

Clinically, the oral mucosa appears erythematous and edematous in the areas of contact with the dentures. Occasionally, vesicles and erosions may be observed (**Fig. 9.6**). The patients complain of an intense burning sensation. The allergic reaction may spread to other oral sites that are not in direct contact with the dentures. The skin patch test is usually positive to acrylic. Additionally, removal of the dentures usually results in improvement or complete resolution of the symptoms and signs. The diagnosis is mainly based on the history and the clinical features.

Differential diagnosis

- Contact stomatitis due to other allergens
- Plasma cell stomatitis
- Denture stomatitis
- Erythematous candidiasis
- Drug-induced lesions

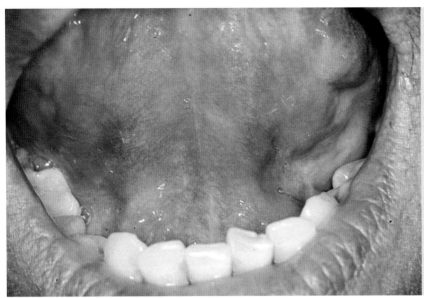

Fig. 9.4 Allergic stomatitis following contact with spearmint-containing chewing gum.

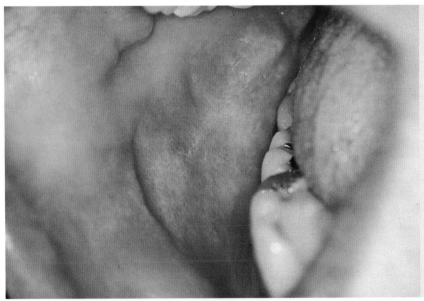

Fig. 9.5 Allergic stomatitis following contact with mint-containing chewing gum.

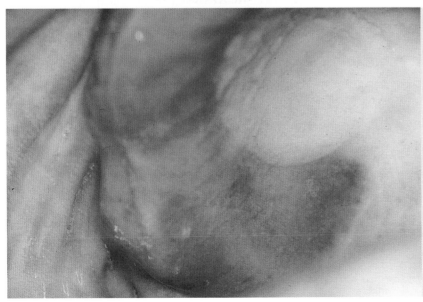

Fig. 9.6 Allergic reaction of the palatal mucosa caused by the denture acrylic.

Pathology

Histopathologic examination reveals a prominent inflammatory reaction in the lamina propria mainly by lymphocytes, plasma cells, and eosinophils. Vasodilation is also observed. Cutaneous patch test is usually positive to acrylic.

Treatment

During the acute phase antihistamines or systemic steroids in low dose may help improve the symptoms and signs. Construction of new dentures with fully polymerized monomer is recommended.

Eugenol Contact Stomatitis

Key points
- It is a rare phenomenon.
- The lesions can be localized or generalized.
- They quickly regress after the removal of eugenol.

Introduction

Eugenol has many uses in dentistry (antiseptic, cement, surgical paste, etc.). In sensitized patients it may cause *localized* or *generalized* allergic reactions after direct contact with the oral mucosa.

Clinical features

Clinically, prominent erythema and edema and rarely erosions are observed (**Fig. 9.7**). The patients complain of intense burning sensation and pain. The skin patch test is usually positive. The diagnosis is based on the history and clinical features.

Differential diagnosis
- Dental resin contact stomatitis
- Contact stomatitis due to other substances
- Plasma cell stomatitis
- Cinnamon contact stomatitis

Treatment

Avoidance of eugenol is recommended. The use of antihistamines can be helpful.

Cinnamon Contact Stomatitis

Key points
- Observed in individuals that consume artificially flavored cinnamon-containing products.
- It is rarely caused by using unprocessed cinnamon.
- The lesions may be located where the cinnamon contacts the oral mucosa for a prolonged period.
- The disorder has unique clinical and histologic features compared with the other types of oral allergies.

Introduction

Artificial cinnamon products are widely used as a flavoring substance in cooking and confectionary manufacture and can be found in sweets, chewing gums and toothpastes, dental floss, and mouthwashes. The release of the cinnamon ethereal oils and their constant contact with the oral mucosa, usually in the form of chewing gums, sweets, toothpaste, dental floss, and mouthwash can cause various hypersensitivity reactions. The clinical and histopathologic features of this process are unique and different than other forms of contact stomatitis.

Clinical features

Clinically, erythema of the oral mucosa and white hyperkeratotic striation or plaques and erosions can be noticed (**Figs. 9.8–9.11**). The most commonly affected sites are the lateral aspects of the tongue, buccal mucosa, and gingiva. An atypical, nonspecific gingivitis can be a common finding in individuals using cinnamon-containing toothpaste. Exfoliative cheilitis and perioral dermatitis have also been described. A burning sensation and pain are also commonly reported. The lesions may be *localized* or *diffuse* and mimic hairy leukoplakia when they develop on the lateral border of the tongue and lichen planus when they occur on the buccal mucosa. The diagnosis is mainly based on the history and the clinical features.

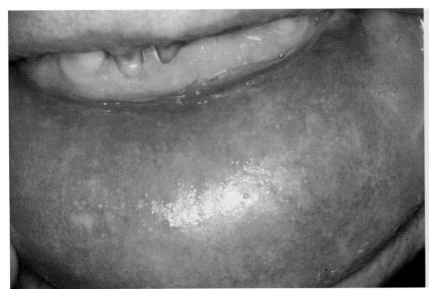

Fig. 9.7 Edema and erythema of the lower lip caused by eugenol.

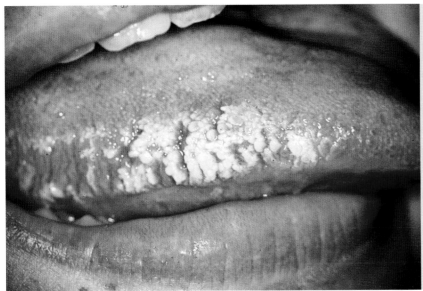

Fig. 9.8 Cinnamon contact stomatitis, prominent, characteristic white lesions on the lateral border of the tongue.

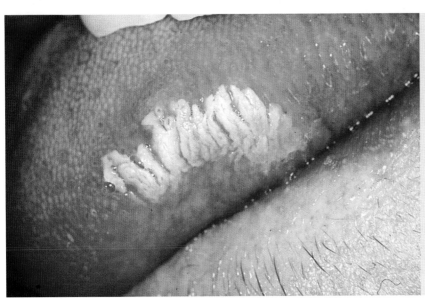

Fig. 9.9 Cinnamon contact stomatitis of the lateral border of the tongue.

Differential diagnosis

- Candidiasis
- Hairy leukoplakia
- Leukoplakia
- Lichen planus
- Plasma cell stomatitis
- Uremic stomatitis
- Chronic biting
- Amalgam contact stomatitis

Pathology

Histopathologic examination reveals hyperkeratosis and acanthosis of the epithelium as well as elongation and expansion of the rete ridges. There is a dense inflammatory infiltrate in the superficial lamina propria mainly by lymphocytes, plasma cells, eosinophils, and histiocytes. Perivascular lymphocytic infiltrate is also a common finding, accompanied by plasmocytes and eosinophils.

Treatment

Discontinuing the use of substances containing cinnamon is the first step. In those cases with persistent severe erosions, systemic steroids in low dose (10–15 mg of prednisolone for 5–7 days) can help the lesions to heal sooner. Topical rinses with chamomile four to five times daily improve the symptoms.

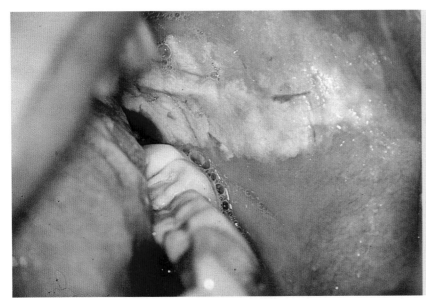

Fig. 9.10 Cinnamon contact stomatitis of the buccal mucosa.

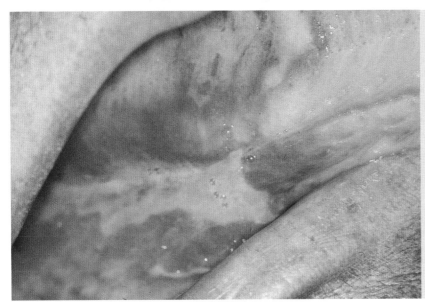

Fig. 9.11 Cinnamon contact stomatitis, erosions of the ventral aspect of the tongue.

10 Oral Lesions due to Drugs

Key points

- The oral mucosa and the skin are often targets of side effects from medication.
- Mucocutaneous drug reactions occur in 0.1 to 1% of patients who receive systemic treatments.
- Over 5% of hospitalized patients for mucocutaneous disease are due to adverse drug reaction.
- High-risk groups include the elderly, females, and those receiving several medications at the same time.
- Simultaneous use of two different medications bears a 5% risk of side effects. This increases to 50% when the number of medication is 5 and to 90 to 100% when the different medications received are over 10.
- High-risk patients are also those receiving certain categories of medication such as sulphonamides, nonsteroidal anti-inflammatories, antiepileptics, and antibiotics.
- Association of the lesions or condition with a specific medication is based on the chronological order of their appearance, the clinical features and literature confirmation.
- Most common oral reactions start as solitary lesions that may then become generalized and sometimes be accompanied by severe systemic manifestations.
- Early withdrawal of the suspected medication is the first step toward treatment.

Principles

Following the cutaneous drug reactions, oral adverse side effects from medication are high in frequency. In theory, every drug can cause side effects. Over 200 different types of medication have been implicated in the development of oral and perioral complications. The list remains open as reactions always need to be recorded and studied. The epidemiology in many cases is based on inpatients.

The association of an adverse reaction to a specific medication is based on three parameters: (a) *the chronological order*, (b) *the clinical features*, and (c) *bibliographic confirmation and search* (**Table 10.1**). Despite the fact, the exact pathogenesis remains elusive; three mechanisms seem to take part in drug reactions. In the *first category* immunologic reaction is responsible and it is unpredictable. In the *second category* nonimmunologic reaction is responsible, that can sometimes be predicted, and in the *third category* genetic predisposition with a possible immunologic and unpredictable participation is included (**Table 10.2**).

In general, assigning causality to a specific agent is complicated, using several different methods to verify it (Naranjo's algorithm, Venulet's algorithm, World Health Organization [WHO] causality term assessment criteria) and a challenge/dechallenge/rechallenge protocol.

Intraorally, the spectrum of adverse drug reactions is great. There are some well-described reactions caused by specific drug categories, such as xerostomia and gingival enlargement. However, the majority of the lesions are characterized by erosion and ulceration of the oral mucosa. The medications implicated in the most frequent oral drug reactions (high risk) are described in **Table 10.3**.

Angioedema

Introduction

Angioedema is characterized by transient edema that involves the dermis, subcutaneous tissue, and submucosa. It mainly affects the skin, oral and laryngeal mucosae, and more rarely the intestinal mucosa. It is commonly associated with urticaria. It is classified into *hereditary*, which is very rare and is usually transmitted via the autosomal dominant pattern of inheritance and *acquired*.

The hereditary type is divided into three types: I and II that are caused by mutations in the *SERPING1* gene and III that has been linked with mutations in the *F12* gene (which encodes the coagulation protein factor XII). Mutation in the *SERPING1* gene results in either reduced levels of C1-esterase inhibitor (*type I hereditary angioedema*) or dysfunctional forms of C1-esterase inhibitor (*type II hereditary angioedema*). All forms of hereditary angioedema lead to abnormal activation of the complement system. Acquired angioedema can be *immunologic, nonimmunologic,* or *idiopathic*. Both hereditary and acquired angioedema are characterized by urticaria on the skin and mucous membranes, while in the hereditary form visceral involvement may also occur. The acquired type is more common and may be caused by foods, medication, infections, high levels of antigen–antibody complexes, immunodeficiency, malignancies, local anesthetics, and other substances. However, in many cases no causative factor can be identified. The allergens can cause an anaphylactic reaction with the participation of mast cells and immunoglobulin E (IgE) that leads to the release of histamine and other vasoactive substances.

Clinical features

Clinically, angioedema of all forms is characterized by edema of the skin, the mucous membranes, and the subcutaneous tissues. The disease has sudden onset and usually lasts 24 to

Table 10.1 Framework of relationship between drugs and reactions[a]

I. **Chronological order**
• Record all medication taken and when
• Time of appearance of the drug eruption
• Time interval between receipt of medication and drug reaction
• Improvement of the reaction after medication discontinuation
• Reappearance of the reaction after taking the medication again
II. **Clinical features**
• Type of initial lesion
• Distribution and number of lesions
• Mucosal/cutaneous involvement
• Existence of general symptoms and signs
• Lymph node enlargement and visceral involvement
III. **Bibliographic confirmation and search**
• Existence of similar reaction from the same medication

[a] *Adapted from Bolognia JL, Jorizzo JL, Schaffer JV. Dermatology. 3rd ed. 2012; Elsevier, partly modified.*

Table 10.2 Pathogenesis of mucosal and cutaneous drug-induced reaction[a]

I. **Immunologic reaction**
• IgE-related drug reactions (anaphylactic stomatitis, angioedema, urticaria)
• Cytotoxic reactions (pemphigus, thrombocytopenia)
• Immune complex–associated reactions (vasculitis, types of urticaria)
• Delayed hypersensitivity reactions (lichenoid manifestations, Stevens-Johnson syndrome, Lyell's syndrome)
II. **Nonimmunologic reaction**
• Drug overdose (i.e., methotrexate toxicity)
• Side effects (mucositis, xerostomia, alopecia, pancytopenia)
• Toxicity from accumulation (methotrexate, minocycline, gold)
• Drug interactions (cyclosporine and azoles, tetracycline and calcium, methotrexate and sulphonamides)
• Metabolic alterations (isoniazid and pellagra)
• Exacerbation of existing disease
III. **Genetic predisposition to medication with possible immunologic reaction**
• Stevens-Johnson syndrome
• Lyell's syndrome
• Lupus erythematosus
• Lichenoid reactions or exacerbation of existing lichen planus
• HIV infection
• Drug eruption with eosinophilia and systemic symptoms (DRESS)

[a] *Adapted from Bolognia JL, Jorizzo JL, Schaffer JV. Dermatology. 3rd ed. 2012; Elsevier, partly modified.*

Table 10.3 Medication groups with high level of oral reactions

• Antibiotics (penicillin, ampicillin, β-lactams)	• Heparin
• Sulphonamides	• Analgesics
• Trimethoprim-sulfamethoxazole	• Allopurinol
• Nonsteroidal anti-inflammatory	• Phenobarbital
• Antiepileptics	• Dapsone
• Barbiturates	• Gold salts
• Diazepam	• Isoniazid
• Captopril	• Indomethacin
• D-Penicillamine	• Cytostatics
• Bisphosphonates	• Anticholinergics
• Nicorandil	• Monoclonal antibodies

72 hours. The skin and mucous membranes are completely normal after the acute episode. There is a predilection for loose tissue areas such as the periocular area, lips, tongue, genitals, hands, feet, or any other area (**Figs. 10.1, 10.2**). The lesions are rarely symmetrical. Clinically, oral lesions present as a sudden, painless, and smooth swelling mainly involving the lips, tongue, and soft palate. Involvement of the gastrointestinal system in severe cases may lead to acute abdomen with abdominal pain and vomiting, while involvement of the respiratory system may lead to edema of the larynx, blocking of the upper airways, and occasionally death. The most severe cases of angioedema may start within a few minutes after drug administration and usually last 24 to 48 hours and may recur. The diagnosis is mainly based on the history and the clinical features.

Differential diagnosis

- Granulomatous cheilitis
- Cheilitis glandularis
- Surgical emphysema
- Trauma

Treatment

Management starts with the withdrawal of the suspected drug or other substances as soon as possible. Antihistamines for 4 to 5 days are usually the first line of treatment. Systemic steroids or intramuscular epinephrine should be administered in more severe cases and in cases where laryngeal angioedema is suspected and the airway is compromised. Hospital admission should be considered in severe life-threatening cases.

In patients with known hereditary angioedema C1-esterase inhibitor concentrate, ecallantide or icatibant, should be administered as soon as an attack is recognized.

Stomatitis Medicamentosa

Introduction

Systemic administration of medication may induce allergic reaction in the oral mucosa characterized as stomatitis medicamentosa. It is caused by the connection of the allergen with the mast cell–IgE complex. The medication most commonly implicated include antipyretics, nonsteroidal anti-inflammatory drugs (NSAIDs), sulphonamides, antibiotics, barbiturates, and others. Fixed drug eruption is inflammatory reaction of the skin or mucosa that characteristically recurs at the same site after the administration of a medication.

Clinical features

Clinically, the disorder is characterized by diffuse or patchy erythema of the oral mucosa, purpuric patches, small vesicles, and painful erosions or ulcers (**Fig. 10.3**). The lesions are of sudden onset and can affect any area of the mouth. They appear during or shortly after the administration of the medication responsible and may recur. The diagnosis is based on the history and the clinical features.

Differential diagnosis

- Drug-induced erosions and ulcers
- Erythema multiforme
- Erosive lichen planus
- Mucous membrane pemphigoid
- Pemphigus
- Herpetic stomatitis
- Discoid lupus erythematosus

Treatment

Cessation of the responsible medication is imperative. Antihistamines or steroids in low doses are administered therapeutically.

Antibiotic-Induced Stomatitis

Introduction

Systemic long-term administration of broad-spectrum antibiotics, especially tetracyclines, may cause a form of stomatitis. However, as nowadays the use of long-term tetracyclines is not as extensive, this form of stomatitis is not frequently encountered.

Clinical features

Clinically, antibiotic-induced stomatitis is characterized by diffuse erythema and ulceration of the oral mucosa with no specific characters. The tongue is very red with apoptosis of the filiform papillae and sometimes microerosions. There is a prominent burning sensation. Similar lesions may be observed in other oral sites (**Fig. 10.4**). Hairy tongue and candidiasis may also occur as a result of changes in the oral microbial

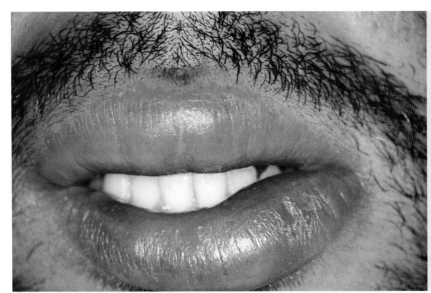

Fig. 10.1 Angioedema, swelling of the lips.

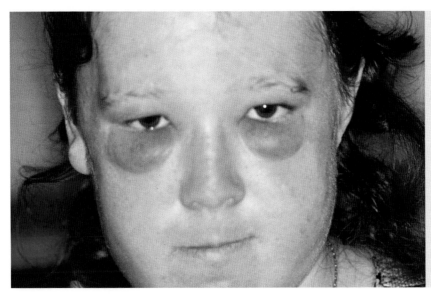

Fig. 10.2 Angioedema, edema of the face.

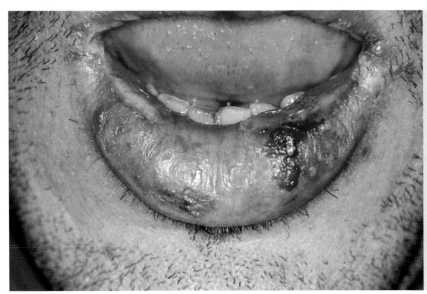

Fig. 10.3 Stomatitis medicamentosa, edema, and erosions of the lower lip following the use of an analgesic.

flora. Coexistence of balanitis and skin rash is not uncommon (**Fig. 10.5**). The diagnosis is based on the history and clinical features.

Differential diagnosis

- Stomatitis medicamentosa
- Erythema multiforme
- Herpetic stomatitis
- Pellagra
- Ariboflavinosis

Treatment

Discontinuation or change of the specific antibiotic and administration of high-dose B-complex vitamins are recommended. Antifungal medication may be required.

Gold-Induced Stomatitis

Introduction

Gold compounds are used mainly in patients with rheumatoid disorders and can cause an adverse toxic reaction. Gold is excreted very slowly, mainly through the kidneys, and also through the saliva. It is possible for it to remain stored in the tissues for a long time. Traces can be detected in the urine 8 to 10 months after cessation of the drug.

Clinical features

Gold toxicity may manifest with headache, fever, pruritus, proteinuria, skin rashes, and oral lesions. More severe adverse reactions include agranulocytosis, thrombocytopenia, or aplastic anemia. Clinically, the oral mucosa appears red, with painful erosions that are covered by a yellowish pseudomembrane (**Fig. 10.6**). Intense burning sensation and increased salivation accompany the lesions. The diagnosis is based on the history and the clinical features.

Differential diagnosis

- Stomatitis medicamentosa
- Erosions due to other medication
- Erythema multiforme
- Erosive lichen planus
- Mucous membrane pemphigoid
- Pemphigus
- Erythematous candidiasis

Treatment

Cessation of gold therapy. Antihistamines and low-dose steroids may be helpful.

Ulcerations due to Methotrexate

Introduction

Methotrexate is a folic acid antimetabolite that is used in the treatment of leukemia, solid tumors, autoimmune diseases, certain types of psoriasis, and as a steroid-sparing agent. It reduces folic acid which is a necessary cofactor in the synthesis of thymidylate and purine nucleotides, required for DNA and RNA synthesis. Side effects occur by inhibiting the formation of DNA and RNA synthesis in both malignant and normal cells.

Clinical features

The most common and severe side effects of methotrexate are pancytopenia and hepatotoxicity and less commonly nausea, vomiting, loss of appetite, alopecia, photosensitivity, infections, and oral lesions. Clinically, the oral mucosa presents with erythematous areas and irregular ulcers that are covered by a whitish slough (**Fig. 10.7**). The lips, buccal mucosa, and tongue are the most commonly affected sites. The lesions appear 2 to 3 weeks after the initiation of treatment and are an indication to lower the dose or cease the use of the drug. The diagnosis is based on the history and the clinical features.

Differential diagnosis

- Ulceration due to other medication
- Erythema multiforme
- Herpetic stomatitis
- Mucous membrane pemphigoid
- Pemphigus

Treatment

Folic acid supplementation and vitamin B–complex administration in high doses can be very helpful. Review of the dose and lowering it if possible is suggested.

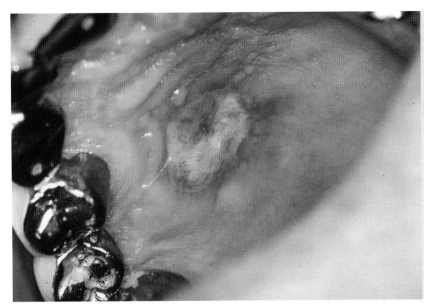

Fig. 10.4 Antibiotic-induced ulceration of the palate.

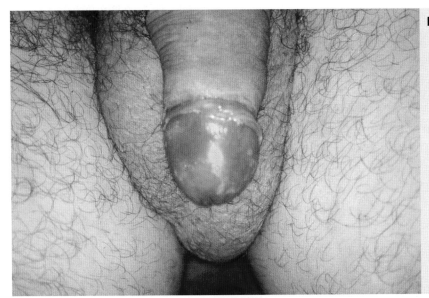

Fig. 10.5 Antibiotic-induced balanitis.

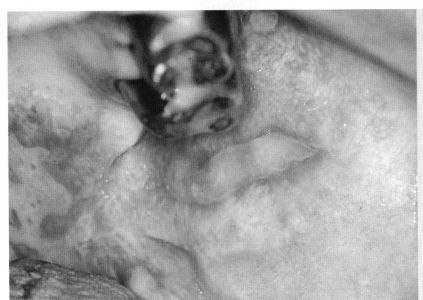

Fig. 10.6 Gold-induced erosions of the palate and buccal mucosa.

Ulcerations due to Azathioprine

Introduction

Azathioprine is an antimetabolite widely used as an immunosuppressive and anti-inflammatory drug for autoimmune and other diseases and also in transplant patients.

Clinical features

Major side effects include leukopenia, thrombocytopenia, immunosuppression, infections, and increased risk of malignancies. Minor side effects are nausea, vomiting, alopecia, gastrointestinal disorders, and oral lesions. Rarely, limited atypical ulcers of the oral mucosa may develop, especially after long-term and high-dose administration (**Fig. 10.8**).

Differential diagnosis
- Ulceration due to other medication
- Traumatic ulceration
- Thermal burn
- Secondary herpes simplex
- Aphthous ulceration

Treatment

Lowering the dose of the drug and vitamin B–complex administration in high dose are recommended.

D-Penicillamine–Induced Oral Lesions

Introduction

D-penicillamine is an agent used in the treatment of hepatolenticular degeneration (Wilson's disease), rheumatoid arthritis, scleroderma, primary biliary cirrhosis, cystinuria, heavy metal poisoning, etc. It has many side effects upon the pulmonary, hematopoietic, gastrointestinal, and renal systems. On occasion, it is responsible for autoimmune mucocutaneous diseases, e.g., pemphigus or bullous pemphigoid.

Clinical features

The most common cutaneous side effects of penicillamine are autoimmune-type disorders (pemphigus, bullous pemphigoid, mucous membrane pemphigoid, systemic lupus erythematosus) and acute sensitivity reaction. The most common oral manifestation is penicillamine-induced pemphigus, which is characterized by vesiculobullous lesions and erosions of the oral mucosa that are clinically, histopathologically, and immunologically identical to those seen in pemphigus vulgaris and pemphigus foliaceus. In many cases, involvement of the oral mucosa is the first sign of the disease (**Fig. 10.9**). D-penicillamine–induced pemphigus usually appears 4 to 8 months after initiation of treatment and in most cases resolves a few months after the cessation of the medication. Penicillamine contains sulfhydryl groups that are speculated to interact with the sulfhydryl groups of Dsg1 and Dsg3. This interaction may modify the antigenicity of the desmogleins which may lead to pemphigus autoantibody production. Other oral manifestations include bullous pemphigoid, mucous membrane pemphigoid, aphthous ulcers, and loss of taste. Mucocutaneous lesions are more common in D-penicillamine–treated patients for rheumatoid arthritis. The diagnosis is based on clinical and laboratory findings.

Differential diagnosis
- Ulceration due to other medication
- Pemphigus vulgaris
- Mucous membrane pemphigoid
- Bullous pemphigoid
- Erosive lichen planus
- Erythema multiforme

Treatment

Discontinuation of the medication is required. Systemic steroids for 3 to 6 weeks are recommended and follow-up is done due to the risk of a relapse.

Ulcerations due to Indomethacin

Introduction

Indomethacin is a nonsteroidal anti-inflammatory agent with analgesic and antipyretic actions. It is used in the treatment of rheumatoid arthritis and other musculoskeletal disorders.

Clinical features

The most common adverse effects of indomethacin include gastrointestinal disorders, headache, vertigo, mucocutaneous allergic reactions, angioedema, and less frequently, thrombocytopenia, agranulocytosis, and aplastic anemia. Clinically, the oral lesions present as painful irregular ulcers usually covered by a pseudomembrane (**Fig. 10.10**). The most frequently affected sites are the tongue, palate, and buccal mucosa. In rare cases, indomethacin can be responsible for the development of pemphigus and mucous membrane pemphigoid with oral manifestations. The diagnosis is mainly based on the history and the clinical features. Histopathologic and immunologic examination is required in persistent cases to rule out chronic bullous diseases.

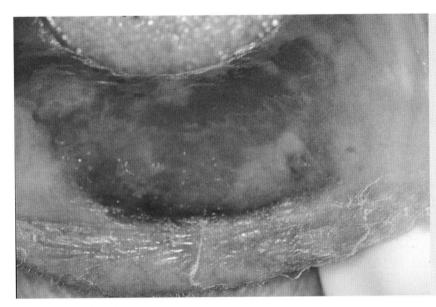

Fig. 10.7 Prominent erythema and extensive ulceration of the lower lip caused by methotrexate.

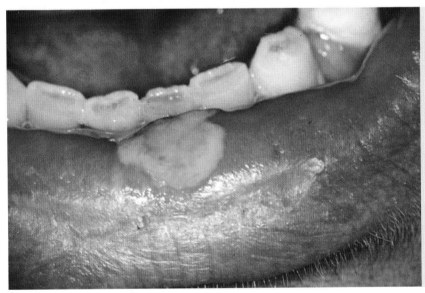

Fig. 10.8 Ulcer of the lower lip caused by azathioprine.

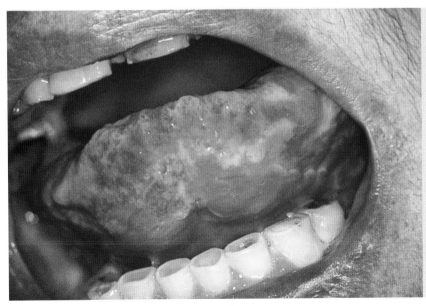

Fig. 10.9 D-penicillamine–induced oral pemphigus manifesting as extensive erosions of the tongue.

Differential diagnosis

- Ulceration due to other medication
- Erythema multiforme
- Mucous membrane pemphigoid
- Pemphigus
- Lupus erythematosus

Treatment

Discontinuation of the drug and systemic administration of low-dose steroids for about a week with subsequent tapering is recommended.

Ulcerations due to Nicorandil

Introduction

Nicorandil is a potassium-channel activator used for the treatment of angina pectoris. The most common side effects are cutaneous and rarely oral lesions occur.

Clinical features

Clinically, oral lesions present as multiple, irregular, painful, superficial ulcers covered by a whitish-yellow pseudomembrane (**Fig. 10.11**). The most commonly affected sites are the tongue, lips, buccal mucosa, and gingiva. The severity and duration of the ulcers is dose-dependent. The diagnosis is based on the history and the clinical features.

Differential diagnosis

- Ulceration due to other medications
- Erythema multiforme
- Mucous membrane pemphigoid
- Pemphigus

Treatment

Cessation of the medication and administration of low-dose systemic corticosteroids for about a week is recommended.

Erosions due to Hydroxyurea

Introduction

Hydroxyurea is a cytotoxic agent that inhibits the M2 subunit of ribonucleotide reductase, thus blocking DNA synthesis. It is used as an antineoplastic agent mainly in the treatment of psoriasis, chronic myeloproliferative disorders, and in patients with sickle cell anemia for prophylaxis against crises. The most serious adverse reactions are bone marrow suppression, anemia, megaloblastic changes, gastrointestinal, renal, and neurologic disorders. Oral and cutaneous side effects are relatively rare.

Clinical features

Clinically, oral lesions present as erythema and multiple, irregular painful erosions. The tongue, palate, lips, and buccal mucosa are the most commonly affected sites (**Fig. 10.12**). The cutaneous lesions are diffuse hyperpigmentation, allergic vasculitis, maculopapular eruption, leg and foot ulcerations, alopecia, and xeroderma (**Fig. 10.13**). The diagnosis is based on the history and the clinical features.

Differential diagnosis

- Ulceration due to other medications
- Erythema multiforme
- Lupus erythematosus
- Erosive lichen planus
- Mucous membrane pemphigoid
- Pemphigus

Treatment

Discontinuation of the medication is recommended. Vitamin B complex and low-dose systemic steroids for a short period of time can be helpful.

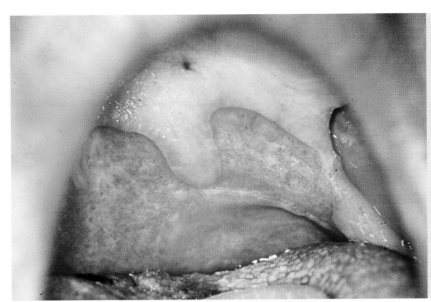

Fig. 10.10 Ulceration of the soft palate caused by indomethacin.

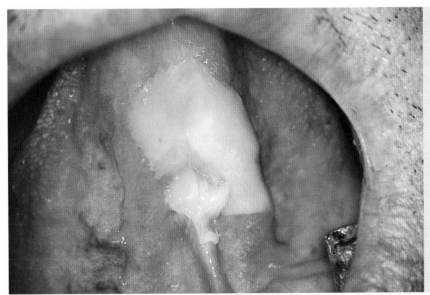

Fig. 10.11 Extensive ulceration of the tongue due to nicorandil.

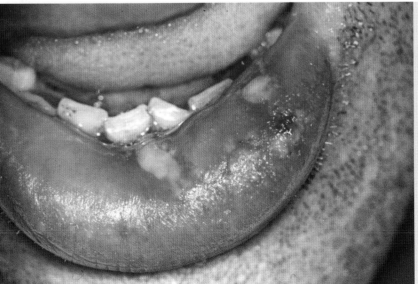

Fig. 10.12 Erosions of the lower lip due to hydroxyurea.

Bisphosphonate-Related Oral Lesions

Introduction

Bisphosphonates are agents that inhibit bone resorption via osteoclastic activity by attaching to hydroxyapatite binding sites, especially on bony surfaces that undergo active resorption. Additionally, they promote osteoclast apoptosis by decreasing the osteoclast progenitor development and recruitment. This interferes with bone remodeling and often reduces bone formation. Nitrogen-containing bisphosphonates (alendronate sodium, neridronate, ibandronate, pamidronate, risedronate, and zoledronic acid) have a different mechanism of action. They exert their effects on osteoclasts and tumor cells by inhibiting a key enzyme (farnesyl diphosphate synthase). They also inhibit angiogenesis and are toxic for the epithelium. Bisphosphonates can be administered orally or intravenously. Intravenous administration leads to greater deposition. They are widely used in the treatment of osteoporosis and osteopenia. They are also used to slow osseous involvement of several malignancies (multiple myeloma, metastatic prostate, or breast carcinoma) by inhibiting tumor cell adhesion to the extracellular bone matrix and other osseous conditions (Paget's disease, osteogenesis imperfecta). The most common side effects of bisphosphonates include headache, dizziness, vertigo, esophagitis, indigestion, constipation, musculoskeletal pain, and osteonecrosis of the jaws. Less common are oral mucosal ulceration, urticaria, angioedema, uveitis, esophageal stenosis, pruritus, skin eruption, Stevens-Johnson syndrome, and Lyell's disease.

Clinical features

The prevalence of bisphosphonate-induced osteonecrosis of the jaws varies greatly and depends on the route of administration and the potency of the agent used. Risk factors are intravenous route of administration, use of more potent bisphosphonates, longer treatment regimes, and higher dose. Other factors include other drugs received (systemic steroids, chemotherapy, estrogen therapy), underlying systemic diseases, dental surgery, and dental infections. Recent studies suggest that up to 29% of cancer patients receiving high potency, intravenous bisphosphonates could present with osteonecrosis of the jaw, compared with less than 0.3% of patients receiving oral bisphosphonates.

Osteonecrosis can occur spontaneously or more frequently and can follow surgical dental treatment or minor trauma. Initially, there is painful exposure of bone with inflammation and edema of the surrounding soft tissues (**Fig. 10.14**). Progressively, it can lead to osteomyelitis, necrosis, and sequestration (**Fig. 10.15**). Less frequently, irregular painful oral ulceration may be observed (**Fig. 10.16**). Although a mandibular predominance has been recorded, involvement of the maxilla or both jaws may occur. Dental panoramic tomography usually reveals a marked radiodensity of the crestal parts of the jaws and periosteal hyperplasia. The diagnosis is based on the history, clinical and radiographic findings.

Differential diagnosis

- Radiotherapy-induced osteonecrosis of the jaws
- Osteomyelitis
- Actinomycosis
- Ulceration due to other medications
- Erythema multiforme

Treatment

There needs to be careful evaluation of the risk of osteonecrosis in patients receiving bisphosphonates prior to oral surgical interventions. The implementation of alternative extraction techniques has also been suggested. Wherever possible treatment should be performed prior to the commencement of bisphosphonate therapy, especially in those patients receiving intravenous bisphosphonates, or oral bisphosphonates but with concomitant risk factors. When surgical intervention has to take place, the trauma to the bone should be minimal as well as trying to minimize the risk of infection. All patients who receive bisphosphonates should be warned of the risks and instructed to maintain a high level of oral hygiene. The use of long-term topical antimicrobial agents and systemic antibiotics has been suggested to be of benefit, but it is not well supported by literature.

Oral Lesions due to Anticoagulants

Introduction

Heparin and warfarin are the most commonly used anticoagulants in the treatment of cardiac, pulmonary, and vascular diseases. Other medication such as aspirin and clopidogrel are used as antiplatelet agents. Heparin essentially deactivates thrombin and other proteases involved in blood clotting. Warfarin inhibits the vitamin K–dependent synthesis of clotting factors II, VII, IX, and X.

Oral anticoagulant therapy predisposes to hemorrhagic lesions in the skin, mucous membranes, and internal organs.

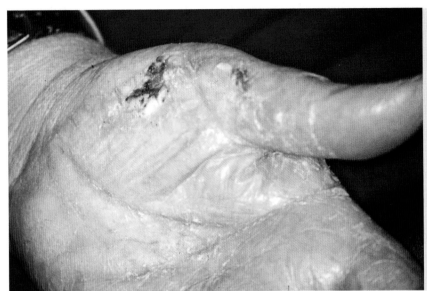

Fig. 10.13 Xeroderma and erosions of the palm due to hydroxyurea.

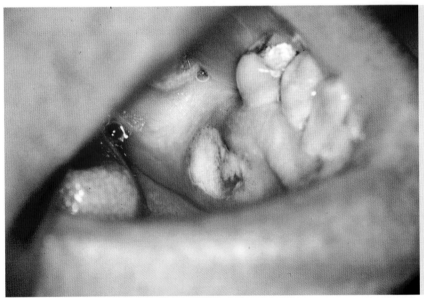

Fig. 10.14 Bisphosphonate-associated osteonecrosis of the mandible, early stage.

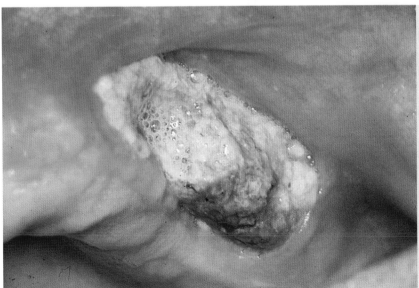

Fig. 10.15 Bisphosphonate-associated extensive osteonecrosis with sequestration of the maxilla.

Clinical features

Oral manifestations may occur either in the form of gingival bleeding or as ecchymoses or hematomas of the oral mucosa (**Fig. 10.17**). Clinically, the lesions may appear spontaneously, or more commonly following mild friction or pressure. They are painless and usually have a deep red color. The diagnosis is based on the history and the clinical features.

Differential diagnosis
- Thrombocytopenia
- Thrombasthenia
- Leukemia
- Aplastic anemia
- Drug-induced platelet dysfunction
- Traumatic hematoma

Treatment

No topical treatment is required. The findings need to be communicated to the treating specialist.

Palatal Perforation due to Cocaine

Introduction

Cocaine is a powerfully addictive stimulant drug that is very widely taken. The most common way of use is inhalation through the nose, known as "snorting." Other ways of administration include intravenous injection, smoking, anal or vaginal insertion, and oral use. Cocaine use leads to serious complications from the cardiovascular, pulmonary, gastrointestinal and genital systems, and the central nervous system (CNS). Additionally, psychological side effects can be seen. Rarely, oral lesions can occur.

Clinical features

Clinically, necrosis and ulceration affecting the anterior labial gingiva have been described after rubbing cocaine on the site. Other oral complications include angular cheilitis, candidiasis, glossodynia, xerostomia, periodontitis, bruxism, and extensive dental caries. In chronic use through nasal inhalation, palatal and nasal septum perforation may occur (**Fig. 10.18**). The perforation of the palate is really an extension of the necrotic lesions of the nasal mucosa toward the palatine bones and the musculature of the soft palate. It is sometimes referred to as cocaine-induced midline destructive lesion and is the result of vasoconstriction and ischemia. The diagnosis is mainly based on the history and the clinical features.

Differential diagnosis
- Tertiary syphilis (gumma)
- Systemic mycoses
- Carcinoma of the nasal mucosa
- Carcinoma of the palate
- Non-Hodgkin's lymphoma
- Postoperative bone deficit

Treatment

Cessation of cocaine use is important. Plastic surgery reconstruction may be helpful. Prosthetics can be used for palatal perforation defects.

Oral Adverse Effects of Retinoids

Introduction

Retinoids are structural and functional analogues of vitamin A that exert multiple effects on cellular differentiation and proliferation, the immune system, and embryonic development. They have a wide use mainly in dermatology either topically or systemically. Oral retinoids are used in the treatment of severe acne, psoriasis, pityriasis rubra pilaris, cutaneous T-cell lymphoma, disorders of keratinization, and some other dermatoses.

Clinical features

Major side effects of systemic retinoids include teratogenicity, muscle effects, bone toxicity, ocular disorders, CNS and psychiatric effects, gastrointestinal, renal mucocutaneous, and many others. Exfoliative cheilitis is the earliest and the most common finding (**Fig. 10.19**). Xerostomia and dryness of the nasal mucosa and eyes are also common. The cutaneous side effects include diffuse hair loss, thinning of the skin, palmoplantar scaling, paronychia, as well as thinning, fragility and shedding of the nail plate, xeroderma, pruritus, epistaxis, and vomiting.

The diagnosis is based on the history and the clinical features.

Differential diagnosis
- Exfoliative cheilitis due to other causes
- Contact cheilitis
- Sjögren's syndrome
- Drug-induced xerostomia

Treatment

The lesions regress after discontinuation of the medication. Topical application of steroid or tacrolimus cream quickly improves exfoliative cheilitis.

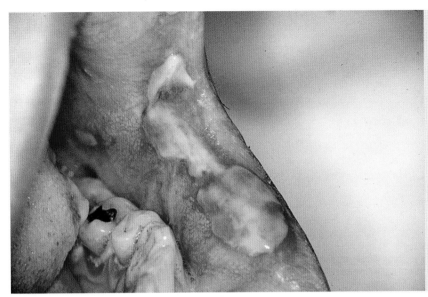

Fig. 10.16 Bisphosphonate-associated erosions of the commissures.

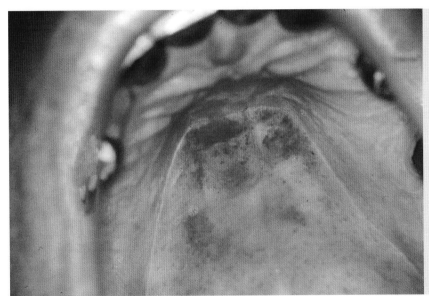

Fig. 10.17 Ecchymoses and hematomas of the palate due to anticoagulants.

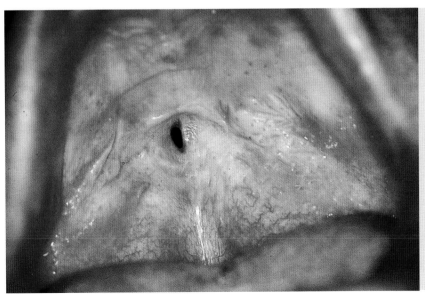

Fig. 10.18 Palatal perforation caused by chronic use of cocaine topically.

Pigmentation due to Antimalarials

Introduction

Antimalarials (quinacrine, chloroquine, hydroxychloroquine, etc.) are nowadays used in the therapy of collagen and skin diseases as well as malaria. Long-term use may lead to pigmentation of the oral mucosa.

Clinical features

Clinically, localized irregular macules or plaques of brown, black, or black-brown color can be observed on the soft palate, buccal mucosa, tongue, or other areas of the oral cavity (**Fig. 10.20**). These lesions are caused by an increase in melanin, are asymptomatic, and usually regress after discontinuation of the medication. The diagnosis is based on the history and the clinical features.

Differential diagnosis
- Normal pigmentation
- Other drug-induced pigmentation
- Smoking pigmentation
- Addison's disease
- Peutz-Jeghers syndrome

Treatment

No treatment is required.

Pigmentation due to Zidovudine

Introduction

Zidovudine (ZDV), also known as azidothymidine, is an antiretroviral medication drug used in the management of patients with HIV infection. The most important of its side effects include bone marrow suppression, nausea, and vomiting. Cutaneous, ungual, and oral mucosal pigmentation have also been described.

Clinical features

Clinically, oral pigmentation appears as irregular macules of brown or black-brown color. The most commonly affected sites are the tongue and palate (**Fig. 10.21**). The diagnosis is predominantly based on the history and less on the clinical presentation.

Differential diagnosis
- Normal pigmentation
- Other drug-induced pigmentation
- Smoking pigmentation
- Peutz-Jeghers syndrome

Treatment

No treatment is required.

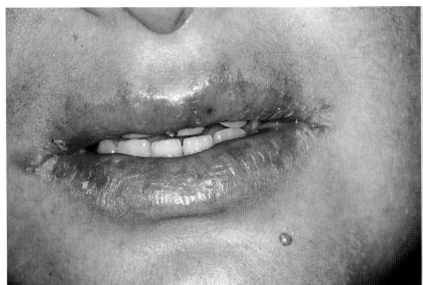

Fig. 10.19 Exfoliative cheilitis caused by systemic retinoids.

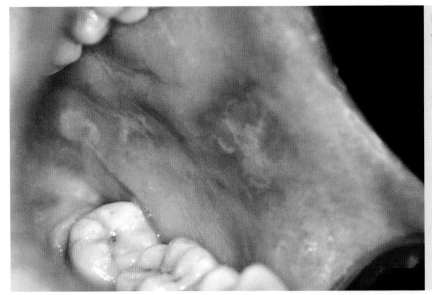

Fig. 10.20 Pigmentation of the buccal mucosa caused by an antimalarial.

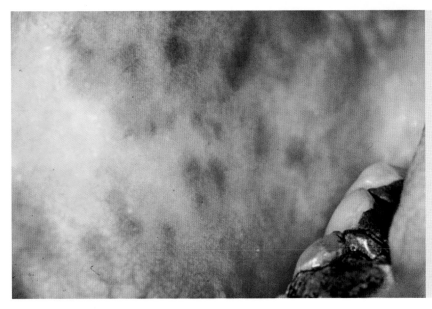

Fig. 10.21 Pigmentation of the buccal mucosa caused by zidovudine.

Oral Pigmentation due to Other Drugs

Introduction

Many different medications may cause oral pigmentation. They include minocycline, sedatives, ketoconazole, clofazimine, hormones (estrogen, thyroxine, contraceptives, adrenocorticotropic hormone [ACTH]/melanocyte-stimulating hormone [MSH]), heavy metals (bismuth, lead), cyclophosphamide, busulfan, various chemotherapeutic agents, and anti-HIV medication.

Clinical features

The clinical presentation is similar to that of other medications causing oral mucosal pigmentation. The diagnosis is therefore mainly based on the history, trying to identify the suspected medication (**Figs. 10.22, 10.23**).

Differential diagnosis
- Other drug-induced pigmentation
- Normal pigmentation
- Smoking pigmentation

Angina Bullosa Hemorrhagica

Key points
- Use of steroid inhalers and mechanical trauma are considered as predisposing factors.
- Hemorrhagic bullae that burst leaving superficial ulceration.
- Soft palate and buccal mucosa are the most commonly affected sites.

Introduction

Angina bullosa hemorrhagica is a benign, principally subepithelial, blood blistering disease. It is characterized by the formation of blood-filled blisters. A genetic predisposition has been suggested, which affects the adhesion between the epithelium and underlying lamina propria, or the anchorage of the mucosal vessels. Another predisposing factor is the long-term use of steroid inhalers. The latter and diabetes mellitus (that has also been implicated as a possible risk factor) lead to vascular fragility. Finally, injury of the oral soft tissues (i.e., from the consumption of hard food) has been associated with the occurrence of blood-filled blisters.

Clinical features

Clinically, the characteristic lesion consists of asymptomatic, single or multiple hemorrhagic bullae that mostly occur on the soft palate and/or the buccal mucosa (**Fig. 10.24**). The bullae then rupture spontaneously leaving superficial ulceration that heals without scarring within 4 to 6 days. The condition is more common in 50- to 60-year-old patients. The diagnosis is based on the history and the clinical features. A biopsy should be performed if a vesiculobullous disease is suspected.

Differential diagnosis
- Mucous membrane pemphigoid
- Bullous pemphigoid
- Linear IgA disease
- Epidermolysis bullosa acquisita
- Pemphigus
- Amyloidosis
- Idiopathic thrombocytopenic purpura

Pathology

Special tests are usually not required. Histopathologic examination reveals a subepithelial, blood-filled bulla. Direct and indirect immunofluorescent is negative.

Treatment

Usually, the bullae regress spontaneously within 4 to 6 days. In the case of multiple lesions a short regime of systemic steroids (i.e., prednisolone 10–20 mg/d for 6–8 days) shortens the healing period of the ulcers.

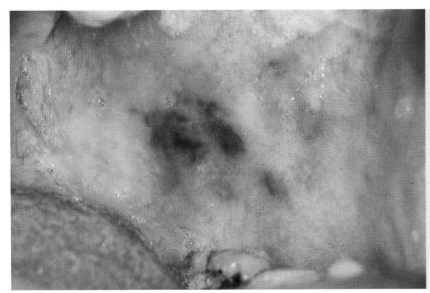

Fig. 10.22 Pigmentation of the buccal mucosa caused by ketoconazole.

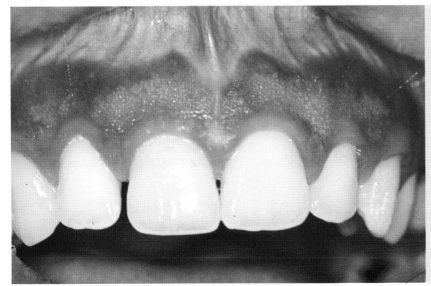

Fig. 10.23 Pigmentation of the gingiva and alveolar mucosa caused by chronic use of thyroxine.

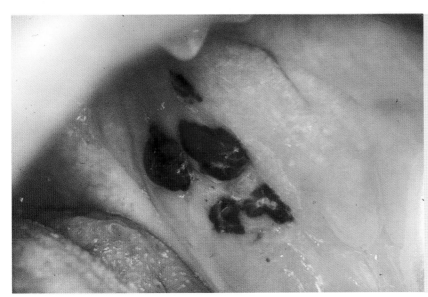

Fig. 10.24 Angina bullosa hemorrhagica, multiple hemorrhagic bullae on the buccal mucosa.

11 Gingival and Periodontal Diseases

Plaque-Related Gingivitis

Key points

- It is the most common form of gingival disease.
- It is caused by plaque accumulation around the gingival margin.
- Systemic and local predisposing factors are implicated.
- The host's immunologic response plays an important role in its development.
- The first line of treatment is the removal of the dental plaque and maintenance of high levels of oral hygiene.

Introduction

Plaque-related gingivitis is an inflammatory disease of the gingiva in the absence of clinical attachment loss. It is caused by the accumulation of microbial plaque, which is a biofilm. Factors contributing to the development of the biofilm include local ones such as poor oral hygiene, malocclusion, ill-fitting prostheses, calculus, smoking, mouth breathing, and food impaction. Systemic factors include diabetes mellitus, some metabolic diseases, immunologic disorders, disorders of leukocyte function, medication, etc. These modify the host's immunologic response to the plaque, contributing to the development of gingivitis.

Clinical features

Plaque-related gingivitis begins at the gingival margin and may spread throughout the gingiva. Clinically, the gingiva become erythematous and edematous, losing their characteristic surface stippling (**Figs. 11.1, 11.2**). Any of the following clinical findings may indicate the presence of plaque-related gingivitis: erythema, edema, bleeding upon even mild provocation, and changes in gingival consistency. Periodontal pockets and radiographic crestal bone loss are not present. However, in cases with great gingival hyperplasia, pseudopockets may develop (**Fig. 11.3**). Plaque-related gingivitis is usually chronic, but acute or subacute forms may occur. If left untreated, it may progress to periodontitis. The diagnosis is made on clinical and radiographic criteria.

Differential diagnosis

- Linear gingival erythema
- Plasma cell gingivitis
- Desquamative gingivitis
- Granulomatous gingivitis
- Periodontitis
- Mouth breathing gingivitis
- Drug-induced gingival enlargement
- Pregnancy-associated gingivitis

Pathology

Histopathologic examination reveals a mild inflammatory reaction in the early stages by polymorphonuclear leukocytes. Gradually, as the inflammation progresses, lymphocytes, plasma cells, and some eosinophils are observed. There is also edema in the lamina propria with vascular dilatation and hemorrhage.

Treatment

Plaque control, good oral hygiene, and elimination of the causative factors are the therapeutic goals of plaque-related gingivitis. The latter may include interventions such as repair or replacement of restorations and prostheses, as required.

Chronic Periodontitis

Key points

- The disease affects all the periodontal tissues.
- A key clinical characteristic is the presence of periodontal pockets.
- The causative factors are the same as in plaque-induced gingivitis.
- Microbes play an important role.
- The most common form of destructive periodontal disease in adults and the most common cause of tooth loss.

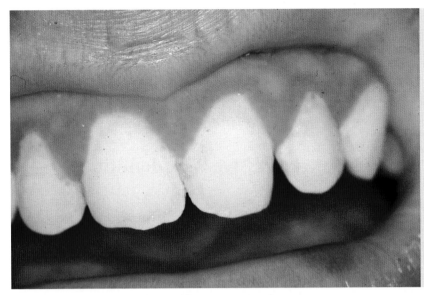

Fig. 11.1 Plaque-related gingivitis, early stage.

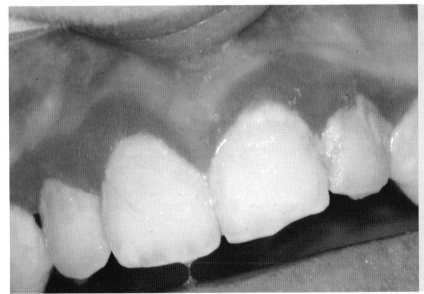

Fig. 11.2 Plaque-related gingivitis, later stage.

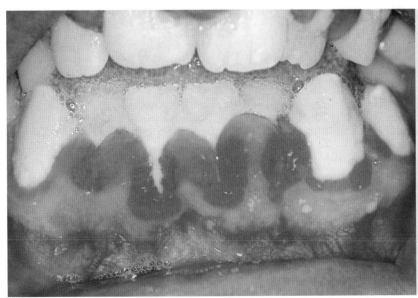

Fig. 11.3 Plaque-related gingivitis with prominent gingival hyperplasia.

Introduction

Chronic periodontitis is an inflammatory disease that affects all the periodontal tissues (gingiva, periodontal membrane, cementum, and alveolar bone). It can be a progression of plaque-related gingivitis. Loss of clinical attachment and apical migration of the junctional epithelium along the root leads to the formation of periodontal pockets. The topical etiologic factors that are implicated in chronic gingivitis are associated with the etiology of periodontitis with emphasis on the role of microbes. The main microorganisms involved in the biofilm formation and the development of periodontitis are *Aggregatibacter actinomycetemcomitans*, *Porphyromonas gingivalis*, *Prevotella intermedia*, and others. The host's defense mechanisms play an important role in the pathogenesis of periodontitis. The classification used for periodontal disease was decided in 1999 and is beyond the scope of this book. In this chapter, two main types of periodontitis will be analyzed: *chronic* and *aggressive*.

Clinical features

Clinically, chronic periodontitis is characterized by loss of clinical attachment and destruction of the periodontal ligament and periodontal pockets formation with probing depths of over 3 to 4 mm. Other clinical signs may include erythema, edema, gingival enlargement, gingival recession, suppuration, bleeding on probing, halitosis, and in more advanced cases, teeth displacement, mobility, and loss (**Figs. 11.4–11.6**). The signs and symptoms may start around the age of 30 years and get progressively worse if remain untreated. The disease can be *localized* or *generalized*. The diagnosis is based on clinical and radiographic criteria.

Differential diagnosis

- Chronic plaque-related gingivitis
- Necrotizing ulcerative periodontitis
- Langerhans cell histiocytosis
- Cyclic neutropenia
- Agranulocytosis
- Leukemia
- Hypophosphatasia
- Acatalasia
- Papillon-Lefévre syndrome
- Chédiak-Higashi syndrome
- Ehlers-Danlos syndrome (some types)
- Glycogen storage disease type 1

Pathology

Histopathologic examination reveals a similar picture to that of chronic gingivitis. However, in chronic periodontitis there is additionally hyperplastic epithelium extending to the depth of the periodontal pocket. There is a reduction of the collagen content and extent of the inflammatory infiltrate apically and laterally. Radiographic examination can be helpful, as it reveals the presence and pattern of bone reduction.

Treatment

There are many aspects in the successful treatment of periodontal disease. Plaque control is important. Supra- and subgingival scaling and root planning should be performed as per the needs of each case. Antimicrobial agents may be used as an adjunct. Surgery can be performed in more advanced cases. There should be an attempt to control any systemic, contributing factors if possible and eliminate any local factors.

Aggressive Periodontitis

Key points

- It affects adolescents and younger adults that are otherwise healthy and has a rapid progression.
- It is classified into localized and generalized forms.
- Its development and progression do not correlate with the amount of dental plaque or calculus.
- The main microbe responsible is *Aggregatibacter actinomycetemcomitans*.

Introduction

Aggressive periodontitis is an inflammatory disease of the periodontal tissues with distinct characteristics. It usually affects children, adolescents, and young adults under 30 years that are otherwise healthy. It has a rapid progression and leads to premature teeth loss. The pathogenesis is not very clear. However, recent research suggests that there is a genetic component for the increased predisposition to the disease. X-linked dominant and autosomal recessive patterns of inheritance have been proposed. The microbes that seem to play an important role in its pathogenesis include *A. actinomycetemcomitans*, *P. intermedia*, *P. gingivalis*, *Fusobacterium nucleatum*, *Tannerella forsythensis*, and others. Specific immunologic dysfunction of the host regarding topical immunologic factors in the periodontium plays an important role in combination with the presence of the microbial flora. Using clinical, microbiological, immunologic, and radiographic criteria, aggressive periodontitis is classified into two categories: *localized* and *generalized*.

Clinical features

The localized form is characterized by circumpubertal onset, developing usually between 10 and 15 years, and has a familial predisposition. Clinically, there are deep periodontal pockets and rapid osseous destruction, with mild or no gingival inflammation. Classically, the lesions are localized around the permanent first molars and incisors with absence of calculus and minimal dental plaque. It leads to mobility and tooth displacement and eventually premature teeth loss. The generalized form may represent progression of the localized form, or may occur spontaneously. It affects adolescents and young adults, usually under 30 years. The main characteristic is attachment loss affecting at least three permanent teeth

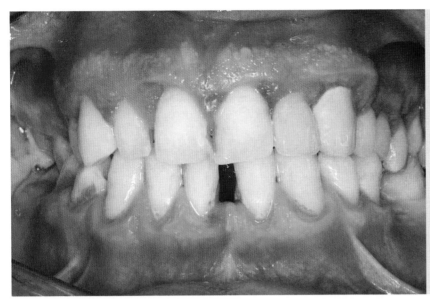

Fig. 11.4 Chronic periodontitis, early stage.

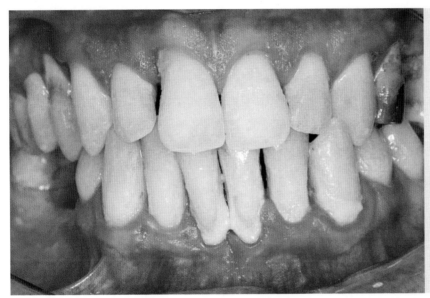

Fig. 11.5 Chronic periodontitis with gingival recession.

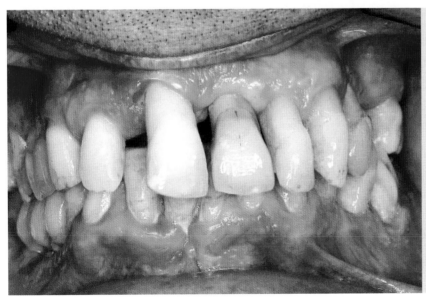

Fig. 11.6 Chronic periodontitis with prominent gingival recession and teeth displacement.

other than first molars and incisors (**Fig. 11.7**). The diagnosis is based on clinical, radiographic, and microbiological criteria.

Differential diagnosis

- Langerhans cell histiocytosis
- Glycogen storage disease type 1b
- Cyclic neutropenia
- Agranulocytosis
- Necrotizing ulcerative periodontitis
- Acatalasia
- Hypophosphatasia
- Papillon-Lefévre syndrome
- Ehlers-Danlos syndrome (some types)
- Chédiak-Higashi syndrome

Pathology

Histopathologic examination reveals findings similar to those of chronic periodontitis. Radiographic and microbiological examination can be useful toward diagnosis, as well as detection of problems in leukocyte function.

Treatment

Periodontal therapy alone is often ineffective in aggressive periodontitis. However, in the early stages of the disease, scaling and root planning, with or without surgical treatment can be combined with antimicrobial therapy. Microbiological identification and subsequent antibiotic sensitivity tests may be useful. The treatment and maintenance of the disease have to be decided by an experienced specialist periodontist. Evaluation and counseling of family members have to be considered due to the potential familial nature of aggressive disease.

Periodontal Abscess

Key points

- A complication of periodontal disease.
- Causative factors include changes in the subgingival microflora and the host's response in combination with local factors.
- Characteristically, the adjacent teeth are usually vital.
- Occasionally, a periodontal abscess can be associated with endodontic pathology.

Introduction

Periodontal abscess is an accumulation of pus within a preexisting periodontal pocket. When the depth of the periodontal pocket exceeds 5 to 8 mm, the soft, edematous gingival tissues may approximate around the cervix of the tooth, causing stenosis or complete obliteration at the pocket opening. The above in combination with changes in the subgingival microflora and the host's response can lead to abscess formation in the area.

Clinical features

Clinically, a periodontal abscess appears as a painful, soft, gingival enlargement of erythematous or normal color. On pressure, pus exudes from the cervical area of the tooth. The teeth involved are tender to percussion and occasionally mobile (**Fig. 11.8**). When the abscess is limited in the free gingiva or the interdental papilla, without extension in the adjacent periodontal tissues, it is characterized as *gingival abscess*. Other symptoms and signs include bleeding, halitosis, and in more severe cases even fever, malaise, and regional lymphadenopathy. A characteristic finding is that the adjacent teeth are usually vital. However, sometimes a periodontal abscess can be associated with endodontic pathology.

The diagnosis is mainly based on clinical criteria.

Differential diagnosis

- Dental abscess
- Gingival cyst of adults
- Lateral periodontal cyst
- Incisive papilla cyst
- Nasolabial cyst
- Actinomycosis

Pathology

Radiographic examination often demonstrates bone loss associated with the previous periodontal defect.

Treatment

Drainage and debridement of the periodontal pocket should be performed during the acute phase. Systemic antibiotics can also be administered if necessary. Following the above periodontal evaluation, periodontal treatments are recommended.

Periodontal Fistula

Key points

- A complication of a periodontal abscess.
- It can cause diagnostic problems.

Introduction

A periodontal fistula forms when pus from a periodontal abscess bores through the gingival tissues and alveolar mucosa.

Clinical features

Clinically, the orifice of the fistula appears red or has granulation tissue. On pressure, pus is released (**Fig. 11.9**). The adjacent teeth are usually vital.

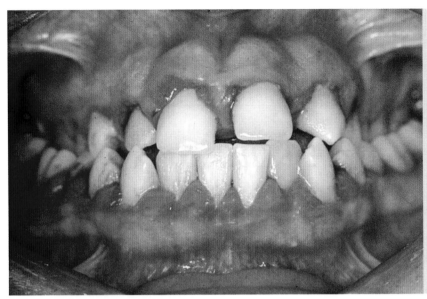

Fig. 11.7 Aggressive periodontitis, generalized form.

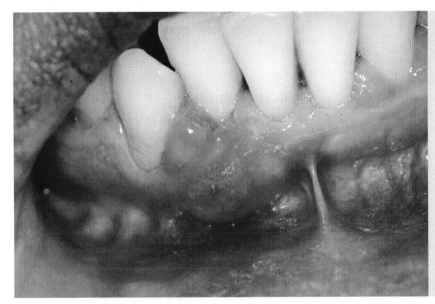

Fig. 11.8 Periodontal abscess on a background of periodontitis.

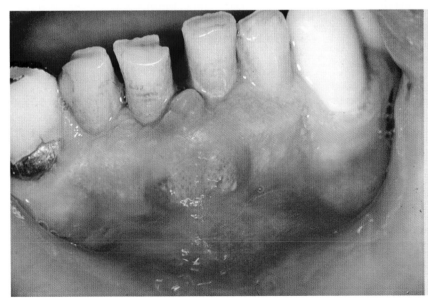

Fig. 11.9 Periodontal fistula on a background of advanced periodontitis.

Differential diagnosis

- Fistula from a dental abscess
- Actinomycosis with fistula formation
- Fistula from osteomyelitis affecting the jaw

Pathology

Radiographic imaging reveals bone destruction in the area.

Treatment

Consists of treatment of the periodontal abscess.

Mouth Breathing Gingivitis

Key points

- Observed in mouth breathers, usually due to nasal problems.
- Common in children and adolescents.
- It mostly affects the upper anterior gingiva.

Introduction

Mouth breathing is usually the result of nasal septum defects or large adenoids in the nasopharynx. It predisposes to gingivitis that has some specific clinical features. It is observed in young patients and affects mainly the upper anterior gingiva.

Clinical features

Clinically, the gingiva and predominantly the interdental papillae are enlarged, dry, erythematous, and shiny and cover part of the teeth crown (**Fig. 11.10**). There is usually a considerable amount of dental plaque in the area. The diagnosis is based on the history and the clinical features.

Differential diagnosis

- Drug-induced gingival enlargement
- Leukemia
- Mucopolysaccharidoses

Pathology

The histologic features are similar to those of plaque-related gingivitis.

Treatment

Restoration of nasal breathing, plaque control, and, if required, gingivectomy are recommended.

Plasma Cell Gingivitis

Key points

- A distinctive pattern of gingival inflammation.
- It usually has a sudden onset.
- The main features are erythema, edema, and a burning sensation.
- It can affect both the free and attached gingiva.

Introduction

Plasma cell gingivitis is a specific type of gingivitis that is histopathologically characterized by dense plasma cell infiltration of the gingival connective tissue. The condition presents with clinical and histopathologic similarities to plasma cell balanitis. The exact cause remains unknown. It is, however, believed to represent a hypersensitivity reaction to an allergen (ingredients in toothpastes, chewing gum, foods, mint, and pepper). Specific mention is made to cinnamon aldehyde and cinnamon flavoring. The disease affects equally both sexes, usually between 20 and 40 years of age. It can last for several months or even years, is resistant to treatment, and tends to relapse.

Clinical features

Clinically, both free and attached gingiva appear erythematous and edematous with loss of normal stippling (**Figs. 11.11, 11.12**). The lesions can be *localized* or more *generalized* and can be accompanied by a burning and itching sensation. Similar lesions have been described on edentulous areas, the tongue, and the lips. The diagnosis can be based on clinical criteria, but has to be confirmed by biopsy and subsequent histopathologic examination.

Differential diagnosis

- Desquamative gingivitis
- Granulomatous gingivitis
- Chronic plaque-related gingivitis
- Linear gingival erythema
- Cinnamon contact stomatitis
- Gingival plasmacytoma
- Erythematous candidiasis
- Erythroplakia
- Leukemia
- Psoriasis on the gingiva

Pathology

Histopathologic examination reveals features that are encountered in psoriasis, including epithelial spongiosis and exocytosis, infiltration by inflammatory cells, apoptotic keratinocytes, and neutrophilic microabscesses. There is prominent inflammatory infiltration in the underlying lamina propria that is dominated by polyclonal plasma cells. Marked vascular dilatation is also observed.

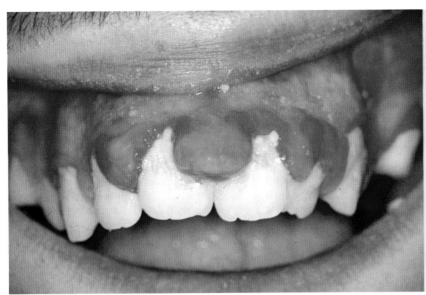

Fig. 11.10 Gingivitis caused by mouth breathing with dental plaque deposits dominating.

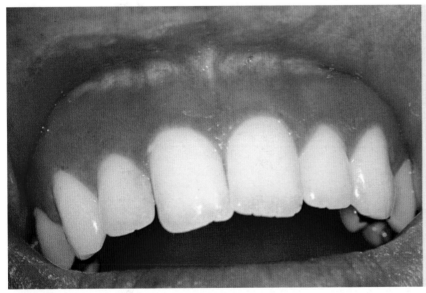

Fig. 11.11 Plasma cell gingivitis, generalized.

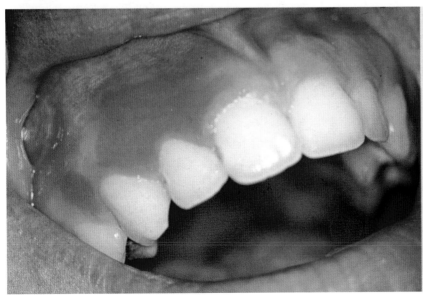

Fig. 11.12 Plasma cell gingivitis, localized.

Treatment

There is no specific therapy, but various treatment modalities have been tried. These include topical and systemic corticosteroids, antihistamines, and topical antifungals. Patients with plasma cell gingivitis should be instructed to keep a dietary history with records of everything taken orally.

Granulomatous Gingivitis

Key points

- A rare and unique form of gingivitis.
- It can be an isolated finding or part of orofacial granulomatosis.
- The clinical features are not specific.
- The diagnosis is confirmed by biopsy and subsequent histopathologic examination.

Introduction

The etiology of the disease remains unknown. It has been associated with foreign body, be it dental material or not, bacterial or fungal infection in the area, or reaction to food additives. In several occasions it represents a local manifestation of a systemic granulomatous disease (Crohn's disease, sarcoidosis, tuberculosis, Melkersson-Rosenthal syndrome, chronic granulomatous disease). There are, however, cases where there is no association with local or systemic disorders.

Clinical features

Granulomatous gingivitis can affect both sexes at any age. However, it more commonly occurs in adulthood. It presents mostly on the free gingiva (gingival margins and interdental papillae) and can be *localized* (involving 2–3 teeth) or *generalized*, extending to a larger area. Clinically, the gingiva appear red and mildly elevated associated with tenderness during mastication and toothbrushing (**Figs. 11.13, 11.14**). The clinical characteristics are not specific. Detailed history and further investigations are required to exclude the presence of a systemic granulomatous disease. The clinical diagnosis should be confirmed by a biopsy followed by histopathologic examination.

Differential diagnosis

- Plaque-related gingivitis
- Plasma cell gingivitis
- Desquamative gingivitis
- Gingival plasmacytoma
- Cinnamon contact stomatitis
- Candidiasis, erythematous

Pathology

Histopathologic examination reveals focal collections of histiocytes, lymphocytes, and multinucleated giant cells (granulomas). On occasions, foreign body materials are detected. The epithelium exhibits hydropic degeneration of the basal cell layer and mild acanthosis. Specific stains for microorganisms should be negative.

Treatment

If granulomatous gingivitis is part of a systemic granulomatous disease, the treatment is the treatment for the systemic condition. If a foreign body is detected, topical excision of the lesions is recommended.

Desquamative Gingivitis

Key points

- It is not an independent disease entity, but a gingival manifestation of some mucocutaneous bullous diseases.
- In over 80 to 90% of the cases, it is caused by mucous membrane pemphigoid or lichen planus.
- The diagnosis is based on clinical, histologic, and immunologic criteria.
- The treatment is the same with that of the underlying disease.

Introduction

Desquamative gingivitis does not represent a specific disease entity, but is a *descriptive term* used for a rather nonspecific gingival manifestation of several disease processes. During the last few decades, research has demonstrated that the majority of cases of desquamative gingivitis represent a manifestation of chronic bullous dermatosis, such as mucous membrane pemphigoid, lichen planus, pemphigus vulgaris, and bullous pemphigoid. In a study of 453 patients with these disorders, we found desquamative gingivitis in 63.6% of those with mucous membrane pemphigoid, 25% in lichen planus, 18.4% in pemphigus vulgaris, and 3.2% in bullous pemphigoid patients. Other diseases that may manifest as desquamative gingivitis include linear IgA disease, epidermolysis bullosa acquisita, psoriasis, systemic lupus erythematosus, and erythema multiforme.

Clinical features

Clinically, desquamative gingivitis is characterized by erythema, edema, and painful erosions of mainly the anterior part of the marginal and attached gingiva, predominantly labially and bucally. A characteristic sign is peeling of the epithelium or elevation with subsequent formation of a hemorrhagic blister after mild friction of the gingiva (**Figs. 11.15–11.17**). The gingival lesions can be either *localized* or *generalized*. Desquamative gingivitis may be the only oral manifestation

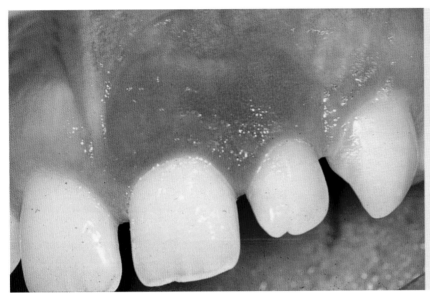

Fig. 11.13 Granulomatous gingivitis, localized.

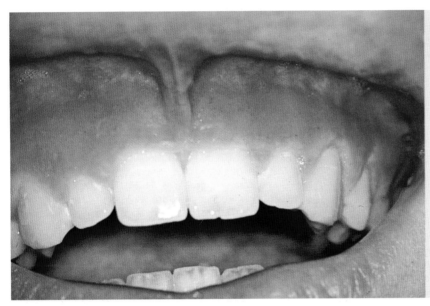

Fig. 11.14 Granulomatous gingivitis, generalized.

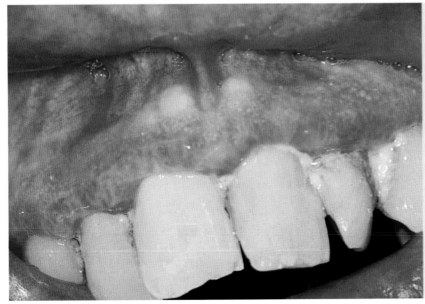

Fig. 11.15 Desquamative gingivitis as a manifestation of mucous membrane pemphigoid.

or may be associated with other oral lesions of a chronic bullous dermatosis. In the presence of desquamative gingivitis, the identification of the underlying disease is based on the following criteria: (a) careful clinical observation of all intraoral and extraoral lesions, (b) histopathologic examination of gingival biopsy, (c) direct and indirect immunofluorescence, and (d) clinical follow-up of the patients.

Desquamative gingivitis is more common in females, usually over 40 years. It does not have a direct impact on the periodontal tissues. However, due to the discomfort and pain that may be caused, it can be indirectly the cause of poor oral hygiene, setting the conditions for the development of periodontal disease.

Differential diagnosis

- Mucous membrane pemphigoid
- Lichen planus
- Pemphigus
- Bullous pemphigoid
- Linear IgA disease
- Dermatitis herpetiformis
- Epidermolysis bullosa acquisita
- Erythema multiforme
- Chronic ulcerative stomatitis
- Drug-induced stomatitis
- Oral psoriasis
- Plasma cell gingivitis
- Granulomatous gingivitis
- Plaque-related chronic gingivitis

Pathology

Laboratory investigations are required for definitive diagnosis. Histopathologic examination will reveal features similar to the underlying disease. Direct and indirect immunofluorescence also give findings like those of the underlying diseases (see mucous membrane pemphigoid, lichen planus, pemphigus, bullous pemphigoid, linear IgA disease).

Treatment

Avoidance of mechanical pressure during toothbrushing and good oral hygiene are of paramount importance. Topical corticosteroids are used and in severe cases systemic corticosteroids have been tried. The general framework of treatment follows the principles of treatment of the underlying disease. Follow-up by a specialist periodontist and oral medicine specialist is recommended to ensure maintenance of high levels of oral hygiene and detection of relapse.

Necrotizing Ulcerative Gingivitis

Key points

- Anaerobic bacteria play an important role in the pathogenesis.
- Predisposing factors include emotional stress, poor oral hygiene, smoking, and HIV infection.
- The age group usually affected are young adults (18–30 years).
- A characteristic clinical sign is necrosis and crater-like formation of the interdental papillae and the marginal gingiva.
- The diagnosis is based on the clinical features.

Introduction

Necrotizing ulcerative gingivitis is an acute, painful, inflammatory disease. The exact etiopathogenesis remains unclear. Anaerobic bacteria (*Borrelia vincentii, Bacillus fusiformis, P. intermedia, P. gingivalis*) and spirochetes are important in its development. Predisposing factors include physical and psychological stress, smoking, poor oral hygiene, HIV infection, and some other forms of immunosuppression.

Clinical features

Necrotizing ulcerative gingivitis is more common in adolescents and young adults. Clinically, it is characterized by crater-like necrosis and ulceration of the interdental papillae and the free gingiva, which are covered by a yellow-grayish pseudomembrane (**Figs. 11.18–11.20**). The gingiva appear erythematous and edematous, are very painful, and may bleed spontaneously. Halitosis and salivation are common. In addition, regional lymphadenopathy, mild fever, and malaise may also occur. The lesions may be *localized* or *generalized*. If the disease is left untreated and the tissue destruction is great, it can progress to *necrotizing ulcerative periodontitis* or may spread to the adjacent soft tissues (*necrotizing ulcerative stomatitis*). The diagnosis is based on the clinical features.

Differential diagnosis

- Necrotizing ulcerative periodontitis
- Primary herpetic gingivostomatitis
- Agranulocytosis
- Neutropenia
- Acute leukemia
- Langerhans cell histiocytosis
- Glycogen storage disease, type 1b
- Scurvy

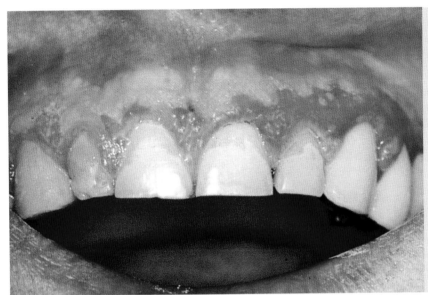

Fig. 11.16 Desquamative gingivitis as a manifestation of lichen planus.

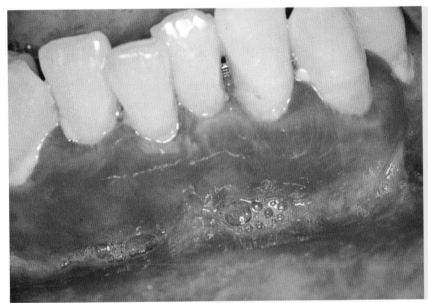

Fig. 11.17 Desquamative gingivitis as a manifestation of lichen planus.

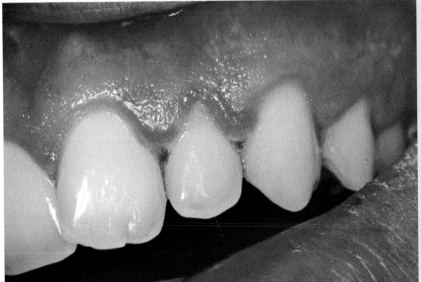

Fig. 11.18 Necrotizing ulcerative gingivitis, early stage.

Pathology

Special investigations are not required. The clinician has to establish, however, whether there is a possibility for underlying immunodeficiency. Histopathologic examination reveals necrosis covered by a fibrin membrane populated with bacteria. The underlying lamina propria demonstrates an intense inflammatory infiltrate. Necrotic material and bacterial colonization are common findings. The histopathologic features are not specific.

Treatment

In severe cases or immunocompromised patients, metronidazole 500 mg three times daily for 6 to 8 days is the treatment of choice. Antibacterial mouthwashes and mouthwashes with oxygen-releasing compounds can also be used alone or in combination with metronidazole. Plaque control measures, scaling, and root planning after the acute stage are necessary.

Gingival Overgrowth due to Drugs

Key points

- The medication mainly implicated is phenytoin, cyclosporine, and calcium channel blockers.
- Common clinical characteristic is potentially great gingival enlargement.
- Predisposing factors are poor oral hygiene and subsequent plaque accumulation.
- The diagnosis is based on the history and the clinical features.

Introduction

Phenytoin, cyclosporine, and calcium channel blockers are the main medications causing gingival enlargement as a side effect. The frequency ranges between 30 and 70%. These drugs are widely used as antiepileptic, immunosuppressive, and antihypertensive agents, respectively. Less frequently, other medication can also be implicated in gingival enlargement such as contraceptives and erythromycin. The frequency and degree of enlargement depends on the treatment regime and its duration. However, important risk factors seem to be the levels of oral hygiene and presence of dental plaque and other local and systemic factors. The exact pathogenesis remains elusive.

Clinical features

The overgrowth usually begins in the interdental papillae and gradually involves the free and attached gingiva. With gradual progression, the gingival enlargement may cover the crowns of the teeth partially or entirely. Clinically, the gingiva are firm, lobulated or smooth, normal or red in color, and painless with little or no tendency to bleed (**Figs. 11.21–11.25**). The enlargement is usually *generalized*, but it *can be limited* to a few teeth and is more prominent in the anterior areas. Phenytoin-induced gingival enlargement mainly affects younger individuals, while the one induced by cyclosporine and calcium channel blockers affects middle-aged and older patients. The medical history and clinical features are important for correct diagnosis.

Differential diagnosis

- Chronic hyperplastic gingivitis
- Pregnancy-associated gingivitis
- Hereditary gingival fibromatosis
- Leukemia
- Wegener's granulomatosis
- Amyloidosis
- Crohn's disease
- Hurler's syndrome
- Zimmermann-Laband syndrome

Pathology

The histologic features are not pathognomonic. Histopathologic examination reveals increase of the collagen and the connective tissue in the lamina propria. The overlying surface may demonstrate epithelial hyperplasia with elongation of the rete ridges. The degree of chronic inflammation varies.

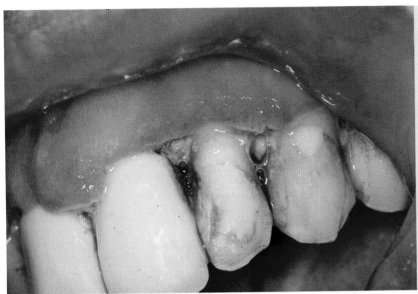

Fig. 11.19 Necrotizing ulcerative gingivitis with extensive destruction of the interdental papillae.

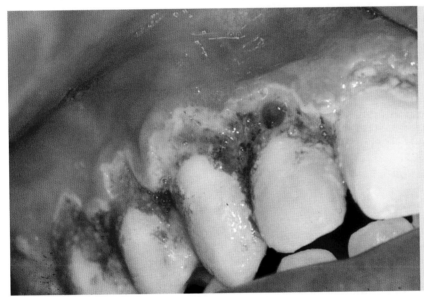

Fig. 11.20 Severe necrotizing ulcerative gingivitis with great destruction of the interdental papillae and the free gingiva.

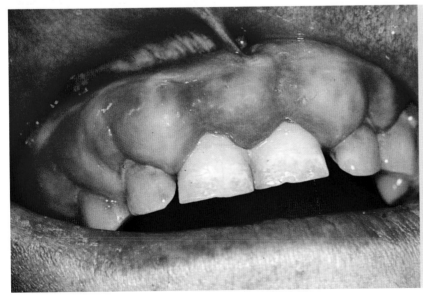

Fig. 11.21 Gingival enlargement caused by phenytoin.

Treatment

Surgical excision of the enlarged gingiva and maintenance of high levels of oral hygiene is the first line of treatment. Discontinuation of the offending drug often results in cessation of the gingival enlargement, but this should be decided by the attending physician.

Hereditary Gingival Fibromatosis

Key points

- It can be idiopathic or familial.
- Most of the isolated cases are inherited in an autosomal dominant pattern of inheritance.
- It may be part of genetic syndromes.

Introduction

Gingival fibromatosis is characterized by progressive gingival enlargement due to fibrous connective tissue hyperplasia. The mutation of son-of-sevenless (*SOS1*) gene is responsible. The mutation may occur on chromosome 2p21-p22, or on 5q13-q22. Another mutation on chromosome 2 has been identified. *SOS1* gene is an oncogene involved in cell growth and the Ras oncogene pathway. The disease is most commonly associated with an autosomal dominant pattern of inheritance. Gingival fibromatosis can also be part of a syndrome such as Zimmermann-Laband, Rutherfurd's, Murray-Puretic-Drescher, and others. The enlargement usually begins by the age of 10 years and affects both the sexes equally.

Clinical features

Clinically, the gingival enlargement may be *generalized* or *localized* to one or more quadrants. The enlargement progressively leads to partial or full coverage of the clinical crown of the teeth (**Fig. 11.26**). The gingival surface appears smooth and rarely nodular. The consistency is firm and the color usually normal. Either jaw may be affected, but the enlargement tends to be more prominent in the maxilla and can cause delayed eruption of the deciduous and permanent teeth, as well as malocclusion. In many cases, the patients also have hypertrichosis. The diagnosis is mainly based on the medical history and the clinical features.

Differential diagnosis

- Drug-related gingival overgrowth
- Gingival enlargement due to mouth breathing
- Leukemias
- Mucopolysaccharidoses (Hurler's syndrome)
- Zimmermann-Laband syndrome
- Chronic hyperplastic gingivitis

Pathology

Histopathologic examination reveals dense collagenous connective tissue, with very few cells and poor vascularity, which forms numerous interlacing bundles in various directions. The surface epithelium is thin with elongated rete ridges that extend into the underlying connective tissue. Molecular tests could be performed to identify the specific mutations.

Treatment

Surgical excision (gingivectomy) of the enlarged gingiva and maintenance of high levels of oral hygiene are the first-line treatment.

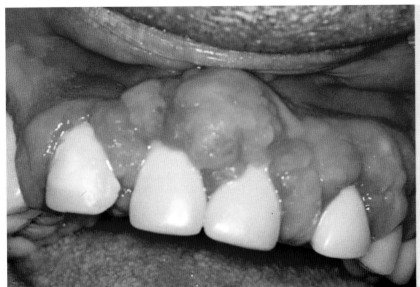

Fig. 11.22 Gingival enlargement caused by cyclosporine.

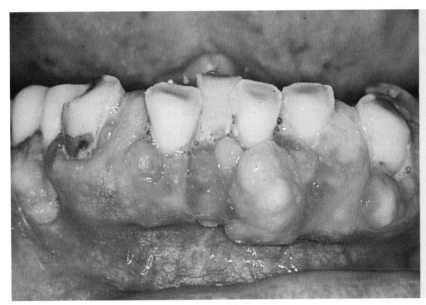

Fig. 11.23 Gingival enlargement caused by cyclosporine.

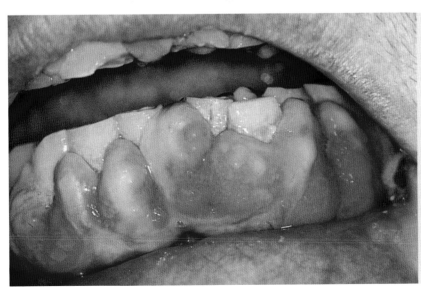

Fig. 11.24 Gingival enlargement caused by nifedipine.

Gingival Deformity

Key points

- Observed in both free and attached gingiva.
- It affects the anterior, labial part of the gingiva.
- Genetic and acquired factors may contribute to the development.

Introduction

Normally, the anterior attached gingiva have a characteristic stippling appearance that many times is compared with that of the surface of an orange. In certain individuals, this can be very prominent. Additionally, friction from toothbrushing can exacerbate this appearance.

Clinical features

The anterior attached gingiva (labial surface) present with an erythematous and prominently stippling, micronodular surface, with depressions and elevations (**Fig. 11.27**). The lesions are usually asymptomatic. The diagnosis is based on clinical and histopathologic criteria.

Differential diagnosis

- Granulomatous gingivitis
- Plasma cell gingivitis
- Wegener's granulomatosis
- Desquamative gingivitis

Pathology

Histopathologic examination usually reveals normal gingiva with more prominent rete ridges and mild hyperkeratosis. The lamina propria exhibits mild inflammatory infiltrate.

Treatment

Mild toothbrushing techniques are recommended. In severe cases, surgical correction may be required.

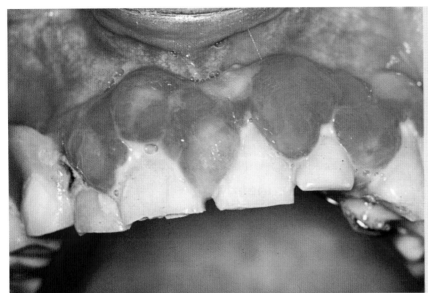

Fig. 11.25 Gingival enlargement caused by felodipine.

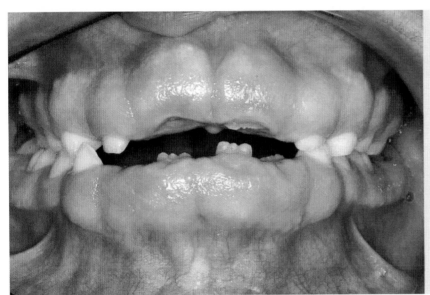

Fig. 11.26 Hereditary gingival fibromatosis. Prominent gingival enlargement that covers the crowns of the teeth.

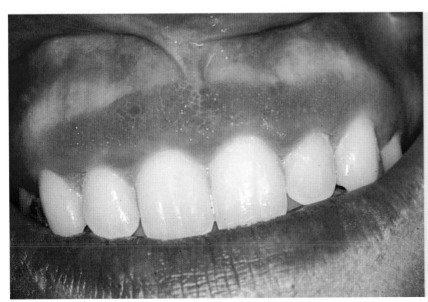

Fig. 11.27 Micronodular surface of the free and attached gingiva.

12 Diseases of the Tongue

Geographic Tongue

Key points

- A relatively common benign disorder of unknown cause.
- Usually coexists with fissured tongue.
- The dorsal surface and the lateral borders of the tongue are the sites of predilection.
- Rarely, the buccal mucosa, floor of the mouth, lips, and palate may be affected.
- No treatment is necessary.

Introduction

Geographic tongue or benign migratory glossitis is a relatively common benign disorder of unknown etiology and pathogenesis, although an inherited gene pattern has been suggested. The prevalence is estimated at least at 1 to 2% or more of the population. Geographic tongue frequently (20–30%) coexists with fissured tongue. In addition, geographic tongue may occur in association with psoriasis and Reiter's syndrome.

Clinical features

Geographic tongue appears in all ages and is slightly more common in females. Clinically, the disorder is characterized by multiple or rarely solitary, usually asymptomatic, circinate erythematous patches, surrounded by a thin, raised whitish border (**Figs. 12.1, 12.2**). This characteristic pattern is caused by desquamation of the filiform papillae, whereas the fungiform papillae remain intact and prominent. The lesions vary in size from several millimeters to several centimeters, persist for a few days or weeks and then heal completely and reappear at other sites of the tongue. Geographic tongue is a benign condition persisting for weeks or months, or even years and is usually restricted to the dorsum and lateral borders of the tongue. Rarely, similar lesions may occur on the buccal mucosa, floor of the mouth, lips, and palate and have been described as *geographic stomatitis* (**Fig. 12.3**). The diagnosis is based on the clinical features.

Differential diagnosis

- Oral psoriasis
- Reiter's syndrome
- Lichen planus
- Candidiasis
- Erythroplakia
- Mucous patches of secondary syphilis
- Drug reactions

Pathology

It is not required. Microscopically, it is characterized by numerous neutrophil collections forming small abscesses (*Munro's abscesses*). Parakeratosis, acanthosis, elongation of the rete ridges, and spongiosis are common findings.

Treatment

Treatment is not required, but the patients should be reassured. In symptomatic cases, homemade mouth rinse with chamomile and avoidance of commercial mouthwashes are recommended.

Fissured Tongue

Key points

- A benign condition of unknown cause and pathogenesis.
- Usually coexists with geographic tongue.
- Multiple fissures on the dorsal surface of the tongue are the prominent clinical pattern.
- No treatment is required.

Introduction

Fissured tongue or plicated tongue is a common developmental disorder with possibly a heredity pattern with a polygenic trait of transmission or an autosomal dominant trait with incomplete penetration. The prevalence rate ranges from 2 to 7%.

Clinical features

Clinically, fissured tongue is characterized by multiple fissures or grooves on the dorsal surface of the tongue and occasionally on the lateral borders as well. Some patients exhibit a deep and wide central fissure and several minor transverse

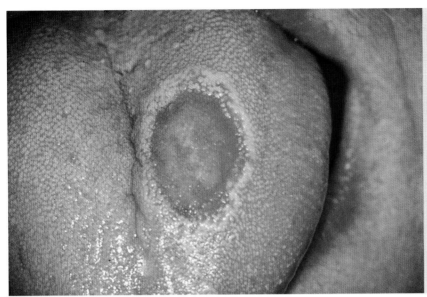

Fig. 12.1 Geographic tongue.

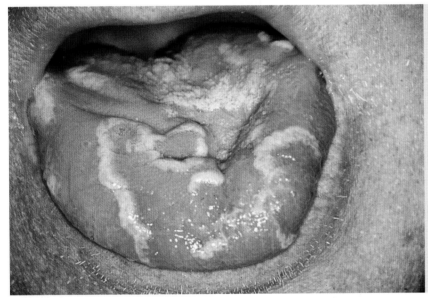

Fig. 12.2 Geographic tongue, multiple lesions.

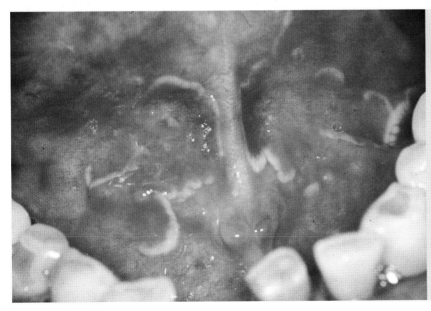

Fig. 12.3 Geographic stomatitis. Geographic tongue–like lesions on the floor of the mouth.

fissures that stem from the central one (**Fig. 12.4**). The fissures may vary in depth, size, and number and usually have a symmetrical distribution. The condition is usually asymptomatic, although food debris, microorganisms, and fungi may be retained in the deeper fissures and may cause mild symptoms such as burning or soreness. Fissured tongue is often associated with geographic tongue (20–30%) and is one of the clinical diagnostic criteria of Melkersson-Rosenthal syndrome and also a common feature of Down's syndrome.

Differential diagnosis

- Melkersson-Rosenthal syndrome
- Sjögren's syndrome
- Interstitial syphilitic glossitis

Pathology

It is not required.

Treatment

No treatment is recommended.

Median Rhomboid Glossitis

Key points

- A developmental abnormality associated with *Candida albicans* infection.
- The disorder develops on the posterior central aspect of the dorsum of the tongue.
- Clinically, it presents in two main forms: flat and lobulated.
- The diagnosis is based on the clinical features.

Introduction

Median rhomboid glossitis is a benign disorder characterized by rhomboid or oval shaped changes on the dorsal surface of the tongue. The etiology is not clear although a developmental defect along with *C. albicans* infection is the most probable theory. The prevalence varies from 0.01 to 1.4%.

Clinical features

Clinically, medium rhomboid glossitis appears as a well-demarcated lesion of rhomboid or oval shape which is localized along the midline of the dorsum of the tongue just anteriorly to the foramen cecum. Two main clinical varieties are recognized, (a) *a smooth*, well-circumscribed red plaque that is devoid of filiform papillae, slightly below the level of the surrounding normal mucosa (**Fig. 12.5**), and (b) a raised

multinodular, firm, reddish mass with a smooth surface without papillae (**Fig. 12.6**). The size of the lesion usually varies from 1 to 3 cm in diameter.

Median rhomboid glossitis is usually asymptomatic, although occasionally secondary *C. albicans* infection may rarely cause a burning sensation or slight soreness.

The diagnosis is based on the clinical features.

Differential diagnosis

- Erythematous candidiasis
- Interstitial syphilitic glossitis
- Geographic tongue
- Lymphangioma
- Hemangioma
- Thyroglossal duct cyst
- Non-Hodgkin's lymphoma

Pathology

It is usually not required. Microscopically, nonspecific, mild inflammatory reaction and loss of the lingual papillae are seen. Parakeratosis and acanthosis with irregular rete ridges may be present. Hypha of *C. albicans* is a common finding.

Treatment

Usually, no treatment is required. However, in cases with *C. albicans* infection, systemic itraconazole or fluconazole 100 mg/d for 7 days improve the subjective symptoms.

Hairy Tongue

Key points

- A relatively common disorder due to elongation of the filiform papillae.
- Predisposing factors are emotional stress, heavy smoking, poor oral hygiene, antibiotics, and radiation of the head and neck area.
- The color may be yellowish-white, brown, or black.
- The diagnosis is based on the clinical features.

Introduction

Hairy tongue is a relatively common, benign disorder characterized by marked hypertrophy and elongation of the filiform papillae due to accumulation of keratin. The cause is not well understood, although several predisposing factors have been implicated such as emotional stress, heavy smoking, use of metronidazole and other antibiotics, long time use of mouthwashes, poor oral hygiene, *C. albicans*, radiotherapy of the head and neck area, etc.

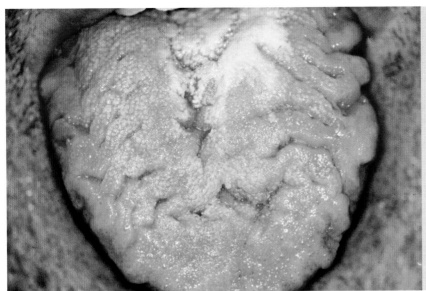

Fig. 12.4 Fissured tongue.

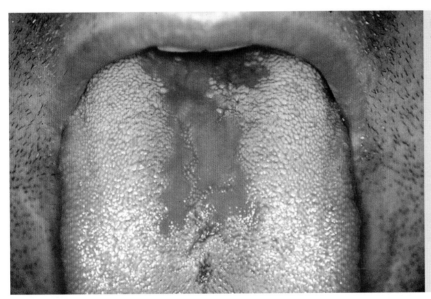

Fig. 12.5 Median rhomboid glossitis, flat type.

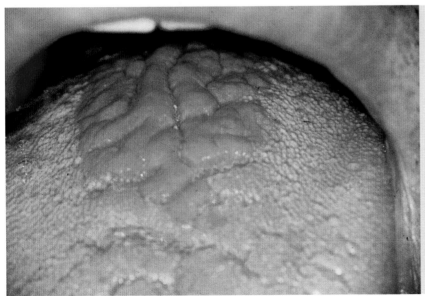

Fig. 12.6 Median rhomboid glossitis, nodular type.

Clinical features

Hairy tongue usually develops in the midline of the dorsum of the tongue just anterior to the circumvallate papillae. Clinically, the disorder is characterized by hypertrophy and elongation of the filiform papillae, resulting in a hair-like appearance. The color of the elongated papillae is usually brown or yellowish-white or even black when pigment-producing bacteria colonize the lesion (**Figs. 12.7, 12.8**). The disorder is usually asymptomatic although the excessive length of the papillae may cause an unpleasant feeling of gagging, bad taste, discomfort, and malodor. Even though hairy tongue is a benign condition, it may cause significant distress to the patients. The diagnosis is based on the clinical features.

Differential diagnosis
- Furred tongue
- Candidiasis
- Acanthosis nigricans

Pathology

It is not required. On histologic examination, marked elongation with hyperkeratosis and parakeratosis of the filiform papillae are present. Colonization of the epithelium by bacteria and *C. albicans* hyphae is a common finding.

Treatment

Excellent oral hygiene, brushing of the dorsum of the tongue by a tongue cleaner and elimination or cessation of any predisposing factors, is the treatment of choice. However, in cases of extreme papillary elongation, topical use of keratolytic agents (e.g., trichloroacetic acid 30%, podophyllin in alcohol, salicylic acid) have been used with success.

Furred Tongue

Key points
- Accumulation of desquamated dead epithelial cells along with debris and bacteria is the cause.
- Poor oral hygiene is also an important predisposing factor.
- The disorder usually resolves, without treatment, in a short time.

Introduction

Furred or coated tongue is a relatively uncommon disorder in healthy individuals. It is common in patients with febrile illnesses, particularly associated with painful oral lesions (e.g., scarlet fever, primary herpetic gingivostomatitis, multiple aphthous ulcers, bullous diseases, etc.). The cause is accumulation of debris, bacteria, and desquamated epithelial cells, along with poor oral hygiene and dehydration.

Clinical features

Clinically, furred tongue presents as a white or whitish-yellow, asymptomatic thick coating on the dorsal surface of the tongue (**Fig. 12.9**). In contrast to hairy tongue, the length of the filiform papillae is almost normal. Bad breath is a common sign. Characteristically, furred tongue occurs and then resolves in a short time. The diagnosis is based exclusively on the clinical features.

Differential diagnosis
- Hairy tongue
- Candidiasis

Pathology

It is not required.

Treatment

Treatment of any underlying illnesses, good oral hygiene, and brushing with a tongue cleaner are recommended.

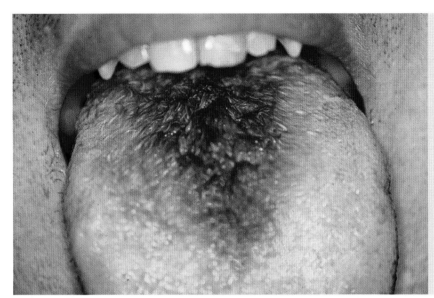

Fig. 12.7 Hairy tongue.

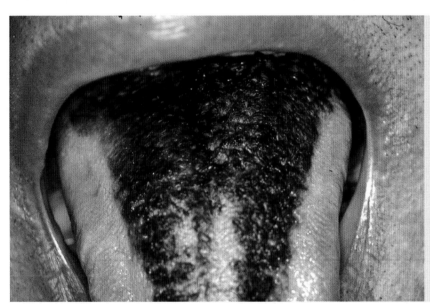

Fig. 12.8 Black hairy tongue.

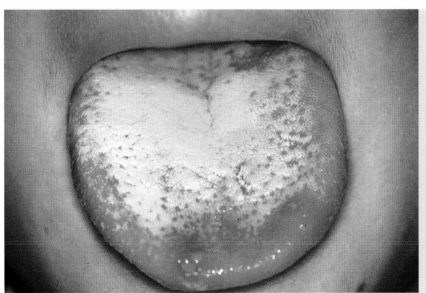

Fig. 12.9 Furred tongue.

Tongue Staining

It is not a pathology but results from covering and staining of the filiform papillae of the dorsum of the tongue. This phenomenon is common, for a very short time, in individuals who use colored mouthwashes, chewing gum, sweets, and drinks (**Figs.12.10, 12.11**).

Plasma Cell Glossitis

Key points

- A rare disorder characterized by erythematous lesions on the tongue.
- The etiology remains unknown.
- Histologically, plasma cell infiltration is the prominent feature.
- Similar lesions can occur on the lips and gingiva.

Introduction

Plasma cell glossitis is a relatively rare disorder of the dorsal and lateral borders of the tongue characterized by persistent erythematous patches, with characteristic plasma cell infiltration on histologic examination. The exact etiology is unknown, although predisposing factors, such as allergic local reactions (mint sweets, cinnamon, peppers, dentifrice, mouthwashes, foods, chewing gum), medications, *C. albicans*, and some endocrine disorders have been implicated. Similar lesions have been described on the gingiva, lips, and other oral sites.

Clinical features

Clinically, plasma cell glossitis has a rapid onset and appears as a localized or diffuse bright erythema and loss of filiform papillae, usually on the dorsal, lateral borders and the ventral surface of the tongue (**Fig. 12.12**). Rarely, extension of the lesions on the palate, floor of the mouth, and buccal mucosa may occur. Typically, edentulous areas are usually free of lesions. The lesions persist for a prolonged period of time and are usually accompanied by a burning sensation.

The clinical diagnosis should be confirmed by histologic examination.

Differential diagnosis

- Geographic tongue
- Cinnamon contact stomatitis
- Allergic reactions
- Candidiasis
- Plasmacytoma
- Granulomatous glossitis
- Reiter's syndrome

Pathology

Histologically, the lesions are mainly characterized by dense polyclonal plasma cell infiltration intermixed with other chronic inflammatory cells. The lamina propria contains multiple dilated vascular channels. The surface epithelium usually exhibits spongiosis and hyperplasia and occasionally exocytosis and neutrophilic microabscesses.

Treatment

The treatment is usually symptomatic. However, in severe symptomatic cases, systemic corticosteroids, e.g., oral prednisolone in a dose of 20 to 30 mg/d for 1 to 2 weeks, then tapered for 2 to 4 weeks is the first-line treatment. The patients should be instructed to keep a dietary history to avoid possible allergens. Recurrences are common.

Glossodynia

Key points

- Glossodynia is not a specific disease entity but a symptom of burning sensation of the tongue.
- Several local and systemic diseases may cause glossodynia.
- In the majority of patients (75–80%) with glossodynia, no local cause can be identified.
- It is one of the most common reasons for patients visiting oral medicine departments and private surgeries.

Introduction

Glossodynia, glossopyrosis, or burning tongue is a common symptom of burning sensation of the tongue and not a specific disease entity. During the last decades, it has become a very common problem, particularly in women over 45 years. In the great majority (75–80%), glossodynia represents a manifestation of an underlying psychological problem with no clinical visible changes. However, several local and systemic diseases may cause glossodynia. Among local disorders, the most common are fissured and geographic tongue, xerostomia, lichen planus, candidiasis, cinnamon contact stomatitis, mouthwashes, mechanical tongue irritation, etc. Systemic diseases that may be associated with glossodynia are iron deficiency anemia, pernicious anemia, hypertension, diabetes mellitus, Sjögren's syndrome, allergic reactions, drugs, and neurologic and nutritional disorders.

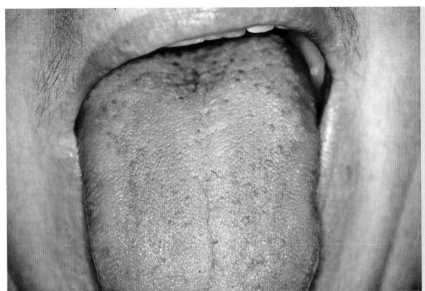

Fig. 12.10 Green staining of the tongue due to chlorophyll-containing sweets (Cloret).

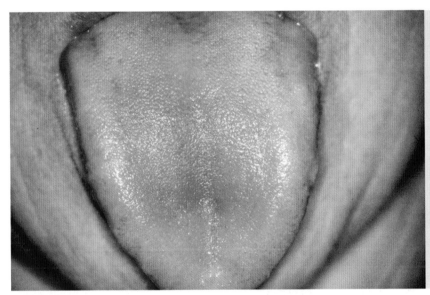

Fig. 12.11 Red staining of the tongue due to local use of antiseptic sweets (Strepsil).

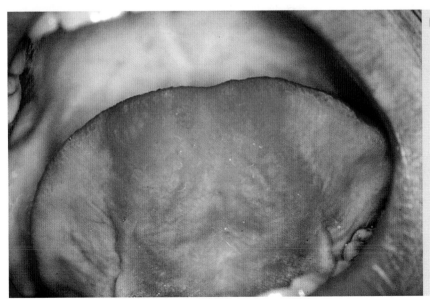

Fig. 12.12 Plasma cell glossitis.

Clinical features

Clinically, in glossodynia of psychological origin, the tongue is usually normal, although slight erythema and mild elongation of fungiform papillae at the tip of the tongue may occasionally occur (**Fig. 12.13**). Characteristically, the patient complains of a burning sensation or itching usually at the tip and the lateral borders of the tongue. Similar symptoms may appear at any area of the mouth (*stomatodynia*). Frequently, xerostomia and taste disorders may occur. As a rule, glossodynia is associated with cancerophobia and microbiophobia, shows remissions and exacerbations, and may persist for months or years. The diagnosis is based on the medical history and the clinical features.

Differential diagnosis

- Local oral diseases
- Systemic diseases associated with glossodynia

Pathology

It is not usually required. In case of suspicion of a systemic disease the proper laboratory tests should be performed.

Treatment

Counseling of patients may be appropriate. This can help them identify that psychological factors may be responsible for their symptoms. In patients with cancerophobia and microbiophobia, the clinician can assure against their presence/cause of their symptoms. Homemade chamomile mouthwash four to five times daily over a long period may improve the symptoms. Avoidance of commercial mouthwashes is recommended as they can exacerbate the symptoms. Mild tranquilizers and antidepressants may be helpful in more severe cases although such agents should be prescribed by the appropriate specialist.

Tongue Varices

Key points
- Varices are abnormally dilated veins.
- The disorder is associated with older age.
- The ventral surface of the tongue is most frequently involved.

Introduction

Tongue varices are abnormal dilations of veins and are a common finding in individuals over 60 years. The disorder is usually not related with any other systemic vascular disease.

Clinical features

Clinically, tongue varices typically appear as multiple, tortuous, sublingual, widened, and elevated, nodule-like, blue-purple lesions, usually bilaterally, on the ventral surface and the lateral borders of the tongue, and less frequently on the floor of the mouth (**Figs. 12.14, 12.15**). Rarely, solitary varices may develop on the buccal mucosa, lips, alveolar mucosa, and soft palate. Oral varices may occasionally become thrombosed. They are benign and asymptomatic. The diagnosis is based on the clinical features.

Differential diagnosis

- Hemangiomas
- Maffucci's syndrome
- Other vascular syndromes
- Melanotic nevi
- Malignant melanoma
- Congenital telangiectasia

Pathology

It is not required.

Treatment

No treatment is required. The patients can be informed of the benign nature of the lesions.

Crenated Tongue

Key points
- There are shallow impressions on the lateral margins of the tongue.
- It is usually a normal asymptomatic phenomenon.
- Systemic diseases which may cause megaloglossia may be associated with crenated tongue.

Introduction

Crenated tongue is a normal phenomenon frequently developed in individuals with misaligned teeth or in those who have the habit of pressing their tongue against the teeth.

Clinical features

Clinically, crenated tongue consists of shallow impressions on the lateral borders of the tongue from the adjacent teeth (**Fig. 12.16**). The disorder is asymptomatic and the mucosa is usually normal, but may rarely be slightly red if there is intense pressure or friction against the teeth.

Systemic diseases such as myxedema, acromegaly, primary systemic amyloidosis, and lipoid proteinosis may cause megaloglossia and subsequently a crenated tongue. The diagnosis is based on the clinical features.

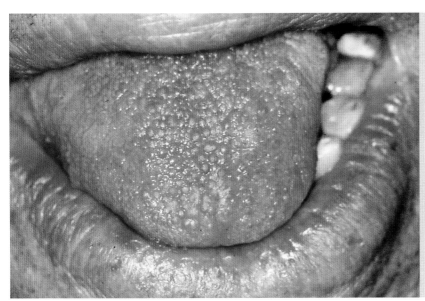

Fig. 12.13 Glossodynia. Redness and swelling of the fungiform papillae of the tongue.

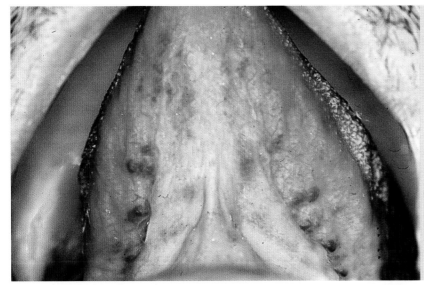

Fig. 12.14 Multiple sublingual varices.

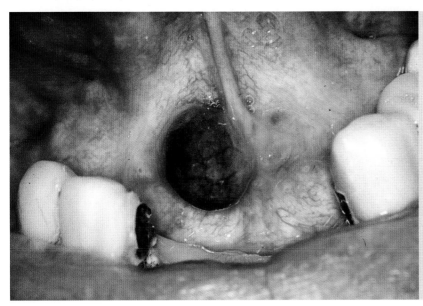

Fig. 12.15 Globular expansion (varice) of the sublingual tuberculum.

Differential diagnosis

- Myxedema
- Angioedema
- Amyloidosis
- Lipoid proteinosis
- Acromegaly

Pathology

It is not required.

Treatment

No therapy except reassurance is required.

Fungiform Papillae Hypertrophy

Key points

- Normal red nodules on the dorsum of the tongue.
- Inflammation of fungiform papillae (papillitis) may cause burning of the tongue.
- Local factors are usually responsible for papillitis.

Introduction

The fungiform papillae are normal, multiple small, round, and slightly elevated red nodules along the anterior portion of the dorsum of the tongue. They consist of vascular and connective tissue and multiple thin neural ends.

Clinical features

Fungiform papillae sometimes become inflamed and enlarged (*papillitis*) and may cause a burning sensation or mild pain, mainly at the tip of the tongue (**Fig. 12.17**).

Excessive smoking, alcohol consumption, hot foods, mechanical friction, irregular tooth surfaces, spices, mouthwashes, etc. may predispose to inflammation and enlargement of the fungiform papillae. The diagnosis is exclusively based on the clinical features.

Differential diagnosis

- Viral oral infections
- Oral drug reactions

Pathology

It is not required.

Treatment

Elimination of the responsible factors is indicated. Homemade mouthwashes with chamomile can be helpful. Avoidance of antiseptic mouthwashes is recommended.

Foliate Papillae Hypertrophy

Key points

- Foliate papillae are a normal anatomical element of the tongue.
- Their size may vary from 0.5 to 2 cm or more.
- Inflammation of the papillae is relatively common.

Introduction

The foliate papillae are localized, bilateral, and symmetrical, on the posterior lateral borders of the tongue and may be small in size or may appear as large protruding nodules 1 to 3 cm in diameter.

Clinical features

The substratum of foliate papillae is lymphoid tissue. Hypertrophy of lymphoid tissue may follow an infection or chronic mechanical irritation from the teeth, resulting to foliate papillitis (**Fig. 12.18**). Clinically, the patients complain of a burning sensation and may frequently be alarmed by the enlarged papillae fearing a malignancy. The diagnosis is based on the clinical features.

Differential diagnosis

- Multiple fibromas
- Multiple papillomas
- Lymphoepithelial cyst
- Non-Hodgkin's lymphoma

Pathology

It is not required, except to rule out other lesions.

Treatment

Reassuring the patient is the best course of action.

Circumvallate Papillae Hypertrophy

Key points

- These are normal anatomical signs at the posterior dorsal surface of the tongue.
- Numerous taste buds are present in the groove surrounding the papillae.

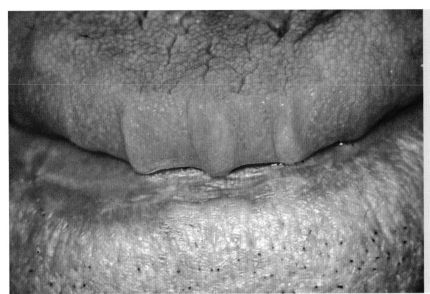

Fig. 12.16 Crenated tongue.

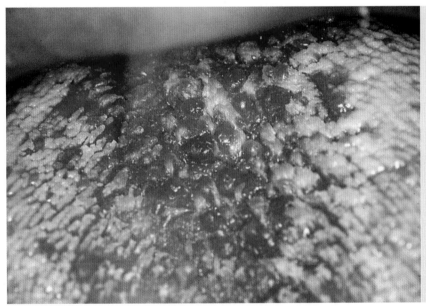

Fig. 12.17 Hypertrophic fungiform papillae on the center of the dorsum of the tongue.

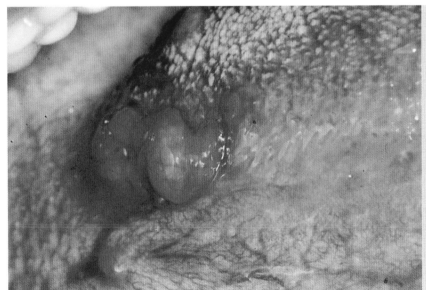

Fig. 12.18 Hypertrophic foliate papillae of the tongue.

Introduction

Circumvallate papillae are located on the posterior aspect of the dorsum of the tongue. These are 8 to 12 in number, arranged in a V-shaped pattern. In the groove surrounding the papillae, numerous taste buds are present.

Clinical features

Clinically, circumvallate papillae present as flattened oral structures of 1 to 3 mm in diameter. Hypertrophy of the papillae results in red, well-circumscribed, raised asymptomatic nodules (**Fig. 12.19**) which, when discovered by the patient, may cause fear of a malignancy. The diagnosis is based on the clinical features.

Differential diagnosis

- Median rhomboid glossitis
- Multiple fibromas
- Multiple papillomas
- Focal epithelial hyperplasia
- Lingual thyroid

Pathology

It is not required.

Treatment

No treatment is indicated apart from reassurance.

Macroglossia

Key points

- Macroglossia means large tongue.
- It is classified into two forms: *congenital* and *acquired*.
- Local and systemic disorders may cause macroglossia.
- Usually, the disorder is asymptomatic.

Introduction

Macroglossia is a large tongue. It is classified into two forms: *congenital* and *acquired*. The congenital form is uncommon and is usually caused by developmental disorders of the tongue (extensive lymphangioma, hemangioma, neurofibromas, or cysts) or may be part of several syndromes (Down's syndrome, Beckwith-Wiedemann syndrome, Hurler's syndrome, Sturge-Weber syndrome, Klippel-Trénaunay-Weber syndrome, neurofibromatosis type 1, and multiple endocrine neoplasia syndrome type 2B).

The acquired form may be caused by several disorders such as hypertrophy of the muscles of the tongue, acromegaly, myxedema, angioedema, amyloidosis, tuberculosis, tertiary syphilis, actinomycosis, tongue malignancies, and orofacial granulomatosis.

Clinical features

Clinically, the tongue is enlarged and can protrude beyond the teeth (**Fig. 12.20**). In many cases, teeth impressions are developed at the lateral borders of the tongue (crenated tongue). Severe enlargement of the tongue may cause functional difficulties in speaking, eating, swallowing, and breathing. Depending of the cause macroglossia may be accompanied by pain or not.

Differential diagnosis

- The list includes all the congenital and acquired causes of macroglossia.

Pathology

It is directed to the causes of macroglossia.

Treatment

It depends on the cause of the disorder.

Microglossia

Key points

- Microglossia means a small tongue.
- It may occur as an isolated disorder or as a part of a genetic syndrome.
- It may be *congenital* or *acquired*.

Introduction

Microglossia is a rare condition where the size of the tongue is abnormally small. The abnormality may occur as an isolated disorder or as part of a syndrome, such as oromandibular agenesia, hypoglossia-hypodactylia syndrome, Pierre Robin syndrome, hemifacial atrophy or developmental disorders, or as an acquired condition (surgery, tumors).

Clinical features

Clinically, the tongue is small with or without symptoms (**Fig. 12.21**). In severe cases of microglossia, difficulties related to speech, swallowing, and breathing may occur.

Differential diagnosis

- All syndromes or developmental disturbances are associated with microglossia.

Pathology

Laboratory investigation is directed to the cause of microglossia.

Treatment

It depends on the cause.

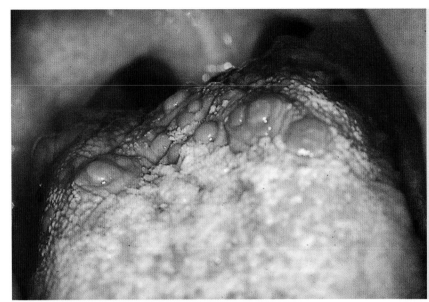

Fig. 12.19 Hypertrophic circumvallate papillae of tongue.

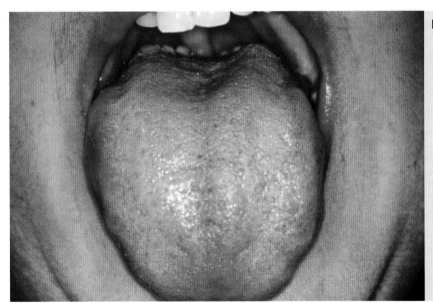

Fig. 12.20 Macroglossia.

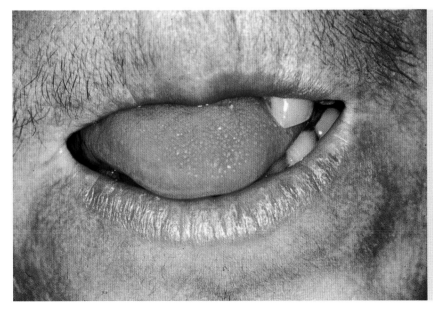

Fig. 12.21 Microglossia.

13 Diseases of the Lips

Median Lip Fissure

Key points
- An uncommon condition that affects approximately 0.6% of the population.
- It occurs in the middle of the lower or upper lip.
- It is of a persistent nature and tends to recur.

Introduction

Median lip fissure is a relatively rare disorder that may appear in both the lower and upper lip and is more common in males than females. The cause of the lesion is not clear, although mechanical irritation, maceration, cold, windy, and dry weather, and sun exposure have been suggested as predisposing factors. In addition, chronic conditions such as human immunodeficiency virus (HIV) infection, Crohn's disease, metabolic disorders, and Down's syndrome may predispose toward lip fissure development. A hereditary predisposition has been proposed for causing weakness in the first branchial arch fusion.

Clinical features

Clinically, median lip fissure presents as a deep, inflamed, persistent vertical fissure in the middle of the lip (**Figs. 13.1, 13.2**). It is usually infected by bacteria and *Candida albicans*. Spontaneous bleeding, discomfort, and pain are common findings. Characteristically, the disorder is persistent and tends to recur. The diagnosis is based on the clinical features.

Differential diagnosis
- Mechanical and thermal trauma
- Cleft lip
- Systemic conditions, e.g., Crohn's disease, metabolic disorders, HIV infection

Laboratory tests

Special tests are not required.

Treatment

Topical corticosteroids with or without antibiotics and nystatin may be helpful. In persistent severe cases, surgical excision with surgical reconstruction.

Angular Cheilitis

Key points
- Usually presents bilaterally.
- It is of multifactorial etiology.
- Reduction of the vertical height and the presence of microbes play a pivotal role.
- Common clinical characteristics are erythema, linear erosions, and white plaques.

Introduction

Angular cheilitis or perlèche is a disorder of the lips that manifests on the corners of the mouth unilaterally or bilaterally. The most common cause is a reduction of the vertical height which results in the development of a skin furrow or fold in the area. Subsequently, saliva flows in the area that can then be superimposed by microorganisms such as *C. albicans*, streptococci, staphylococci, and others. Mechanical trauma has also a role in the development of the disorder. Angular cheilitis is commonly observed in iron deficiency anemia, megaloblastic anemia, Plummer-Vinson syndrome, riboflavin deficiency, Crohn's disease, sarcoidosis, and HIV infection.

Clinical features

Clinically, the condition is characterized by erythema and fissuring starting at the corners of the mouth and then extending in a radial pattern beyond the mucocutaneous border, toward the skin in more severe cases (**Figs. 13.3, 13.4**). Occasionally, crusts and white plaques cover the fissures. A burning sensation and feeling of dryness may be experienced that makes the patient lick the affected areas that in turn results in perpetuating the situation. If untreated, angular cheilitis may last for a long time, showing remissions and exacerbations. The diagnosis is based on the clinical features.

Differential diagnosis
- Iron deficiency anemia
- Megaloblastic anemia
- Plummer-Vinson syndrome
- Riboflavin deficiency
- HIV infection
- Crohn's disease

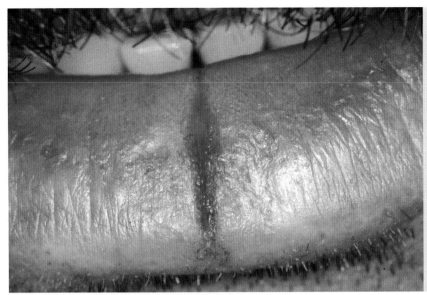

Fig. 13.1 Median lip fissure of the lower lip.

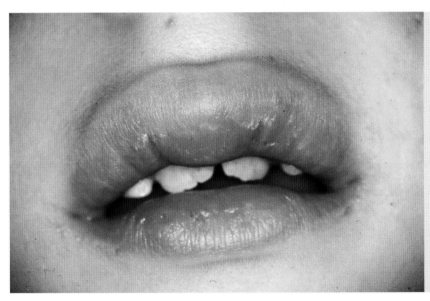

Fig. 13.2 Two fissures on either side of the midline of the upper lip in a patient with Crohn's disease.

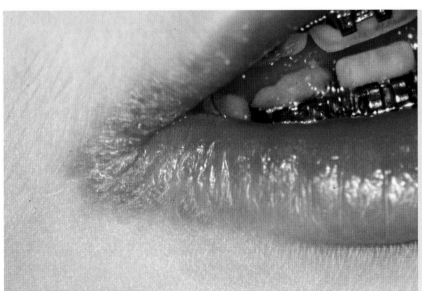

Fig. 13.3 Angular cheilitis.

Laboratory tests

Special tests are not required for the condition itself. However, they might be necessary to reveal a possible underlying systemic condition or disease.

Treatment

Treatment of angular cheilitis consists of treatment of the underlying cause such as correction of the occlusal vertical dimension, vitamin administration, treatment of underlying anemia, etc. Topical treatments including local steroids along with antifungal or antibiotic ointments can be helpful.

Exfoliative Cheilitis

Key points

- An uncommon condition of unknown cause.
- It usually affects younger individuals (under 30 years) of both sexes.
- Characteristically, a thickened surface layer occurs.
- Recurrences are common.

Introduction

Exfoliative cheilitis is a chronic inflammatory disorder of the vermilion border of the lips. It is characterized by the persistent formation of scales and crusts, caused by increased production and apoptosis of keratin. It is more common in young women. A stressful event or stress in general can trigger an obsessive-compulsive tendency to lick the lips. Although exfoliative cheilitis is of unknown cause, factitious activity is mentioned in the literature. Personality disorders associated with depression have also been associated with the condition. Other triggers, deteriorating factors include mouth breathing, lip licking, lip sucking, use of topical agents (cosmetics, lipstick, toothpaste, mouthwashes), very cold or hot weather, prolonged sun exposure, and superinfection (bacterial, fungal).

Clinical features

Clinically, a burning sensation and mild edema precede, followed by thick scales that detach leaving a painful, erythematous area. *Candida albicans* superinfection is common. The lesions are confined to the vermilion border of one or both lips (**Fig. 13.5**). They may persist with varying severity for months or years, with remissions and exacerbations, and may cause a significant cosmetic problem to the patient.

Differential diagnosis

- Contact cheilitis
- Retinoid cheilitis
- Actinic cheilitis
- Lip-licking cheilitis

Laboratory tests

Special tests are not required.

Treatment

Lip licking should be avoided. Topical therapies that have been tried include moistening agents, such as cocoa butter, topical steroids, antifungal agents, tacrolimus, *Calendula officinalis*, etc. Topical use of tacrolimus ointment (Protopic) 0.1 or 0.03% twice a day for 1 or 2 weeks, followed for 2 to 3 weeks once a day application seems to have the best results.

Contact Cheilitis

Key points

- A type of allergic reaction to topical allergens.
- It is of sudden onset and recedes after the causative factor is removed.
- Clinically, it is characterized by erythema, edema, and scaling of the lips.

Introduction

Contact cheilitis is an inflammatory disorder of the lips that is attributed to allergy. Some authors make the distinction between irritant contact cheilitis, when the inflammation is caused by a local irritant, or allergic contact cheilitis to describe allergic contact dermatitis that affects the lips. The most common causes include lipsticks, lip balms, toothpaste, dentifrices, mouthwashes, spices and aromatic substances (cinnamon, mint, vanilla), and foods.

Clinical features

Clinically, contact cheilitis is characterized by mild edema and erythema, followed by the formation of thick, white-brown scales that can detach (**Fig. 13.6**). A burning sensation and mild pain are often reported by the patients. It is usually confined to the vermilion border of the lips and recedes quickly with the removal of the causative agent. The diagnosis is based on the history and the clinical features.

Differential diagnosis

- Exfoliative cheilitis
- Plasma cell cheilitis
- Lip-licking cheilitis
- Actinic cheilitis

Laboratory tests

Patch test can be useful in identifying the causative agent.

Treatment

Treatment consists of discontinuation of all contact with the offending substance, if this is identified. The use of topical steroids can be helpful.

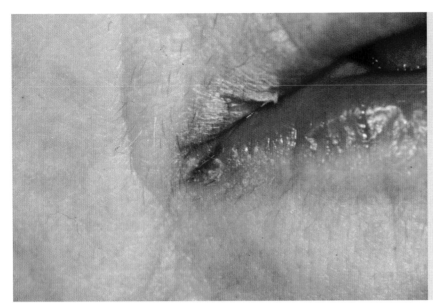

Fig. 13.4 Angular cheilitis.

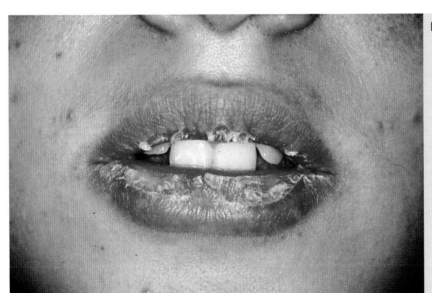

Fig. 13.5 Exfoliative cheilitis.

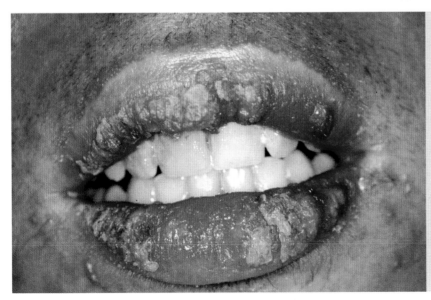

Fig. 13.6 Contact cheilitis caused by contact with an aromatic agent (cinnamon).

Licking Cheilitis and Dermatitis

Key points
- Constant licking of the lips is the cause.
- It commonly occurs in children and can affect both lips and the perioral skin.
- A chronic problem that recedes if the patient stops licking the lips.

Introduction

Licking cheilitis is an inflammatory reaction that almost exclusively occurs in children that have a habit of continuously licking the area.

Clinical features

Clinically, prominent erythema affecting the vermilion border, the commissures, and the perioral skin is developed. This can be accompanied by crusts, scales, and fissures (**Figs. 13.7, 13.8**). The patients complain of pruritus, a burning sensation, and dryness. The diagnosis is based on the history and the clinical features.

Differential diagnosis
- Perioral dermatitis
- Exfoliative cheilitis
- Contact cheilitis

Laboratory tests

Special tests are not required.

Treatment

Discontinuation of the licking habit is the key to treatment. Topical steroid creams or topical tacrolimus might be of help.

Actinic Cheilitis

Key points
- Usually affects the lower lip.
- It is more common in individuals over 50 years with fair skin.
- The main etiologic factor is chronic sun exposure.
- It is classified in the potentially malignant disorders.

Introduction

Actinic cheilitis is a chronic inflammatory process usually affecting the vermilion border of the lower lip. It occurs mostly in males, over 50 years, that have been subjected to years of sun exposure (i.e., farmers, sailors, outdoor workers, etc.).

Clinical features

Clinically, mild edema and erythema are observed, characteristically on the vermilion border of the lower lip. Fine scaling may also occur (**Figs. 13.9, 13.10**). Progressively, the epithelium becomes thin and atrophic with small whitish-gray areas intermingled with red regions. Later the lip becomes dry and scaly with fissuring and microerosions. Actinic cheilitis is considered a potentially malignant disorder as there is an increased risk of development of leukoplakia and squamous cell carcinoma.

The diagnosis is based on the history and the clinical features. However, a biopsy is highly recommended to define the possible presence of malignant transformation.

Differential diagnosis
- Exfoliative cheilitis
- Contact cheilitis
- Discoid lupus erythematosus
- Scleroderma
- Lichen planus
- Leukoplakia
- Squamous cell carcinoma

Pathology

Histopathologic examination reveals hyperkeratosis and epithelial atrophy. Frequently, epithelial dysplasia is present that can be mild, moderate, or severe. Carcinoma in situ or even squamous cell carcinoma may be observed. The underlying lamina propria has dense connective tissue with abundant and often degenerated collagen.

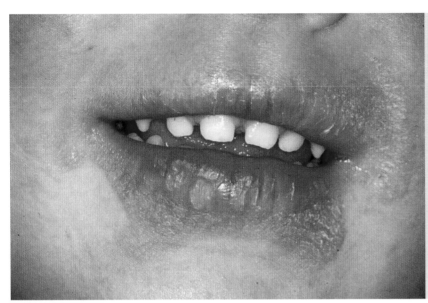

Fig. 13.7 Mild licking cheilitis.

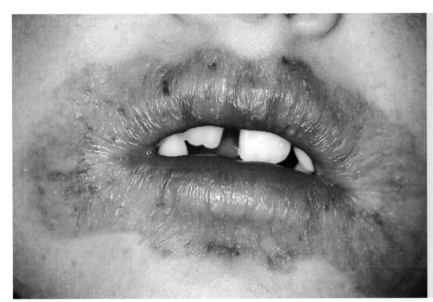

Fig. 13.8 Prominent licking cheilitis and dermatitis.

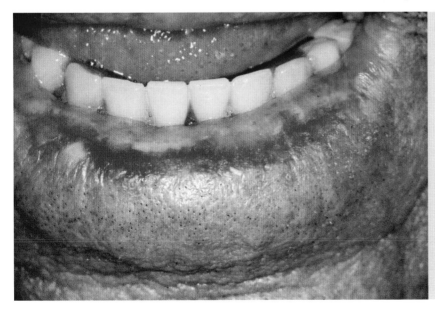

Fig. 13.9 Actinic cheilitis.

Treatment

Protection from prolonged sun exposure is important. Treatments that have been tried include laser ablation, imiquimod cream, 5-fluorouracil cream, topical retinoids, cryotherapy, photodynamic therapy, etc. In severe cases, surgical excision of the involved areas of the lip is recommended. Regular monitoring of the patients is suggested.

Cheilitis Glandularis

Key points
- It classically affects the lower lip.
- It is the result of minor salivary gland inflammatory hypertrophy.
- Clinically, three forms are recognized.

Introduction

Cheilitis glandularis is a rare chronic inflammatory disorder of the lower lip. The cause remains unknown, although several etiologic factors have been suggested such as chronic irritation, actinic changes, smoking, and heredity. It mostly affects individuals over 40 years, although it has also been observed in teenagers. It is caused by hypertrophy and inflammation of the minor salivary glands. Cheilitis glandularis can lead to actinic changes of the lip through chronic exposure to the external environment of the delicate lower labial mucosa.

Clinical features

Clinically, it consists of enlargement of the lower lip which characteristically results in dilation and inflammation of the orifices of the minor salivary glands' secretory ducts. They appear as numerous, pinhead red openings from which mucus or mucopustular fluid may be expressed on pressure (**Fig. 13.11**). Crusting, erosions, and microabscesses may also occur.

Traditionally, three forms of cheilitis glandularis have been recognized, depending on its severity: (a) *simple*, which is the most common, (b) *superficial suppurative*, and (c) *deep suppurative*. The last two forms are a result of microbial infection, and the clinical signs and symptoms are more severe. It is believed that the three types represent a continuous cycle and disease progression if the simple form is left untreated.

Diagnosis is based on the clinical features but has to be confirmed by a biopsy and subsequent histologic examination.

Differential diagnosis
- Cheilitis granulomatosa
- Crohn's disease
- Sarcoidosis
- Tuberculosis
- Lymphangioma
- Lymphoedema

Pathology

Histopathologic examination reveals dense, chronic inflammatory infiltrates within and around the glandular parenchyma, mucous/oncocytic metaplasia, and ductal dilatation. The epithelium may appear normal, but epithelial maturation disturbance may be present.

Treatment

Topical steroids are commonly used but can be of limited value. If bacterial infection is present, antibiotic treatment is required. Some cases may require plastic surgery. In persistent cases with actinic changes, vermilionectomy is indicated.

Cheilitis Granulomatosa

Key points
- Cheilitis granulomatosa is considered a localized type of orofacial granulomatosis.
- It may be solitary or part of other systemic diseases.
- It clinically presents as a persistent, nontender lip swelling.
- Noncaseating granulomatous inflammation is present.

Introduction

Cheilitis granulomatosa, also known as Miescher's cheilitis, is an uncommon chronic disorder of unknown cause. It usually affects young adults of either sex. It may occur either as an isolated disorder or as part of an underlying granulomatous systemic disease, such as the Melkersson-Rosenthal syndrome, sarcoidosis, and Crohn's disease. Some authors believe that the isolated cases are a monosymptomatic form of the Melkersson-Rosenthal syndrome, or orofacial granulomatosis. Its etiology remains unknown although dietary or other allergens have been implicated in some cases.

Clinical features

Clinically, granulomatous cheilitis is a chronic process that presents as diffuse swelling of the lower lip and/or the upper lip (**Figs. 13.12–13.14**). The surrounding skin and oral mucosa may be normal or erythematous. Small vesicles, erosions, and scaling may occasionally appear. The disease usually has a sudden onset and a chronic course, with remissions and exacerbations, finally leading to permanent enlargement of the lips. Rarely, cheilitis granulomatosa may be associated with facial nerve palsy and fissured tongue resulting in Melkersson-Rosenthal syndrome. The clinical diagnosis has to be confirmed by biopsy and histopathologic examination.

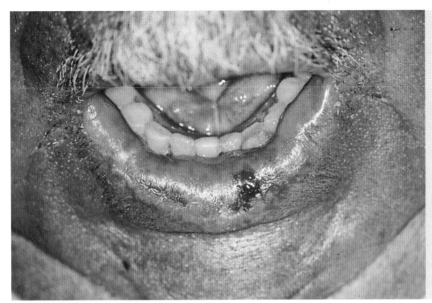

Fig. 13.10 Actinic cheilitis.

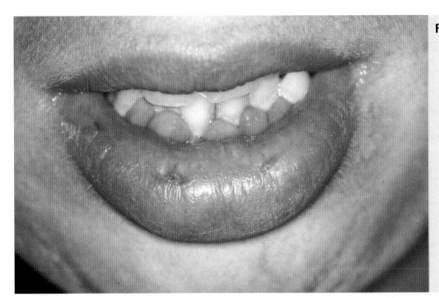

Fig. 13.11 Cheilitis glandularis.

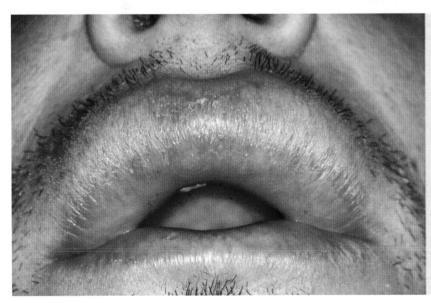

Fig. 13.12 Cheilitis granulomatosa of the upper lip.

Differential diagnosis

- Cheilitis glandularis
- Crohn's disease
- Sarcoidosis
- Melkersson-Rosenthal syndrome
- Angioedema
- Lymphoedema
- Lymphangioma

Pathology

Histopathologic examination reveals a noncaseating granulomatous, inflammatory process. The noncaseating granulomas are formed of epithelioid histiocytes, lymphocytes, and multinucleated giant cells. There can also be edema and diffuse lymphocytic infiltration. Special stains for bacterial and fungal detection are negative.

Treatment

Treatments that have been tried with varying results include intralesional corticosteroids, long-term anti-inflammatory agents, antibiotics (tetracycline, erythromycin), clofazimine, dapsone, sulfasalazine, thalidomide, etc. In severe cases, systemic corticosteroids, e.g., prednisolone 20 to 30 mg/d for 2 to 3 weeks along with minocycline 100 to 150 mg/d for 1 to 2 months have been effective in controlling the disease. In advanced cases, surgical reduction may be indicated.

Plasma Cell Cheilitis

Key points

- A rare inflammatory disorder of unknown etiology.
- Clinically, it is characterized by edema and erythema of the lip.
- The diagnosis is confirmed by biopsy and histopathologic examination.

Introduction

Plasma cell cheilitis is a rare inflammatory disorder of the lips, characterized by a dense infiltration of mature plasma cells. The cause remains unknown; however, in some cases, allergic reaction to chemical substances and food has been implicated. It usually occurs in middle-aged individuals.

Clinical features

Clinically, plasma cell cheilitis presents with diffuse erythema and mild edema of the vermilion border, usually of the lower lip (**Fig. 13.15**). Similar lesions may be observed on the gingiva and the tongue. As the clinical features are not pathognomonic, histopathologic confirmation of the clinical diagnosis is required.

Differential diagnosis

- Contact cheilitis
- Actinic cheilitis
- Erythematous candidiasis
- Discoid lupus erythematosus
- Erythroplakia
- Lichen planus

Pathology

Histopathologic examination reveals a dense inflammatory infiltrate in the lamina propria, predominantly by polyclonal plasma cells with no light chain restriction. Edema and vascular dilatation are also seen. The epithelium might show mild hyperplasia and spongiosis.

Treatment

The treatment of plasma cell cheilitis is symptomatic and includes topical corticosteroids, tacrolimus ointment, and intralesional and systemic steroids. The condition tends to relapse.

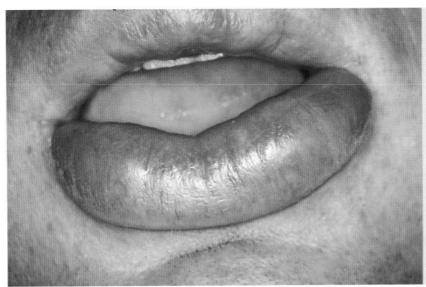

Fig. 13.13 Cheilitis granulomatosa of the lower lip.

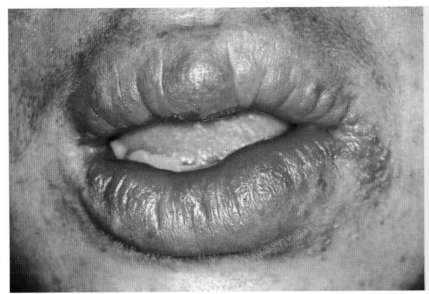

Fig. 13.14 Cheilitis granulomatosa affecting both upper and lower lips.

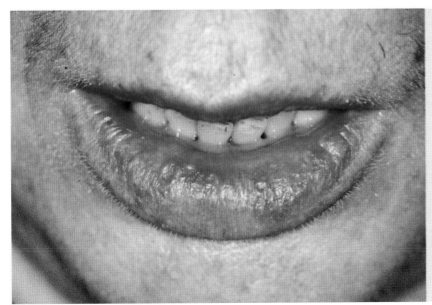

Fig. 13.15 Plasma cell cheilitis.

Crenated Lip

Key points

- It is usually observed on the lower lip.
- It is asymptomatic.

Introduction

Crenated lip may be observed when there are large interdental spaces, teeth rotations, and labial edema.

Clinical features

Clinically, areas of asymptomatic, mild indentations are observed interspaced with elevations that correspond to the teeth and interdental spaces, respectively (**Fig. 13.16**). The oral mucosa is usually normal, but can also become slightly erythematous. The diagnosis is made on a clinical basis.

Differential diagnosis

- Angioedema
- Lymphoedema
- Myxoedema
- Amyloidosis
- Lipoid proteinosis

Laboratory tests

Special tests are not required with the exception of suspicion of systemic disease.

Treatment

Treatment is not required.

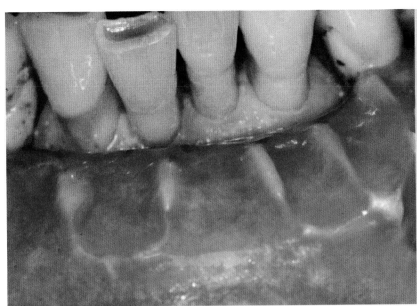

Fig. 13.16 Crenated lower lip.

14 Soft Tissue Cysts

Mucocele

Key points

- Common lesion that originates from the minor salivary glands.
- Three types are recognized using pathogenetic criteria.
- Most commonly seen on the lower lip of children and adolescents.
- Surgical excision is the treatment of choice.

Introduction

Mucocele, or mucous cyst, is one of the common lesions that originate from the minor salivary glands and are formed by the collection of mucous. While the majority of mucoceles are developed in children and adolescents, the lesion can occur at any age.

Depending on the pathogenesis, three types of mucoceles, are recognized: (a) extravasation mucoceles that are the most common and their pathogenesis is related to duct rupture following mechanical trauma (usually biting), (b) retention mucoceles, that are rare and their pathogenesis is related to partial obstruction of the duct, probably due to infection, calculus, or sialoliths, and (c) superficial mucoceles, that is a variant of mucous extravasation cyst. The latter is related to collection of mucous at the epithelial-connective tissue junction, causing epithelial detachment and formation of a small vesicle of 1 to 3 mm in diameter.

Most frequently, mucoceles occur on the lower labial mucosa (70–85% of the cases), usually at the level of the canines and less commonly on the floor of the mouth, ventral surface of the tongue, buccal mucosa, palate, and retromolar area.

Clinical features

Clinically, mucoceles present as a painless, well-defined, swelling that fluctuates and is of bluish, normal, or mildly red color and soft consistency (**Figs. 14.1, 14.2**). They vary in size from a few millimeters to several centimeters in diameter and can be located superficially or deeper in the tissues. They usually are of sudden onset, reaching their final size quickly, and then retaining it for a few weeks. Sometimes they empty partially, either spontaneously, or following trauma, and then reform due to accumulation of fresh fluid. The more superficial types are commonly observed on the soft palate, the retromolar area, and the posterior third of the buccal mucosa. Clinically, this form appears as one or more vesicles, containing cloudy liquid. They tend to burst within 1 to 3 days, leaving small superficial ulceration that heal within 2 to 4 days (**Fig. 14.3**). The diagnosis is mainly based on clinical criteria.

Differential diagnosis

- Pyogenic granuloma
- Lymphangioma
- Hemangioma
- Fibroma
- Lipoma
- Myxoma
- Mucoepidermoid carcinoma
- Cystadenoma

Pathology

Histopathologic examination of extravasation mucoceles reveals a well-circumscribed cavity that is filled with mucous and is surrounded by granulation tissue response. Characteristically, it lacks epithelial lining. In the surrounding tissue, inflammatory cells and foamy histiocytes are observed as well as elements of minor salivary glands. In the retention form of mucoceles, the cavity wall is lined by the ductal glandular epithelium.

Treatment

Conservative surgical excision is the treatment of choice. Occasionally, a mucocele may recur after surgery.

Ranula

Key points

- A variety of mucocele.
- Occurs on the floor of the mouth.
- Marsupialization is the surgical treatment of choice.
- Recurrences are relatively common.

Introduction

Ranula is a variety of mucocele that characteristically occurs in the floor of the mouth. The source of mucin spillage arises from the ducts of the submandibular gland, sublingual gland, or the minor, accessory salivary glands of the floor of the mouth. It is caused by trauma or obstruction of the duct and are seen most frequently in children and young adults.

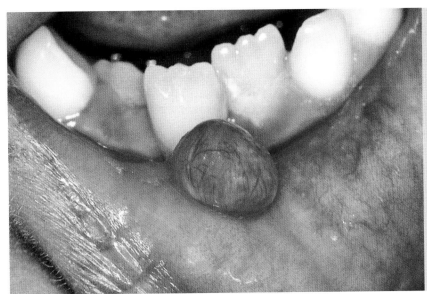

Fig. 14.1 Mucocele on the lower lip.

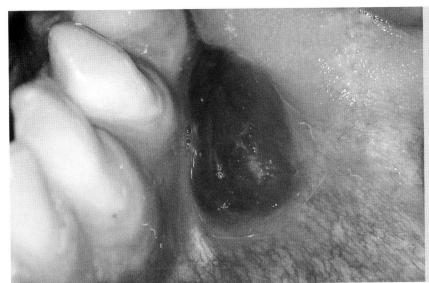

Fig. 14.2 Mucocele on the buccal sulcus.

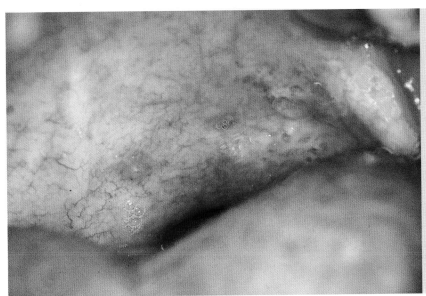

Fig. 14.3 Mucocele on the soft palate.

Clinical features

Clinically, the ranula appears as painless, dome-shaped, fluctuant swelling in the floor of the mouth. The color ranges from normal to translucent blue. It fluctuates on palpation and is of soft consistency (**Fig. 14.4**). The lesion is usually located lateral to the midline, on either side. The average size is 1 to 2 cm, but larger lesions may form, reaching several centimeters in diameter, causing speech, mastication, and swallowing problems. The diagnosis is mainly based on clinical criteria.

Differential diagnosis
- Dermoid cyst
- Lymphoepithelial cyst
- Lymphangioma
- Hemangioma

Pathology

The histopathologic examination reveals features similar to those of mucocele.

Treatment

The treatment of choice is surgical marsupialization. However, this procedure is occasionally unsuccessful for large ranulas originating from the body of sublingual gland; in such cases removal of the offending gland is suggested to prevent recurrences.

Lymphoepithelial Cyst

Key points
- The cyst is formed by entrapment of glandular epithelium within oral lymphoid tissue.
- The floor of the mouth, and the posterior third of the lateral aspects of the tongue are the most common sites of development.
- The diagnosis is based on the clinical and histologic features.

Introduction

Lymphoepithelial cyst of the oral mucosa is an uncommon developmental lesion that is probably caused by cystic degeneration of glandular or surface mucosal epithelium entrapped within oral lymphoid tissue during embryogenesis. The lesion usually becomes apparent between the ages of 20 and 50 and can affect either sex. It is histologically similar to the cervical lymphoepithelial cyst.

Clinical features

Clinically, lymphoepithelial cyst presents as a mobile, submucosal asymptomatic nodule of yellowish or whitish color, and rubbery consistency. The diameter is usually a few millimeters, but can rarely reach 1 to 2 cm. It most commonly occurs in the floor of the mouth (**Fig. 14.5**), followed by the ventral and posterior lateral aspects of the tongue, soft palate, and tonsillar area (**Fig. 14.6**). The clinical diagnosis has to be confirmed by histologic examination.

Differential diagnosis
- Lipoma
- Mucocele
- Dermoid cyst
- Lymphoid hyperplasia
- Lymphangioma

Pathology

Histopathologic examination reveals a cystic cavity, that is lined by a thin, flattened, stratified squamous epithelium without rete ridges that may contain degenerated keratinized cells. Characteristically, the cyst wall contains dense lymphoid tissue.

Treatment

Conservative surgical excision is the treatment of choice.

Cervical Lymphoepithelial Cyst

Key points
- A variant of lymphoepithelial cyst.
- It occurs on the lateral cervical aspect.
- The clinical diagnosis should be confirmed by histology.

Introduction

Cervical lymphoepithelial cyst or branchial cleft cyst is an uncommon developmental lesion of the lateral aspect of the neck. The pathogenesis remains unclear. There are two aspects regarding the origin: (a) remnants from branchial clefts (particular from the second 95%) and (b) it represents cystic alteration of embryologic or tonsillar epithelium within cervical lymphoid tissue. The cyst becomes evident usually during the second or third decade of life.

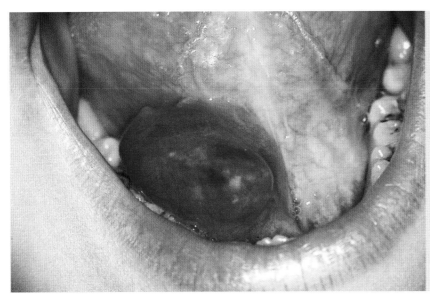

Fig. 14.4 Ranula.

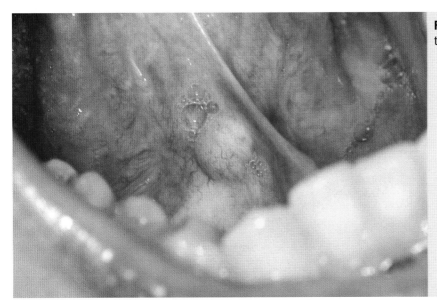

Fig. 14.5 Lymphoepithelial cyst on the floor of the mouth.

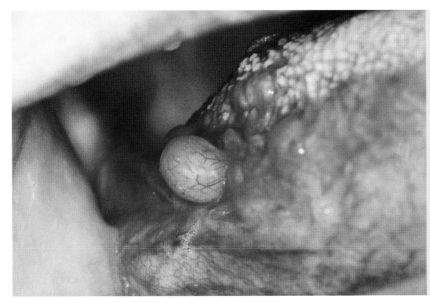

Fig. 14.6 Lymphoepithelial cyst between the foliate papillae of the tongue.

Clinical features

Clinically, cervical lymphoepithelial cyst appears as a soft, spherical, and fluctuant enlargement usually on the upper part of the lateral aspect of the neck, anterior to the sterno-cleidomastoid muscle (**Fig. 14.7**). The size varies between 2 and 10 cm in diameter. It is usually asymptomatic, but patients may complain of tension in the area, or even mild pain if secondary infection occurs. The clinical diagnosis has to be confirmed by histologic examination.

Differential diagnosis
- Lymph node enlargement
- Thyroglossal duct cyst
- Cystic hygroma
- Hodgkin's disease
- Non-Hodgkin's lymphoma
- Lymph node metastases

Pathology

Histologically, the cyst cavity is lined by stratified squamous or ciliated columnar epithelium surrounded by dense lymphoid tissue.

Treatment

The treatment of choice is surgical excision.

Dermoid Cyst

Key points
- A developmental cystic malformation.
- Classified histologically into three types: *epidermoid*, *dermoid*, and *teratoma*.
- It usually occurs in the floor of the mouth.

Introduction

Dermoid cyst is an uncommon developmental lesion arising from inclusion of embryonic epithelial remnants during embryological development. The cystic wall is lined by squamous-like epithelium and might contain dermal adnexal structures in the cyst wall (hair follicles, sebaceous and sweat glands, and rarely teeth). Using histologic criteria, it is classified into three types: *epidermoid*, *dermoid*, and *teratoma*. Most common types are the dermoid and epidermoid. The main site of occurrence is the midline of the floor of the mouth and more rarely the lips. It usually appears before 35 years and has no sex predilection.

Clinical features

Clinically, dermoid cyst presents as an asymptomatic enlargement of a few millimeters and up to 10 cm in diameter (**Fig. 14.8**). Characteristically, it has a soft dough-like consistency on palpation and normal or slightly reddish color. When the cyst is located above the geniohyoid muscle, it displaces the tongue upward, causing difficulties in mastication, speech, swallowing, or even breathing. If located between the geniohyoid and mylohyoid muscles, it protrudes submentally with a "*double-chin*" pattern. When a dermoid cyst develops in the lips, it appears as a spherical or linear enlargement with rubbery consistency (**Fig. 14.9**). The diagnosis is based on clinical and histopathologic criteria.

Differential diagnosis
- Lymphoepithelial cyst
- Ranula
- Cystic hygroma
- Salivary duct inflammation
- Abscess
- Lymph node enlargement

Pathology

Histopathologic examination reveals a cystic cavity that is lined by stratified squamous epithelium with a prominent granular layer, containing mainly keratin. The cystic wall is made of connective tissue and may contain hair follicles, sebaceous and sweat glands, and very rarely teeth.

Treatment

Surgical excision is the treatment of choice.

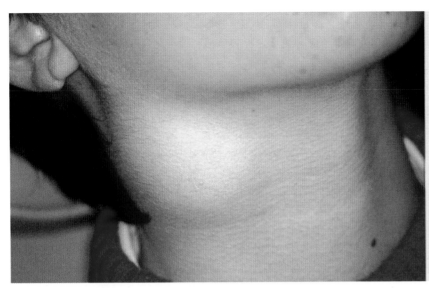

Fig. 14.7 Cervical lymphoepithelial cyst.

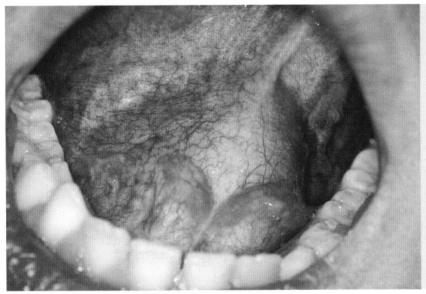

Fig. 14.8 Dermoid cyst protruding on the floor of the mouth.

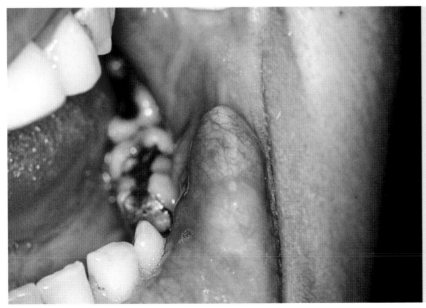

Fig. 14.9 Epidermoid cyst of the lower lip.

Eruption Cyst

Key points
- A type of dentigerous cyst.
- Characteristically, it develops around the crown of an erupting tooth.
- Clinically, it appears as a soft, spherical enlargement of blue/black color.

Introduction

Eruption cyst is a variant of dentigerous cyst that is associated with an erupting deciduous or permanent tooth, located just above the tooth crown. It is relatively common and usually occurs at the site of eruption of the central incisors and molars, usually in children younger than 10 years. Mechanical trauma may result in a considerable amount of blood in the cystic cavity forming the bluish color.

Clinical features

Clinically, eruption cyst appears as well-demarcated, soft fluctuant swelling directly overlying the crown of an erupting deciduous or permanent tooth. Very often, the color is blue, or black (**Figs. 14.10, 14.11**). The diagnosis is usually based on the history and the clinical features.

Differential diagnosis
- Hematoma
- Hemangioma
- Oral pigmented nevi
- Malignant melanoma
- Amalgam tattoo

Pathology

Histopathologic examination reveals a cystic cavity lined by a thin, nonkeratinized squamous epithelium, while the wall consists of connective tissue with mild inflammatory infiltrate.

Treatment

The majority of eruption cysts do not require intervention. However, in cases with symptoms or secondary infection, a simple excision of the roof of the cyst is recommended.

Gingival Cysts of the Newborn

Key points
- Become apparent at birth or during the first 1 to 3 weeks of life.
- Characteristically, occur on the alveolar mucosa.
- These are small, white nodules of 1 to 3 mm in diameter.
- These regress spontaneously.

Introduction

Gingival cysts of the newborn are quite common. These become apparent at birth or shortly after. They arise from remnants of the dental lamina.

Clinical features

Clinically, present as multiple or solitary, superficial and raised whitish asymptomatic nodules of 1 to 3 mm in diameter (**Figs. 14.12, 14.13**). The cysts occur along the alveolar ridge, usually of the maxilla. The gingival cysts of the newborn contain keratin and regress spontaneously within a few weeks or months. Similar lesions may occur along the median palatal raphe (*Epstein's pearls*) or scattered in the hard palate (*Bohn's nodules*). The diagnosis is based on the clinical features and usually histologic confirmation is not required.

Differential diagnosis
- Various hamartomas
- Granular cell tumor of the newborn

Pathology

Histopathologic examination reveals that the cyst is lined by a thin and flattened parakeratinized epithelium. The cavity contains keratin remnants.

Treatment

Treatment is not required as the lesions regress spontaneously.

Gingival Cyst of the Adult

Key points
- Originates from the remnants of the dental lamina.
- Characteristically, it occurs in the area between the lower lateral incisor and premolar (70–80%).
- The cyst appears as a spherical enlargement of normal color.

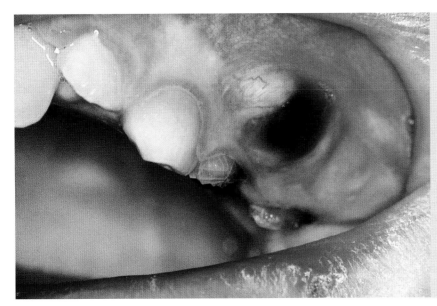

Fig. 14.10 Eruption cyst.

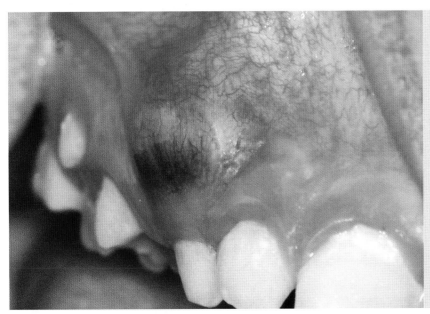

Fig. 14.11 Eruption cyst.

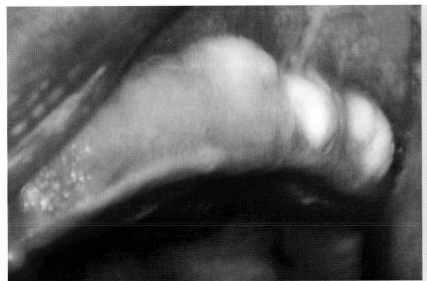

Fig. 14.12 Gingival cysts of the newborn, multiple white nodules on the upper alveolar mucosa.

Introduction

Gingival cyst of the adult is an uncommon lesion. It originates from the remnants of the dental lamina and can occur on the free or the attached gingiva.

Clinical features

Clinically, gingival cyst of the adult appears as a well-circumscribed and painless swelling on the gingiva, covered by normal mucosa (**Fig. 14.14**). The size varies from a few millimeters to 1 cm in diameter. The adjacent teeth are vital on examination. It is more common in patients older than 40 years, in the mandibular vestibule, between the lateral incisor and first premolar. There are no radiographic findings. The diagnosis is based on the clinical features and the histologic examination.

Differential diagnosis

- Lateral periodontal cyst
- Dental or periodontal abscess
- Mucocele
- Lipoma
- Fibroma

Pathology

Histopathologic examination reveals a cystic cavity lined by a thin and flattened epithelium, that is thicker in places and contains clear cells. The wall of the cyst consists of dense connective tissue that does not usually show any inflammatory reaction.

Treatment

The treatment of choice is surgical excision.

Incisive Papilla Cyst

Key points

- Variant of incisive canal cyst.
- It occurs in the incisive papillary area without osseous involvement.
- There are no radiographic findings.

Introduction

Incisive papilla cyst is a rare variant of incisive canal cyst that arises from epithelial rests of the nasopalatine foramen.

Clinical features

Clinically, it appears as a spherical soft swelling of the incisive papilla covered by normal mucosa (**Fig. 14.15**). Often, it may become inflamed and painful due to infection. There are no radiographic findings. The diagnosis is based on the clinical features but has to be confirmed by histology.

Differential diagnosis

- Dental or periodontal abscess
- Trauma of the palatine papilla
- Fibroma
- Lipoma

Pathology

Histopathologic examination reveals a cystic cavity lined by a thin squamous, cylindrical, or columnar epithelium. The cavity wall is formed by dense connective tissue with mild-to-moderate inflammation.

Treatment

Surgical removal is the treatment of choice.

Nasolabial Cyst

Key points

- Occurs on the upper lip, either side of the midline.
- Clinically, appears as a spherical enlargement inferior to the nasal alar region.
- There are no radiographic findings.

Introduction

Nasolabial cyst is a rare soft tissue dysplastic cyst with unclear pathogenesis. It has been suggested that the cyst develops from epithelial remnants of the nasolacrimal duct or from epithelial remnants entrapped along the line of fusion of the maxillary, lateral, and medial nasal processes.

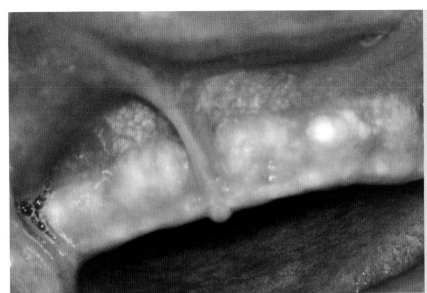

Fig. 14.13 Gingival cyst of the newborn, solitary white nodule.

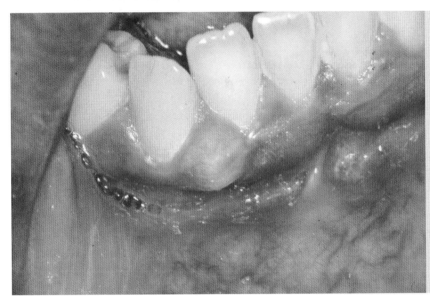

Fig. 14.14 Gingival cyst of the adult between the lower lateral incisor and canine.

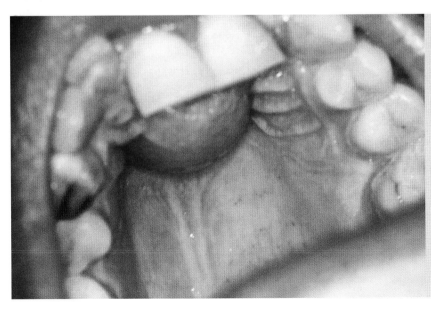

Fig. 14.15 Incisive papilla cyst.

Clinical features

The cyst is more common in females, usually between 40 and 50 years, and it is usually unilateral and very rarely bilateral.

Clinically, nasolabial cyst appears as a painless, spherical, soft swelling of the nasolabial fold of the upper lip lateral to the midline resulting in elevation of the ala of the nose. Extraorally, the enlargement is noticed on the upper lip and the ala of the nose (**Fig. 14.16**). The patients may complain of a feeling of tension in the area, nasal obstruction, and difficulty placing their upper denture. The diagnosis is mainly based on the clinical features, but has to be confirmed by histology.

Differential diagnosis
- Soft tissue abscess
- Dental or periodontal abscess
- Mesenchymal neoplasms
- Minor salivary glands' neoplasms
- Mucocele

Pathology

Histopathologic examination reveals that the cystic cavity is lined by pseudostratified ciliated columnar epithelium usually with intermingled goblet cells and occasional foci of squamous metaplasia. The cyst wall consists of dense connective tissue with usually mild inflammation.

Treatment

Surgical excision is the treatment of choice.

Thyroglossal Duct Cyst

Key points
- It arises from epithelial remnants of the thyroglossal duct.
- It may form anywhere along the thyroglossal duct between the thyroid and the foramen cecum on the base of the tongue.
- Intraorally, it can appear on the dorsum of the tongue close to the foramen cecum.
- Fistula formation is common.

Introduction

Thyroglossal duct cyst is a rare developmental anomaly that may form anywhere along the thyroglossal duct from the foramen cecum of the tongue to the thyroid gland. It is formed by epithelial remnants of the thyroglossal duct. It is more frequent in children and young patients (up to 50% of the cases appear before the age of 20). However, a significant proportion (15%) arises in patients older than 50 years of age. There is no sex predilection. Approximately, in 70 to 80% of cases the thyroglossal duct cyst develops below the hyoid bone.

Clinical features

Clinically, thyroglossal duct cyst presents as a circumscribed painless, fluctuant swelling, a few millimeters to several centimeters in diameter on the anterior neck. Intraorally, it is usually found on the dorsum of the tongue close to the foramen cecum and very rarely in the floor of the mouth (**Fig. 14.17**). It can usually form near the thyroid gland, protruding in the neck (**Fig. 14.18**). A fistula may form opening on the skin or intraorally on mucosal surface. The cyst grows slowly without symptoms except in the cases where it can be significantly enlarged, where it can cause dysphagia and difficulty in swallowing. Rarely, thyroid carcinoma may originate in a thyroglossal duct cyst (0.5–1%). The diagnosis is based on clinical criteria but has to be confirmed by further investigations.

Differential diagnosis
- Median rhomboid glossitis
- Fibroma
- Leiomyoma
- Lipoma
- Squamous cell carcinoma

Laboratory tests

To aid the diagnosis, computed tomography (CT) scanning is more useful for lesions close to the hyoid bone, while magnetic resonance imaging (MRI) is preferred for lesions near the tongue base. Ultrasound and scintiscanning can be helpful in certain cases. Radioisotope examination is recommended adjunct, especially preoperatively. Histopathologic examination reveals a cystic cavity lined by stratified squamous epithelium, or/and columnar and cuboidal epithelium. In the cystic wall, the presence of thyroid tissue is not uncommon.

Treatment

Surgical excision of the cyst and the thyroglossal duct, known as *Sistrunk procedure*, is usually undertaken.

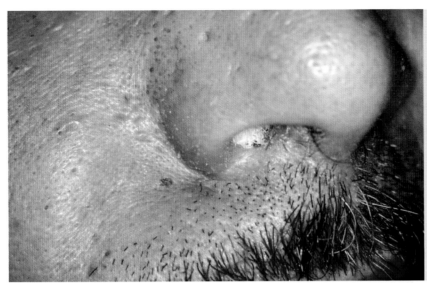

Fig. 14.16 Nasolabial cyst, swelling at the nasolabial area.

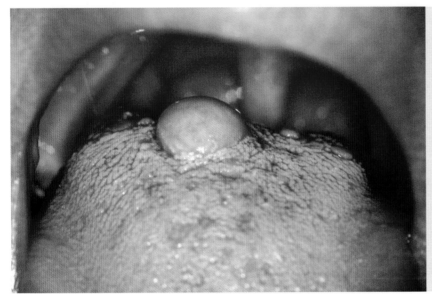

Fig. 14.17 Thyroglossal duct cyst on the midline of the dorsum of the tongue.

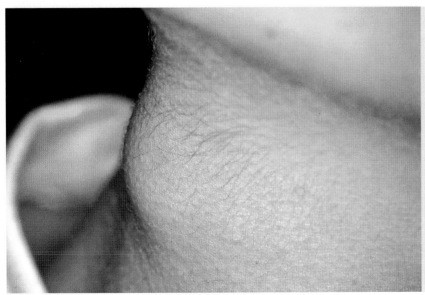

Fig. 14.18 Thyroglossal duct cyst, enlargement close to the thyroid gland.

15 Viral Infections

Primary Herpetic Gingivostomatitis

Key points

- It is caused by herpes simplex virus, type 1 (HSV-1).
- The onset is abrupt.
- Numerous oral vesicles and erosions, high fever and bilateral, cervical lymphadenopathy are the main clinical features.
- Chills, nausea, anorexia, malaise, irritability, sore mouth, and headache are common.
- Often starts as pharyngitis or tonsillitis.
- Resolves spontaneously in 10 to 15 days leaving partial immunity.

Introduction

Human herpes virus (HHV) family has eight members: herpes simplex virus, type 1 (HSV-1) and type 2 (HSV-2); varicella-zoster virus, type 3 (VZV or HHV-3); Epstein-Barr virus, type 4 (EBV or HHV-4); cytomegalovirus (CMV or HHV-5); type 6 (HHV-6); type 7 (HHV-7); and herpes virus, type 8 (HHV-8). The pathogenesis of herpetic infections follows the course: *primary infection—latent phase—reactivation*. Primary herpetic gingivostomatitis is an acute infectious disease mainly affecting children (1–6 years), adolescents, and rarely adults. The cause is HSV-1 or, less often HSV-2, the latter being the most common cause of genital herpes. Type 1 is transmitted through direct contact with saliva or other secretions, while type 2 is sexually transmitted. Initial contact with HSV-1 may produce either acute primary disease (3–5%) or, most often, a subclinical asymptomatic infection. They both lead to partial immunity.

Clinical features

Clinically, primary herpetic gingivostomatitis is characterized by systemic and local symptoms (high fever, 38–39°C, headache, malaise, loss of appetite, dysphoria, pain and a burning sensation in the mouth, and difficulty in swallowing), that precede the oral lesions by 1 to 2 days. The oral mucosa is red and edematous, with numerous coalescing vesicles. Within 24 hours, the vesicles rupture, leaving painful, small, round ulcers, covered by a yellowish-gray pseudomembrane and surrounded by an erythematous halo. New vesicles continue to appear over 3 to 5 days. Lesions are painful and cause sialorrhea. The ulcers gradually heal in 10 to 14 days without scarring. Bilateral painful, mandibular, and cervical lymphadenopathy is a typical clinical sign. Although localized involvement may be seen, oral lesions are usually widespread (**Fig. 15.1**). Both the movable and attached oral mucosa can be affected. Involvement of free and attached gingiva is a constant feature (**Fig. 15.2**). Quite often the disease initially presents as pharyngitis and/or tonsillitis, spreading later to the oral mucosa. Limited involvement of the lips and perioral skin may be seen (**Fig. 15.3**). Lesions on the fingers, eyes, nose, ears, and the genitals may develop due to autoinoculation (**Fig. 15.4**). Serious complications are rare, but include keratoconjunctivitis, pharyngitis, esophagitis, pneumonitis, meningitis, and encephalitis. In immunocompromised patients, clinical presentation of herpetic stomatitis is distinct, characterized by larger ulcers that spread laterally and are surrounded by a circinate, raised, white-yellow border. Diagnosis is made on clinical grounds and only rarely laboratory confirmation is required.

Differential diagnosis

- Herpetiform aphthous ulcers
- Herpangina
- Drug-induced stomatitis
- Erythema multiforme
- Stevens-Johnson syndrome
- Hand-foot-and-mouth disease
- Acute necrotizing ulcerative gingivitis

Pathology

This is rarely necessary. Histologic examination reveals ballooning degeneration of the epithelial cells (edematous, round, multinuclear cells with large clear nuclei), intercellular edema, acantholysis, and intraepithelial vesicle formation. Cytology (material is obtained from the base of a vesicle) may show multinuclear epithelial giant cells (*Tzanck cells*). Detection of HSV antigens by direct immunofluorescence or polymerase chain reaction (PCR) confirms the diagnosis in difficult cases. Elevated serum antibody titer is evident 5 to 8 days after the infection. Lastly, isolation of the virus by viral culture is available, but 3 to 6 days are required for results—and is now rarely undertaken.

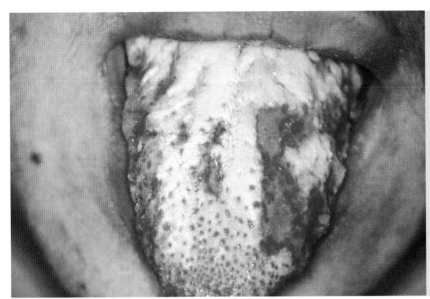

Fig.15.1 Primary herpetic gingivo-stomatitis. Extensive erosions on the tongue.

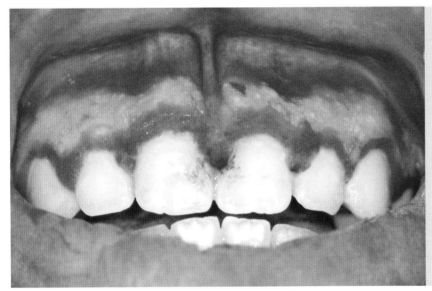

Fig. 15.2 Primary herpetic gingivo-stomatitis. Marked erythema, edema, and erosions on the gingiva.

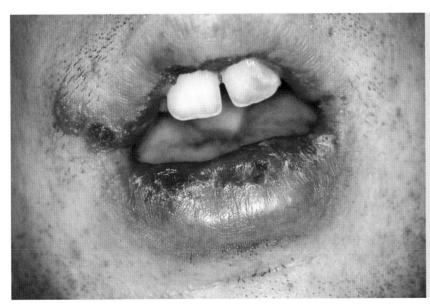

Fig. 15.3 Primary herpetic gingivo-stomatitis. Lesions on the lips and the perioral skin.

Treatment

Antiviral agents (acyclovir, famciclovir, valacyclovir) are the first-line therapy. Treatment should be initiated during the first 3 to 4 days after the onset of symptoms. In children, oral suspension of acyclovir is administered. Concurrent administration of systemic corticosteroids, e.g., dexamethasone oral solution 2 mg/5 mL twice a day for 3 to 4 days, may offer rapid alleviation of symptoms. Dexamethasone should be avoided in children less than 5 years of age, as well as in immunosuppressed individuals. Valacyclovir is given at a dose of 500 mg twice a day for 5 days, and famciclovir at a dose of 250 mg twice a day for 5 to 7 days. Topical application of oral solutions with anti-inflammatory and anesthetic actions, such as ketoprofen (Solu-Ket 1.6%), contributes to pain relief. Lastly, the treatment of herpetic infection in the immunocompromised host requires higher doses of antivirals over longer periods of time.

Secondary Herpetic Stomatitis

Key points

- This is caused by reactivation of HSV-1.
- It develops mainly on keratinized areas of the mouth (gingiva, hard palate, alveolar mucosa), as well as on the lips.
- In transplant recipients and immunosuppressed patients, it may mimic primary herpetic gingivostomatitis.
- Lesions self-heal in 4 to 6 days.

Introduction

Secondary herpetic stomatitis results from the reactivation of HSV-1 and follows primary herpetic infection. As antibodies against HSV-1 are present, symptoms are mild. Predisposing factors include emotional or physical stress, febrile illness, cold, minor trauma of the oral mucosa, tooth extraction, or local anesthesia. In individuals with active HIV infection, transplant recipients, and immunocompromised patients severe forms of recurrent herpetic oral lesions are relatively common.

Clinical features

Clinically, localized, closely grouped vesicles develop. These later rupture, leaving superficial erosions that heal in about 1 week (**Fig. 15.5**). However, in the immunosuppressed patients (leukemia, non-Hodgkin's lymphoma, transplant recipients, active HIV infection) recurrent herpetic infection may persist for several weeks or months. In such cases the erosions are of larger size with tendency to spread laterally and are surrounded by a whitish-yellow, raised halo (**Fig. 15.6**). Secondary herpetic stomatitis most commonly affects adults. It is usually localized on the palate, gingiva, and lips. Because of acquired immunity during the primary infection, the symptoms are usually mild and signs, such as fever and lymphadenopathy, are characteristically absent or mild. The diagnosis is based exclusively on the history and the clinical features.

Differential diagnosis

- Primary herpetic gingivostomatitis
- Early herpes zoster
- Aphthous ulcers
- Hand-foot-and-mouth disease
- Streptococcal stomatitis
- Primary and secondary syphilis (chancre, syphilitic plaques)
- Traumatic erosions

Pathology

It is not required.

Treatment

It is symptomatic. Lesions heal spontaneously in 4 to 6 days.

Herpes Labialis

Key points

- The most common form of HSV-1 reactivation.
- It is located on the vermilion border and the adjacent skin of the upper or lower lip.
- It recurs frequently.

Introduction

Herpes labialis is by far the most common form of secondary herpetic infection in the oral and perioral region. It is caused by reactivation, usually, of HSV-1. It involves the upper or the lower lip with equal frequency, and affects women more often than men in a ratio of approximately 2:1.

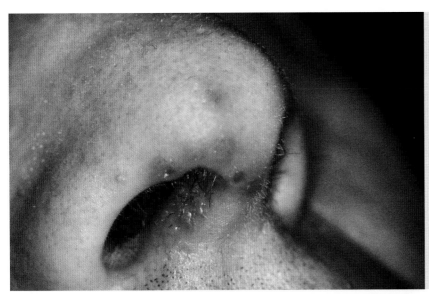

Fig. 15.4 Primary herpetic gingivo-stomatitis. Lesions on the nose due to inoculation of the virus from the mouth.

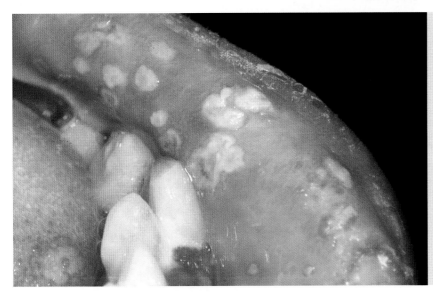

Fig. 15.5 Secondary herpes. Grouped vesicles on the mucosa of the lower lip.

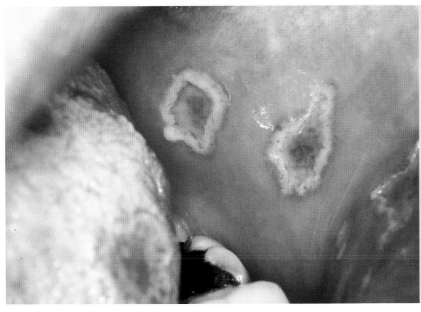

Fig. 15.6 Secondary herpes in an immunosuppressed patient. Typical, persisting lesions on the buccal mucosa.

Clinical features

Clinically, herpes labialis is initially characterized by initial itching and burning, followed by edema and redness and the development of clusters of small vesicles located on the vermilion border and the adjacent perioral skin. The vesicles soon rupture, within 2 to 3 days, leaving small ulcers covered by crusts (**Fig. 15.7**) that heal spontaneously without scarring in 5 to 8 days. In immunocompromised individuals, lesions can be more severe and extensive and may last for 1 to 3 months (**Fig. 15.8**). Recurrences are a typical feature of herpes labialis and may be associated with fever, emotional or physical stress, menstruation, sun exposure, cold weather, or local trauma. The diagnosis is exclusively made on clinical grounds.

Differential diagnosis
- Syphilitic chancre
- Traumatic erosions
- Impetigo

Pathology

It is not required.

Treatment

Topical application of acyclovir or penciclovir cream or ointment, during the early stages, may be helpful.

Herpes Zoster

Key points
- It is caused by the reactivation of herpes virus, type 3 (VZV).
- It usually affects sensory nerves, more often a single dermatome.
- Involvement of the trigeminal nerve represents 20 to 30% of the cases.
- Lesions characteristically exhibit a unilateral distribution.
- It is most common among the elderly and the immuno-suppressed individuals.
- Systemic antiviral drugs are the first line of treatment.

Introduction

Herpes zoster is an acute vesicular disease that is caused by the reactivation of latent VZV, also referred as *herpes virus, type 3*, in the partially immune host. It mostly affects older individuals, over 50 years, and is very rare in infants and children. There is no gender predilection. An increased incidence of herpes zoster is observed in patients under long-term therapy with corticosteroids or other immunosuppressants, or during radiotherapy, as well as in patients with underlying malignancy, especially of the lymphoid tissue (Hodgkin's disease, non-Hodgkin's lymphoma, leukemia). Herpes zoster can be common in patients with active HIV disease. These cases are characterized by severe and extensive involvement and are seen among younger individuals. The thoracic, cervical, trigeminal, and lumbosacral dermatomes are most frequently affected. Trigeminal involvement occurs in approximately 15 to 20% of the cases.

Clinical features

Clinically, the first symptom of the disease is usually tenderness and pain in the involved dermatome. Constitutional symptoms such as fever, malaise, and headache may also occur. After 2 to 4 days the eruptive phase follows, characterized by grouped maculopapules on an erythematous base, which rapidly form vesicles and in 2 to 3 days evolve into pustules. Within 5 to 10 days the pustules crust and persist for 10 to 20 days. New lesions continue to appear for several days. The regional lymph nodes are usually tender and enlarged. The unilateral distribution of the lesions is the most characteristic clinical feature of herpes zoster. Oral manifestations may occur when the second and third branches of the trigeminal nerve are involved. Frequently, intraoral involvement is associated with unilateral skin lesions on the face (**Fig. 15.9**). Oral mucosal lesions are almost identical to the cutaneous lesions.

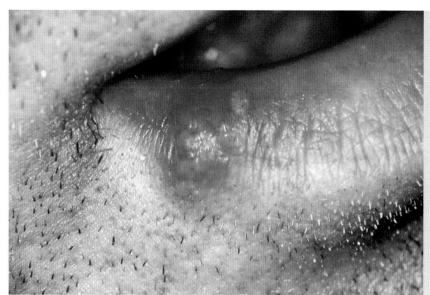

Fig. 15.7 Herpes labialis.

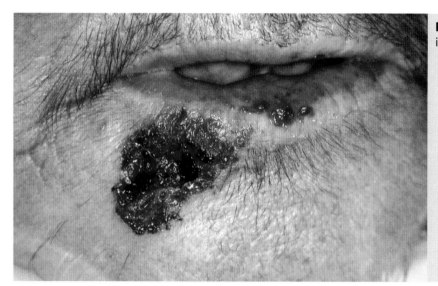

Fig. 15.8 Severe herpes labialis in an immunocompromised patient.

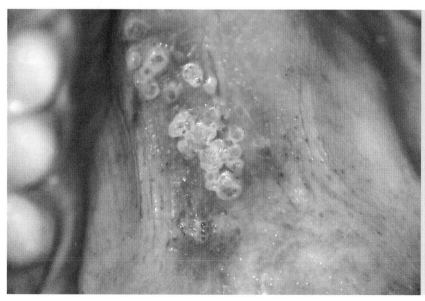

Fig. 15.9 Herpes zoster, unilateral cluster of vesicles on the right aspect of palate.

An itching sensation and pain, which may simulate pulpitis, precede the oral lesions. These begin as unilateral clusters of vesicles which in 2 to 3 days rupture, leaving ulcers surrounded by a broad erythematous zone (**Figs. 15.10, 15.11**). The ulcers heal without scarring in 2 to 3 weeks. Postherpetic trigeminal neuralgia is the most common complication of oral herpes zoster. Rarely, osteomyelitis, jaw bone necrosis, or loss of teeth may occur in immunocompromised patients. The diagnosis is based on clinical criteria.

Differential diagnosis
- Secondary herpetic stomatitis
- Varicella
- Erythema multiforme
- Herpangina

Pathology

Cytologic examination confirms virally modified epithelial cells with acantholysis and formation of multiple, free-floating Tzanck cells with nuclear margination of chromatin and multinucleation. The immunoglobulin G (IgG) antibody titer to VZV may risk between the acute and convalescent phases.

Treatment

Antiviral therapy is effective if started early, within 3 to 4 days from the onset of symptoms. Oral valacyclovir (e.g., 1.0–1.5 g, three times a day for 7 days) or oral famciclovir (e.g., 500 mg, three times a day for 7 days) are the treatments of choice. Brivudin (Brivir, 125 mg once daily for 7 days) has increased efficacy with a simplified dosage schedule. Prednisolone (20–30 mg for 1 week, tapered for a further week) may alleviate acute symptoms and reduce the risk for postherpetic neuralgia. Analgesics, anticonvulsants, and sedatives are also administered to control the pain.

Varicella (Chickenpox)

Key points
- Contagious disease of childhood.
- Represents the primary infection by VZV or HHV-3.
- Outbreaks occur in winter and spring.
- The oral mucosa is frequently involved, but the involvement is mild.

Introduction

Varicella (chickenpox) is an acute exanthematous, highly contagious disease of childhood, caused by VZV or HHV-3. It develops following first contact with VZV in a previously nonimmunized host. The disease has an increased prevalence during winter and spring. The virus is transmitted by airborne droplets as well as by direct contact with active lesions.

Clinical features

The incubation period lasts 10 to 20 days, followed by the prodrome phase which is characterized by malaise, headache, pharyngitis, and low-grade fever. In 2 to 3 days a maculopapular, erythematous skin rash develops that rapidly evolves into vesicles and pustules that rupture leaving small erosions, covered by crusts. New lesions appear in successive waves over 2 to 4 days. As a result, lesions at different stages of evolution are present simultaneously, representing a characteristic clinical feature. The lesions heal within 10 to 15 days. The trunk, face, and scalp are most commonly involved (**Fig. 15.12**). The oral mucosa is often affected, but the lesions are asymptomatic and fewer in number, thus remaining inconspicuous. Clinically, small vesicles appear that soon rupture, leaving shallow erosions, covered by whitish material and surrounded by a red halo (**Fig. 15.13**). Oral lesions show a predilection for the palate and lips. In addition, gingivitis is commonly present. In healthy children, the disease is self-limited (usually 7–10 days) and uncomplicated. Complications may occur, including secondary bacterial infection of the cutaneous lesions and, very rarely, neurologic disorders and pneumonia. Varicella may occur rarely in adulthood. In these cases, the signs and symptoms are more severe, as well as the complications, e.g., pneumonitis, central nervous system involvement, and encephalitis. Affected people are contagious 2 days before the skin rash appears and until the lesions crust. Diagnosis is based on the history and the clinical features.

Differential diagnosis
- Primary herpetic gingivostomatitis
- Aphthous ulcers
- Herpangina
- Hand-foot-and-mouth disease
- Drug eruption
- Measles

Pathology

In most cases, it is not required. In difficult cases, the same tests as in herpes zoster may occasionally be useful.

Treatment

This is symptomatic. Antipyretics, antihistamines, and topical treatment for the skin lesions are used. In children less than 2 years and in adults, administration of valacyclovir, famciclovir, or acyclovir is recommended. Vaccination between 2 and 6 years is an important prevention strategy. The management of the disease belongs to the pediatrician.

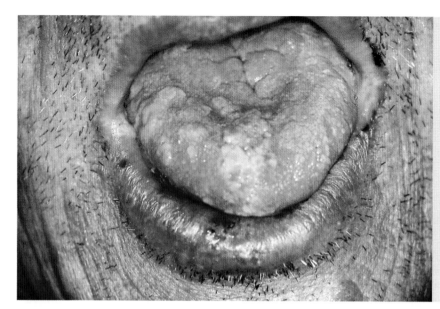

Fig. 15.10 Herpes zoster. Unilateral distribution of oral and skin lesions.

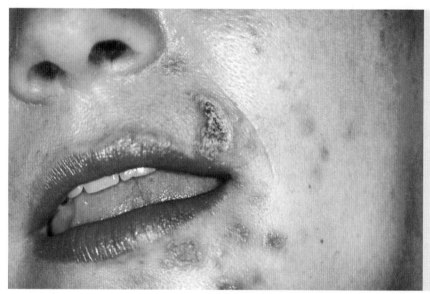

Fig. 15.11 Herpes zoster. Typical facial skin lesions in unilateral distribution.

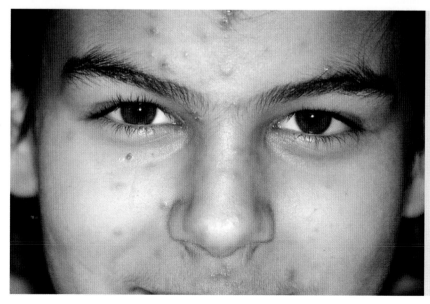

Fig. 15.12 Varicella. Maculopapular rash and vesicles on the skin of the face.

Infectious Mononucleosis

Key points

- EBV or HHV-4 is the cause.
- Transmitted by saliva.
- Palatal petechiae, uvular edema, oral lymphoid enlargement, and ulcerative gingivitis are the most common oral lesions.

Introduction

Infectious mononucleosis is an acute, self-limited disease, caused by the EBV or HHV-4 that is transmitted via saliva transfer. It is more common in children and young adults, aged 15 to 25 years. Intrafamilial spread of the virus is frequent. In a healthy host, EBV remains latent in B cells, after the primary infection, for life. The incubation period is long, approximately 30 to 50 days, and the clinical presentation is variable. EBV appears to be implicated in the pathogenesis of Burkitt's lymphoma, some other types of non-Hodgkin's lymphoma, nasopharyngeal carcinoma, and lymphoepithelial carcinoma, as well as in other lymphohyperplastic disorders in transplant recipients and other immunosuppressed patients. It is also the causative agent of hairy leukoplakia.

Clinical features

Infectious mononucleosis is clinically characterized by low-grade fever, which persists for 1 to 2 weeks, sore throat, malaise, headache, generalized lymphadenopathy (mostly cervical and auricular), splenomegaly, and hepatomegaly. A maculopapular eruption, mostly located on the trunk, head and neck, and the extremities, may appear on day 4 to 6 and lasts for about 1 week (**Fig. 15.14**). It is very characteristic that ampicillin causes exacerbation of the skin eruption in 80 to 100%. Oral manifestations are common and the most constant feature is palatal petechiae, solitary or grouped (**Fig. 15.15**). In addition, uvular edema, inflammation of the oral lymphoid tissue, erosions, ulcerative gingivitis, and diffuse mucosal erythema may be observed. Sore throat, tonsillitis, and pharyngitis are also present in association with the oral lesions. Signs and symptoms subside in 3 to 4 weeks. The diagnosis is usually based on clinical grounds but should be confirmed by special laboratory tests.

Differential diagnosis

- Leukemia
- Secondary syphilis
- Streptococcal oropharyngitis
- Diphtheria
- Drug reaction
- Palatal erythema from fellatio
- HIV infection
- Viral hepatitis
- Cytomegalovirus infection
- Toxoplasmosis

Pathology

Identification of serum heterophile antibodies (monospot test) confirms the diagnosis. Increased titers of EBV DNA in serum are of diagnostic help.

Treatment

The disease is self-limited and the treatment is symptomatic. Combination of acyclovir, valacyclovir, or famciclovir with low doses of systemic corticosteroids has been used with partial success for infectious mononucleosis.

Cytomegalovirus Infection

Key points

- CMV or HHV-5 is the cause of the infection.
- Newborns and immunosuppressed adults are the most susceptible.
- CMV may reside latently in salivary glands, macrophages, lymphocytes, and endothelium.
- It is the main cause of congenital deafness and intellectual disability, as well as retinopathy and blindness in patients with AIDS.
- The oral mucosa and salivary glands may be affected, when immunosuppression is present.

Introduction

CMV or HHV-5 exhibits common features with the other herpes viruses: primary infection—latent phase—reactivation. It represents one of the most common intrauterus fetal infections in humans. In immunocompetent individuals, the infection is asymptomatic in more than 95% of the cases. Newborns, patients with AIDS, transplant recipients, and other immunosuppressed patients with AIDS are at an increased risk for CMV infection. It is transmitted through biological fluids (saliva, blood, urine, semen, breast milk, vaginal secretions), transplant tissue, and feces. Following primary infection, CMV can remain in latent state throughout the host's life and very rarely becomes symptomatic. Reactivation of the virus results in recurrent infection. Most commonly involved structures include the lymphoid tissue, lungs, liver, gastrointestinal tract, retina, as well as salivary glands and central nervous system, particularly in the newborns.

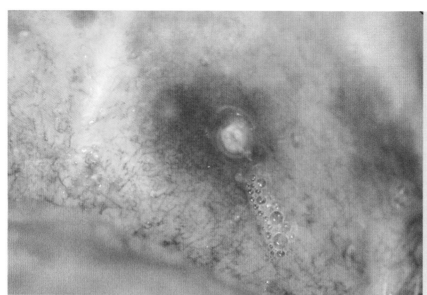

Fig. 15.13 Varicella. Small vesicle with erythematous halo on the palate.

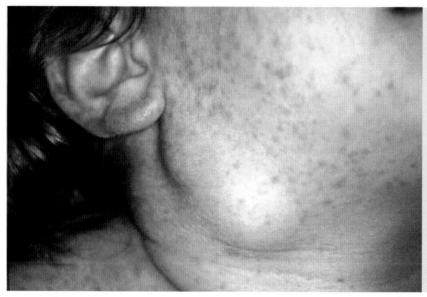

Fig. 15.14 Infectious mononucleosis. Characteristic skin lesions on the cheek associated with auricular and cervical lymphadenopathy.

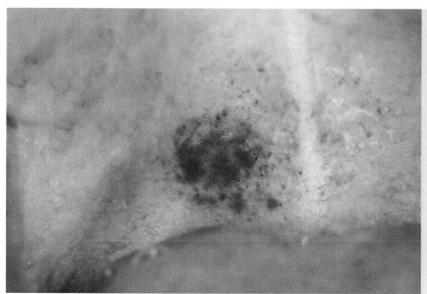

Fig. 15.15 Infectious mononucleosis. Characteristic petechiae located at the border between hard and soft palate.

Clinical features

The majority of acute CMV infections are asymptomatic and only 5 to 10% may present a variety of signs and symptoms, similar to those of infectious mononucleosis. The most common signs and symptoms are fever, sore throat, cough, pharyngitis, malaise, myalgia, joint pain, abdominal pain, diarrhea, lymphadenopathy, hepatosplenomegaly, adenopathy, and meningeal irritation. Occasionally, a maculopapular, pruritic cutaneous eruption and petechiae may be seen. In addition, genital and perianal ulceration has been described. Oral lesions are rare and occur mainly in patients with AIDS, immunocompromised transplant patients, and in other immunosuppressed individuals. Clinically, in the oral mucosa atypical ulcers, 0.5 to 1.0 cm in diameter, appear, without specific clinical features that persist for a long time (**Fig. 15.16**). Additionally, painful sialadenitis of the minor and major salivary glands has been observed. In such cases, enlargement of the major salivary glands and xerostomia may occur. The course of CMV infection is usually mild and self-limited. Rarely, complications may occur including eye disorders, pneumonia, myocarditis, gastrointestinal and hematologic disorders, CNS involvement, etc. The clinical diagnosis should always be confirmed by laboratory tests.

Differential diagnosis
- Infectious mononucleosis
- Herpes simplex
- Traumatic ulcer
- Chancre
- Nonspecific oral ulceration
- HIV disease
- Toxoplasmosis

Pathology

Viral culture was previously the most reliable diagnostic method. Recently, this technique has been improved and has become faster with the use of monoclonal antibodies directed against CMV antigens. Other available techniques include PCR and enzyme-linked immunosorbent assay (ELISA). Histologic examination is characterized by large, CMV-infected cells that have been described as "*owl eye-like*" and are considered pathognomonic for CMV infection.

Treatment

Management of active CMV infection falls under the remit of infectious disease specialists. The main agents used are intravenous ganciclovir and oral valanciclovir.

Human Papilloma Virus Infection

See Chapter 34, 1a, p. 480.

Herpangina

Key points
- It is caused by Coxsackie enteroviruses, group A, usually types 1 to 6, 8, 10, and 22.
- The disease has a peak incidence during summer and autumn.
- Typically, oral lesions are localized on the soft palate, uvula, and tonsils.
- Diagnosis is based on the history and the clinical features.

Introduction

Herpangina is an acute infection caused by Coxsackie virus group A, types 1 to 6, 8, 10, and 22 and occasionally other types. It has a peak incidence during summer and autumn and affects, more frequently, children and young adults.

Clinical features

Clinically, the disease has an acute onset, characterized by sudden fever, ranging from 38 to 40°C, headache, dysphagia, sore throat, nausea, and malaise. Within 24 to 48 hours, an acute inflammation of the posterior oral mucosa and oropharynx develops with concurrent appearance of numerous small vesicles, 2 to 5 mm in diameter. The vesicles become confluent and soon rupture, leaving painful shallow ulcers (**Figs. 15.17, 15.18**). The lesions characteristically involve the soft palate and uvula, tonsils, faucial pillars, posterior pharyngeal wall, and, rarely, the posterior tongue. The absence of lesions on the lips, gingiva, buccal mucosa, and the floor of the mouth is highly characteristic. The systemic symptoms resolve in 4 to 6 days while the oral ulceration heals in approximately 8 to 10 days. The diagnosis is based on the history and the clinical features.

Differential diagnosis
- Primary herpetic gingivostomatitis
- Herpetiform aphthous ulcers
- Hand-foot-and-mouth disease
- Streptococcal stomatitis and pharyngitis
- Gonococcal stomatitis
- Acute lymphonodular pharyngitis
- Erythema multiforme

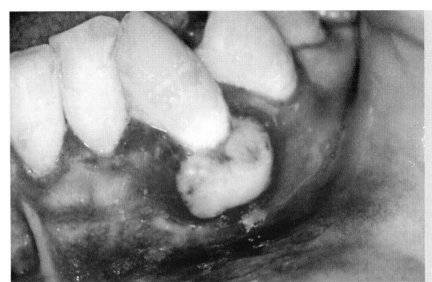

Fig. 15.16 Cytomegalovirus infection. Atypical ulcer of the gingiva.

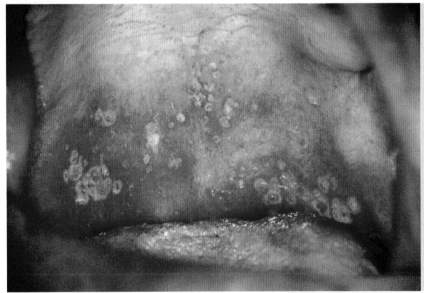

Fig. 15.17 Herpangina. Numerous vesicles and shallow ulcers on the soft palate.

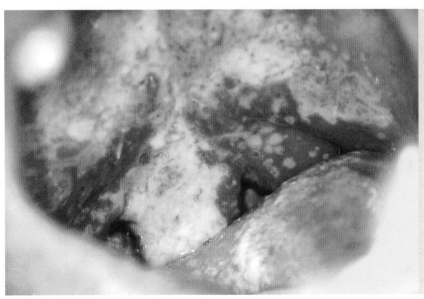

Fig. 15.18 Herpangina. Numerous shallow ulcers on the soft palate and uvula.

Pathology

Diagnostic investigations are rarely warranted. Histologic examination reveals intraepithelial vesicle formation with intracellular edema and spongiosis. Epithelial necrosis and ulceration follows the vesicles' rupture. Serology for antibody titers, PCR assay, and viral culture for the isolation of the virus are useful diagnostic tests particularly in questionable cases.

Treatment

It is symptomatic. In most cases, the disease resolves spontaneously without complications.

Hand-Foot-and-Mouth Disease

Key points

- It is caused by Coxsackie enteroviruses, mainly type A16.
- The disease may occur in epidemics or isolated cases.
- Clinical presentation and sites of involvement are typical.

Introduction

Hand-foot-and-mouth disease is an acute infection caused by various types of Coxsackie virus, mainly A16 and, less often, A5, A9, and A10. It usually affects children and young adults. The disease may occur in *epidemics* or *isolated cases.*

Clinical features

Clinically, small vesicles appear on the oral mucosa, 5 to 30 in number, that soon rupture, leaving slightly painful, shallow ulcers (2–6 mm in diameter), surrounded by a red halo (**Fig. 15.19**). Any site on the oral mucosa may be involved, except the gingiva. The skin lesions consist of small, turbid vesicles, 1 to 50 in number, surrounded by a narrow red halo and are localized on the lateral and dorsal aspects of the fingers, toes, palms, and soles (**Fig. 15.20**). However, lesions may appear on the buttocks, knees, and extremities (**Fig. 15.21**). The course is usually mild. Low-grade fever and general symptoms may be present. The disease lasts 5 to 8 days and resolves spontaneously without treatment. The diagnosis is based on clinical criteria.

Differential diagnosis

- Herpangina
- Herpetiform aphthous ulcers
- Minor aphthous ulcers
- Secondary herpetic stomatitis

Pathology

This is usually not necessary. Viral isolation from culture of skin lesions and PCR assay are useful laboratory diagnostic tests in doubtful cases.

Treatment

This is symptomatic.

Acute Lymphonodular Pharyngitis

Key points

- The disease is caused by Coxsackie virus, A10.
- Frequently affects children and young adults.
- Lesions characteristically develop on the soft palate, uvula, and tonsillar pillars.
- Multiple, raised, discrete papules are the prominent clinical features.

Introduction

Lymphonodular pharyngitis is an uncommon acute febrile disease caused by Coxsackie virus, A10, with characteristic location.

Clinical features

The disease frequently affects children and young adults. Clinically, acute lymphonodular pharyngitis presents with fever, ranging from 38 to 41°C, mild headache, loss of appetite, and sore throat, followed, after 2 to 3 days, by a characteristic nonvesicular eruption on the uvula, soft palate, anterior tonsillar

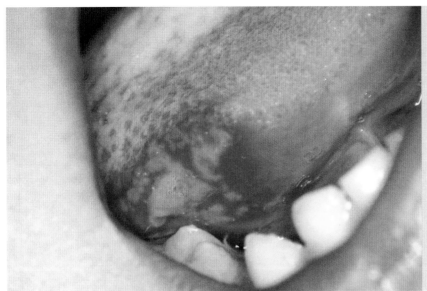

Fig. 15.19 Hand-foot-and-mouth disease. Shallow ulcers on the lateral margin of the tongue.

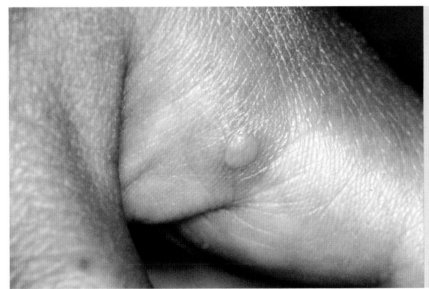

Fig. 15.20 Hand-foot-and-mouth disease. A small vesicle on the finger.

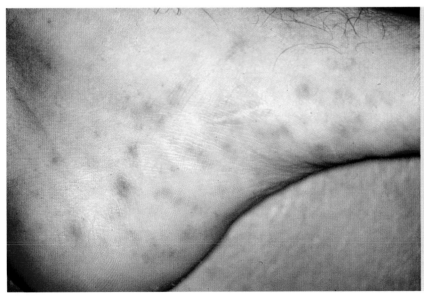

Fig. 15.21 Hand-foot-and-mouth disease. Multiple vesicles on the sole and the lateral aspect of the foot.

pillars, and posterior pharynx (**Fig. 15.22**). The lesions consist of multiple, raised, discrete papules, whitish to yellowish in color surrounded by an erythematous halo. The size of the lesions varies from 3 to 6 mm in diameter. They last 4 to 8 days. The papules represent hyperplastic lymphoid aggregates. The diagnosis is based on the history and the clinical features.

Differential diagnosis

- Herpangina
- Herpes simplex
- Herpetiform aphthous ulcers
- Other viral infections

Pathology

This is usually not required. The isolation of the virus, serologic examination, and PCR assay may be used in doubtful cases.

Treatment

This is symptomatic as the disease is self-limited.

Measles

Key points

- An acute, contagious infection of childhood, caused by a *Paramyxovirus*, genus *Morbillivirus*.
- Most cases develop during winter.
- It is spread through respiratory droplets.
- Koplik's spots are the more characteristic oral lesion, on the buccal mucosa.
- The diagnosis is based on the history and the clinical features.

Introduction

Measles is an acute, contagious infection of childhood, caused by a specific *Paramyxovirus*, genus *Morbillivirus*. The disease is more common during winter and is transferred by respiratory droplets. Measles vaccine has been widely used in many continents, resulting in dramatic restriction of the prevalence and rate of infection.

Clinical features

Clinically, after an incubation period of 8 to 12 days, the patient presents with fever, malaise, chills, cough, and conjunctivitis. Three to four days later a characteristic maculopapular

rash appears behind the ears and on the forehead, and spreads within 24 hours to the rest of the face, the neck, the trunk, and the extremities (**Fig. 15.23**). The rash starts fading from the 6th to 10th day onward. Characteristic bluish-white specks with bright red areolae (*Koplik's spots*) may appear on the buccal mucosa at the level of the first and second molars, 1 to 2 days before the onset of the rash. A diffuse erythema, petechiae and, rarely, small round erosions on the oral mucosa may also be observed (**Figs. 15.24, 15.25**). Complications such as encephalitis, otitis media, pneumonia, and enteritis are rare. The diagnosis is based on clinical criteria.

Differential diagnosis

- Acute candidiasis
- Minor aphthous ulcers
- Herpetic lesions
- Infectious mononucleosis
- Varicella

Pathology

Serologic tests are useful in the diagnosis of atypical cases.

Treatment

It is symptomatic. Bed rest during the febrile period, fluids and antipyretics are recommended. Routine prophylactic vaccination against measles is recommended for all children between 12 and 16 months.

Mumps

Key points

- Acute viral infection, commonly of childhood.
- It is caused by a *Paramyxovirus*, genus *Rubulavirus*.
- The virus is transmitted through respiratory droplets, saliva, and urine.
- The parotid gland is most frequently involved.
- Vaccination protects from infection.

Introduction

Mumps or epidemic parotitis is an acute viral infection, most commonly of childhood, caused by a *Paramyxovirus*, genus *Rubulavirus*. The virus can be transmitted through respiratory droplets, saliva, and urine. The parotid gland is more frequently affected, followed by the submandibular and sublingual salivary glands.

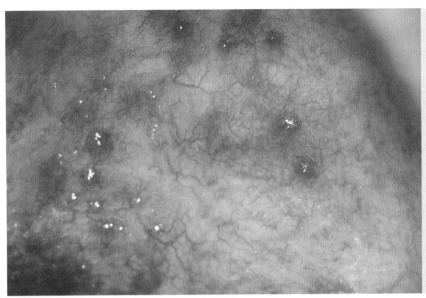

Fig. 15.22 Acute lymphonodular pharyngitis, multiple lesions on the soft palate.

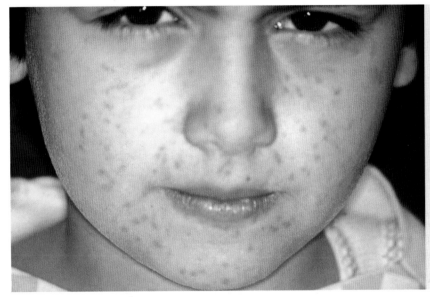

Fig. 15.23 Measles, typical maculopapular lesions on the face.

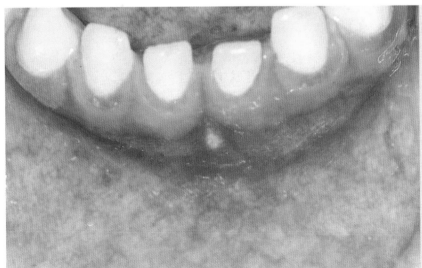

Fig. 15.24 Measles, small erosion on the labial sulcus.

Clinical features

Clinically, after an incubation period of 14 to 21 days, variable fever, chills, headache, loss of appetite, malaise, and myalgia are the symptoms experienced, followed by pain in the parotid area. Tender, rubbery swellings, usually of one, or rarely both, of the parotids, are the presenting signs that last for approximately 7 days (**Fig. 15.26**). Characteristically, the salivary gland duct orifices *Stensen's* and *Wharton's* are swollen and red. Movements of the mandible and saliva stimulating foods increase the pain from the parotids. Epididymitis, orchitis, meningoencephalitis, and pancreatitis are the most common, albeit rare, complications. The diagnosis is based on the history and the clinical features.

Differential diagnosis

- Acute suppurative parotitis
- Calculi in the salivary glands
- Buccal cellulitis
- Angioedema
- Sjögren's syndrome
- Mikulicz's syndrome
- Heerfordt's syndrome
- Salivary gland neoplasms
- Lymph node enlargement

Pathology

Usually, it is not required. However, the diagnosis can be confirmed by serologic examination and isolation of the virus from saliva. Elevated serum amylase and relative lymphocytosis may be present.

Treatment

This is symptomatic. Bed rest during the febrile period, analgesics, and antipyretics are the suggested measures. Vaccination for children of 12 to 16 months is the best preventive measure.

Molluscum Contagiosum

Key points

- A poxvirus-induced benign skin lesion.
- It is usually transmitted via sexual contact and less often from contaminated clothing, bath, and swimming water.
- An increased prevalence of molluscum contagiosum has been observed in HIV-infected patients.
- The most common skin areas involved are the head, eyelids, trunk, and genitalia.
- Oral involvement is extremely rare.

Introduction

Molluscum contagiosum is a benign lesion usually seen on the skin and caused by a poxvirus. The virus is transmitted via sexual contact and contaminated clothes, baths, and swimming pools. The lesions may develop at any age, but most cases are found in children and young adults. Males are affected more frequently than females. An increased incidence of molluscum contagiosum has been observed in patients with HIV infection.

Clinical features

Clinically, the lesions are characterized by grouped, minute (usually 3–6 mm), dome-shaped, sessile, papules, often with central umbilication. Small amounts of whitish fluid may exude on pressure from these lesions. Any skin region may be involved, but the head, eyelids, trunk, and genitalia are most often affected (**Fig. 15.27**). In AIDS patients, the lesions may be large with a verrucous surface. Molluscum contagiosum is extremely rare in the oral cavity. The clinical picture of oral lesions is similar to that of skin lesions and is characterized by multiple small hemispheric reddish papules with a central

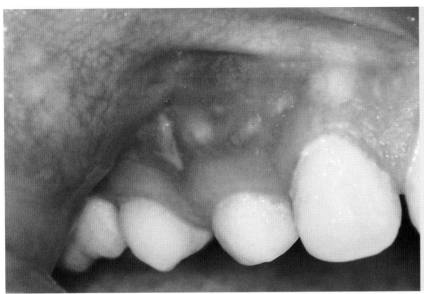

Fig. 15.25 Measles, multiple erosions on the alveolar mucosa.

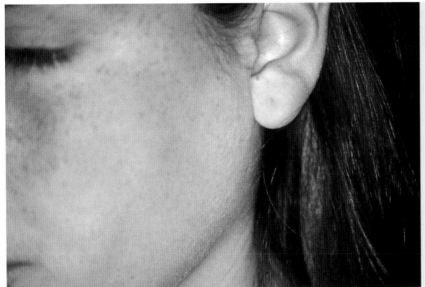

Fig. 15.26 Mumps, swelling of the left parotid.

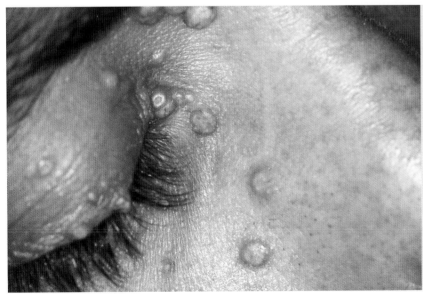

Fig. 15.27 Molluscum contagiosum, multiple typical lesions on the skin.

umbilication (**Fig. 15.28**). The buccal mucosa, labial mucosa, and palate are the sites of involvement in the reported cases. The diagnosis is based on the clinical features.

Differential diagnosis

- Lymphangioma
- Hemangioma
- Pyogenic granuloma
- Condyloma acuminatum

Pathology

Histopathologic examination establishes the final diagnosis. Microscopically, areas of enlarged epidermal cells, which contain multiple intracytoplasmic inclusion bodies (*molluscum bodies* or *Henderson-Paterson bodies*) are seen. The dermis shows little or no inflammatory infiltration.

Treatment

Conservative surgical excision or cryotherapy are the preferred treatment modalities of the oral lesions. Sharp curettage, liquid nitrogen or topical keratolytics, imiquimod, and laser for the skin lesions are suggested.

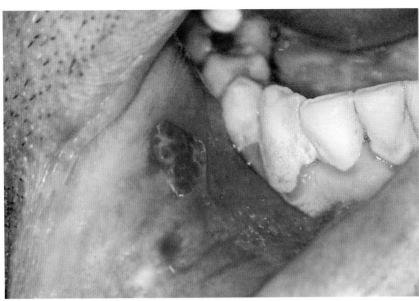

Fig. 15.28 Molluscum contagiosum, multiple lesions on the labial mucosa.

16 Oral Manifestations of HIV Infection

Key points

- The most important epidemic of the late 20th and the early 21st century.
- Human immunodeficiency virus (HIV) is the cause.
- Various oral lesions may occur at any stage of the infection; however, these lesions are indicative and not specific for HIV disease.
- Alarming oral clinical manifestations suggestive of HIV infection are oral hairy leukoplakia (OHL), necrotizing ulcerative gingivitis, necrotizing ulcerative periodontitis, and severe herpes zoster in young patients.
- The current therapeutic protocol of combination antiretroviral therapy (cART) has effectively reduced the oral and cutaneous manifestations of HIV infection.
- The clinical manifestations depend on the CD4+ T-lymphocyte count and the viral load of HIV.
- Some HIV-related infections may become apparent or worsen when the immune status improves during the cART therapy, such as herpes zoster, condyloma acuminatum—cytomegalovirus (CMV), *Mycobacterium avium*, a phenomenon termed *immune reconstitution syndrome*.
- cART prolongs the overall survival of patients; hence, HIV infection may not be a lethal but rather a chronic infection.

Introduction

Since the onset of HIV infection in the 1980s, oral lesions have been recorded during all stages of the infection. HIV infection is a disease caused by the HIV. It is transmitted through sexual contact, through blood or blood products and during labor, or from the mother to the fetus. The main target of the virus is CD4+ T lymphocytes. Their depletion results in immune deficiency. HIV infection is still considered a pandemic. Since the beginning of the epidemic, 71 million people have been infected with HIV virus and approximately 34 million have died.

The clinical spectrum of HIV infection is extremely broad, ranging from full-blown AIDS to clinically healthy individuals who carry HIV antigens or antibodies. Between these two extremes are patients who exhibit various clinical and laboratory manifestations of HIV infection. In 1993, the Centers for Disease Control and Prevention (CDC) suggested a revised classification system for HIV infection for adolescents and adults. Patients were categorized on the basis of clinical conditions associated with HIV infection and CD4+ T-lymphocyte counts. The main high-risk group for HIV infection remains, in most areas, homosexual and bisexual men (50–60%), but also injection drug users and heterosexual contacts of high-risk individuals. Since the disease was first recognized in the 1980s, remarkable progress has been made in improving the quality and duration of life of HIV-infected people.

The oral and perioral manifestations are mainly the result of cellular immunodeficiency induced by HIV infection and may be divided into five major groups: *infections, neoplasms, neurologic disturbances, drug-induced lesions*, and *lesions of unknown cause*.

In 1993, the EC-Clearinghouse[1] of oral problems related to HIV infection and World Health Organization (WHO) Collaborating Center on Oral Manifestations of the Immunodeficiency Virus classified the oral lesions, according to relevance to HIV infection, in three major groups: Group 1—*strongly associated lesions*, Group 2—*less commonly associated lesions*, and Group 3—*rarely associated lesions* (**Table 16.1**).

These oral lesions may represent early or late manifestations of the disease. A strong correlation exists between viral load and HIV-related oral lesions.

In the last two decades, the management of HIV disease has undergone major changes with the introduction of cART. This therapy works by decreasing the viral load, hence lessening any fall in CD4+ T-lymphocyte numbers. cART has been so effective in the management of HIV infection that the history of HIV/AIDS can be considered as pre- and post-cART periods. The latest clinical observations show a dramatic decrease in the prevalence of oral lesions in the era of cART therapy, compared with the earlier period. In addition, the laboratory tests for the viral load count and specific T4-cell count are currently very reliable indicators for the disease's control and therapeutic decisions. A disadvantage of cART is the development or worsening of certain HIV-related infections (such as herpes zoster, condyloma acuminatum, *M. avium intracellulare*) during the phase of immune reconstitution. Some of the oral lesions and diseases may also be present in non-HIV patients; hence, they are only considered indicative (markers) of possible HIV infection and should be evaluated in correlation with the medical history and other clinical and laboratory findings, particularly in cases where the HIV status is unknown.

---

[1] In the group participated: T. Axell, A.M. Azul, S. Challacombe, G. Ficarra, S. Flint, D. Greenspan, C. Hammerle, G. Laskaris, I. Loeb, M. Lucas-Tomas, P.A. Monteil, J.J. Pindborg, P. Reichart, P. Robinson, C. Scully, P. Swango, S. Syrjanen, M.H. Thornhill, I. van der Waal, D.M. Williams and D. Wray

Table 16.1 EC-Clearinghouse classification of oral manifestations of HIV infection

Group 1 Strongly associated lesions	Group 2 Less commonly associated lesions
Candidiasis • Erythematosus • Pseudo-membranous Hairy leukoplakia Linear gingival erythema Necrotizing ulcerative gingivitis Necrotizing ulcerative periodontitis Kaposi's sarcoma Non-Hodgkin's lymphoma	Bacterial infections • *Mycobacterium avium intracellulare* • *Mycobacterium tuberculosis* Melanosis Noma Salivary gland disorders • Xerostomia • Salivary gland swelling Thrombocytopenic purpura Nonspecific ulcerations Viral infections • Herpes simplex • Herpes zoster Chickenpox • Condyloma acuminatum • Verruca vulgaris • Focal epithelial hyperplasia

Group 3
Rarely associated lesions

Bacterial infections

• *Actinomyces israelii*
• *Escherichia coli*
• *Klebsiella pneumoniae*
• Bacillary angiomatosis

Drug-induced lesions (ulcers, lichenoid reactions, erythema multiforme, Stevens-Johnson syndrome, Lyell's syndrome)

Fungal infections

• *Cryptococcus neoformans*
• *Geotrichum Candidum*
• Histoplasmosis
• Mucormycosis
• *Aspergillus flavus, fumigatus*

Neurologic disorders

• Bell's palsy
• Trigeminal neuralgia

Viral infections

• Cytomegalovirus (CMV)
• Molluscum contagiosum

Recurrent aphthous stomatitis

Bacterial Infections

The three most common infections are linear gingival erythema, necrotizing ulcerative gingivitis, and necrotizing ulcerative periodontitis.

a. *Linear gingival erythema* in the pre-cART era was identified in 5 to 10% of patients, while nowadays seems to be very rare. Clinically, linear gingival erythema is characterized by a fiery red band along the margin of the gingiva. The lesion does not respond to plaque control measures or root planning and scaling. Gingival bleeding may occur spontaneously or on probing (**Fig. 16.1**). The lesions are often infected with *Candida albicans.*

Differential diagnosis

- Dental plaque-related gingivitis
- Plasma cell gingivitis

Treatment

High level of oral hygiene, scaling, polishing of teeth and possibly antifungal drugs.

b. *Necrotizing ulcerative gingivitis* used to be common (5–16%) and was classified as a highly suspicious lesion for HIV infection. Today its frequency is much lower. The clinical presentation is similar to non-HIV–infected patients (**Figs. 16.2, 16.3**). Sometimes the ulceration exceeds the attached gingival margins and oral mucosa and is then considered necrotizing ulcerative stomatitis.

c. *Necrotizing ulcerative periodontitis* is a late manifestation of HIV and used to be recorded in 5 to 17% of patients. Clinically, necrotizing ulcerative periodontitis is characterized by soft tissue ulceration and necrosis and rapid destruction of the periodontal attachment apparatus, which results in tooth loss (**Fig. 16.4**). Spontaneous bleeding and severe deep pain are common. The condition does not respond to conventional periodontal treatment. HIV-associated periodontitis is usually localized, although severe cases may be generalized.

Differential diagnosis

- Agranulocytosis
- Aplastic anemia
- Leukemia
- Aggressive periodontitis

Treatment

Local conservative treatment for periodontitis, topical antiseptic mouthwashes, systemic metronidazole, and oral hygiene instructions for maintenance of the therapeutic results are recommended.

Other infections: Other rare bacterial infections causing oral lesions are bacillary angiomatosis, ulceration due to common bacterial infection (**Fig. 16.5**), and more rare other bacterial infections from bacteria such as *M avium intracellulare, Enterobacter cloacae, Klebsiella pneumoniae, Pseudomonas aeruginosa* (**Fig. 16.6**). In addition, tuberculosis and syphilis may coexist with HIV infection (**Figs. 16.7, 16.8**).

Viral Infections

Oral viral infections are common in HIV-infected individuals. They may present in any stage of the disease. The cART treatment has significantly reduced the frequency of oral viral infections.

a. OHL was previously considered to be a reliable clinical sign that the patient is HIV-infected, but it must be reported that OHL can occur in other immunocompromised patients (e.g., drug-induced immunosuppression). During the pre-cART era, the frequency of OHL was 20 to 30%, while currently it is significantly lower. In HIV, the lesion is observed in patients with a CD4 count less than 500 cells/mm^3. Epstein-Barr virus is the cause of OHL. Clinically, OHL presents as an asymptomatic, whitish, slightly elevated, nonremovable lesion of the tongue, often bilaterally. Characteristically, the surface of the lesion is corrugated with a vertical orientation, but flat and smooth lesions may also be seen (**Figs. 16.9, 16.10**). The lesions may extend to the ventral and dorsal aspects of the tongue. Other sites are very rarely affected. The lesion can be superinfected with *C. albicans*. OHL is not a precancerous lesion.

Differential diagnosis

- Candidiasis
- Chronic tongue biting
- Leukoplakia
- Leukoedema
- Cinnamon contact stomatitis
- Oral lichen planus
- Discoid lupus erythematosus
- Geographic tongue
- Oral psoriasis
- White sponge nevus
- Uremic stomatitis

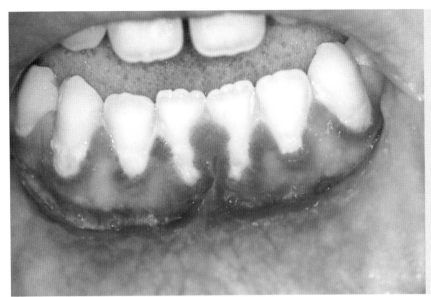

Fig. 16.1 Linear gingival erythema.

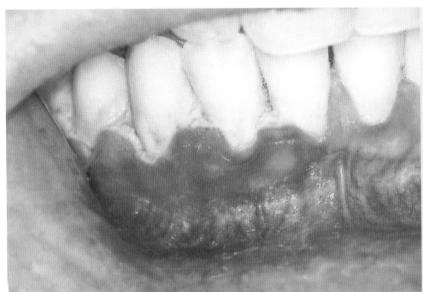

Fig. 16.2 Necrotizing ulcerative gingivitis, mild lesions.

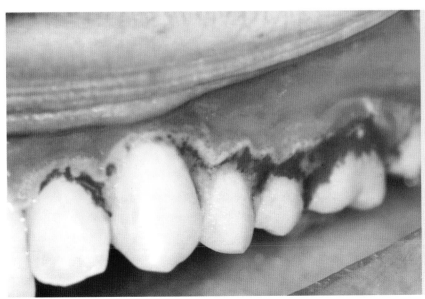

Fig. 16.3 Necrotizing ulcerative gingivitis, severe lesions.

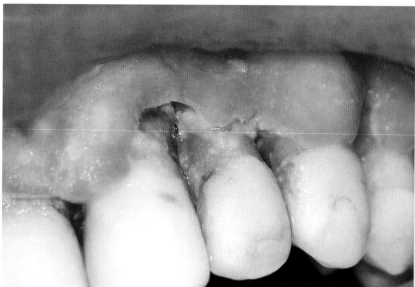

Fig. 16.4 Necrotizing ulcerative periodontitis.

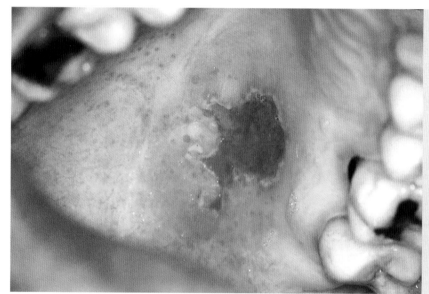

Fig. 16.5 Palatal ulceration due to viridans streptococci.

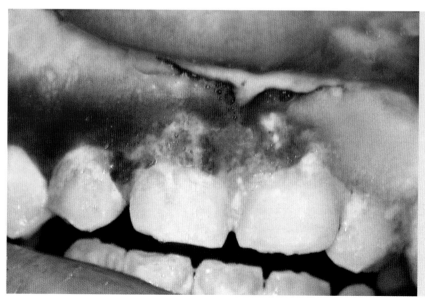

Fig. 16.6 Gingival necrosis due to *Pseudomonas aeruginosa*.

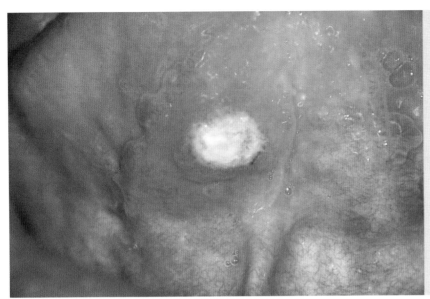

Fig. 16.7 Syphilitic ulceration.

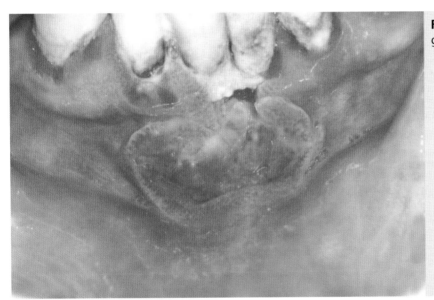

Fig. 16.8 Tuberculous ulcer on the gingiva and sulcus.

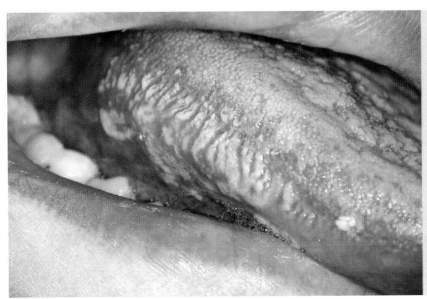

Fig. 16.9 Marked hairy leukoplakia.

Pathology

Microscopically, the epithelium exhibits acanthosis with balloon cells in the upper part of the epithelium and parakeratosis, while dysplasia is absent. Demonstration of Epstein-Barr virus (e.g., by in situ hybridization) confirms the diagnosis.

Treatment

Usually is not warranted, although regression with acyclovir, valacyclovir, or ganciclovir can occur. OHL usually regresses during the cART therapy.

b. *Other viral infections*: Herpes simplex, in severe HIV disease, is very common (**Fig. 16.11**) while herpes zoster and herpangina are less common. Some rare cases of CMV ulceration have also been reported (**Fig. 16.12**), which are clinically atypical and require identification of the virus to be diagnosed. Human papilloma virus (HPV) infections are common in the oral mucosa and may present as condyloma acuminatum, verruca vulgaris, and focal epithelial hyperplasia. Perioral molluscum contagiosum may also occur.

Fungal Infections

Fungal infections are common in patients with HIV infection. Candidiasis is the most common while more rarely systemic mycoses may develop.

a. *Candidiasis*: Oral candidiasis is common in HIV patients and is reported in 70 to 95% of patients not receiving cART. The clinical features of oral candidiasis in HIV patients include extensive appearance of the lesions, frequent recurrences, and resistance to treatment. Moreover, apart from *C. albicans*, other species such as *Candida krusei*, *Candida glabrata*, *Candida tropicalis*, and *Candida parapsilosis* have been identified in oral candidiasis in HIV patients.

The most common clinical types of oral candidiasis are pseudomembranous (**Fig. 16.13**) and erythematous (**Fig. 16.14**). The treatment consists of long-term administration of azoles (i.e., fluconazole, itraconazole) or even amphotericin B.

b. *Systemic fungal infections*: There is a higher incidence of histoplasmosis, cryptococcosis, mucormycosis, geotrichosis, and aspergillosis among HIV patients. These infections usually appear later in the disease when the CD4+ T-cell count is below 100 cells/mm³.

Neoplasms

The development of neoplasia is among the serious complications of HIV disease. Common HIV-related neoplasms of the oral cavity are Kaposi's sarcoma and Non-Hodgkin's lymphoma (NHL).

a. *Kaposi's sarcoma*: Four types of Kaposi's sarcoma have been described: (a) *classic*, (b) *endemic or African*, (c) *iatrogenic*, and (d) *epidemic or AIDS-Kaposi*. The AIDS-Kaposi is the most common, usually diagnosed in homosexual HIV-infected patients. It has been diagnosed in 15 to 20% of HIV patients. The lesions of the skin are more common (**Fig. 16.15**), while 50 to 60% of such patients also have oral lesions. Rarely, Kaposi's sarcoma affects only the oral mucosa. Human herpes virus 8 (HHV-8) is the causative agent of Kaposi's sarcoma. Since the introduction of cART, a marked decrease was reported in the incidence of Kaposi's sarcoma (3–5%). Clinically, in early stages the lesions present as asymptomatic macules, flat plaques, or red papules (**Fig. 16.16**). The lesions grow slowly and form tumor-like masses. A characteristic clinical sign is the deep red color of the lesions. They are usually multiple and painless. The palate and gingiva are the most commonly affected sites and less commonly the buccal mucosa, tongue, floor of the mouth, and the lips. Simultaneously, lesions may exist on the eye (**Fig. 16.17**).

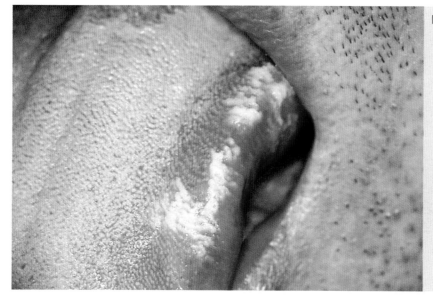

Fig. 16.10 Oral hairy leukoplakia.

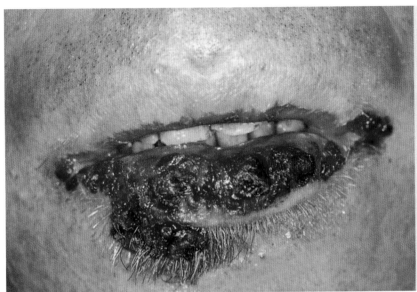

Fig. 16.11 Severe lesions of herpes labialis.

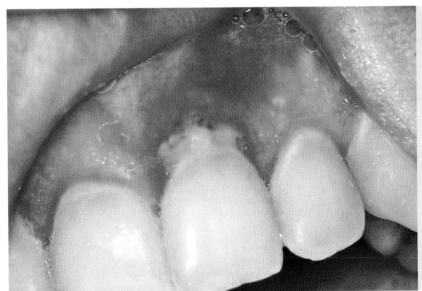

Fig. 16.12 Intense erythema and ulceration due to cytomegalovirus (CMV).

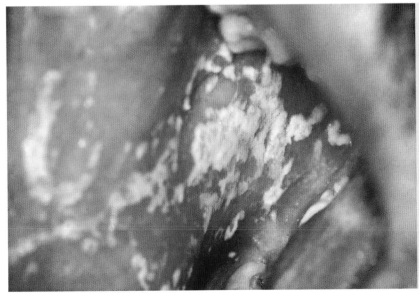

Fig. 16.13 Pseudomembranous candidiasis on the buccal mucosa.

Differential diagnosis

- Bacillary angiomatosis
- Pyogenic granuloma
- Peripheral giant cell granuloma
- Angiosarcoma
- Hemangioma and other vascular tumors

Pathology

Biopsy and histologic examination (see p. 596).

Treatment

Therapy is typically based on radiotherapy and/or chemotherapy, although previously suggested (and not commonly used) approaches include intralesional interferon, laser excision, and surgical removal (see p. 598).

b. NHL is the second most common neoplasm of the oral cavity in HIV patients. After the introduction of highly active antiretroviral therapy (HAART), NHL's frequency significantly fell. The NHL is usually of B-cell origin and rarely of T cell. Clinically, it appears as a lump or inflammatory enlargement with or without ulceration. Common sites are the posterior gingiva, soft palate, posterior tongue, and rarely the perioral area (**Fig. 16.18**). Cases of oral Burkitt's lymphoma have been reported (**Fig. 16.19**). Finally, very rarely, intraoral Hodgkin's disease has been described in HIV disease (**Fig. 16.20**).

Iatrogenic Lesions

Drug-induced iatrogenic lesions are common among HIV patients. **Table 16.2** summarizes the most common cART-induced lesions affecting the oral and perioral area. The frequency of these lesions is not precise. The ones most commonly seen are drug-induced stomatitis, erythema multiforme, Stevens-Johnson syndrome, Lyell's syndrome, ulcers (**Fig. 16.21**), and neutropenia (**Fig. 16.22**). Moreover, melanotic pigmentation of the oral mucosa and lichenoid lesions may also develop. Finally, facial lipodystrophy, a characteristic skin lesion, is a possible complication (**Fig. 16.23**).

Neurologic Disorders

Neurologic disorders of the oral cavity are very rare. Bell's palsy and trigeminal neuropathy are the ones that usually manifest at the late stages of the disease.

Lesions of Unknown Etiology

This group comprises of several atypical lesions with unclear etiology. The most common lesions are aphthous ulcers (**Figs. 16.24, 16.25**), ulcers of unknown etiology (**Figs. 16.26, 16.27**), salivary gland lesions (**Fig. 16.28**), exfoliative cheilitis, desquamation of the lingual papillae, hairy tongue, thrombocytopenic purpura (**Fig. 16.29**), and Reiter's syndrome. Furthermore, unusual lesions such as eyelid elongation (**Fig. 16.30**), leukonychia (**Fig. 16.31**), and finger clubbing (**Fig. 16.32**) have been described.

From the wide range of lesions of the oral cavity, those that are closely related to HIV infection are candidiasis, OHL, linear gingival erythema, necrotizing ulcerative periodontitis, Kaposi's sarcoma, and NHL.

However, it should be recalled that because of the advent of cART, oral HIV-related lesions have decreased significantly and are less severe than the past.

Table 16.2 Adverse oral reactions to antiretroviral therapy drugs

Drugs	Oral and facial adverse reactions
I. Nucleoside reverse transcriptase inhibitors (NRTIs)	
• Didanosine (Videx)	Xerostomia
• Stavudine (Zerit)	Lipodystrophy
• Zidovudine (Retrovir)	Lipodystrophy
• Zalcitabine (Hivid)	Lipodystrophy, ulcers, melanosis, CMV infection Ulcers
II. Nonnucleoside reverse transcriptase inhibitors (NNRTIs)	
• Delavirdine (Rescriptor) and Efavirenz (Sustiva)	Stevens-Johnson syndrome, toxic epidermal necrolysis
III. Protease inhibitors	
• Amprenavir (Agenerase)	Glossodynia, metallic taste
• Fosamprenavir	Exfoliative cheilitis
• Ritonavir (Norvir)	Lipodystrophy

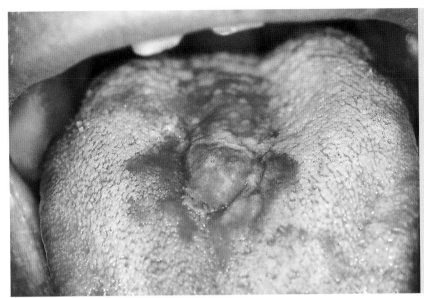

Fig. 16.14 Erythematous candidiasis on the dorsum of the tongue.

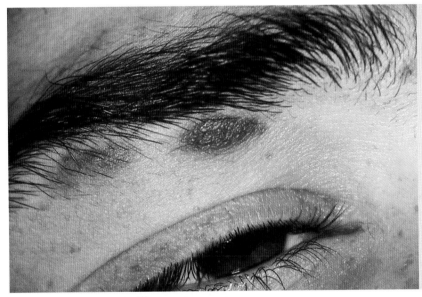

Fig. 16.15 Kaposi's sarcoma, two melanotic plaques on the skin.

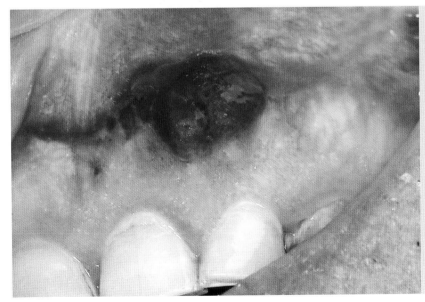

Fig. 16.16 Kaposi's sarcoma on the maxillary sulcus.

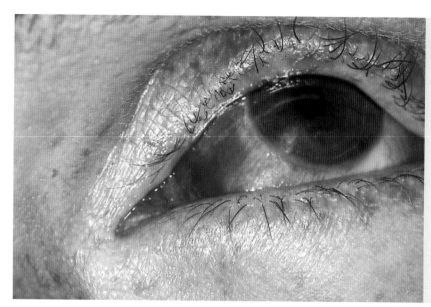

Fig. 16.17 Kaposi's sarcoma of the eye.

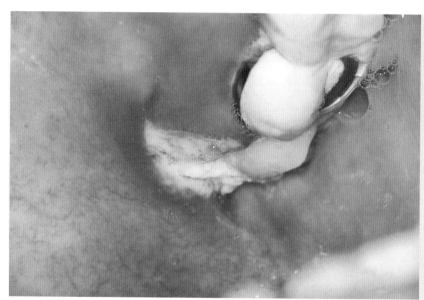

Fig. 16.18 Non-Hodgkin's lymphoma, ulceration on the posterior gingiva.

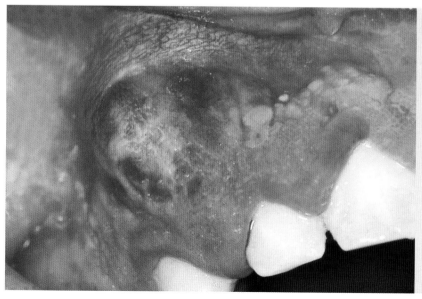

Fig. 16.19 Burkitt's lymphoma in the sulcus.

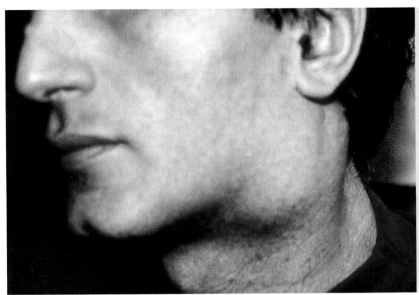

Fig. 16.20 Hodgkin's disease, enlarged submandibular lymph nodes.

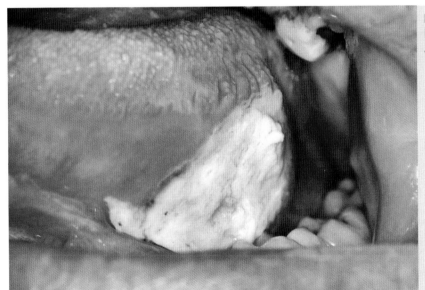

Fig. 16.21 Large ulcer on the left border of the tongue due to azidothymidine.

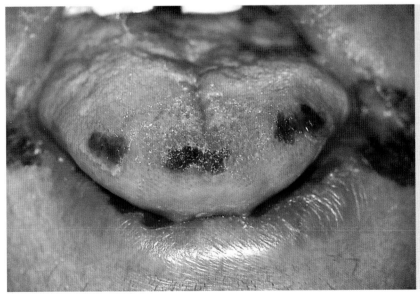

Fig. 16.22 Ulceration of the tongue due to chemotherapy.

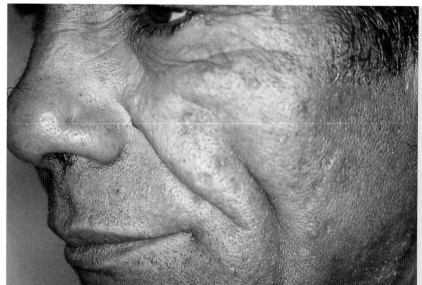

Fig. 16.23 Facial lipodystrophy due to ritonavir.

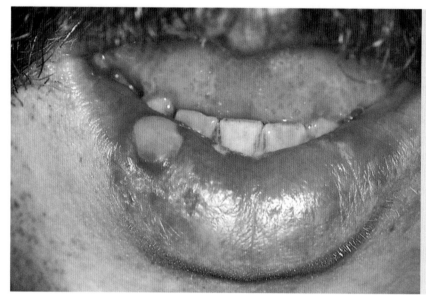

Fig. 16.24 Aphthous ulcers on the lower lip.

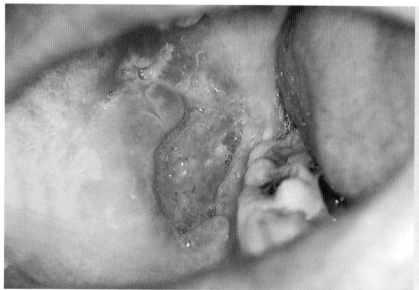

Fig. 16.25 Major aphthous ulcer on the buccal mucosa.

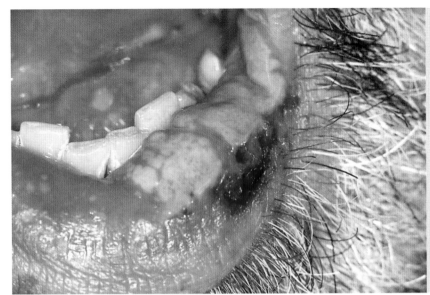

Fig. 16.26 Multiple atypical ulcers on the lower lip and the floor of the mouth.

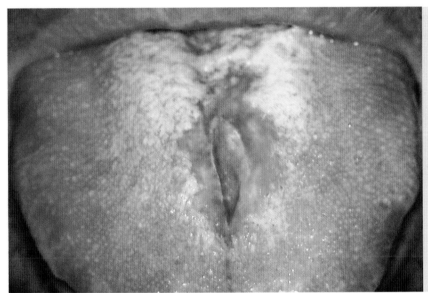

Fig. 16.27 Atypical ulceration on the dorsum of the tongue.

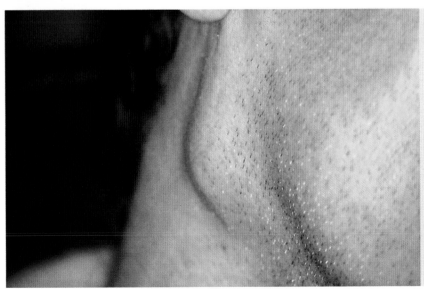

Fig. 16.28 Cystic enlargement of the parotid.

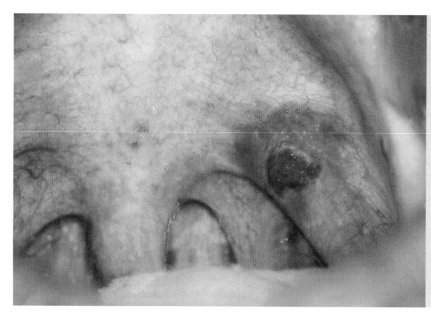

Fig 16.29 Thrombocytopenic purpura and petechiae on the soft palate.

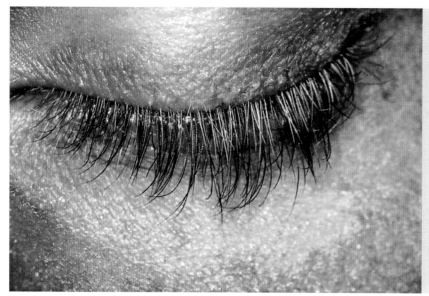

Fig. 16.30 Eyelids, elongation.

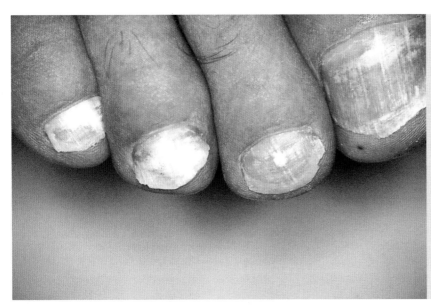

Fig. 16.31 Leukonychia.

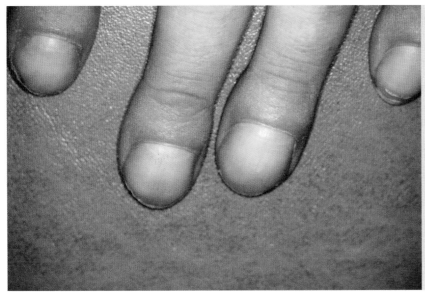

Fig. 16.32 Finger clubbing.

17 Bacterial Infections

Necrotizing Ulcerative Stomatitis

Key points

- A rare complication of necrotizing ulcerative gingivitis.
- *Fusiform bacillus*, *Borrelia vincentii*, and other anaerobic microorganisms are the most common associated bacteria.
- It is more common in immunocompromised individuals and HIV-infected people.

Introduction

Necrotizing ulcerative gingivitis may on occasion extend beyond the gingiva and involve other areas of the oral mucosa. In such cases, the term necrotizing ulcerative stomatitis is used. Rarely, the disease may occur in the absence of ulcerative gingivitis.

Clinical features

Clinically, the oral mucosa is red, ulcerated, with ulcers with irregular margins, and may be covered with a dirty, white-grayish smear (**Figs. 17.1, 17.2**). In these cases, the subjective complaints and objective general phenomena associated with ulcerative gingivitis may be more intense. The buccal mucosa, opposite the third molar, is the most commonly affected area. Rarely, it may involve the tongue, lips, and palate. The onset of the disease can be sudden or insidious. Necrotizing ulcerative stomatitis can be a manifestation of HIV infection, but rarely appears in non–HIV-infected patients. The presence of gingival lesions is of diagnostic significance (**Fig. 17.3**). The diagnosis is based on the history and the clinical features.

Differential diagnosis

- Agranulocytosis
- Neutropenia
- Leukemia
- Major aphthae
- Wegener's granulomatosis
- Langerhans cell histiocytosis
- Syphilis, second stage
- Tuberculosis
- Noma
- Scurvy

Pathology

Laboratory tests are not recommended. Relevant tests should be applied only if it is necessary to exclude other diseases.

Treatment

In addition to debridement of local deposits, systemic metronidazole 500 mg every 8 hours, for 6 to 7 days is the most common therapeutic scheme. Other antibiotics can be used. Mouthwashes with oxygen-producing elements are also helpful. If the patients do not respond to antibiotics, an underlying systemic disease should be suspected and investigated.

Cancrum Oris

Key points

- A multifactorial, rare, rapidly progressive disease.
- Spirochete and anaerobic infection together with local and systemic predisposing factors are the cause.
- Gangrenous necrosis is the presenting clinical feature.
- Occasionally, the lesions may perforate the facial skin and jaw bones.

Introduction

Cancrum oris or noma is a rare, rapidly progressive, and severely destructive disease, usually involving the oral tissues. It more commonly affects children and rarely adults, particularly in socioeconomically deprived areas of Africa, Asia, and South America. It is extremely rare in Europe and North America. *Fusospirochetal microorganisms*, *Staphylococcus aureus*, *Streptococcus species*, and *Pseudomonas aeruginosa* are almost always present in the lesions. Predisposing factors may be local or systemic and include poor oral hygiene, severe protein malnutrition, systemic infections and parasitic diseases, diabetes mellitus, leukemia, HIV infection and AIDS, malignancies, and immune defects.

Clinical features

Clinically, cancrum oris frequently begins as acute necrotizing ulcerative gingivitis that quickly spreads to the neighboring oral tissues. Gangrenous necrosis involves the buccal mucosa, lips, and the underlying bone, producing catastrophic lesions

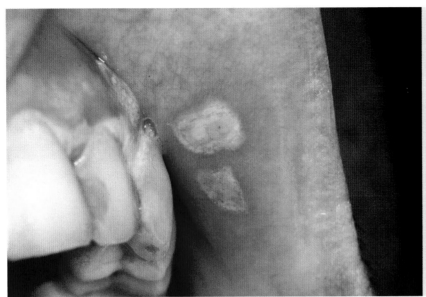

Fig. 17.1 Acute necrotizing ulcerative stomatitis, ulcerations in buccal mucosa.

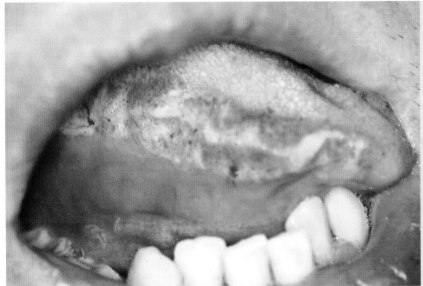

Fig. 17.2 Acute necrotizing ulcerative stomatitis, ulcerations on the lateral borders of the tongue.

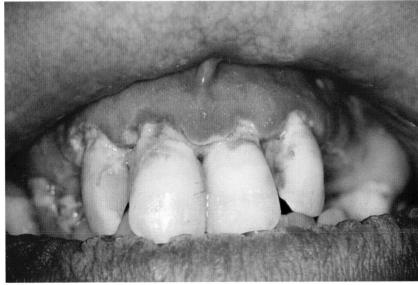

Fig. 17.3 Acute necrotizing ulcerative gingivitis on the upper gingiva. The same patient as in **Fig. 17.2**.

of the face (**Figs. 17.4, 17.5**). The gangrenous ulcers have an irregular border and are covered with whitish-brown fibrin and debris. Hypersalivation, halitosis, malaise, fever, and regional lymphadenopathy are always present. The diagnosis is usually based on clinical criteria.

Differential diagnosis
- Malignant granuloma
- Burkitt's lymphoma
- Malignant tumors
- Leukemia
- Agranulocytosis
- Systemic fungal infections
- Tuberculosis
- Late syphilis

Pathology

Microbiological culture of exudates may be necessary to determine the choice of antibiotics in resistant cases.

Treatment

Without treatment, the disease is frequently fatal. Antibiotics, e.g., high-dose penicillin IV (10–20 MIU daily) and metronidazole 2 to 3 g/d are the medications of choice. Hydration and a nutritious diet as soon as possible are important. Surgical reconstruction should follow after stabilization of tissue destruction. This may sometimes even be undertaken when there is acute disease.

Pericoronitis

Key points
- Commonly located on the gingiva covering a partially erupted lower third molar.
- Mechanical trauma and bacteria are the cause.
- The diagnosis is based on clinical criteria.

Introduction

Pericoronitis is an inflammatory reaction that develops in the tissues surrounding an impacted or partially erupted tooth, usually the lower third molar. The tissues involved are the gingiva and the mucosal flap overlying the crown of the tooth. Continuous mechanical trauma of the overlying mucosa and gingiva and accumulation of bacteria and debris beneath the overlying mucosal flap are the causes of the lesion.

Clinical features

Clinically, there is redness and swelling of the gingiva and the mucosal flap (the operculum) overlying and surrounding the semi erupted tooth (**Fig. 17.6**). Frequently, ulceration and

abscess formation may occur. Pericoronitis is usually accompanied by intense pain, halitosis, low-grade fever, malaise, and regional lymphadenopathy. The diagnosis is based exclusively on clinical criteria.

Differential diagnosis
- Necrotizing ulcerative gingivitis
- Herpetic gingivitis
- Non-Hodgkin's lymphoma
- Leukemia

Pathology

This is not required. Microscopically, the epithelium is hyperplastic while the connective tissue exhibits dense inflammatory infiltration by polymorphonuclear leukocytes, lymphocytes, eosinophils, and plasma cells.

Treatment

During the acute phase, local antiseptics, analgesics, and good local oral hygiene are the recommended measures. In the presence of fever and other systemic signs and symptoms, systemic use of antibiotics such as metronidazole 250 to 500 mg three times daily for 4 to 6 days or penicillin 1 to 2 MIU/d for 4 to 5 days is recommended. Surgical removal of the overlying gingival flap or extraction of the offending tooth may be performed after the acute phase to avoid recurrence.

Staphylococcal Infection

Key points
- Rare in the oral mucosa.
- *Staphylococcus aureus* and *Staphylococcus epidermidis* are the cause.
- Various systemic diseases and immunodeficiency states predispose to the infection.
- Nonspecific ulceration is the main clinical feature.
- The diagnosis should be confirmed by microbiological tests.

Introduction

Staphylococcal infections are rare in the oral mucosa and are caused by strains of *S. aureus* and *S. epidermidis*. Predisposing factors include trauma, poor oral hygiene, and systemic diseases such as diabetes mellitus, tuberculosis, immune deficiencies, e.g., HIV disease.

Clinical features

Clinically, there is a round or oval ulcerative lesion with raised borders covered by a whitish or brown-white necrotic exudate

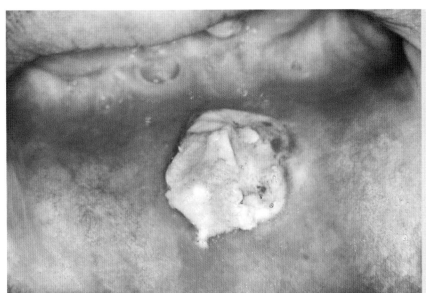

Fig. 17.4 Noma, early mucosal ulceration of the lower lip.

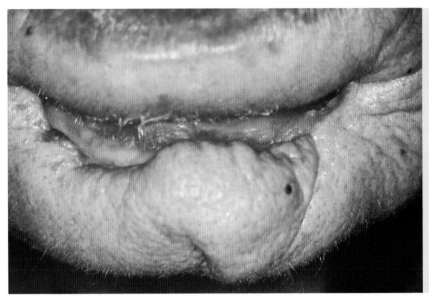

Fig. 17.5 Noma, perforation of the lower lip with extension to the skin and scarring at a late stage.

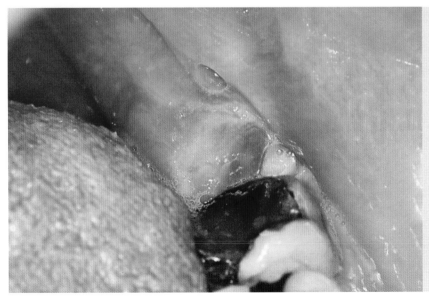

Fig. 17.6 Pericoronitis.

(**Figs. 17.7, 17.8**). Intense inflammation surrounds the ulcer. Regional lymphadenopathy and fever may be present.

Differential diagnosis

- Aphthous ulcer
- Trauma
- Streptococcal oral infection
- Tuberculosis
- Syphilitic ulcer
- Wegener's granulomatosis
- Cyclic neutropenia
- Myelodysplastic syndromes

Pathology

Gram staining and microbiological culture are necessary to confirm the diagnosis.

Treatment

Local antiseptics, e.g., 0.2% chlorhexidine gluconate may be used as mouthwash three times daily. Systemic antibiotics may be used in severe, persistent cases such as erythromycin 250 to 500 mg every 8 hours or clarithromycin 250 to 500 mg twice daily for 4 to 6 days. Oral cephalosporins may also be used.

Impetigo

Key points

- The most common bacterial skin infection in children.
- *Staphylococcus aureus* and less often *Streptococcus pyogenes* are the causes.
- Clinically, two types have been described: bullous and nonbullous.
- The perioral area is a commonly affected site.
- The diagnosis is based on clinical examination.

Introduction

Impetigo is a common, highly contagious, superficial skin infection that primarily affects children. Mainly, *S. aureus* and rarely *S. pyogenes* are the cause. The infection is transmitted by direct skin contact. Predisposing factors are warm and wet weather, minor skin trauma, and states of immunosuppression. The disease is classified in two clinical types: (a) *bullous type* which is rare and usually affects infants, (b) *nonbullous* which is more common (> 70%) and affects usually children between 5 and 15 years.

Clinical features

Clinically, the nonbullous type appears as red macules, 2 to 4 mm in diameter, which quickly evolve into a vesicle or pustule, then rupture, leaving a superficial erosion covered with "*honey-colored*" yellow crust. The lesions extend to the surrounding healthy skin. The most frequently affected areas are the face, around the mouth, and nose (**Fig. 17.9**). Mild lymphadenopathy may be present. The disease is self-limited and the lesions heal without treatment within 2 to 3 weeks without scarring. In the bullous type, patients present with superficial bullae of 1 to 5 cm in size, which later rupture leaving erosions covered with a thin crust (**Fig. 17.10**). The lesions heal quicker than those of the nonbullous type. The diagnosis is based on clinical criteria.

Differential diagnosis

- Herpetic infection
- Chickenpox
- Candidiasis
- Eczema
- Insect bite
- Pemphigus

Pathology

Usually, not required. Microscopically, spongiosis and neutrophilic vesicles and pustules develop within the epidermis, while the dermis exhibits infiltration by neutrophils, lymphocytes, and eosinophils. Microbiological testing may be necessary in some cases.

Treatment

Topical antibiotic treatment with mupirocin or fusidic acid, cream or ointment, is effective and consists the first line of treatment. In patients with extensive disease, oral antibiotics such as erythromycin and penicillinase-resistant penicillin (e.g., flucloxacillin) are indicated. Other choices are first- or second-generation cephalosporins.

Staphylococcal Scalded Skin Syndrome

Key points

- It usually affects children under 6 years.
- The exfoliative staphylococcal toxins ETA and ETB are responsible.
- The toxins bind to desmoglein-1 causing cleavage of the epidermis, resulting in bullae formation.
- The clinical presentation includes erythema, skin scaling, bullae, and skin exfoliation.
- Perioral lesions are common, while the oral mucosa is unaffected.

Introduction

The staphylococcal scalded skin syndrome (SSSS) is a rare staphylococcal, toxin-mediated infection of *S. aureus*. The

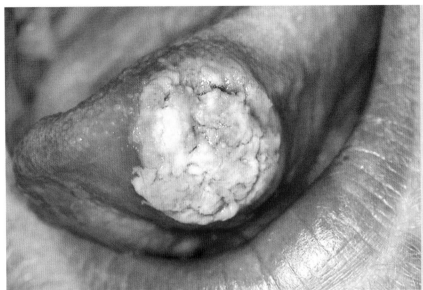

Fig. 17.7 Staphylococcal ulceration on the tongue.

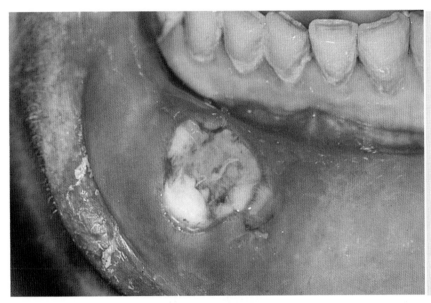

Fig. 17.8 Staphylococcal ulceration of the lower lip.

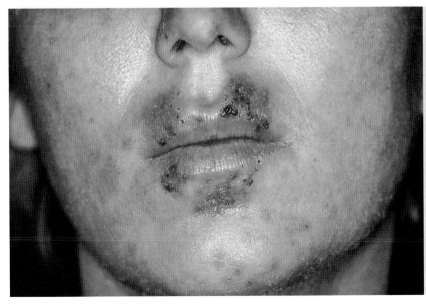

Fig. 17.9 Impetigo in perioral area, not bullous type.

exfoliative toxins ETA and ETB bind to desmoglein-1 (Dsg1), at the granular layer, causing cleavage of the epidermis. As a result, the bonds between the superficial skin keratinocytes rupture and bullae are formed. The disease generally affects children less than 6 years and rarely adults, with chronic renal insufficiency or immunosuppression.

Clinical features

The disease begins with mild symptoms such as fever, malaise, irritability, weakness, photophobia, and tenderness of the skin. After 2 to 3 days, generalized skin erythema is observed. Later, flaccid, endoepidermal bullae appear which rupture, leaving moist erosions and crusts which cover almost the whole-body surface (**Fig. 17.11**). The oral mucosa is usually not affected. The common facial clinical features include facial edema, perioral fissures, and lip crusting. The Nikolsky's sign is positive. The skin lesions heal without scarring in 10 to 15 days. The diagnosis is mainly based on clinical criteria.

Differential diagnosis

- Toxic epidermal necrolysis
- Stevens-Johnson syndrome
- Impetigo, bullous type
- Kawasaki's disease
- Severe drug reaction
- Pemphigus foliaceus
- Graft-versus-host disease

Pathology

The definitive diagnosis of SSSS relies on culture and biopsy results. Histologic findings include intraepidermal cleavage, with splitting, that occurs beneath and within the stratum granulosum. The cleavage space may enclose free-floating or partly attached acantholytic cells. What is left of the epidermis appears normal and the dermis shows no inflammation. With the use of examination of frozen sections of the lesions and slide latex agglutination, double immunodiffusion, and enzyme-linked immunosorbent assay (ELISA) tests, we can easily confirm the diagnosis and identify the toxins responsible for the disease. Microbiological culture is indicated in all patients for identification and antibiotic sensitivity of the causative organism. *Staphylococcus aureus* can be cultured from the conjunctiva, nasopharynx, feces, or pyogenic foci on the skin.

Treatment

Patients should be hospitalized under the care of pediatric and dermatology specialists. The treatment aims at the eradication of the staphylococcal foci of infection. It generally requires intravenous penicillinase-resistant, antistaphylococcal antibiotics. The current treatment of choice is cloxacillin or dicloxacillin. Supportive care is also very important with appropriate attention to fluid and electrolyte management as the disrupted epidermal barrier function may cause dehydration.

Streptococcal Infection

Key points

- A debatable infectious oral disease.
- The infection is usually caused by β-hemolytic *Streptococcus*.
- The gingiva and tongue are common oral sites of involvement.
- The oral lesions can be preceded by streptococcal tonsillitis.

Introduction

Streptococcal oral infection is a debatable disease caused by β-hemolytic *Streptococcus*. It is a rare entity. The causative role of streptococci is controversial because it is not clear whether streptococcal infection is the primary cause or whether it represents a secondary infection of pre-existing lesions.

Clinical features

The disease is usually localized on the gingiva, tongue, and rarely in other oral areas (**Fig. 17.12**). Frequently, the oral lesions follow tonsillitis or upper respiratory tract infection. Clinically, redness, edema of the gingiva, and patchy superficial, round, or linear erosions covered with a white-yellowish smear are observed. The interdental papillae remain intact. The disease is localized and rarely involves the entire gingival tissues. Mild fever and submandibular lymphadenopathy are also present. The clinical diagnosis should be confirmed by laboratory tests.

Differential diagnosis

- Herpetic gingivostomatitis
- Necrotizing ulcerative gingivitis
- Staphylococcal infection

Pathology

Gram staining and culture may confirm the clinical diagnosis.

Treatment

It consists of oral antibiotics, primarily oral penicillin 500 to 750 mg/d for 6 to 8 days. Erythromycin 250 to 500 mg every 8 h/d or clarithromycin 250 to 500 mg twice a day for 4 to 6 days may be used.

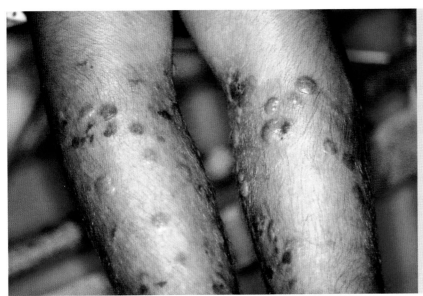

Fig. 17.10 Impetigo on the skin of the lower limbs, bullous type.

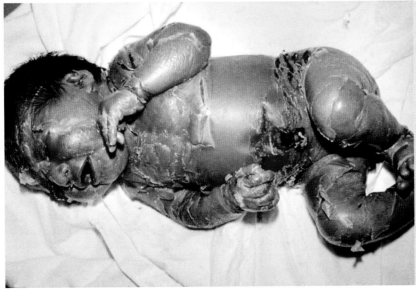

Fig. 17.11 Staphylococcal scalded skin syndrome, total destruction of the skin and lips.

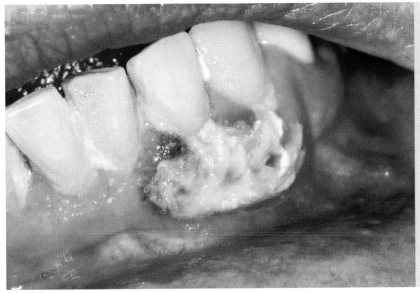

Fig. 17.12 Ulceration on the gingiva and alveolar mucosa of the mandible by β-hemolytic *Streptococcus*.

Erysipelas

Key points

- Common cause is *S. pyogenes* (group A).
- The infection usually affects the face and the lower extremities.
- The oral mucosa is not involved.
- The diagnosis is based on clinical criteria.

Introduction

Erysipelas is an acute skin bacterial infection primarily involving the dermis and lymphatic vessels. The disease is nearly always caused by group A *streptococci* (*S. pyogenes*). The sites of predilection are the lower extremities and the face.

Clinical features

The oral mucosa is not involved. However, in cases of facial erysipelas, the redness and edema may extend to the vermilion border and the lip mucosa (**Figs. 17.13, 17.14**). After an incubation period of 3 to 5 days, abrupt onset of fever, chills, nausea, malaise, and headache usually occur. Soon after, the skin lesion appears. Clinically, erysipelas is characterized by a shiny, hot, edematous, bright red, and slightly elevated plaque, which is sharply demarcated from the surrounding healthy skin and may show small vesicles. The disease may recur and cause permanent edema of the lips. The diagnosis is made on clinical grounds.

Differential diagnosis

- Cellulitis
- Herpes zoster
- Angioedema
- Contact dermatitis
- Sweet's syndrome
- Discoid lupus erythematosus
- Other facial infections

Pathology

There is usually no need for laboratory tests. Histologically, diffuse edema with neutrophilic and eosinophilic infiltration of the dermis along with lymph vessels dilatation are the principal features. The detection of *Streptococcus* with direct immunofluorescence and latex agglutination tests or culture could prove helpful in some cases. The circulating antibodies against *Streptococcus* could be useful.

Treatment

Oral antibiotics, especially penicillin for 10 to 15 days, or alternatively, erythromycin for 7 to 12 days are the first-line choice for treatment.

Scarlet Fever

Key points

- Primarily, a disease in children usually between 1 and 10 years.
- It is caused by the erythrogenic toxins A, B, and C produced by group A *β-hemolytic Streptococci*.
- Main clinical features are fever, malaise, and punctate erythema.
- Oral lesions are nonspecific; the most distinctive feature is the hypertrophy of the fungiform papillae.

Introduction

Scarlet fever or scarlatina is an acute infection caused by group A *β-hemolytic Streptococci*, which produces erythrogenic toxins, types A, B, and C. It is usually a disease of childhood (1–10 years). More than 80% of children over 10 years have antibodies for *Streptococcus*. The seasonal peaks are observed in winter and spring.

Clinical features

Scarlet fever, after an incubation period of 2 to 4 days, begins with pharyngitis, fever, chills, headache, malaise, vomiting, nausea, anorexia, abdominal pain, and lymphadenopathy. The rash appears 1 to 2 days later and is characterized by tiny papules on a diffuse, punctate, erythema giving a rough sandpaper appearance to the skin. It first appears on the upper trunk and quickly spreads within 6 to 12 hours to the whole body. The face is infrequently involved, with few papules and a characteristic perioral pallor. The oral mucosa is red, edematous, and the tongue may be covered by a thick white coating (**Fig. 17.15**). Later, hypertrophy of the fungiform papillae follows, giving the tongue a characteristic "*strawberry*" appearance. Other oral lesions include palatal petechiae. Cervical lymph nodes may be enlarged. Complications of the disease include peritonsillar abscess, sinusitis, otitis, pneumonia, acute glomerulonephritis, myocarditis and meningitis, and rheumatic fever. The diagnosis is usually made on clinical grounds.

Differential diagnosis

- Infectious mononucleosis
- Measles
- Drug reactions
- Scarlatiniform eruption
- Kawasaki's disease
- Staphylococcal scalded skin syndrome

Pathology

Histologic examination reveals dilated capillaries and lymphatic vessels. Edema and perivascular inflammatory infiltration and hemorrhage may occur.

The isolation of group A *streptococci* confirms the diagnosis.

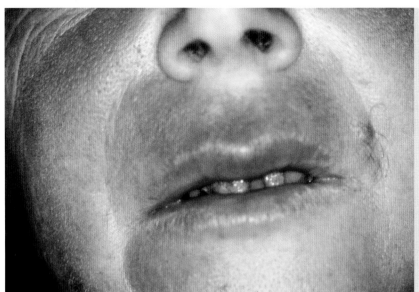

Fig. 17.13 Erysipelas of facial skin with extension on the upper lip.

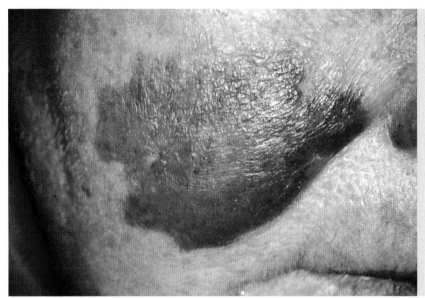

Fig. 17.14 Erysipelas on the skin of the cheek.

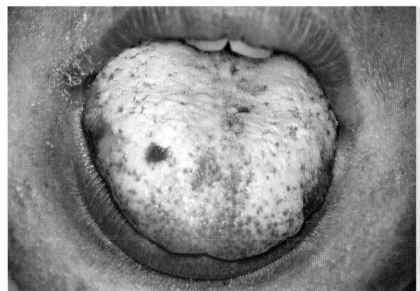

Fig. 17.15 Scarlet fever, furry tongue, swollen fungiform papillae, and mild erosion.

Treatment

Penicillin VK, 500 mg orally four times a day, is the drug of choice for 10 to 15 days or erythromycin, 500 mg orally four times a day for 7 to 12 days, is indicated, but the therapy is best left to the pediatrician.

Oral and Cutaneous Sinus of Tooth Origin

Key points

- It is the result of nonvital tooth and periapical abscess formation.
- The abscess may be symptomatic or asymptomatic.
- The fistula is usually asymptomatic and may generate intraorally or extraorally in the surrounding skin area.

Introduction

Necrosis of the pulp of the tooth frequently leads to the creation of periapical abscess. By the time the abscess (pus) diffuses along the path of lesser resistance of the bone, it creates a fistulous resource that flows either intraorally or extraorally in skin. The lesion may be symptomatic or asymptomatic.

Clinical features

Clinically, there is the opening of the fistula from which pus is discharged either automatically or upon pressure of the surrounding tissues. Often in the ejection, orifice is created, an eminence of reactive granulation tissue, with erythema in the periphery (**Fig. 17.16**). Chronic lesions are usually asymptomatic. Typically, the test of the pulp vitality of the offending tooth is negative, while the entrance of gutta-percha cone or dental probe at the opening of the canal fistula leads to the responsible tooth. Occasionally, dental abscesses can eject extraorally to the skin and drain via a cutaneous sinus (**Figs. 17.17, 17.18**). The diagnosis is made clinically and radiographically.

Differential diagnosis

- Periodontal abscess and fistula
- Soft tissue abscess
- Cellulitis
- Osteomyelitis
- Actinomycosis

Pathology

Intraoral or panoramic X-ray reveals the responsible tooth.

Treatment

Endodontic treatment of the responsible tooth or extraction leads to spontaneous resolution of the fistula.

Cellulitis

Key points

- An acute infectious process of the dermis and subcutaneous soft tissues.
- *Staphylococcus aureus* and β-hemolytic *S. pyogenes* are the most common causative organisms.
- Clinically, it is characterized by flushing, heat, pain, and edema of the affected area.
- In children, it is frequent in the head and neck, while in adults, it is more frequent at the hands and feet.
- The diagnosis is based mainly on clinical criteria.

Introduction

The cellulitis is a relatively common acute bacterial infection of the skin and underlying soft tissues. The responsible microorganisms are mainly *S. aureus*, β-hemolytic *Streptococci*, and, less often, gram-negative and anaerobic bacteria. Cellulitis, caused by *Haemophilus influenzae*, type B occurs commonly in the facial soft tissues in infants and children and is the result of odontogenic infection. Predisposing factors are immune deficiency, diabetes mellitus, and vascular disease.

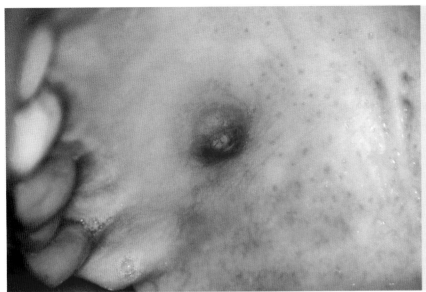

Fig. 17.16 Dental fistula on the palate.

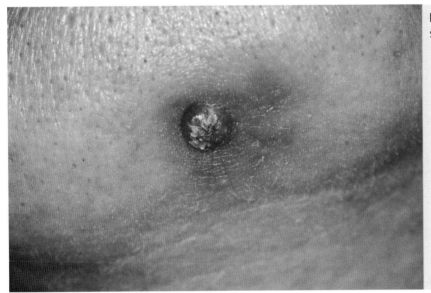

Fig. 17.17 Cutaneous fistula on the submandibular area, of dental origin.

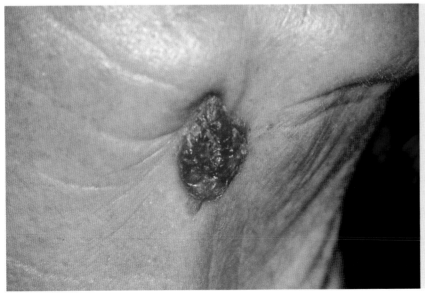

Fig. 17.18 Cutaneous fistula and dermatitis in submandibular region, of dental origin.

Clinical features

Clinically, cellulitis has a variable onset and presents as a diffuse, firm, ill-defined erythematous, swelling associated with warmth and pain (**Figs. 17.19, 17.20**). The overlying skin shows a deep purplish discoloration. Usually, there are associated systemic symptoms of fever, chills, malaise, and lymphadenopathy. The diagnosis is usually based on the clinical features.

Differential diagnosis

- Erysipelas
- Acute parotitis
- Angioedema
- Panniculitis
- Venous thrombosis
- Dental and periodontal abscess
- Insect bites

Pathology

Usually, it is not needed.

Treatment

Systemic administration of oral cloxacillin 250 to 500 mg every 6 hours for 6 days or oral flucloxacillin 250 to 500 mg every 6 hours or oral amoxicillin 500 mg every 8 hours for 6 days are the drugs of choice. Oral ciprofloxacin 500 to 750 mg twice daily alone or in combination with metronidazole 500 mg every 8 hours for 6 days may also be used in more severe cases.

Oral Soft Tissue Abscess

Key points

- Mainly due to *S. aureus* and β-hemolytic *Streptococcus*.
- The tongue and buccal mucosa are the most frequent sites affected.
- Painful round swelling which may raise or may be circumscribed deep into muscle layers.
- The diagnosis is based on clinical criteria.

Introduction

Oral soft tissue abscesses are relatively uncommon resulting from infections of nondental and periodontal origin.

Staphylococcus aureus and *β-hemolytic Streptococcus* and, rarely, other microorganisms are responsible for creating the abscess. The transfer of bacteria is usually hematogenously, while the origin of the infection is usually difficult to determine.

Clinical features

Clinically, the soft tissue abscess occurs with an acute or subacute form and is characterized by soft or fairly hard painful swelling with irregular borders. The swelling is usually within the muscle layers and rarely relies on the mouth. The size ranges from a few to several centimeters. The tongue, lip, and buccal mucosa are the most frequent sites of involvement (**Figs. 17.21, 17.22**). The diagnosis is based on clinical features and the findings of the microbiological examination.

Differential diagnosis

- Actinomycosis
- Tuberculosis
- Lipoma
- Mucocele
- Lymphoepithelial cyst
- Dermoid cyst
- Foreign body reaction

Pathology

Smear staining and bacterial cultures may be useful.

Treatment

Surgical incision and drainage of pus along with systemic administration of appropriate antibiotics, e.g., dicloxacillin 500 mg every 8 hours for 6 to 8 days or erythromycin 500 mg three times a day for 4 to 6 days are the treatment of choice. Metronidazole 500 mg three times a day for approximately 6 days may be used either alone or in combination with one of the above antibiotics.

Peritonsillar Abscess

Key points

- An infectious complication of tonsillitis.
- It is mainly due to *pyogenic streptococci* and *anaerobes* in the area.
- Pain, dysphagia, difficulty in swallowing, fever, swelling of the tonsils, and lymphadenitis are the main signs and symptoms.
- The diagnosis is based on clinical criteria.

Introduction

The peritonsillar abscess is usually a complication of recurrent infection of the tonsils and is mainly due to *pyogenic streptococci* and *anaerobic bacteria* and, more rarely, other gram-positive or gram-negative microorganisms.

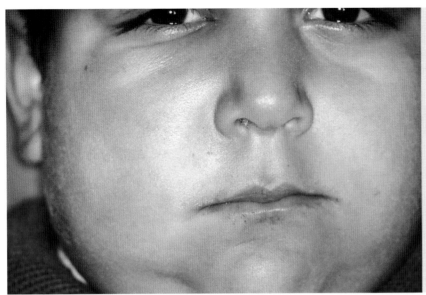

Fig. 17.19 Facial cellulitis on the right side due to dental abscess.

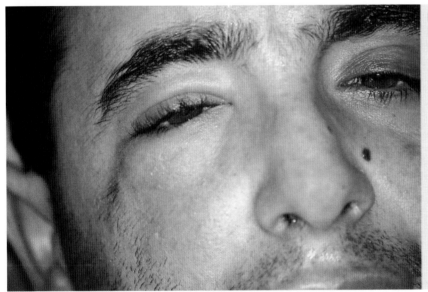

Fig. 17.20 Cellulitis and swelling below the right eye and cheek caused by dental abscess.

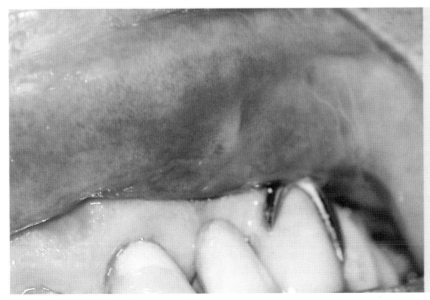

Fig. 17.21 Abscess on the upper lip.

Clinical features

Clinically, peritonsillar abscess appears as a soft swelling in the tonsillar and adjacent area. The lesion coexists with intense inflammation and often automatic drainage and discharge of pus (**Fig. 17.23**). Pain, dysphagia, fever, and lymphadenitis of the cervical area are additional signs and symptoms. The diagnosis is based mainly on clinical features.

Differential diagnosis
- Ludwig's angina
- Herpetic infection
- Tuberculosis
- Actinomycosis
- Syphilis
- Non-Hodgkin's lymphoma
- Systemic mycoses

Pathology

Usually, it is not required. In some cases, the microbiological examination helps in the diagnosis and the identification of the causative bacteria.

Treatment

Surgical incision and drainage of pus along with systemic administration of antibiotics, e.g., erythromycin 500 mg three times daily for 6 to 8 days or second-generation cephalosporins in combination with metronidazole 500 mg three times a day for 6 to 8 days, are the treatment of choice.

Acute Suppurative Parotitis

Key points
- Mainly due to *S. aureus* and *S. viridans*.
- The transfer of bacteria occurs either hematogenously or through the duct of the gland.
- Painful swelling of the parotid gland with characteristic inflammation and secretion of pus mixed with salivary fluid from the duct opening.
- The diagnosis is based mainly on clinical criteria.

Introduction

Acute suppurative infection of the parotid glands is usually unilateral and most frequently appears in patients over 60 years, although it may also occur during childhood. *Staphylococcus aureus*, *S. viridans*, and other bacteria of the oral flora are usually responsible for the infection, which may be hematogenous or spread by oral bacteria via the salivary ducts.

Clinical features

Clinically, the disease is characterized by induration, tenderness, and painful swelling of the parotid gland (**Fig. 17.24**).

Stensen's papilla is inflamed and pus may be discharged from the duct opening, particularly after pressure on the parotid gland (**Fig. 17.25**). Saliva stimulating foods and chewing movement of the mandible tend to increase the pain. Low-grade fever and weakness may be present. The diagnosis is mainly based on the clinical features.

Differential diagnosis
- Epidemic parotitis
- Obstructive parotitis
- Sjögren's syndrome
- Mikulicz's syndrome
- Heerfordt's syndrome
- Sialadenosis (sialosis)
- Non-Hodgkin's lymphoma
- Parotid tumors
- HIV infection
- Hepatitis C virus (HCV) infection

Pathology

Usually, it is not required. In persistent cases, microbiological examination and culture of pus help to determine the microorganism responsible. Fine-needle aspiration (FNA) can provide important diagnostic information.

Treatment

Systemic administration of an appropriate antibiotic, e.g., second-generation cephalosporins 500 mg three times daily for 4 to 6 days or erythromycin 500 mg three times a day for 4 to 6 days, is the treatment of choice.

Acute Submandibular Sialadenitis

Key points
- Mainly due to *S. aureus* and various strains of streptococci.
- Painful swelling, inflammation, and characteristic outflow of pus and serous fluid from the hypoglossal cusp.
- The diagnosis is mainly based on clinical criteria.

Introduction

Acute suppurative infection of the submandibular gland is relatively rare compared with the frequency of analogous infections of the parotid gland. *Staphylococcus aureus*, *S. pyogenes*, *S. viridans*, and other bacteria of the oral flora are usually responsible. The microorganisms may reach the submandibular gland, either through the gland duct or via the bloodstream.

Clinical features

Clinically, it is characterized by painful swelling, usually unilateral, in the submandibular region, which may be soft or

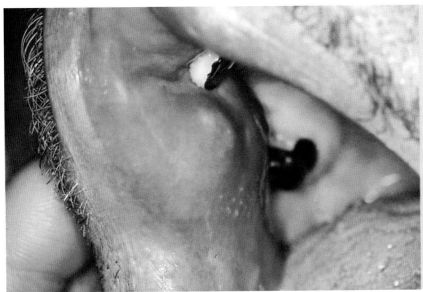

Fig. 17.22 Abscess on the buccal mucosa.

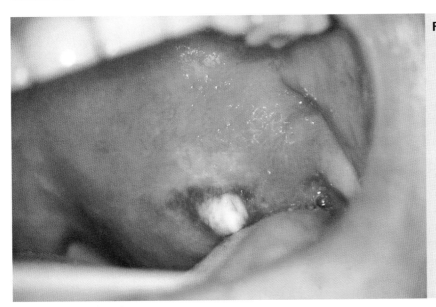

Fig. 17.23 Peritonsillar abscess.

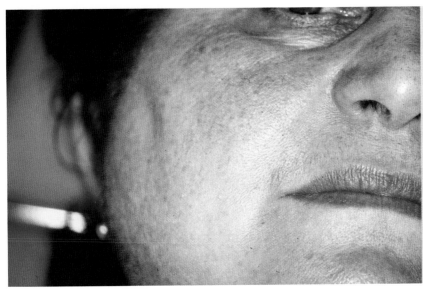

Fig. 17.24 Suppurative parotitis, swelling of the parotid gland.

indurated (**Fig. 17.26**). The overlying skin is red and tense. Intraorally, inflammation at the orifice of the duct and outflow of pus, particularly after pressure in the submandibular salivary gland area are common findings (**Fig. 17.27**). The diagnosis is mainly based on the clinical features.

Differential diagnosis

- Submandibular duct obstruction
- Mumps
- Submandibular lymph nodes swelling
- Sjögren's syndrome
- Mikulicz's syndrome
- Heerfordt's syndrome
- Non-Hodgkin's lymphoma
- HIV infection
- HCV infection

Pathology

Usually, it is not required. Microbiological examination may help in difficult cases. In addition, FNA biopsy may be helpful.

Treatment

Systemic administration of appropriate antibiotics, e.g., second-generation cephalosporins 500 mg three times daily for 4 to 6 days or erythromycin 500 mg three times a day for 4 to 6 days, is the treatment of choice.

Klebsiella Infections

Key points

- It is due to the strain *Klebsiella pneumoniae*.
- The bacillus primarily affects the respiratory and urinary system.
- Infection of the mouth is very rare.
- Oral ulceration is the prominent feature.
- The clinical diagnosis should be confirmed microbiologically.

Introduction

Klebsiella pneumoniae is a gram-negative bacillus, which is part of the normal flora of the mouth and the gastrointestinal tract. Respiratory and urinary tracts are the mainly involved systems while other areas of the body are rarely infected. Predisposing factors of the infection are diabetes mellitus, immunosuppression, and long-term use of antibiotics. Infection in the mouth of *Klebsiella* is very rare and may occur in patients with diabetes mellitus, infection, HIV infection, and in patients with malignant tumors undergoing chemotherapy.

Clinical features

Clinically, the infection appears as an irregular deep ulcer with a necrotic center covered by a thick brown-whitish pseudomembrane (**Fig. 17.28**). Fever and lymphadenopathy may be present. The clinical features are not pathognomonic and microbiological confirmation is necessary.

Differential diagnosis

- Necrotizing ulcerative stomatitis
- Tuberculosis
- Chancre
- *Staphylococcal* infection
- *Streptococcus* infection
- *Pseudomonas* infection
- Major aphthous ulcer
- Eosinophilic ulcer

Pathology

The microbiological examination and isolation of the organism is necessary for a final diagnosis.

Treatment

Drugs of choice are tetracycline and mainly ciprofloxacin, 500 mg three times per day for 6 to 10 days. Alternative drugs are second- and third-generation cephalosporins or aminoglycosides.

Pseudomonas Infections

Key points

- It is mainly due to the strain *P. aeruginosa*.
- An opportunistic pathogen and it mostly affects immunosuppressed individuals.
- The oral and perioral areas are rarely affected.
- The clinical diagnosis should be confirmed microbiologically.

Introduction

Pseudomonas aeruginosa is a gram-negative, strictly aerobic bacillus. It is an opportunistic pathogen. Predisposing disorders of *Pseudomonas* infection are cystic fibrosis, glycogen storage disease type Ib, congenital and acquired neutropenia, leukemias, and premature neonates and debilitated elderly people taking antibiotics, especially in a hospital environment. The respiratory and urinary tract, eyes and ears, sinus, nails, skin, and subcutaneous tissues are more commonly involved. Rarely, mouth, lips, and perioral region infection may occur.

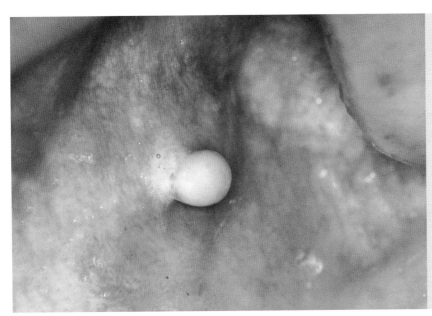

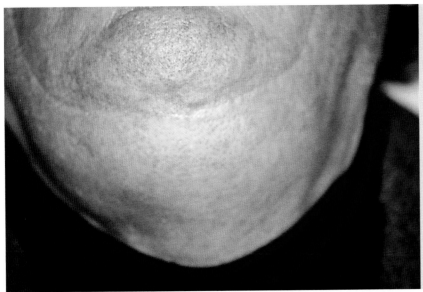

Fig. 17.25 Suppurative parotitis, characteristic exudation of pus from the orifice of the parotid duct.

Fig. 17.26 Submandibular sialadenitis, bilateral swelling of submandibular region.

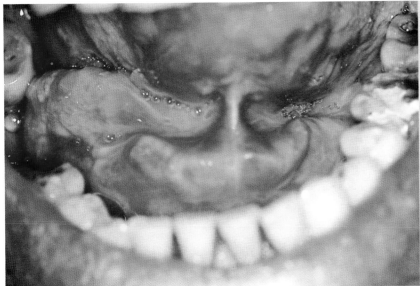

Fig. 17.27 Submandibular sialadenitis, inflammation and swelling of the hypoglossal cusp.

Clinical features

Clinically, oral infection presents as an irregular necrotic ulceration, which tends to expand and is accompanied by intense inflammation (**Fig. 17.29**). Posthealing scarring can occur (**Fig. 17.30**). The clinical features of the infection are not diagnostic and microbiological confirmation of diagnosis is required.

Differential diagnosis
- Infections from other bacteria
- Neutropenia
- Agranulocytosis
- Tuberculosis

Pathology

The microbiological examination and isolation of the microbe is necessary for final diagnosis.

Treatment

First-choice drugs are ciprofloxacin 500 mg twice daily for 6 days or piperacillin-tazobactam or ceftazidime or cefepime. The precise treatment requires liaison with physicians.

Cat-Scratch Disease

Key points
- A bacterial infection that is transmitted from cats to humans as the result of a scratch or bite.
- The cause of the disease is usually *B. henselae* and other executives.
- It affects the skin and lymph nodes.

Introduction

Cat-scratch disease is a bacterial infection caused by the gram-negative bacillus *B. henselae*. The bacterium enters the skin following scratching from the clutches or licking or biting of a cat. In immunocompetent people, it is a benign, self-limited illness characterized by tender regional lymph nodes' enlargement. The disease is primarily seen in young people during autumn and winter.

Clinical features

Clinically, at the inoculation site of the bacteria, a small papule or pustule develops with erythema and mild swelling of the overlying skin in approximately 5 to 15 days. Then 2 to 4 weeks after the scratch, persistent swelling of regional lymph nodes usually presents, which can last up to 2 to 6 months. Fever, headache, weakness, and malaise are common symptoms. Often when most of the signs and symptoms are established, the point of entry of the bacteria on the skin has healed and is no longer visible. If scratching occurs on the facial skin, a symptomatic swelling of the submaxillary lymph nodes arises (**Fig. 17.31**). Patients often visit the dentist thinking that this is a dental or periodontal infection. The diagnosis is based on patient history, clinical features, and serologic tests.

Differential diagnosis
- Dental abscess
- Periodontal abscess
- Various oral infections
- Leukemia
- Other hematologic diseases
- Hodgkin's disease
- Bacillary angiomatosis

Pathology

Histologically, the affected lymph nodes show central necrosis surrounded by epithelioid cells and histiocytes. Staining with Warthin-Starry silver demonstrates the bacillus within necrotic areas. Serologic tests with high specificity and sensitivity of *B. henselae* include indirect immunofluorescence, the ELISA for immunoglobulin M (IgM) antibodies, and polymerase chain reaction (PCR).

Treatment

The disease is usually self-limited within 3 to 4 months. The administration of antibiotics (e.g., azithromycin or doxycycline are the drugs of choice) may be helpful.

Bacillary Angiomatosis

Key points
- It is due to gram-negative bacteria *B. henselae* and *B. quintana*.
- Occurs mainly in patients with AIDS.
- It is the result of intense proliferation of vascular angiostimulating factors generated by bacteria.
- Primarily affects the skin and is uncommon in the oral mucosa.

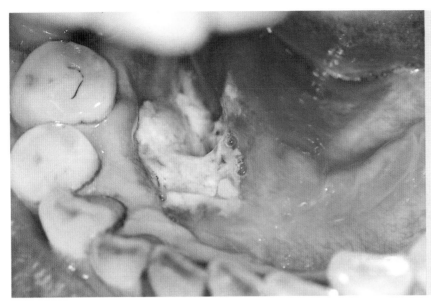

Fig. 17.28 Oral ulcerations on the floor of the mouth caused by *Klebsiella*.

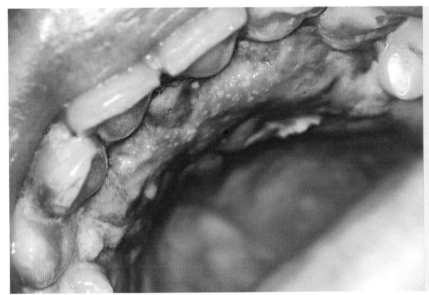

Fig. 17.29 Extensive necrotic lesions on the gingiva and palate due to *Pseudomonas aeruginosa*.

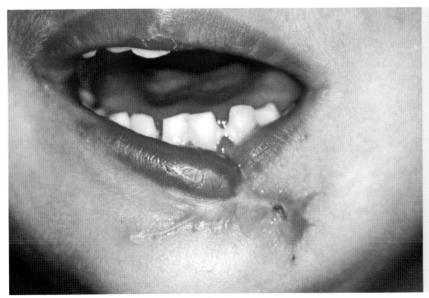

Fig. 17.30 Scars on the lower lip and skin from infection with *Pseudomonas aeruginosa*.

Introduction

Bacillary angiomatosis is a rare, opportunistic bacterial infection produced by intense vascular proliferation. It was first described in 1983 in patients with AIDS. The cause of the disease are *B. quintana* and *B. henselae*—two gram-negative bacteria. The vascular proliferation is believed to result from the production of an angiostimulating factor from the two strains of *Bartonella*.

Clinical features

Clinically, the cutaneous lesions of bacillary angiomatosis appear as asymptomatic erythematous papules or plaques or nodules with a smooth surface (**Fig. 17.32**). The lesion may become ulcerated or covered by crusting. The number of lesions is variable (one to many), and this depends on the degree of the immunosuppression of the patient. Infection of the mouth is rare and clinically manifests as an asymptomatic red nodule or plaque (**Fig. 17.33**). The gingiva, tongue, and palate are the usual sites affected. The clinical picture of the lesions of both the skin and mouth is atypical and not diagnostic. Extracutaneous bacillary angiomatosis may develop in any organ and may occur with or without skin disease. The clinical diagnosis should be confirmed by histologic examination.

Differential diagnosis

- Pyogenic granuloma
- Kaposi's sarcoma
- Hemangioma
- Leiomyoma
- Angiosarcoma
- Amyloidosis

Pathology

On histologic examination, marked proliferation of blood vessels, large swollen endothelial cells, inflammatory cells, especially neutrophils, are the principal features. Bacillary particles appear as dark purple granular material, especially following the Warthin-Starry silver stain.

Treatment

The drug of first choice is erythromycin (e.g., 500 mg every 8 hours per day for at least 3 months). Antibiotics of second choice include doxycycline, azithromycin, and clarithromycin.

Actinomycosis

Key points

- The cause is the gram-positive anaerobic bacterium *Actinomyces israelii*, which is part of the normal flora of the mouth.
- The disease is classified into three forms: *cervicofacial, pulmonary, and abdominal.*
- Characteristic clinical signs of the cervicofacial type are swelling, induration, and fistulas formation with outflow of pus containing the characteristic *sulfur granules.*
- The drug of choice is penicillin.

Introduction

Actinomycosis is a subacute or chronic granulomatous infectious disease due to *A. israelii*, a gram-positive anaerobic bacterium. With anatomical criteria, disease is classified into three forms: (a) cervicofacial, (b) pulmonary/thoracic, and (c) abdominal. Oral lesions develop in the cervicofacial form, which constitutes around 50 to 60% of cases. The infection is endogenous resulting from the bacterium of the normal oral flora entering to the soft tissues following injury, tooth extraction, open nonvital tooth, fracture of the jaw, or tonsillitis, etc. It may then be extended to the salivary glands, bone of the jaw, and skin of the neck and face.

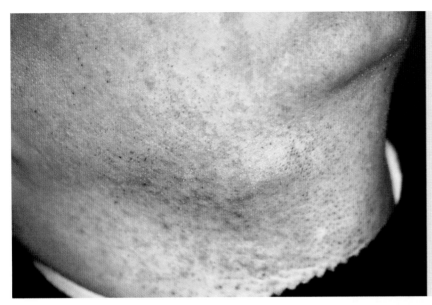

Fig. 17.31 Cat-scratch disease, swelling of the submaxillary lymph nodes.

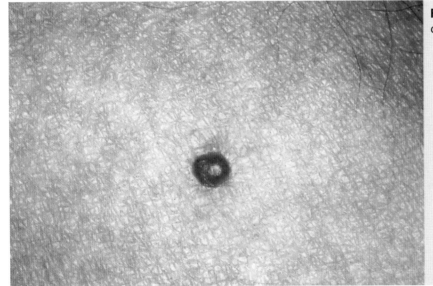

Fig. 17.32 Bacillary angiomatosis, deep colored red lump on the skin.

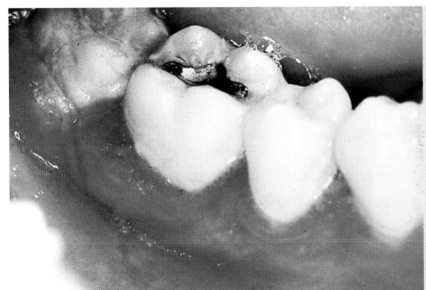

Fig. 17.33 Bacillary angiomatosis, elevated red lesion on the gingiva in the molar region.

Clinical features

Clinically, at the site of inoculation, there is an inflammatory swelling that grows slowly, is usually painless, and characteristically hard on palpation (**Figs. 17.34, 17.35**). As the lesion progresses, multiple abscesses and draining sinuses form, usually on the skin of the face and upper neck (**Fig. 17.36**). Yellow purulent material that represents colonies of *Actinomyces* (*sulfur granules*) may discharge from these sinuses. As the disease becomes chronic, healing of old lesions results in scar formation, but new abscesses and sinuses develop. Mandibular or maxillary involvement may be severe and usually is associated with trismus. Common oral locations of actinomycosis are the tongue, lips, buccal mucosa, submandibular and submental area. The clinical diagnosis should be confirmed by histologic and microbiological examination.

Differential diagnosis

- Tuberculosis
- Systemic mycoses
- Abscess of oral soft tissues
- Dental and periodontal abscess and fistula
- Other bacterial infections
- Benign and malignant tumors

Pathology

The histologic examination reveals a granulomatous reaction with pus collection. Histiocytes, epithelioid cells, plasma cells, and neutrophils can be observed at the periphery of the abscess, while in the center, the characteristic granules of the *Actinomyces* colonies known as "*sulfur granules*" are seen. These granules exhibit basophilic staining centrally and peripherally eosinophilic, with the use of common hematoxylin-eosin stain.

Treatment

Intramuscular penicillin G (e.g., 10–20 MU/d for 4–6 weeks) is the drug of choice for early cervicofacial actinomycosis. This regimen is usually followed by oral penicillin V (e.g., 500 mg four times daily for 1–3 months). Localized, limited disease usually responds well to a combination of surgical removal of the infected tissues and a 2- to 4-week course of penicillin. Tetracycline 500 mg three to four times daily for 2 to 4 months may be used as an alternative drug for patients allergic to penicillin. Intramuscular or intravenous ampicillin 50 mg/kg/d for 4 to 6 weeks, followed by oral amoxicillin 500 mg/d for 6 to 12 additional months can be given to prevent recurrences. Surgical procedures such as drainage and resection can be combined with drug therapy.

Tuberculosis

Key points

- Caused by the *Mycobacterium tuberculosis*.
- Increased morbidity is observed in recent years.
- Fever, night sweats, cough, fatigue, weight loss, and anorexia are the most common constitutional symptoms of pulmonary tuberculosis.
- The oral lesions of tuberculosis are rare and usually manifest as a solitary ulcer.

Introduction

Tuberculosis is one of the world's most widespread chronic infectious disease that primarily affects the lungs and is due to the bacillus *M. tuberculosis*. The morbidity of the disease has increased in recent years with the emergence of HIV infection, the vast movement of populations, increased frequency of immunosuppressive treatments, and relaxation of preventive vigilance. The oral mucosa involvement is relatively rare and the frequency ranges between 0.05 and 1.4%. Tuberculosis of the mouth is normally secondary after primary tuberculosis of the lungs. The transport and inoculation of the bacillus in the oral mucosa occurs either hematogenously or through the lymphatic system or rarely by direct inoculation in individuals with pulmonary tuberculosis and positive sputum for *Mycobacterium*.

Clinical features

Oral tuberculosis appears as a painless or painful ulcer, usually single and rarely multiple. Clinically, the ulcer is irregular at the periphery with thin margins, vegetated base

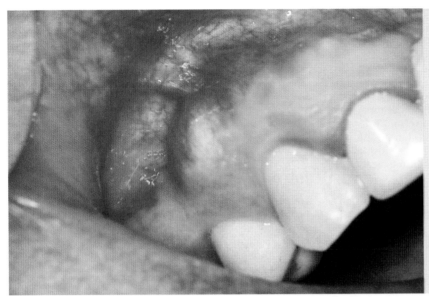

Fig. 17.34 Actinomycosis, swelling in the alveolar mucosa between canine and premolar.

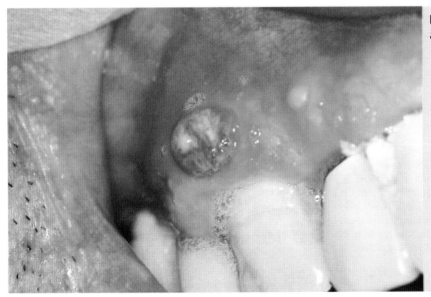

Fig. 17.35 Actinomycosis, abscesses and fistulae on the alveolar mucosa.

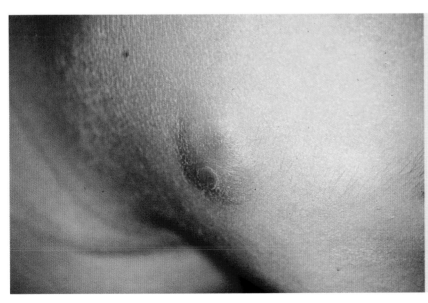

Fig. 17.36 Actinomycosis, skin abscess and fistula on the cheek.

covered by a yellowish-gray exudate and has a soft base. The size ranges from 1 to 5 cm. The dorsal surface of the tongue is most commonly affected (**Figs. 17.37, 17.38**), followed by the buccal mucosa, commissures (**Fig. 17.39**), soft palate, gingiva, and lips. Uncommon sites of involvement are the jaws and the apex of teeth. Regional lymphadenopathy usually accompanies the oral lesions (**Fig. 17.40**). Tuberculosis of submandibular and cervical lymph nodes may lead to *scrofula* with multiple fistula formation (**Fig. 17.41**). Occasionally, the oral ulceration is the first clinical apparent sign of an otherwise silent tuberculosis. The diagnosis of oral tuberculosis is based on clinical features, histologically and microbiologically.

Differential diagnosis

- Major aphthous ulcer
- Traumatic ulcer
- Sarcoidosis
- Wegener's granulomatosis
- Eosinophilic ulcer
- Chancre
- Necrotizing sialadenometaplasia
- Non-Hodgkin's lymphoma
- Squamous cell carcinoma
- Systemic mycoses
- Actinomycosis

Pathology

Histologic examination of oral biopsy specimen shows granulomas with central caseous necrosis and epithelioid histiocytes, Langhans-type giant cells, and lymphocytes. The presence of mycobacteria, with special stain Ziehl-Neelsen, is positive in 30 to 50% of cases. Chest radiology is essential. Culture of sputum, Mantoux, tuberculin skin test, and nuclei acid amplification (DNA and RNA) tests for *M. tuberculosis* are necessary for definite diagnosis.

Treatment

Tuberculosis requires management by appropriate medical teams. Therapy is long term and consists of a multiple-drug administration of streptomycin, isoniazid, ethambutol, rifampin, pyrazinamide, and others.

Lupus Vulgaris

Key points

- A form of cutaneous tuberculosis.
- Often affects the skin of the cheeks, nose, and ears.
- Red-brown papules or nodules are the typical skin lesions.
- Oral lesions are rare.

Introduction

Lupus vulgaris is the most prevalent secondary form of tuberculosis of the skin. It is usually observed in previously sensitized people with a strongly positive delayed-form hypersensitivity reaction to tuberculin.

Clinical features

Clinically, cutaneous lesions present as a red-brown coalescing papules or nodules forming plaques with an "*apple-jelly*" color on diascopy. The plaques progressively increase in size with a central scar formation. The most common cutaneous sites affected are the face, cheeks, nose, ear lobes, and, more rarely, other areas (**Fig. 17.42**). The oral mucosa is rarely affected, although the lips, buccal mucosa, gingiva, and palate are the sites of predilection. The oral lesions are either the result of spreading from facial lesions or may result from hematogenous or lymphatic spread. Clinically, oral lupus vulgaris begins with multiple small red nodules, which coalesce and quickly become necrotic forming extensive, irregular, vegetating ulcerations with soft base (**Figs. 17.43, 17.44**). The untreated ulceration grows slowly, causing tissue damage, such as stricture of the oral opening, uvula destruction, and tooth loss.

Differential diagnosis

- Squamous cell carcinoma
- Systemic mycoses
- Non-Hodgkin's lymphoma
- Wegener's granulomatosis
- Leishmaniasis

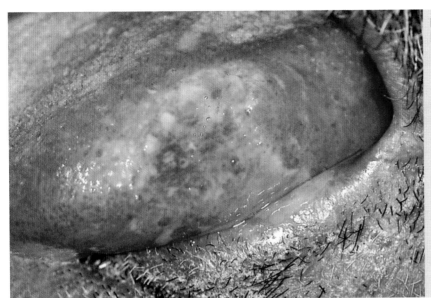

Fig. 17.37 Tuberculosis, ulcer in the lateral edge of the tongue.

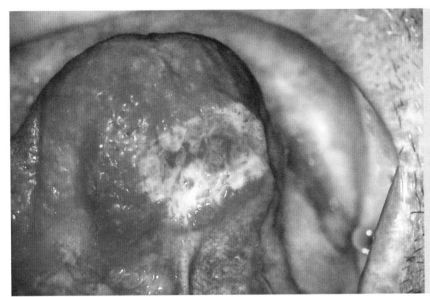

Fig. 17.38 Tuberculous ulcer on the lower surface of the tongue.

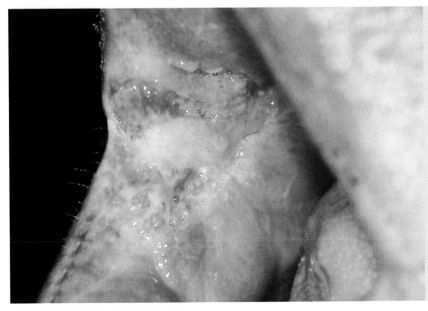

Fig. 17.39 Tuberculous ulcer on the buccal mucosa.

Pathology

The histologic findings are identical to those of tuberculosis.

Treatment

Treatment consists of antituberculous treatment. This should be undertaken by appropriate medical specialists.

Leprosy

Key points

- Chronic infectious disease caused by the bacillus *Mycobacterium leprae.*
- Slowly progressive disease characterized by granuloma formation and neurotropism with a predilection for skin and the peripheral nerves.
- The mouth is affected at a rate of 10 to 20%, mainly in the lepromatous form.
- The drug therapy has greatly improved the disease prognosis.

Introduction

Leprosy is a chronic, systemic granulomatous infectious disease caused by the bacillus *M. leprae.* It is transmitted from person to person and is endemic mainly in Africa, Asia, South America, Japan, and less in Mediterranean countries, including Greece. Transmission of the bacillus is difficult and requires a long period of promiscuity with the patient, while the incubation period ranges from 4 to 10 years. Leprosy affects the skin, mucous membranes, nerves, bones, and viscera. On clinical, bacteriologic, immunologic, and histopathologic criteria it is classified into six forms: two main types with *lepromatous* at one end, *tuberculoid* at the other end, and three *borderline types* (two with features close to the two main types, and one with a mixture of features), and finally *indeterminate leprosy* (unspecified form).

Clinical features

There is a wide spectrum of clinical manifestations of leprosy. The disease primarily involves the peripheral nervous system and the skin. In the tuberculoid form, skin patches or plaques appear which are red or reddish-brown in color, and stand out clearly from healthy skin due to their deep colored halo; they are mainly located in the buttocks and legs. In this form, the main signs are neurologic disorders (loss of sensory, analgesia, neuralgia). The lepromatous form is characterized by patches and papules, but mostly reddish nodules, solitary or confluent, called *lepromata* and identified mostly on the face and ears, creating the characteristic lion-like faces "*leonine facies.*" Neurologic disorders are rarer in this form. The borderline forms are characterized by lesions of both the previous types, while the indeterminate leprosy manifests with discolored unspecified spots or patches on the skin and, neurologic disorders that are rarely present. The mouth is affected, usually in lepromatous form in 10 to 20% and especially in the end stages of the disease.

Clinically, oral lesions appear as multiple small, red nodules (*lepromas*) that progress to necrosis and ulcerations (**Fig. 17.45**) which cause atrophic scars and tissue destruction (**Fig. 17.46**). The palate, dorsum of the tongue, lips, and gingiva are most frequently affected. Rarely, in late stages, the anterior part of the maxilla may be involved resulting in loss of anterior teeth.

Differential diagnosis

- Syphilitic gumma
- Nasal-type non-Hodgkin's lymphoma from natural killer (NK)/T cells
- Systemic mycoses
- Malignant neoplasms
- Traumatic lesions

Pathology

Microbiological testing for bacillus in nasal secretion and a thick drop of blood will assure the diagnosis. Histologic examination and the lepromin or Mitsuda test may be useful.

Treatment

In the recent years, the World Health Organization (WHO) guidelines have been used with great success. A multidrug therapy scheme is used including dapsone, clofazimine, rifampin, ofloxacin, and minocycline.

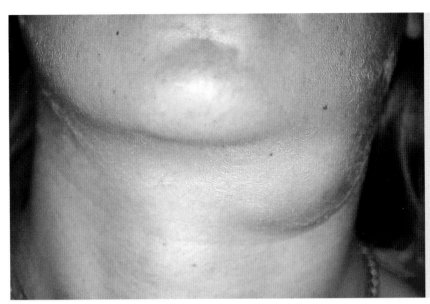

Fig. 17.40 Tuberculosis, swollen cervical and submaxillary lymph nodes.

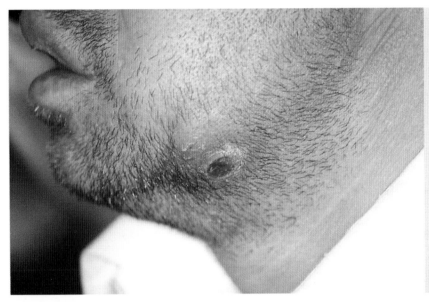

Fig. 17.41 Tuberculosis, submaxillary lymph node swelling and fistula creation.

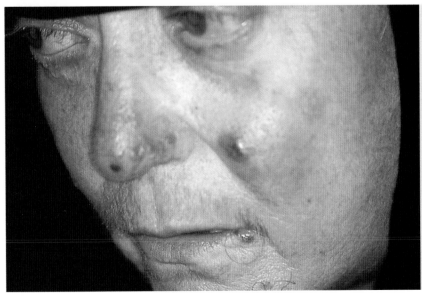

Fig. 17.42 Lupus vulgaris on the facial skin.

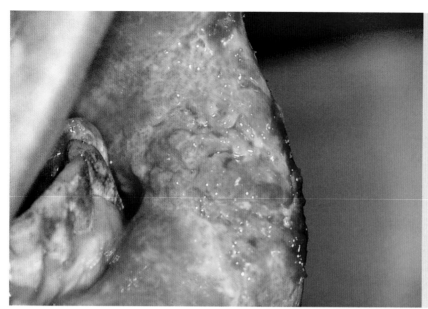

Fig. 17.43 Lupus vulgaris, extensive ulceration with vegetative bottom, on the lower lip.

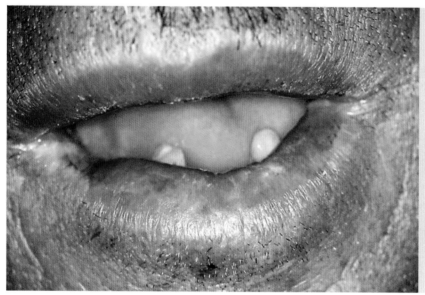

Fig. 17.44 Lupus vulgaris, swelling and edema of the lower lip.

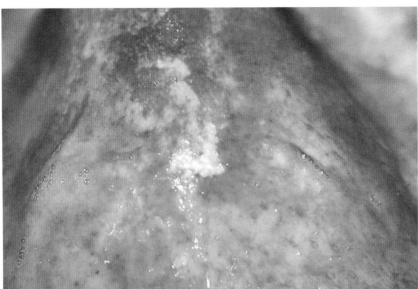

Fig. 17.45 Leprosy, erosions on the palate.

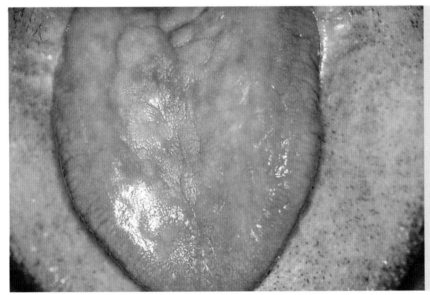

Fig. 17.46 Leprosy, mucosal atrophy on the dorsal surface of the tongue.

18 Sexually Transmitted Bacterial Infections

Syphilis

Key points

- Syphilis is a sexually transmitted infection caused by *Treponema pallidum*.
- The disease may be *congenital* or *acquired*.
- Syphilis is clinically classified into *primary, secondary*, and *tertiary* stages with a *latent* (*early* and *late*) period preceding the tertiary stage.
- Oral manifestations may occur in all clinical stages.
- The diagnosis is based on direct detection of *T. pallidum* and various serologic tests.
- Penicillin G is the treatment of choice for all stages of the disease.

Introduction

Syphilis is a sexually transmitted disease caused by *T. pallidum*. It may be *congenital* or *acquired*. Acquired syphilis is most often transmitted through sexual intercourse, but rarely nonvenereal transmission may occur. Placental transmission of *T. pallidum* from an infected mother to the fetus causes congenital syphilis. The modern classification of syphilis is based on epidemiologic, clinical, and therapeutic criteria, and is as follows: *early syphilis* (which includes primary and secondary stages and clinical relapses due to incomplete treatment and lasts < 1 year), *latent syphilis*, which is subclassified into *early stage* (lasts a year or less) and *late stage* (lasts more than a year), and *late syphilis*, also called *tertiary syphilis* because of untreated disease. The natural history of syphilis is presented in **Table 18.1**. Oral manifestations are common and may develop in all stages of syphilis.

Primary Syphilis

The primary lesion of acquired syphilis is the *chancre*. It is usually localized on the genitalia, but in approximately 10% of the cases, it may occur extragenitally (anus, rectum, fingers, nipples, etc.) and especially in the oral cavity. Direct orogenital contact (fellatio or cunnilingus) is the usual mode of acquisition of an oral chancre, but kissing may also be responsible if

Table 18.1 Natural history of syphilis

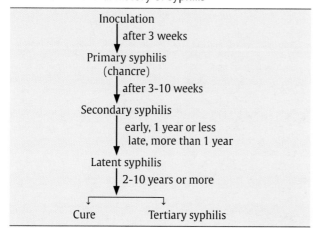

```
                Inoculation
                    │ after 3 weeks
                    ▼
             Primary syphilis
               (chancre)
                    │ after 3-10 weeks
                    ▼
            Secondary syphilis
                    │ early, 1 year or less
                    │ late, more than 1 year
                    ▼
              Latent syphilis
                    │ 2-10 years or more
                    ▼
          ┌──────────┴──────────┐
          ▼                     ▼
        Cure            Tertiary syphilis
```

Table 18.2 Oral lesions of syphilis

I.   **Primary syphilis** (5–10%)
- Chancre
- Regional lymphadenopathy

II. **Secondary syphilis**
- Macular syphilides
- Papular syphilides
- Mucous patches
- Condylomata lata
- Atypical erosions
- Malignant syphilis (lues maligna)—very uncommon
- Systemic lymphadenopathy

III. **Tertiary syphilis**
- Gummas
- Atrophic glossitis
- Interstitial glossitis

one of the partners has infectious oral lesions. The oral lesions of all stages of syphilis are presented in **Table 18.2**.

Clinical features

After an incubation period of 10 to 90 days (average, 21 days), the chancre appears at the site of inoculation (**Fig. 18.1**).

In males, most oral chancres tend to appear on the upper lip, and in females, on the lower lip, followed by the tongue, palate, and tonsillar areas. Clinically, the chancre begins as an inflammatory papule that soon erodes. The classic chancre appears as a round or oval painless ulcer with a smooth surface, raised border, and indurated base. It is often surrounded by a narrow red border and is covered by a grayish serous exudate teeming with *T. pallidum* (**Figs. 18.2–18.4**).

The chancre is usually solitary, although multiple lesions may appear simultaneously or in rapid succession. It varies in size from a few millimeters to 3 cm in diameter. A constant finding is enlarged regional lymph nodes, which are usually unilateral and less often bilateral. The enlarged lymph nodes are discrete, mobile, hard, and nontender. Without treatment, the chancre heals spontaneously within 3 to 8 weeks.

The diagnosis of primary syphilis is based on the history, clinical features, and bacteriologic and serologic tests.

Differential diagnosis

- Traumatic ulcer
- Angular cheilitis
- Aphthous ulcer
- Behçet's disease
- Chancroid
- Tuberculous ulcer
- Herpes simplex
- Eosinophilic ulcer
- Infectious mononucleosis
- Squamous cell carcinoma

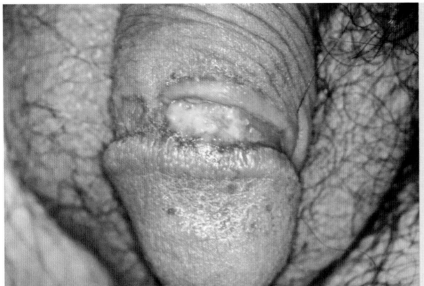

Fig. 18.1 Chancre on the sulcus of the penis.

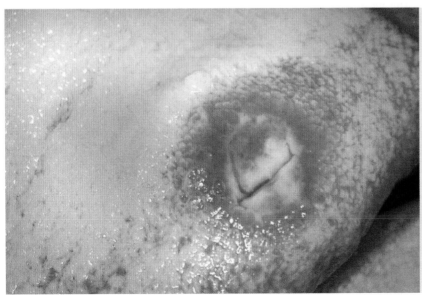

Fig. 18.2 Two chancres on the floor of the mouth.

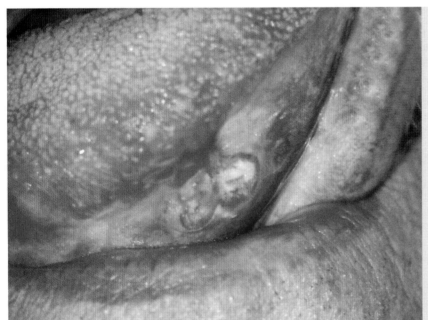

Fig. 18.3 Chancre on the dorsum of the tongue.

Pathology

Dark-field microscopic identification of *T. pallidum* in smears taken from the surface of chancre is the most sensitive and specific test for the diagnosis of primary syphilis. Serologic tests for syphilis must always be performed, but it should be remembered that during the very early primary phase, these tests may be negative.

Secondary syphilis

The signs and symptoms of secondary syphilis begin 6 to 8 weeks after the appearance of the chancre, which may still be present at the time of initiation of this stage.

Clinical feature

The clinical features of secondary syphilis are classified into two major groups: constitutional symptoms and signs and generalized mucocutaneous manifestations. The former may precede or accompany mucocutaneous lesions and include malaise, low-grade fever, headache, lacrimation, sore throat, loss of appetite, weight loss, polyarthralgias and myalgias, systemic lymphadenopathy (which is a classic and constant finding), along with splenomegaly. The enlarged lymph nodes are painless, discrete, mobile, and hard-rubbery on palpation. Generalized mucocutaneous manifestations include pruritus, nail involvement, macular, papular, pustular, nodular, follicular, and other lesions.

Mucous membrane lesions are multiple and frequent and may appear alone or in association with skin lesions. These lesions usually last for 2 to 10 weeks and disappear without scarring.

Macular syphilides: Macular syphilides (roseolas) are the earliest manifestations of secondary syphilis; they last for a few days and usually go unnoticed. In the oral mucosa, macular syphilides are most frequently found in the soft palate. Clinically, they appear as multiple red oval spots (**Fig. 18.5**).

Mucous patches: Mucous patches are by far the most frequent oral manifestation of secondary syphilis. They are flat or slightly raised, painless, oval or round papules with erosions or superficial ulcers covered by a grayish-white membrane (**Figs. 18.6–18.9**). They are teeming with spirochetes and are extremely contagious. The lesions may be surrounded by a red halo and vary in size from 3 to 10 mm or more in diameter. Mucous patches tend to be arranged symmetrically; they are usually multiple and rarely occur as solitary lesions. They occur most frequently on the tongue, palate, tonsils, mucosal surface of the lips, commissures, buccal mucosa, gingiva, and the larynx. Occasionally, mucous patches may be the only manifestation of secondary syphilis for a long period of time.

Papular syphilides: Papular syphilides are the most common and characteristic lesions of secondary syphilis on the skin, but they are rare in the oral mucosa (**Figs. 18.10–18.12**). Alopecia and nail involvement are common (**Fig. 18.13**). The oral lesions usually coalesce, forming slightly raised, painless, firm, and round nodules with a grayish-white color. The lesions have a tendency to ulcerate and are usually located on the commissures and buccal mucosa and rarely in other areas. Papular syphilides and mucous patches are always associated with bilateral, regional lymphadenopathy.

Condylomata lata: In moistened skin areas, the eroded papular syphilides have the tendency to coalesce and hypertrophy, forming elevated, vegetating, or papillomatous lesions, the condylomata lata. The most frequent localizations of condylomata lata are the perigenital and perianal area, axillae, submammary and umbilical areas (**Fig. 18.14**). Condylomata lata rarely appear in the oral cavity, usually at the corners of the mouth and the palate (**Fig. 18.15**). They appear as painless, slightly exophytic, multiple lesions with an irregular surface and are contagious.

Differential diagnosis

- Candidiasis
- Lichen planus
- Leukoplakia
- Aphthous ulcers
- Herpetic stomatitis
- Erythema multiforme
- Trauma
- Infectious mononucleosis
- A plethora of other oral lesions that may mimic secondary syphilis

Pathology

Dark-field microscopic examination and immunofluorescence for the detection of *T. pallidum* may be a helpful diagnostic tool. In addition, serologic tests (Venereal Disease Research Laboratory [VDRL], rapid plasma reagin [RPR], fluorescent treponemal antibody absorption [FTA-ABS], *T. pallidum* immobilization [TPI], *T. pallidum* hemagglutination assay [TPHA]) give more distinctive results in secondary syphilis.

Late syphilis

After a latency period of 2 to 10 years or more, untreated syphilis may progress to severe clinical manifestations of late syphilis. The main manifestations of late syphilis are mucocutaneous lesions, cardiovascular manifestations, central nervous system (CNS), and bone lesions. Late syphilis is rare in many Western countries nowadays. The oral lesions of late syphilis include gummas, atrophic glossitis, and interstitial glossitis.

Gummas: A gumma is a syphilitic granulomatous lesion that originates as a subcutaneous mass secondarily extending both to the epithelium and the deeper tissues. Gummas appear initially as painless elastic swellings that have a tendency to necrose, forming a characteristic stringy mass. A punched-out ulcer forms and finally heals, leaving a scar. The size varies from 1 to 10 cm. The sites of predilection are the legs, scalp, face, and chest (**Fig. 18.16**). Gummas are frequently located on the hard palate, which they may destroy and perforate (**Fig. 18.17**). The lesion may also involve the soft palate and rarely other oral regions.

Differential diagnosis

- Squamous cell carcinoma or other malignant tumors
- Leprosy
- Extranodal natural killer (NK)-/T-cell lymphoma, nasal type
- Other non-Hodgkin's lymphomas

Atrophic glossitis: The tongue is frequently involved in late syphilis. Clinically, there is atrophy of the filiform and fungiform papillae, and the dorsum becomes smooth and atrophic. Vasculitis ending in an obliterative endarteritis is the process of the underlying changes. Atrophic syphilitic glossitis may lead to the development of leukoplakia and squamous cell carcinoma (**Fig. 18.18**).

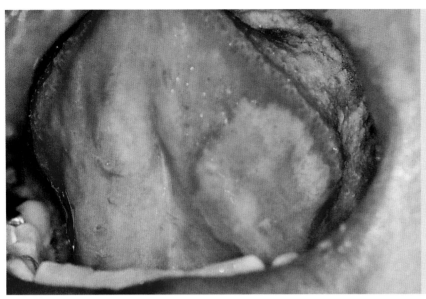

Fig. 18.4 Chancre on the ventrum of the tongue.

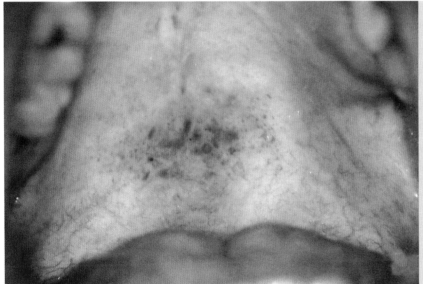

Fig. 18.5 Macular syphilides on the palate.

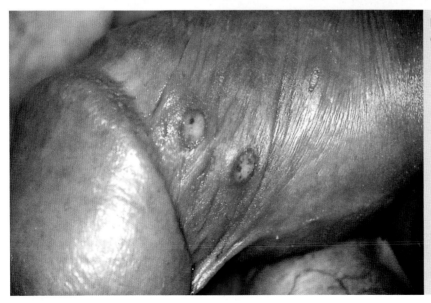

Fig. 18.6 Syphilitic mucous patches on the sulcus of the penis.

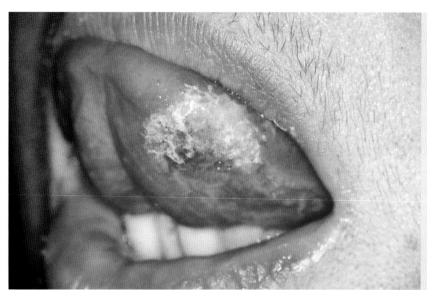

Fig. 18.7 Syphilitic mucous patches on the lateral border of the tongue.

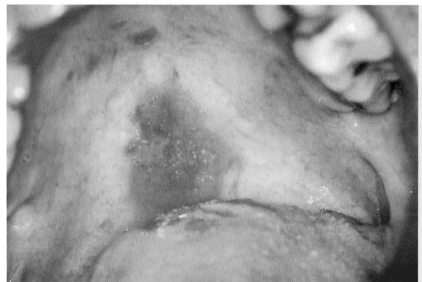

Fig. 18.8 Syphilitic mucous patches of the palate.

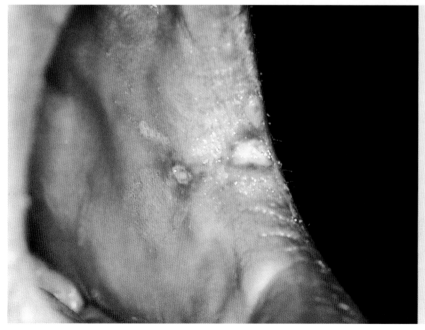

Fig. 18.9 Syphilitic mucous patches on the commissure.

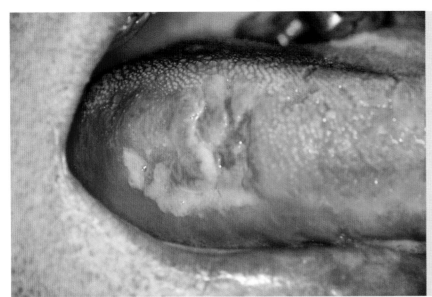

Fig. 18.10 Syphilitic papules and erosions on the tongue.

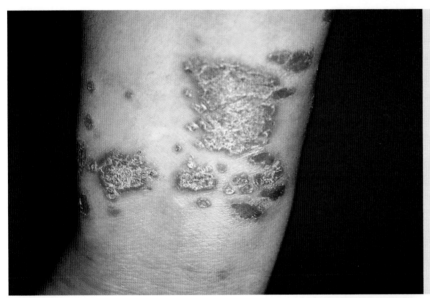

Fig. 18.11 Confluent plaque forming syphilitic papules on the skin.

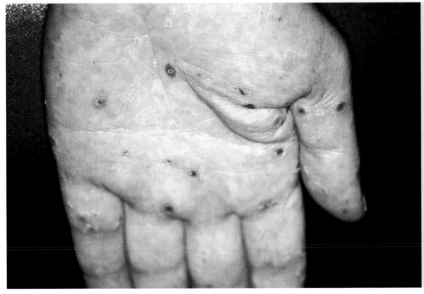

Fig. 18.12 Typical syphilitic papules on the skin of the palm.

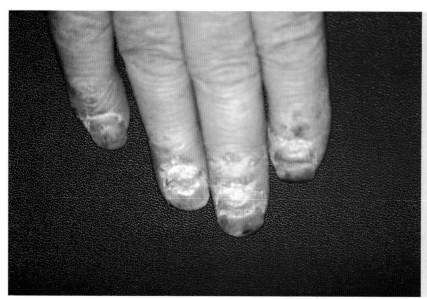

Fig. 18.13 Syphilitic paronychia.

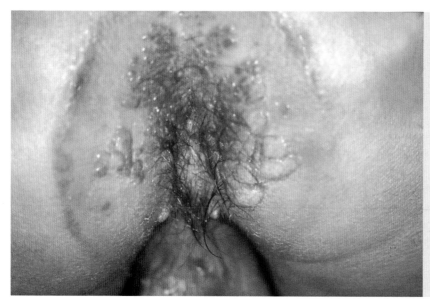

Fig. 18.14 Condylomata lata on the perianal region.

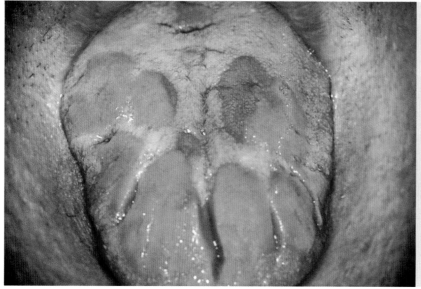

Fig. 18.15 Condyloma lata on the dorsum of the tongue.

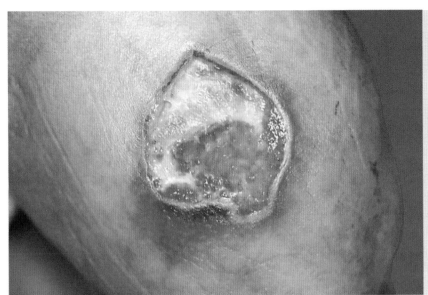

Fig. 18.16 Typical syphilitic gumma of the skin.

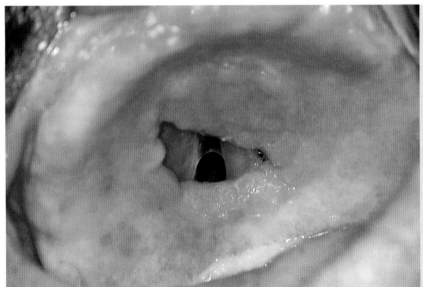

Fig. 18.17 Perforation of the palate by syphilitic gumma.

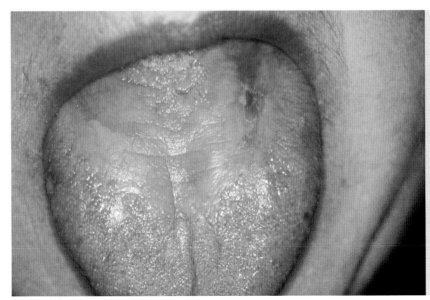

Fig. 18.18 Syphilitic atrophic glossitis.

Differential diagnosis

- Lichen planus, atrophic form
- Leukoplakia
- Plummer-Vinson syndrome
- Megaloblastic anemia

Interstitial glossitis: Late syphilis of the tongue may occur either as a solitary gumma or most commonly as a diffuse gummatous infiltration, which heals spontaneously, leading to interstitial glossitis. This is the result of contracture of the lingual musculature after the gumma has healed. The tongue appears smoothly lobular with irregular deep figures (**Fig. 18.19**). Leukoplakia and squamous cell carcinoma may be a complication.

Differential diagnosis

- Fissured tongue
- Amyloidosis
- Benign and malignant tumors

Treatment

Penicillin G is the treatment of choice for all stages of syphilis. The schedules and dosages are internationally established and depend on the stage of the disease. If penicillin allergy exists, erythromycin or cephalosporins may be administered. In primary and secondary syphilis as well as early latent syphilis (< 1 year in duration), a single intramuscular dose of 2.4 million units of benzathine penicillin is recommended, while for latent syphilis (> 1 year in duration), a dose of 2.4 million units weekly for 3 weeks is the suggested regimen. The treatment of syphilis should be left to appropriate specialists—as medication can vary between units and regions.

Congenital syphilis

Congenital (prenatal) syphilis reflects vertical transmission *in utero*. It is classified as *early* if the disease manifests before the age of 2 years, *late* if it becomes apparent after 2 years, and *stigmata*, which are developmental changes without active infection. The most common stigmata are high-arched palate, short mandible, rhagades at the commissures, saddle nose, frontal bossing, Hutchinson's teeth, and dysplastic molars. The dysplastic permanent incisors, along with interstitial keratitis and eighth nerve deafness, comprise the classic Hutchinson's triad, and are the most common findings of congenital syphilis. Clinically, the upper central permanent incisors are widely spaced and shorter than the lateral incisors. They are conical or barrel-shaped at the incisal edge and are usually smaller at the cervical margins (**Fig. 18.20**). Notched areas of the incisal edge may be present. Similar changes may exist in the lateral incisors and the teeth may be irregularly spaced. The permanent first molars may be dysplastic (*Moon's molars, Fournier's molars, mulberry molars*). Usually, the first lower molars are affected. Affected molars are narrower on their occlusal surfaces and have supernumerary cusps.

Gonococcal Stomatitis

Key points

- The most common sexually transmitted disease caused by the gram-negative diplococcus *Neisseria gonorrhoeae*.
- Primarily involves mucous membranes of genital tract, anus, and rectum.
- The pharynx and oral mucosa are less frequently affected.
- The microorganism is transmitted after direct sexual contact with an infected person.
- Currently, third-generation cephalosporins are the drugs of choice for gonococcal infection.

Introduction

Gonorrhea is a common infectious disease caused by the gram-negative diplococcus *N. gonorrhoeae*. It occurs at all ages and affects both sexes. Gonorrhea is sexually transmitted and involves the mucous membranes of the human genital tract, anal canal, pharynx, and rarely the oral mucosa. Systemic dissemination may cause signs and symptoms in many other organs. Gonococcal stomatitis and pharyngitis are the result of fellatio or cunillingus and are more common in prostitutes and homosexual men.

Clinical features

Gonococcal stomatitis is a rare disease without specific clinical signs. Clinically, the oral mucosa is red, inflamed, and the patient complains of itching and burning. Rarely, erosions covered with a whitish pseudomembrane may occur. The soft palate, buccal mucosa, and gingiva are more frequently affected (**Figs. 18.21, 18.22**). Gonococcal pharyngitis is more common than oral disease and can manifest as a sore throat, a diffuse or patchy erythema and edema, with or without tiny pustules on the tonsillar pillars and uvula. Notably, oral gonococcal infection may be asymptomatic. The clinical diagnosis should be confirmed by laboratory tests.

Differential diagnosis

- Streptococcal stomatitis
- Herpetic infection
- Herpangina
- Candidiasis
- Cinnamon contact stomatitis
- Infectious mononucleosis

Pathology

Identification of the microorganisms by Gram's stain, or culture, or molecular biological techniques establishes the definitive diagnosis.

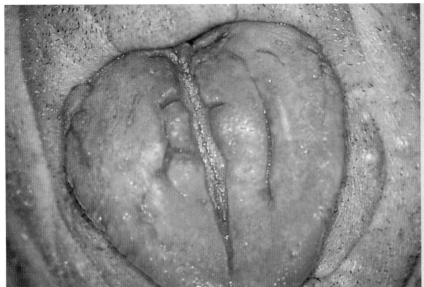

Fig. 18.19 Interstitial syphilitic glossitis.

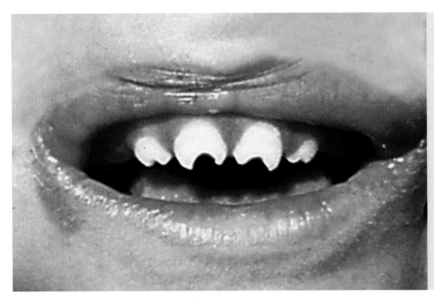

Fig. 18.20 Congenital syphilis, Hutchinson's teeth.

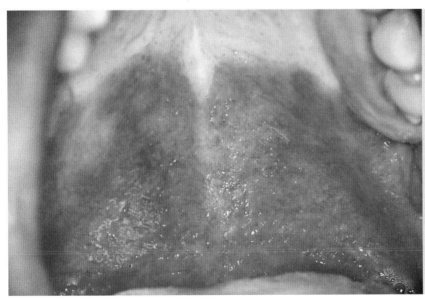

Fig. 18.21 Gonococcal stomatitis, intense redness of the mucous membrane of the palate and the uvula.

Treatment

Oral lesions are self-limited and colonization usually disappears within 3 months. Third-generation cephalosporins (e.g., ceftriaxone 125 mg injection in a single dose or ciprofloxacin, 500 mg as single dose or ofloxacin 400 mg as single dose) are the drugs of choice.

Chancroid

Key points
- Sexually transmitted disease caused by gram-negative, anaerobic bacterium *Haemophilus ducreyi*.
- The disease is common in Africa, Caribbean, and Southeast Asia, and rare in Europe.
- Chancroid clinically presents as acute genital ulcers and regional, inguinal lymphadenopathy.
- Oral lesions are very uncommon.

Introduction

Chancroid is an acute venereal disease caused by *H. ducreyi*, a gram-negative bacillus. The disease is rare in Europe and the United States and occurs most frequently in underdeveloped countries (Africa, Asia, Caribbean), especially in communities with poor hygiene. The disease is almost always sexually transmitted. Genital and perianal regions are most commonly affected.

Clinical features

Classically, chancroid is characterized by acute genital ulcers and painful inguinal lymphadenitis (**Fig. 18.23**). Oral lesions may occur after orogenital contact but are extremely rare. After an incubation period of 3 to 6 days, the disease begins as a small red papule or macule that soon becomes pustular and finally ulcerates. The ulcer is round or oval, 1 mm to 2 cm in diameter with slightly raised border and a soft base (**Fig. 18.24**). It is covered with a gray-whitish exudate and is surrounded by a red halo. It is painful and is usually accompanied by bilateral or unilateral lymphadenopathy. The lesions are not pathognomonic. The diagnosis should be confirmed by laboratory tests.

Differential diagnosis
- Aphthous ulcer
- Traumatic ulcer
- Primary and secondary syphilis

Pathology

Gram's stain of smears and culture in special culture media are necessary for accurate diagnosis.

Treatment

Azithromycin (e.g., 1 g in a single dose) or ciprofloxacin (e.g., 500 mg for 3 days) or erythromycin (e.g., 500 mg three times a day for 7 days) are the drugs of choice.

Donovanosis

Key points
- A rare, chronic, ulcerative bacterial infection caused by Calymmatobacterium (*Klebsiella*) granulomatis.
- The disease is most common in India, South Africa, New Guinea, and Australia.
- It is usually sexually transmitted.
- The glans penis, prepuce, frenulum and coronal sulcus, and the vulvar area are the more frequently affected sites.
- Extragenital locations, including oral lesions are rare.
- The demonstration of *Donovan bodies* in smear or biopsy specimens confirms the diagnosis.

Introduction

Donovanosis or granuloma inguinale is a rare, chronic, relapsing granulomatous, anogenital, bacterial infection due to gram-negative bacillus Calymmatobacterium (*Klebsiella*) granulomatis. The infection is usually sexually transmitted, although it may occur in sexually inactive individuals. Donovanosis is usually restricted in India, Indonesia, South Africa, New Guinea, Papua, and Australia. The lesions usually occur on the skin and mucous membranes of the genitalia or perineal region.

Clinical features

The incubation period ranges from 1 to 10 weeks or more. Clinically, the disease presents as a small, usually painless, papule or nodule. The lesions progressively expand forming a sharply demarcated ulcer, with a beefy-red granulomatous surface and a tendency for bleeding. The anogenital skin, the mucous membranes, and inguinal areas are most commonly affected. Extragenital involvements of the skin, bones, abdominal wall, larynx, pharynx, nose, and oral mucosa may rarely occur. The oral lesions may be primary or more frequently secondary of anogenital disease. Clinically, the oral lesions present as painful or painless chronic granulomatous ulceration or

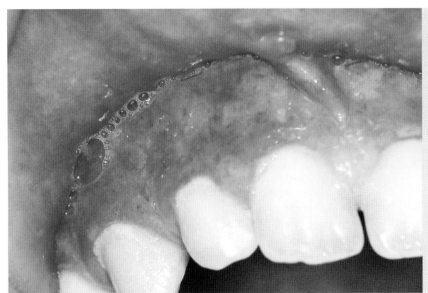

Fig. 18.22 Gonococcal stomatitis, redness, and erosions on the gingival and the alveolar mucosa.

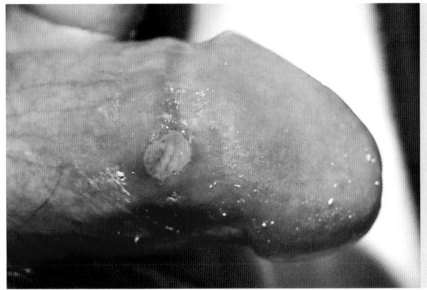

Fig. 18.23 Chancroid on the penis.

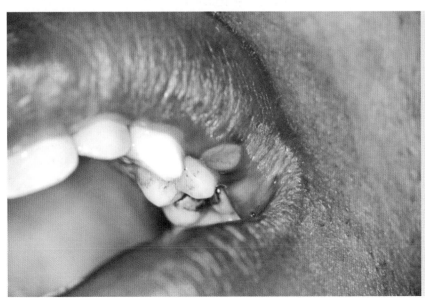

Fig. 18.24 Chancroid on the upper lip.

vegetating granulomatous swelling (**Fig. 18.25**). The gingiva, palate, and buccal mucosa are the sites of predilection.

The diagnosis of oral donovanosis is based on the history, the clinical features, and mainly on the laboratory tests.

Differential diagnosis

- Syphilis
- Chancroid
- Systemic mycoses
- Orofacial granulomatosis
- Pyostomatitis vegetans
- Crohn's disease
- Wegener's granulomatosis
- Tuberculosis
- Leishmaniasis

Pathology

The demonstration of *Donovan bodies* in tissue smear or biopsy specimen by Wright, Giemsa, and Leishman stains are necessary for definite diagnosis.

Treatment

The treatment of choice includes doxycycline (e.g., 100 mg orally twice daily), azithromycin (e.g., 1 g orally once a week), ciprofloxacin (e.g., 750 mg orally twice daily), erythromycin (e.g., 500 mg orally four times a day), or trimethoprim-sulfamethoxazole. All therapeutic regimens are for a minimum of 6 weeks.

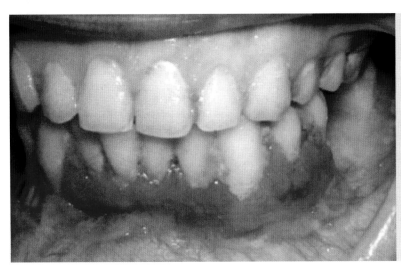

Fig. 18.25 Donovanosis, ulcerated red granulomatous swelling of the lower gingiva.

19 Fungal Infections

Candidiasis

Key points

- *Candida albicans,* which is part of the normal oral flora, is responsible for the majority of such diseases.
- Predisposing factors may be local or systemic.
- Oral mucosal candidiasis is classified into primary and secondary.
- The treatment of choice is the systemic use of azoles with excellent results.

Introduction

Candidiasis is the most frequent fungal infection and is caused by *C. albicans*, a fungus found in 20 to 50% of healthy people and is rarely caused by other strains (*Candida tropicalis, Candida glabrata, Candida krusei, Candida parapsilosis, Candida guilliermondii*). In healthy individuals, without any local predisposing factor, *C. albicans* causes no clinical manifestations. Predisposing factors for candidiasis include *local* ones, such as xerostomia, poor oral hygiene, chronic mucosal trauma, use of local antibiotics, chronic use of inhalational and topical steroids, radiotherapy to the head area, and *systemic* ones, such as iron deficiency anemia, diabetes mellitus, primary immunodeficiency, HIV infection and AIDS, leukemia and other malignancies, neutropenia, use of steroids and immunosuppressive medication, broad-spectrum antibiotics, hypoparathyroidism, cortical adrenal insufficiency, and other endocrine diseases. The newborns and infants are also particularly susceptible to candidiasis. Usually, candidiasis presents as a localized and superficially spreading infection; however, in immunocompromised and neutropenic patients, it has the potential to spread in a systemic fashion with significant mortality.

Oral mucosal candidiasis presents with a wide spectrum of clinical manifestations. It is classified into *primary*, including lesions exclusively in the mouth and the perioral area, and *secondary*, which includes the oral manifestations of the systemic mucocutaneous fungal infections. The diagnosis is mainly based on the history and clinical features with further investigations required only for difficult cases.

Primary Candidiasis

Primary oral candidiasis includes the following clinical varieties:

a. *Pseudomembranous candidiasis* is the most common form of the disease and is usually acute, but chronic involvement may also rarely occur. Clinically, it is characterized by creamy white or whitish-yellow, slightly elevated spots or plaques, which usually can be easily detached, leaving a raw underlying reddish or normal surface. These lesions may be localized or generalized and may appear at any oral site, but more frequently on the buccal mucosa, the tongue, and the soft and hard palates (**Figs. 19.1, 19.2**). Subjective complaints include xerostomia, a slight burning sensation, and difficulty in swallowing. The diagnosis is usually based on the clinical features.

b. *Erythematous candidiasis* is also classified as acute or chronic. It is highly prevalent in HIV-infected individuals (not receiving antiretroviral therapy [ART]), but may rarely be observed in patients receiving broad-spectrum antibiotics, corticosteroids, or other immunosuppressive agents. Clinically, it presents as erythematous patches that have a predilection for the palate (**Fig. 19.3**) and the dorsal surface of the tongue (**Fig. 19.4**). The patients may describe a burning sensation.

c. *Nodular or plaque-like candidiasis* is a rare, chronic form of candidiasis that is characterized by deep infiltration of the oral tissues by fungal hyphae and epithelial hyperplasia. Clinically, it presents as white, firm, and raised plaques occasionally surrounded by erythema (**Fig. 19.5**). The lesions may persist for years, do not detach, and are usually located on the tongue and the commissures. It has been suggested that this type of candidiasis predisposes to squamous cell carcinoma and can therefore be classified as a precancerous lesion.

d. *Papillary hyperplasia of the palate* is a rare chronic form of candidiasis that usually affects people with a high-arched palate who do not wear dentures. Clinically, multiple, small, spherical nodules appear on the palate, which are usually red (**Fig. 19.6**). White lesions might also be observed. This lesion should not be confused with denture stomatitis, which appears in people wearing dentures.

e. *Lesions contaminated with Candida*: The lesions do not have *C. albicans* as their sole etiologic factor, but are caused by a combination of factors. Angular cheilitis (**Fig. 19.7**), median rhomboid glossitis (**Fig. 19.8**), and denture-induced stomatitis (**Fig. 19.9**) are included in this group.

Secondary Candidiasis

Secondary candidiasis includes the following two clinical types:

a. *Chronic mucocutaneous candidiasis*: This form of candidiasis is a heterogeneous group of clinical syndromes that are characterized by chronic lesions of the skin, nails, and mucosae. It usually appears in childhood and is often associated with numerous immunologic abnormalities, predominantly cell-mediated immunity and rarely of humoral immunity. This type mostly appears sporadically, but there have been families reported with autosomal recessive pattern of inheritance. Clinically, the early oral lesions are similar to those seen in pseudomembranous candidiasis, but later white plaques appear that are similar to the lesions of chronic nodular candidiasis. Characteristically, the lesions

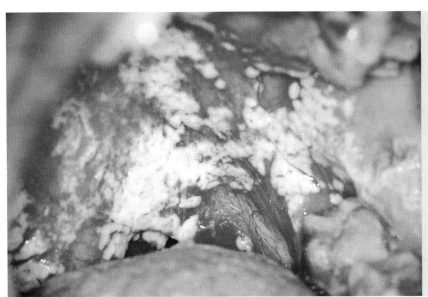

Fig. 19.1 Pseudomembranous candidiasis on the palate.

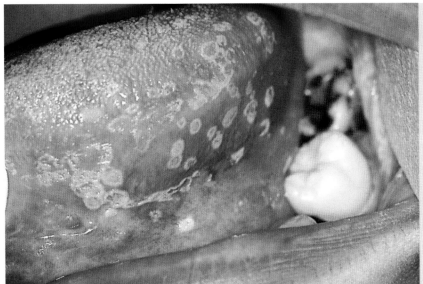

Fig. 19.2 Pseudomembranous candidiasis on the lateral and ventral aspects of the tongue.

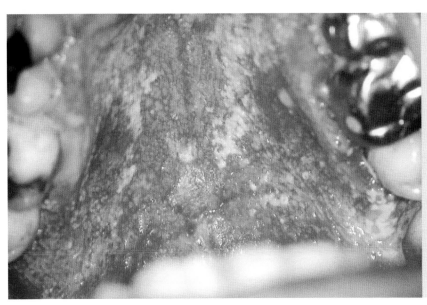

Fig. 19.3 Erythematous candidiasis on the palate.

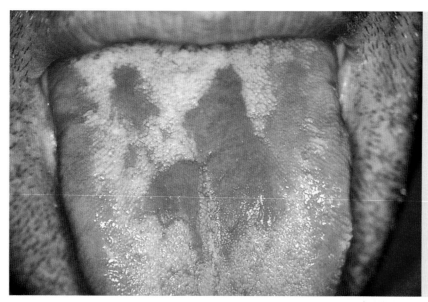

Fig. 19.4 Erythematous candidiasis on the dorsum of the tongue.

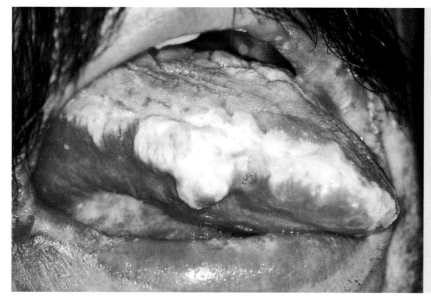

Fig. 19.5 Hyperplastic candidiasis on the lateral border of the tongue.

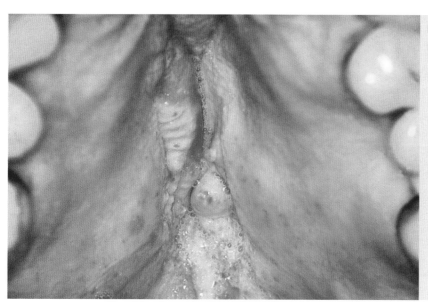

Fig. 19.6 Candidiasis, papillary hyperplasia of the palate.

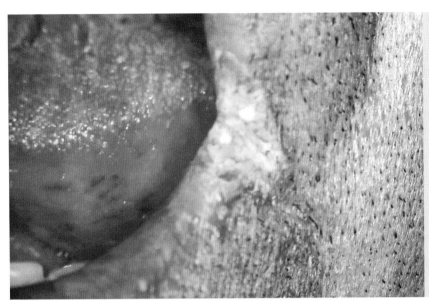

Fig. 19.7 Angular cheilitis contaminated with Candida albicans.

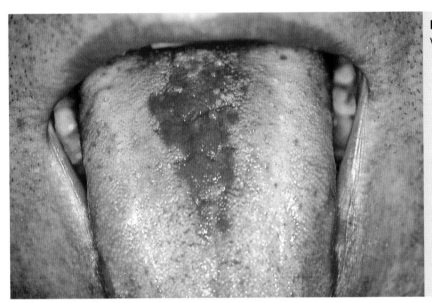

Fig. 19.8 Median rhomboid glossitis with Candida albicans presence.

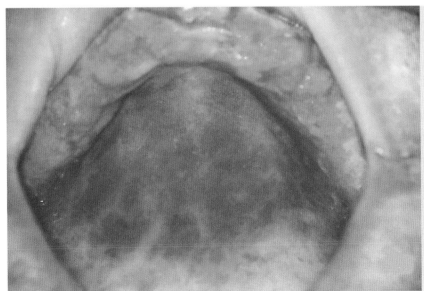

Fig. 19.9 Denture-induced stomatitis with participation of Candida albicans.

are generalized, with a predilection for the buccal mucosa, commissures, tongue, palate, and lips, and may extend to the oropharynx and esophagus (**Figs. 19.10, 19.11**). Cutaneous and nail involvement in varying degrees of severity are associated with the oral lesions (**Fig. 19.12**).

b. *Candida-endocrinopathy syndrome*: This is a unique form of chronic mucocutaneous candidiasis that is accompanied by endocrinopathies, such as hypoparathyroidism, hypoadrenalism, hypothyroidism, or even pancreatic and ovarian hypofunction. Oral manifestations usually arise at the age of 4 to 6 years and then deteriorate, whereas the endocrinopathy may be delayed in onset. Clinically, the oral, skin, and nail lesions are similar to those seen in chronic mucocutaneous candidiasis. Initially, there can be adherent white irregular plaques, but eventually severe atrophic lesions and erosions may be noticed (**Figs. 19.13, 19.14**). Conjunctivitis and alopecia of eyebrows can also be observed (**Fig. 19.15**).

c. The diagnosis of most forms of candidiasis is based on the clinical features. However, occasionally the diagnosis should be confirmed by a smear or culture examination or even histologically.

Differential diagnosis

- Leukoplakia
- Hairy leukoplakia
- Lichen planus
- Cinnamon contact stomatitis
- Chronic biting
- Leukoedema
- Oral epitheliolysis
- Mucous patches of secondary syphilis
- White sponge nevus
- Discoid lupus erythematosus
- Erythroplakia
- Fellatio
- Chemical or thermal burns

Pathology

Direct microscopic examination of smears and microbiological culture are of limited diagnostic use. In chronic forms, as the nodular candidiasis, histopathologic examination with periodic acid-Schiff (PAS) stain shows hyphae of *Candida* within the superficial layer of the epithelium.

Treatment

Identification and possible resolution of local or systemic causative factors are essential for the treatment of candidal infection. Nystatin and miconazole are the drugs of choice for topical use. Topical treatment is usually performed to infants and children. Triazoles (e.g., fluconazole, itraconazole) are useful systemic agents. The dosage and duration of treatment largely depends on the type of candidiasis and the presence of predisposing factors, e.g., a dose of 100 to 200 mg/d for 7 to 14 days after clinical resolution of fluconazole or itraconazole is adequate in most types of candidiasis in patients with intact immunity. In chronic forms of candidiasis and in immunocompromised patients (independent of the candidiasis type), the duration of treatment might reach 2 to 4 months. In patients with hematologic malignancies, AIDS, and transplant patients, oral solutions may ensure good absorption from the gastrointestinal tract, as it is more effective. Prior to treatment of any type of candidiasis, the oral hygiene levels have to be improved and any local or systemic predisposing factors to be dealt with.

Histoplasmosis

Key points

- *Histoplasma capsulatum* is the cause.
- Endemic in some areas with particularly warm and humid climates.
- Transmitted through inhalation of the fungus spores.
- Oral and cutaneous manifestations most commonly result from disseminated disease.

Introduction

Histoplasmosis is a systemic fungal disease caused by the dimorphic fungus *H. capsulatum*. It is transmitted through inhalation of spores or rarely by direct skin inoculation. Birds, fowl, and even bats are significant reservoirs for *H. capsulatum*. The disease is endemic in the United States, in the Mississippi, Ohio River Valleys, and Canada, where approximately 80 to 90% of the adult population may exhibit positive histoplasmin skin testing. Other areas include countries of the South and Central America, Africa, and Asia, while it is rare in European countries. An increased incidence of histoplasmosis has been reported in HIV-infected patients and other immunocompromised patients.

Clinically, histoplasmosis is classified into *acute pulmonary* and *chronic pulmonary*, *disseminated* and *primary cutaneous histoplasmosis*. Oral manifestations usually arise with disseminated disease.

Clinical features

Oral and skin lesions of histoplasmosis are nonspecific making the diagnosis difficult on clinical examination. In chronic disseminated disease, oral lesions occur in approximately 35 to 45% of cases and are clinically characterized by irregular and indurated painful ulceration with a verrucous surface. Rarely, nodules can be observed on the palate, gingiva, tongue, and the lips (**Figs. 19.16, 19.17**). Ipsilateral lymphadenopathy is also present. Constitutional symptoms such as persistent low-grade fever, dyspnea, retrosternal pain, spleen and liver enlargement, lymphadenopathy, and endocrinopathy are common. The clinical diagnosis should be confirmed by a biopsy and histologic examination.

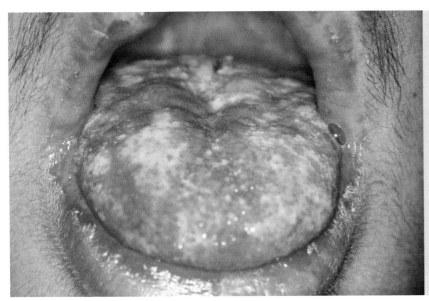

Fig. 19.10 Chronic mucocutaneous candidiasis with extensive lesions on the tongue.

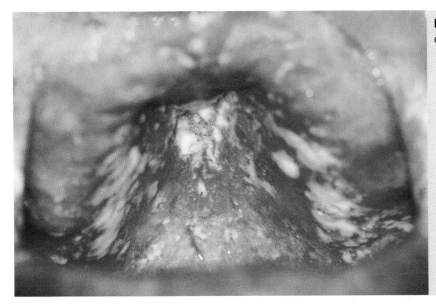

Fig. 19.11 Chronic mucocutaneous candidiasis, lesions on the palate.

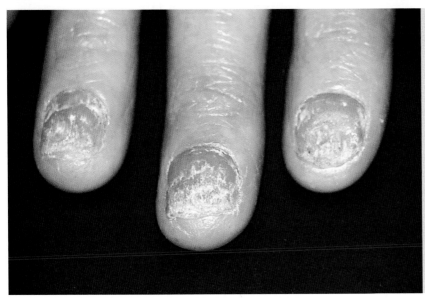

Fig. 19.12 Chronic mucocutaneous candidiasis, lesions on the nails.

Differential diagnosis

- Other systemic fungal infections with oral manifestations
- Major aphthous ulcers
- Tuberculosis
- Syphilis
- Wegener's granulomatosis
- Non-Hodgkin's lymphoma
- Squamous cell carcinoma
- Leishmaniasis

Pathology

Microscopically, multiple histiocytes and giant cells are observed with the characteristic intracellular yeast forms surrounded by a clear rim. For better identification of *H. capsulatum*, tissue should be stained with PAS or Grocott's methenamine silver (GMS). Highly sensitive and specific polymerase chain reaction (PCR)-based assays may be used to detect histoplasmosis in blood and tissue.

Treatment

First line of treatment in severe cases is parenteral administration of amphotericin B (e.g., 1 mg/kg/d for 2–3 weeks), followed by itraconazole per os (e.g., 200–400 mg/d) for 6 to 12 months. In milder forms, the administration of itraconazole or ketoconazole alone is sufficient. Recently, successful treatment with voriconazole or posaconazole has been reported.

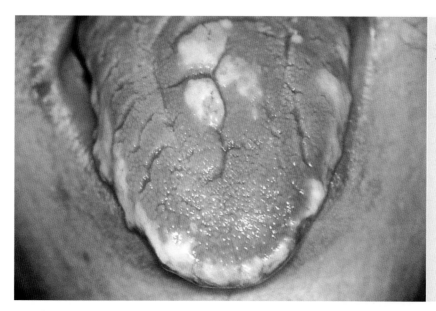

Fig. 19.13 Candida endocrinopathy syndrome, multifocal lesions on the tongue.

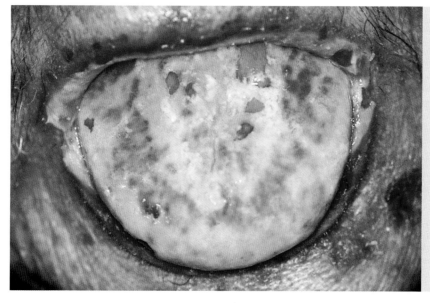

Fig. 19.14 Candida endocrinopathy syndrome, generalized lesions on the tongue and the lips.

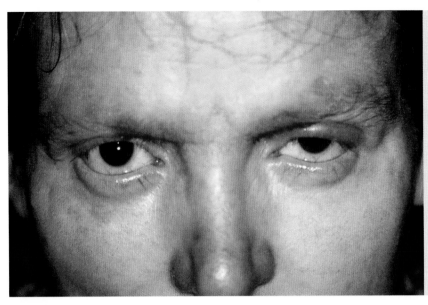

Fig. 19.15 Candida endocrinopathy syndrome, alopecia of the eyebrows, and blepharitis.

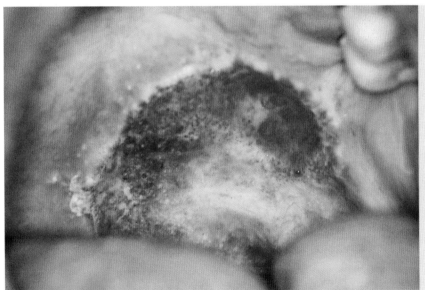

Fig. 19.16 Histoplasmosis on the palate.

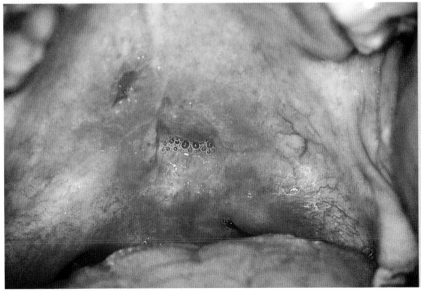

Fig. 19.17 Histoplasmosis on the palate, two small ulcers are noticed.

Blastomycosis

Key points

- The dimorphic fungus *Blastomyces dermatitidis* is the cause.
- Endemic in certain areas of North America.
- The lungs are the first point of entry as the fungus is inhaled.
- The clinical manifestations can be divided into *pulmonary* and *extrapulmonary*.
- The mouth is affected in approximately 20 to 25% of the cases.

Introduction

Blastomycosis is a rare, systemic, fungal infection caused by the dimorphic fungus *B. dermatitidis*. It is endemic in certain areas of North America, whereas sporadic cases have been reported in South America, India, and Africa. Humans can be infected when contaminated soil is disturbed and spores are inhaled. The clinical manifestations can be *pulmonary* and *extrapulmonary*. The main extrapulmonary involvement is the skin. Other extrapulmonary manifestations are less common and include osseous, genitourinary, central nervous system, and other sites.

In approximately 20 to 25% of patients, oral or nasal mucosal lesions occur. These are caused either from direct fungal inoculation and are considered primary, or from spread of pulmonary disease and are then considered secondary.

Clinical features

Clinically, oral blastomycosis presents as solitary or multiple ulcers with a slightly verrucous and irregular surface and thin borders that mimic squamous cell carcinoma. The most commonly oral affected sites are the palate, tongue, lips, and the gingiva (**Fig. 19.18**). The pulmonary disease mimics tuberculosis, manifests with pyrexia, weight loss, nocturnal sweats, and a persistent cough. The cutaneous lesions can be solitary or multiple and appear well-circumscribed papulopustular and verrucous plaques with scale crust. Central ulceration may occur and mimic pyoderma gangrenosum. The clinical diagnosis should be confirmed by histologic examination.

Differential diagnosis

- Squamous cell carcinoma
- Tuberculous chancre
- Syphilitic chancre
- Other systemic fungal infections

Pathology

Microscopically, oral and skin lesions reveal a mixed inflammatory infiltrate with clusters of polymorphonuclear leukocytes and granulomas that have a characteristic broad base (*broad-based budding*) and contain round, fungal hyphae. The presence of pseudoepitheliomatous hyperplasia can mimic squamous cell carcinoma. The detection of the fungus is easier with special stains such as PAS or the GMS. Culture can also be helpful in diagnosis.

Treatment

The treatment of choice is itraconazole (e.g., 200–400 mg/d for 3–6 months), alternatively, fluconazole (e.g., 400–800 mg/d). Voriconazole can also be used. In more severe cases and in immunocompromised patients, parenteral liposomal amphotericin B is administered either alone or in combination with itraconazole or fluconazole.

Paracoccidioidomycosis

Key points

- The dimorphic fungus *Paracoccidioides brasiliensis* is the cause.
- Endemic in Central and South America.
- Transmitted by spore inhalation.
- The lungs, skin, mucosae, gastrointestinal tract, adrenals, spleen, and the lymph nodes are most frequently affected.
- Oral lesions are common.

Introduction

Paracoccidioidomycosis or South American blastomycosis is a rare, systemic, fungal infection caused by the dimorphic fungus *P. brasiliensis*. In most cases, infection occurs by inhalation of the conidia from the environment. It is endemic to South and Central America and mainly affects farmers. The disease starts usually from the lungs and can be spread to the lymph nodes, adrenals, skin, mucosae, and gastrointestinal tract.

Clinical features

Clinically, paracoccidioidomycosis is characterized by weight loss, fever, dyspnea, cough, lymph node enlargement, skin rash and ulcers of the nose, larynx, oropharynx, and oral cavity. Clinically, oral lesions usually present as a painful irregular ulcer with a granulomatous surface. The most commonly affected sites are the palate, alveolar mucosa, gingiva, and tongue (**Figs. 19.19, 19.20**). If untreated, perforation of the hard palate may occur in severe cases. A rare clinical presentation is that of primary mucocutaneous form with oral and perioral distribution due to trauma from chewing contaminated sticks and leaves. The clinical diagnosis should be confirmed by histology.

Differential diagnosis

- Mucocutaneous leishmaniasis
- Tuberculosis
- Sarcoidosis
- Syphilis
- Wegener's granulomatosis
- Squamous cell carcinoma
- Nasal natural killer (NK)-T non-Hodgkin's lymphoma
- Necrotizing sialadenometaplasia
- Other systemic mycoses that affect the mouth

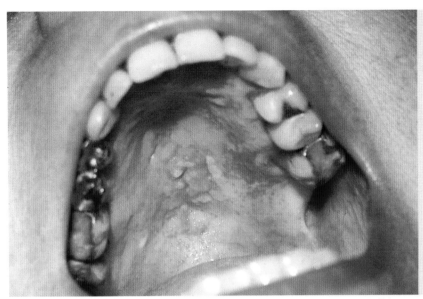

Fig. 19.18 Blastomycosis, ulcers on the palate.

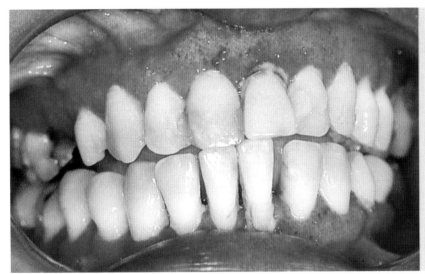

Fig. 19.19 Paracoccidioidomycosis, enlargement and ulceration on the gingiva.

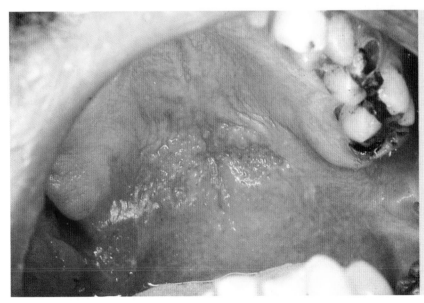

Fig. 19.20 Paracoccidioidomycosis, ulcer on the palate.

Pathology

Histopathologic examination is required for the final diagnosis. Microscopically, pseudoepitheliomatous hyperplasia and ulceration of the epithelium are observed. In the underlying connective tissue, there is prominent granulomatous inflammatory reaction. Yeast forms are found within and outside of multinucleated giant cells and the macrophages. PAS and GMS stains are the best choice for the detection of the organism.

Treatment

First line of treatment is itraconazole (e.g., 200–400 mg/d for 3–6 months). Alternatively, ketoconazole can be used (e.g., 200–400 mg/d for 6–12 months). Finally, in serious disseminated disease, parenteral liposomal amphotericin B is recommended.

Mucormycosis

Key points

- An opportunistic, fungal infection caused by the *Zygomycetes* group of microorganisms and mainly the strains *of Mucor, Rhizopus*, and *Absidia*.
- Main predisposing factors are primary or secondary immunodeficiency and poorly controlled diabetes mellitus.
- Five major clinical forms are *rhino-orbitocerebral, pulmonary, gastrointestinal, cutaneous*, and *disseminated*.
- The mouth is commonly involved in the rhino-orbitocerebral type.
- The prognosis is usually poor.

Introduction

Mucormycosis or zygomycosis is a rare, often fatal, acute opportunistic fungal infection. Fungi of the family Mucoraceae, mainly *Mucor, Rhizopus*, and *Absidia* strains are the cause of the disease. It usually affects debilitated individuals. The most common predisposing condition is poorly controlled diabetes mellitus with ketoacidosis as well as hematologic malignancies, burns, malnutrition, uremia, liver cirrhosis, HIV disease, organ transplantation, cancer chemotherapy, and immunosuppression. The fungus is acquired from the environment through spore inhalation and characteristically erodes arteries, causing thrombosis, ischemia, and finally necrosis of the surrounding tissues.

Clinical features

There are five major clinical forms: *rhino-orbitocerebral, pulmonary, gastrointestinal, cutaneous*, and *disseminated*. The rhino-orbitocerebral form is the most common accounting for 40 to 70% of all cases. Clinically, the disease is characterized by low-grade fever, headache, malaise, sinus pain, bloody nasal discharge, periorbital or perinasal swelling and edema, ptosis of the eyelid, extraocular muscle paresis, vision disturbances, facial nerve palsy and progressive lethargy, and eventually death. Palatal necrotic ulceration are the most characteristic oral lesions. The ulcer is sharply demarcated with a characteristic black necrotic eschar while the bone is exposed. Eventually, the soft and hard tissue destruction leads to perforation of the palate, tooth loss, and collapse of the nasal septum (**Figs. 19.21–19.23**). The mucosa surrounding the ulcer is usually thickened. Orbital and intracranial invasion is a common complication. Early recognition and diagnosis of the disease are crucial for survival. The clinical diagnosis should be confirmed with histology and culture.

Differential diagnosis

- Nasal NK-T non-Hodgkin's lymphoma
- Wegener's granulomatosis
- Syphilitic chancre
- Agranulocytosis
- Malignancies
- Aspergillosis
- Other systemic mycoses that affect the mouth

Pathology

Histopathologic examination reveals broad ribbon-like *Rhizopus* hyphae within the necrotic tissues. Suppuration and necrosis as well as blood vessel invasion by the fungi are common. PAS staining is helpful for the detection of the fungus.

Treatment

Intravenous administration of liposomal amphotericin B and surgical debridement of all the necrotic tissues are the first line of treatment. Posaconazole is currently considered as a second-line drug. Identification and correction of underlying predisposing conditions is also important.

Aspergillosis

Key points

- An opportunistic, fungal infection caused by *Aspergillus*, especially by the strains *Aspergillus fumigatus* and *Aspergillus flavus*.
- Predisposing factors are primary and secondary immunodeficiencies, burn, surgical wounds.
- Five clinical types of aspergillosis are recognized.
- Intraorally, atypical ulceration is observed with a characteristic yellow-black surface.

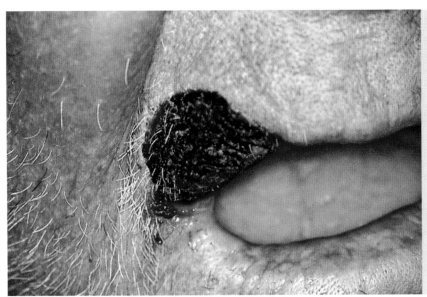

Fig. 19.21 Mucormycosis, early lesion on the upper lip.

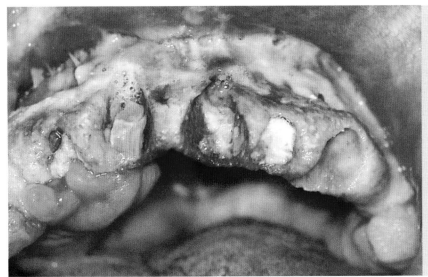

Fig. 19.22 Mucormycosis, established lesions, and extensive destruction of soft and hard tissues.

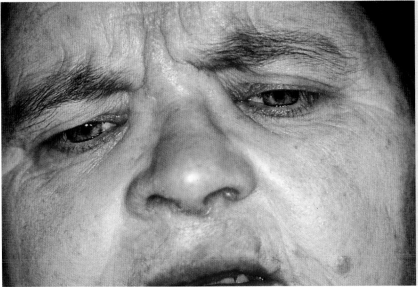

Fig. 19.23 Mucormycosis, collapse of the nasal septum in the patient of **Fig. 19.22**.

Introduction

Aspergillosis is an opportunistic fungal infection, with a broad spectrum of clinical manifestations. *Aspergillus flavus* and *A. fumigatus* are the main pathogenic species implicated. The disease is transmitted by inhalation of spores from the soil, water, organic debris, decaying vegetation, and air-conditioning equipment.

Five types of aspergillosis are recognized: *allergic bronchopulmonary, aspergilloma (fungus balls), invasive, chronic necrotizing pulmonary*, and *cutaneous*. The most common form is invasive pulmonary aspergillosis, which is characterized by high mortality. The most frequent predisposing factors include neutropenia, organ transplantation, hematologic malignancies, AIDS, high-dose steroids, and immunosuppressives. The fungus extends through the epithelial cells eventually invading the vascular endothelial cells, causing necrosis.

Clinical features

The clinical manifestations of invasive pulmonary aspergillosis are fever, dyspnea, dry cough, retrosternal and pleuritic pain, and tachycardia. Oral lesions present as irregular ulcerations with a tendency to spread with a characteristic yellowish-black surface formed by necrotic tissues (**Fig. 19.24**). The lesions are most frequently localized in the palate, gingiva, tongue, and the lips and may be the first clinical signs of the disease. Rarely, the disease begins in the oral cavity following a tooth extraction or endodontic therapy and may spread to the surrounding tissues. Perforation of the nasal septum may be observed (**Figs. 19.25, 19.26**). The clinical diagnosis should be confirmed with appropriate laboratory tests.

Differential diagnosis

- Mucormycosis
- Nasal NK-T non-Hodgkin's lymphoma
- Wegener's granulomatosis
- Agranulocytosis
- Leukemia
- Tuberculosis
- Malignancies
- Other systemic mycoses that affect the mouth

Pathology

The histopathologic examination of lesions demonstrates septate hyphae with 45-degree branching, especially with PAS and GMS staining. Computed tomography (CT) scan of the chest and microbiological culture from biopsy material can also be helpful toward diagnosis.

Treatment

Voriconazole and posaconazole are the drugs of choice. Itraconazole (e.g., 200–400 mg/d for 1–4 months, depending on the type and gravity of the disease) is also the first line of treatment. Alternatively, intravenous amphotericin B can be administered in severe systemic infection.

Cryptococcosis

Key points

- An opportunistic infection caused by *Cryptococcus neoformans*.
- Predisposing factors are primary and secondary immunodeficiencies.
- The disease is classified into *pulmonary* and *disseminated*.
- The mouth is rarely affected, mainly in disseminated disease.

Introduction

Cryptococcosis is a rare, chronic fungal disease caused by *C. neoformans*. It is usually transmitted through airborne fungal spores, usually from dead leaves, stored grain, bird droppings (e.g., pigeons), and compost piles. It is an opportunistically pathogenic microorganism that becomes aggressive in immunocompromised patients. This was the reason behind the association of HIV infection. Other predisposing conditions include hematologic malignancies, organ transplants, poorly controlled diabetes mellitus, and immunosuppressive treatment. The disease is classified into *pulmonary* (which is the most common form) and *disseminated*.

Clinical features

In the pulmonary disease, the signs and symptoms include cough, low-grade fever, dyspnea, sternal pain, hemoptysis, nocturnal sweats, and weight loss. However, most of the times the signs and symptoms are mild and can go undetected. The disseminated form usually involves the central nervous system (CNS) followed by bone, skin, genitourinary tract, lymph nodes, liver, spleen, adrenals, and, rarely, the oral mucosa. Cutaneous lesions occur in approximately 15% of patients as papules and nodules that proceed to ulcerate (**Fig. 19.27**). The oral mucosa is rarely affected with chronic ulceration that can be indurated and tender on palpation (**Fig. 19.28**). The tongue, palate, gingiva, and tooth socket after extraction are the most common sites of involvement. Apart from the history and clinical features, the diagnosis is based on the histopathologic examination.

Differential diagnosis

- Squamous cell carcinoma
- Minor salivary gland adenocarcinoma
- Tuberculosis
- Eosinophilic ulcer
- Non-Hodgkin's lymphoma
- Histoplasmosis
- Aspergillosis
- Mucormycosis
- Leishmaniasis

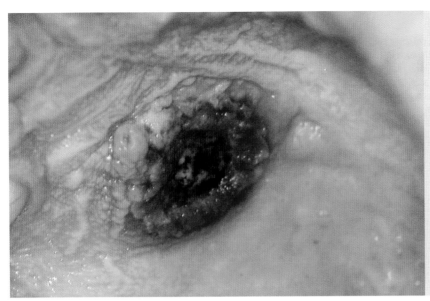

Fig. 19.24 Aspergillosis, ulceration on the palate.

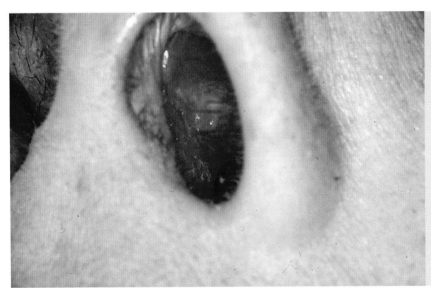

Fig. 19.25 Aspergillosis, prominent erythema and ulceration of the nasal septum mucosa.

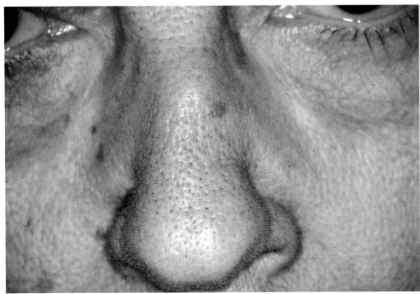

Fig. 19.26 Aspergillosis, nasal disfigurement due to perforation and destruction of the nasal septum.

Pathology

Histopathologic examination is the most reliable test for the final diagnosis. Granulomatous inflammatory reaction of the underlying corium can be seen microscopically, where the fungal hyphae can be detected with special stains such as PAS, Alcian blue, and GMS staining. Culture and detection of cryptococcal antigen in serum or in cerebrospinal fluid (CSF) can also be useful.

Treatment

Systemic amphotericin B parenterally (e.g., 0.5–1 mg/kg/d) which can be combined with 5-fluorocytosine (e.g., 150 mg/kg/d) is the first line of treatment. This regimen should be taken for at least 2 weeks, followed by fluconazole per os (e.g., 400 mg/d) for 6 to 8 weeks. Alternatively, fluconazole (e.g., 20–30 mg/kg/d) or itraconazole (e.g., 200–400 mg/d) can be given. Third-generation triazoles such as posaconazole and voriconazole seem to be effective in treating cryptococcosis.

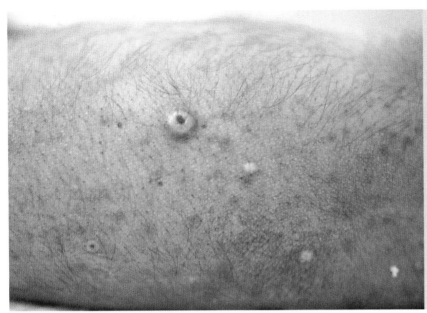

Fig. 19.27 Cryptococcosis, cutaneous nodules.

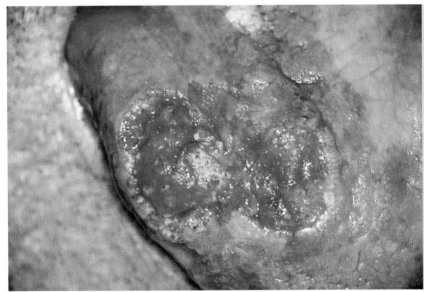

Fig. 19.28 Cryptococcosis, ulceration on the dorsum of the tongue.

20 Protozoal and Parasitic Infections

Leishmaniasis

Key points

- A chronic, parasitic disease where the responsible microorganisms are found within phagolysosomes of mononuclear phagocytes.
- Endemic in the Mediterranean basin, North America, and parts of Africa and Asia.
- Clinically, leishmaniasis is divided into four clinical subtypes: cutaneous, mucocutaneous, diffuse cutaneous, and visceral.
- The disease is rare in the mouth.

Introduction

Leishmaniasis is a parasitic infection with a broad spectrum of clinical manifestations, that is caused by different strains of *Leishmania* protozoan parasites. Clinically, leishmaniasis is divided into four clinical subtypes: (a) *cutaneous* or *Oriental sore* is the most common form of the disease caused by *Leishmania tropica*, (b) *mucocutaneous* caused by *Leishmania braziliensis*, (c) *diffuse cutaneous* by *Leishmania amazonensis*, and (d) *visceral* (*kala-azar*) which is the most serious form of the disease, caused by *Leishmania donovani*. Classification by geographic occurrence divides leishmaniasis into two major groups: 1. *Old world* leishmaniasis, caused by *Leishmania* species found in Africa, Asia, the Middle East, the Mediterranean, and India; 2. *New world* leishmaniasis, caused by *Leishmania* species found in Central and South America. *Leishmania tropica* is endemic in urban areas. In Greece, the most common type is cutaneous leishmaniasis that is endemic in Creta, Euboea, and the rest of the islands. It is transmitted by the bite of infected sandflies of the *Phlebotomus* and *Lutzomyia* species. Major reservoirs of the parasite are humans and dogs. Leishmaniasis has been observed in HIV-infected patients.

Clinical features

The clinical manifestations of cutaneous leishmaniasis usually occur on the face and other exposed parts of the body, but are very rare in the mouth.

Initially, at the inoculation site of the parasite, a small papule is formed of approximately 3 to 4 mm in diameter. This eventually develops into a nodule or tubercle of red or brown-red color which then ulcerates (**Figs. 20.1, 20.2**). A brown-gray crust eventually covers the ulcer, and the surrounding tissues are inflamed. The ulceration has an irregular shape and can grow much bigger, accompanied by mild pain. The lips and commissures are the most frequently involved sites in the oral and perioral area (**Fig. 20.3**). Mucosal leishmaniasis refers to oral and nasal lesions not preceded or accompanied by cutaneous lesions. The diagnosis is based on the history, the clinical features, but should be confirmed by special tests.

Differential diagnosis

- Basal cell carcinoma
- Squamous cell carcinoma
- Insect bite
- Furuncle
- Erysipelas
- Tuberculosis
- Sarcoidosis
- Syphilis
- Systemic fungal infections
- Non-Hodgkin's lymphoma

Pathology

Isolation and culture of the parasite from infected tissue is performed following a biopsy. Histologically, cutaneous and oral mucosa lesions exhibit areas of ulceration, pseudoepitheliomatous hyperplasia, and mixed inflammatory infiltrate consists of lymphocytes, plasma cells, neutrophils, and histiocytes. Amastigotes of the parasite are found within macrophages. Giemsa, Wright, and Feulgen stains are used to demonstrate the parasite in smears and tissue. The skin reaction test (*Leishman reaction*) has been an important diagnostic tool (positive in upto 90% of the cases).

Treatment

First-line treatment for cutaneous leishmaniasis is parenteral pentavalent antimonials (meglumine 20 mg/kg/d for 20 days or sodium stibogluconate 20 mg/kg/d for 20 days or miltefosine 2.5 mg/g/d PO for 28 days). Alternative treatments include pentamidine, fluconazole, and liposomal amphotericin B.

Oral Myiasis

Key points

- Infestation of the oral mucosa by fly larvae.
- Usually, occurs in tropical and subtropical countries and uncommonly in Europe.
- Two main types are *wound* and *furuncular*.
- The nose and skin might be involved but very rarely the mouth.
- The diagnosis is clinical and aided by ultrasound.

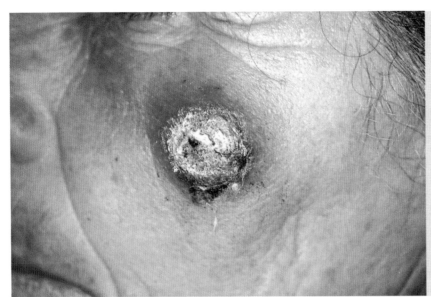

Fig. 20.1 Leishmaniasis of the face.

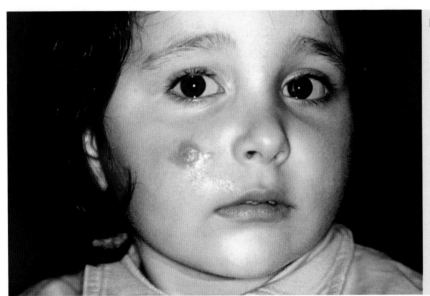

Fig. 20.2 Leishmaniasis of the face.

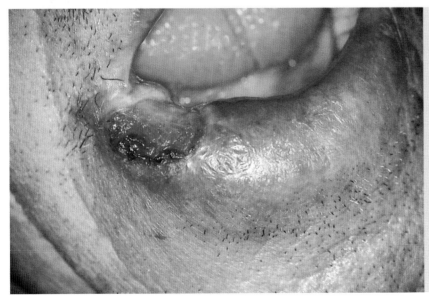

Fig. 20.3 Leishmaniasis ulcer on the lower lip.

Introduction

Cutaneous and oral myiasis are an infestation of the skin and oral mucosa by larvae (maggots) of a variety of species usually of the diptero genus. It is more common in tropical and subtropical areas of Africa and the Americas, particularly with a warm and humid environment and low levels of hygiene. Intraorally, the eggs of various types of flies can be deposited (*Cochliomyia hominivorax, Chrysomya bezziana*) in a postextraction socket, existing ulceration, periodontal disease, or in patients who might be sleeping with open mouth, especially outdoors in the summer months. Predisposing factors include old age, alcohol-related disease, neurologic disease, oral malignancies, mouth breathing, halitosis, and very poor oral hygiene. The flies are drawn by the bad odor of food remnants and debris present due to very poor oral hygiene. The eggs hatch within 24 hours and the developing larvae release toxins that cause tissue destruction. The larvae continuously penetrate into deeper layers in their quest for live, fresh tissue, similar to a "*drilling rig.*" Eventually, after 5 to 7 days, when they reach their maximum size, shrink and fall off the lesion. Myiasis usually develops on the skin, and more rarely on the nose, ears, oral and perioral area, anus, and vagina. Two main clinical types of cutaneous myiasis are recognized, the *wound* and *furuncular.*

Clinical features

Oral myiasis usually occurs in the anterior parts of the mouth, within soft and hard tissues. Clinically, necrotic irregular ulceration is observed within which the larvae can be seen (**Fig. 20.4**). The lesions are painful and purulent associated with edema, bad odor, and lymphadenopathy. The patient is usually malnourished and can have malaise and fever. The diagnosis is based on the history and the clinical features. The discovery of larvae in the lesions is pathognomonic of the disease.

Differential diagnosis
- Osteonecrosis due to drugs or radiation
- Osteomyelitis
- Necrotizing ulcerative stomatitis
- Noma

Pathology

This is usually not necessary. The larvae can be seen macroscopically. Microscopically, an inflammatory reaction occurs with neutrophils, eosinophils, lymphocytes, plasma cells, and giant cells.

Treatment

Surgical debridement and removal of the larvae is the first line of treatment. Care should be taken when removing the larvae as they tend to anchor their spines onto the host. If parts of larvae are left behind, they can cause a significant granulomatous inflammatory reaction. Anesthetizing the larvae with local anesthetic may prevent them from anchoring their spines. Alternatively, local anesthetic can be injected into the lesion to increase local pressure and force the larvae to come to the surface. The wound should be cleaned daily following the above. Alternatively, larvicides such as ivermectin (topically or as an oral dose) mineral turpentine, ethanol spray, and oil of betel leaf, have been used.

Oral Cysticercosis

Key points
- The parasite *Taenia solium* is the cause.
- Humans are the main host and pigs are an intermediate host.
- Mostly affects the brain and rarely the heart, musculature, lungs, eyes, and skin.
- The mouth is rarely affected.

Introduction

Cysticercosis is an infection caused by the parasite *T. solium.* It is caused by ingestion of food contaminated with eggs from human stools, inadequately cooked pork meat, or direct contact with contaminated stools. The parasite eggs develop in the human intestines into larvae called *cysticerci.* These transverse the intestinal walls and enter the bloodstream or lymph, causing cystic spaces in the tissues they land. The disease is endemic in Mexico, Central and South America, Philippines, India, and East Asia. It is more likely in areas of deprivation and low hygiene levels, where humans and animals live together. The disease is very rare in Europe and the United States. Cysticercosis has a worldwide distribution, affecting more than 40 to 50 million people.

Clinical features

In cysticercosis, cysts may develop in any organ or tissue of the body. Central nervous system (CNS) involvement neurocysticercosis presents with epilepsy, neurologic symptoms, and psychological disorders may be affected. It can also lead to hydrocephalus, meningitis, persistent headache, vomiting, loss of vision, and other symptoms depending on the affected organs and systems. A serious complication is the formation of cysts in the base of the brain that leads to early death. In endemic areas, 80 to 90% of the infected patients may have cysts in the subcutaneous tissue, mucous membranes, and muscle, while the CNS is affected in approximately 10%.

The skin is relatively rarely affected by multiple, painless, subcutaneous nodules. The mouth is rarely affected (in ~4.1% of the cases).

The most commonly affected intraoral sites are the buccal mucosa, tongue, and lips. Clinically, a solitary nodule is observed that is usually well demarcated, soft in palpation, and asymptomatic, with a diameter 0.5 to 2 cm and is covered by normal mucosa (**Figs. 20.5, 20.6**). The clinical features are not diagnostic, hence confirmatory histopathology is needed.

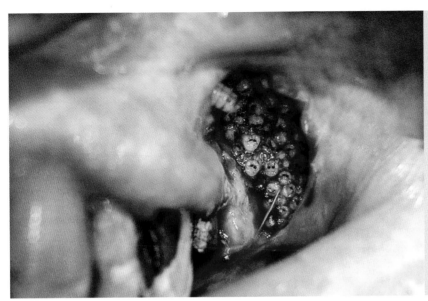

Fig. 20.4 Myiasis, multiple larvae within an ulcerated area of the alveolar mucosa.

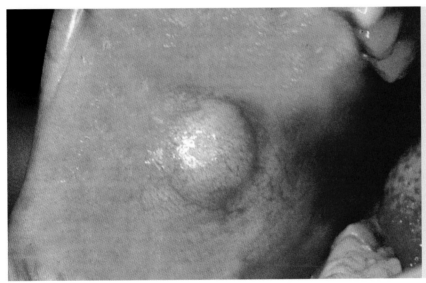

Fig. 20.5 Cysticercosis, nodule in the buccal mucosa.

Differential diagnosis

- Lipoma
- Myxoma
- Fibroma
- Neurofibroma
- Granular cell tumor
- Epidermoid cyst
- Mucocele
- Mucoepidermoid carcinoma

Pathology

Histologically, there are cystic spaces in the lamina propria that contain the parasite and are surrounded by a capsule of connective tissue. An inflammatory infiltrate in the connective tissue mainly consisting of neutrophils, eosinophils, and histiocytes occurs. Granulomas may be present with multinucleated giant cells and calcium mineral deposition.

Stool examination is also recommended. Computed tomography (CT) and magnetic resonance imaging (MRI) can be helpful in the diagnosis of neurocysticercosis. An enzyme-linked immunoblot assay is the test of choice with specificity of 100% and sensitivity of 90%.

Treatment

In patients with active disease, first-line treatments are praziquantel or albendazole. Localized intact oral lesions can simply be surgically excised.

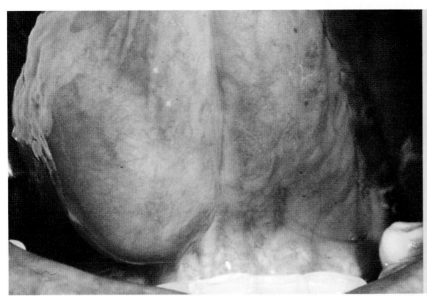

Fig. 20.6 Cysticercosis, large cystic enlargement on the ventral aspect of the tongue.

21 Orofacial Granulomatosis

Orofacial Granulomatosis

Key points
- A heterogeneous group of granulomatous diseases of the mouth and face.
- The diseases are not caused by bacteria and are characterized by granuloma formation without caseation at the microscopic level.
- Clinically, they are characterized by persistent, painless enlargement of the involved areas.

Introduction

Wiesenfeld et al proposed the term "*orofacial granulomatosis*" in 1985. Local and systemic disorders affecting the mouth, lips, and face belong to this group. They are not caused by bacteria and histologically they are characterized by noncaseating granulomas formation. Local diseases such as cheilitis granulomatosa and the Melkersson-Rosenthal syndrome and systemic diseases such as Crohn's disease, sarcoidosis, and tuberculosis are the two main groups of the disorder. However, often the lesions encountered in clinical practice cannot be classified in either subgroup. The precise etiology remains unclear. The prevailing view is that chronic antigenic stimulation, resulting in a cellular immune response, causes the macroscopic lesions. The most frequent causative correlated factors include foodstuffs, dietary complements, aromatic essences (e.g., cinnamon, benzoate), products of dental hygiene, materials used in dentistry, silicone injection, and other foreign bodies.

Clinical features

Orofacial granulomatosis affects both sexes in equal proportions and is most frequent between the ages of 10 and 30.

The common clinical characteristic of all disorders falling under the definition of orofacial granulomatosis is the chronic and recurrent, progressive, usually painless enlargement of the lips, perioral region, gingiva, buccal mucosa, and rarely other areas of the oral cavity (**Figs. 21.1–21.4**). Ulcers may develop occasionally. A high index of suspicion for Crohn's disease is warranted if ulcers are present, particularly in children and young patients.

History and clinical evaluation together with laboratory documentation of the diagnosis are important. Crohn's disease should be ruled out in collaboration with a gastroenterologist where appropriate.

Differential diagnosis
- Cheilitis granulomatosa
- Melkersson-Rosenthal syndrome
- Crohn's disease
- Sarcoidosis
- Angioedema
- Lymphangioma
- Tuberculosis
- Plasma cell gingivitis
- Plasmacytoma

Pathology

Microscopically, in all forms of orofacial granulomatosis, inflammation with granuloma formation without caseation is present. Abundant epithelioid histiocytes, lymphocytes, and often multinucleated giant cells are observed in the granulomas. Dilated lymph and blood vessels surround the granulomas. The search for acid-fast bacteria and fungi using special stains is negative and foreign bodies are absent.

Treatment

A thorough investigation of the gastrointestinal tract for Crohn's disease by a specialist and exclusion of sarcoidosis are necessary before the initiation of treatment. In cases where either of these diseases is present, the primary responsibility for patient care lies with the specialists. If local lesions alone are present, then systemic corticosteroids are the first-choice treatment, e.g., prednisolone 20 to 30 mg/d usually in combination with drugs that inhibit granuloma formation, such as minocycline 100 mg/d or metronidazole 250 to 500 mg/d. The treatment regimen lasts for 1 to 3 months depending on the severity of the lesions. Dapsone, clofazimine, thalidomide, sulfasalazine, and immunosuppressants have also been used as the second-choice treatments. In mild forms of the disease, intralesional corticosteroids such as triamcinolone acetonide or betamethasone dipropionate and sodium phosphate retard are recommended as the initial therapy. A course of three to four intralesional injections may be used. Before any treatment, food additives, flavoring agents, products of oral hygiene, and foreign materials should be excluded. Relapses are frequent.

Melkersson-Rosenthal Syndrome

Key points
- The syndrome is part of the orofacial granulomatosis group.
- Swelling of the face and lips, facial nerve paralysis, and fissured tongue are the main clinical features.
- Cheilitis granulomatosa may be a monosymptomatic form of the syndrome.

Introduction

The Melkersson-Rosenthal syndrome is a clinical variant of orofacial granulomatosis. The syndrome is rare and affects young individuals of both sexes. The etiology is related to that of orofacial granulomatosis.

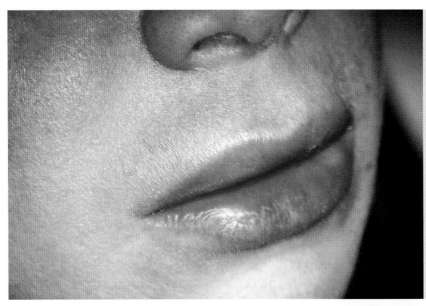

Fig. 21.1 Orofacial granulomatosis, lip swelling due to silicone injection.

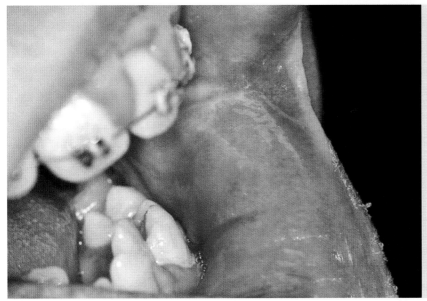

Fig. 21.2 Orofacial granulomatosis of unknown cause on the buccal mucosa and the lower lip.

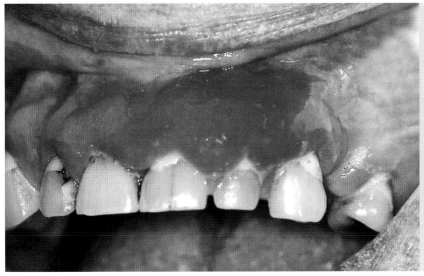

Fig. 21.3 Idiopathic granulomatous lesions on the gingival and the alveolar ridge.

Clinical features

The main clinical features of the syndrome are persistent enlargement of the lips, relapsing enlargement of the face, relapsing unilateral palsy of the facial nerve, and a fissured tongue (**Figs. 21.5, 21.6**). Edematous swelling and rarely ulcers of the gingiva, buccal mucosa, palate, and the mucobuccal fold may also occur. Some investigators consider cheilitis granulomatosa as a monosymptomatic form of Melkersson-Rosenthal syndrome. Clinical and histopathologic criteria are the basis of diagnosis.

Differential diagnosis

- Other forms of orofacial granulomatosis
- Peripheral facial nerve palsy
- Cheilitis glandularis
- Crohn's disease
- Sarcoidosis
- Heerfordt's syndrome
- Angioedema
- Lymphangioma

Pathology

Histopathology of a tissue sample is necessary for diagnosis. The microscopic findings are those described for orofacial granulomatosis.

Treatment

The basic guidelines and the drugs used in the treatment of orofacial granulomatosis are also used in the treatment of the syndrome. Systemic and intralesional corticosteroids are the treatment of choice. Sulfasalazine, clofazimine, chloroquine, dapsone, immunosuppressants, minocycline, and metronidazole usually in combination with steroids have also been used. Surgical reconstruction has been used to improve permanent disfiguration of the lips.

Sarcoidosis

Key points

- Sarcoidosis is a systemic granulomatous disease of unknown etiology.
- It usually affects the lungs and lymph nodes and less often the skin, eyes, bones, and other internal organs, such as the liver, spleen, and endocrine glands.
- Rarely, the disease affects the oral mucosa, salivary glands, and the jaw bones.

Introduction

Sarcoidosis is a chronic, multisystemic granulomatous disease, with unknown etiology. The characteristic histopathologic lesion is a noncaseating granuloma.

The dominant view is that it is the result of cellular immune response against microbial or other antigens (bacteria, viruses, fungi). Some investigators believe that it is an autoimmune disease. The disease attacks mainly the lymph nodes, lungs, eyes, and skin. More rarely, it may involve the bones, spleen, liver, salivary glands, endocrine glands, and oral mucosa.

Clinical features

Sarcoidosis affects more frequently women between 20 and 50 years. Clinically, multiple red or reddish-violaceous papules, nodules, or plaques appear on the skin of the face, extremities, thighs, and fingers. Lupus pernio, erythema nodosum, scars, and persistent plaques are also common skin manifestations. The nails may also be involved. The skin lesions may be dispersed or confluent occurring in 20 to 30% of patients and may be the only manifestation of the disease.

The oral mucosa may also rarely be involved. The most frequent sites of oral localization of sarcoidosis are the lips, tongue, palate, and gingiva (**Figs. 21.7–21.9**). Clinically, small or large red nodules that rarely ulcerate are the main oral manifestations. The salivary glands, jaws, and temporomandibular joints may also be affected. The jaw lesions may mimic periodontitis. Splenomegaly and lymphadenopathy usually accompany the oral lesions. Constitutional symptoms such as fever, malaise, diffuse arthralgias, weight loss, and respiratory symptoms such as dyspnea, cough, and retrorenal pain are common.

The diagnosis is based on clinical and laboratory findings.

Differential diagnosis

- Other forms of orofacial granulomatosis
- Tuberculosis
- Crohn's disease
- Lupus erythematosus
- Amyloidosis
- Non-Hodgkin's lymphoma
- Leishmaniasis

Pathology

Histopathology is essential in making a diagnosis. Microscopically, the tissue specimens show noncaseating granulomas, composed of epithelioid cells, few, if any, lymphocytes, and frequently, multinucleated, Langhans-type giant cells.

Serology shows increased antinuclear antibody (ANA) titers in 30% of patients and increased concentration of angiotensin-converting enzyme (ACE) in 60% of patients. Finally, imaging studies of the bones and lungs may be needed.

Treatment

Systemic steroids and local infiltration of tissues with injectable steroids is the first-line treatment. In systemic disease, prednisolone 1 mg/kg/d is administered for 4 to 6 weeks, with tapering of the dose thereafter. Hydroxychloroquine in a dose of 200 to 400 mg/d or chloroquine 250 to 500 mg/d are usually effective for the control of skin and oral lesions. Second-line drugs in the therapeutic armamentarium include immunosuppressants, thalidomide, and recently, biological agents.

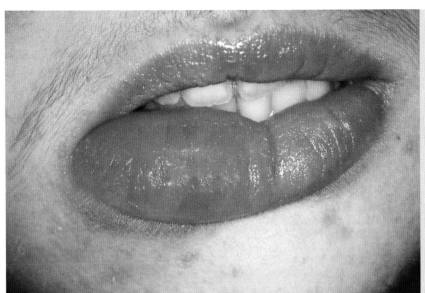

Fig. 21.4 Crohn's disease, cheilitis granulomatosa.

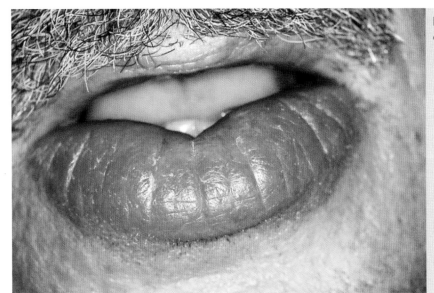

Fig. 21.5 Melkersson-Rosenthal syndrome, cheilitis granulomatosa.

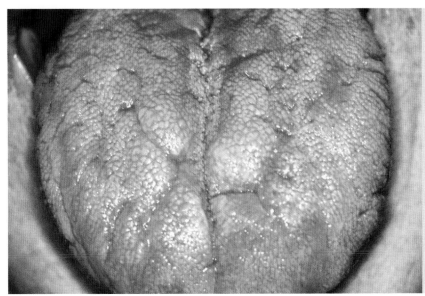

Fig. 21.6 Melkersson-Rosenthal syndrome, fissured tongue.

Heerfordt's Syndrome

Key points
- Heerfordt's syndrome is a clinical variant of sarcoidosis.
- Fever, enlargement of the parotids, uveitis, and facial nerve paresis are the principal clinical manifestations.
- Histopathologic examination is helpful for final diagnosis.

Introduction

Heerfordt's syndrome is also known as uveoparotid fever or uveoparotitis. It is a clinical variant of sarcoidosis characterized by fever, painless enlargement of the parotids, uveitis, and facial nerve palsy.

Clinical features

Clinically, the syndrome is characterized by bilateral, firm, painless enlargement of the parotids which is often the first manifestation of the disease and is present in 80% of patients. The submandibular, sublingual, and lacrimal glands may also be enlarged, but infrequently (**Fig. 21.10**). Subjective complaints include malaise, gastrointestinal upset with nausea and vomiting, low-grade fever, while xerostomia and xerophthalmia are frequently present. Lymph node enlargement, erythema nodosum, and skin nodules of variable size may also be present. Early, frequent, ocular manifestations include uveitis, keratitis, and conjunctivitis that may be unilateral or bilateral. Clinical and histopathologic criteria are essential for diagnosis.

Differential diagnosis
- Sjögren's syndrome
- Mikulicz's syndrome (IgG4 disease)
- Orofacial granulomatosis

Pathology

Histopathology is necessary for definite diagnosis. The histopathologic findings are identical to those of sarcoidosis. All other tests used in the diagnosis of sarcoidosis are also helpful for the diagnosis of Heerfordt's syndrome. Kveim-Siltzbach skin test may also be useful.

Treatment

Corticosteroids and other drugs are used for the treatment of sarcoidosis.

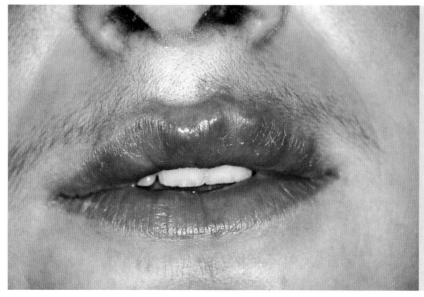

Fig. 21.7 Sarcoidosis, multiple red-violet nodules of the upper lip.

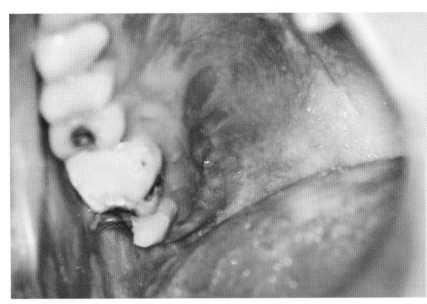

Fig. 21.8 Sarcoidosis, erythema, and erosions on the palate.

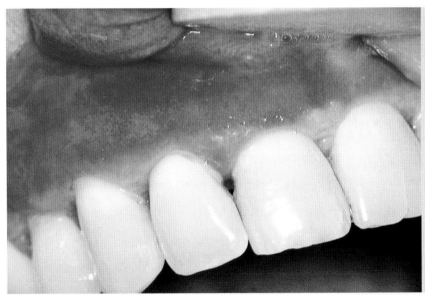

Fig. 21.9 Sarcoidosis, intense erythema, and swelling of the attached gingiva and the alveolar mucosa.

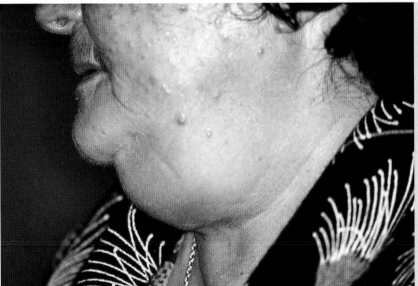

Fig. 21.10 Heerfordt's syndrome, swelling of submandibular and sublingual glands, and sarcoidosis of skin nodules.

22 Diseases with Possible Immunopathogenesis

Aphthous Ulcers

Key points

- The most common diseases of the oral mucosa.
- The most probable mechanism is cellular-type immune response.
- Ulcers usually present in the mobile, nonkeratinized part of the oral mucosa.
- Aphthous ulcers are classified into *minor, major,* and *herpetiform* types.
- It may also represent a manifestation of systemic disease.

Introduction

Aphthous ulcers or recurrent aphthous stomatitis (RAS) is one of the most common diseases of the oral mucosa, affecting 10 to 30% of the population. The exact etiology remains unknown. Several theories have been proposed and have caused confusion rather than shedding light on the pathogenesis. Many predisposing factors have been implicated in the development of aphthous ulcers, including genetic predisposition, allergy, bacteria, viruses, iron deficiency, low levels of vitamin B_{12} and folic acid, hormonal disturbances, trauma, stress, etc. Finally, there is evidence that impaired cell-mediated immune response plays a role in the pathogenesis. According to clinical criteria, based on the size, number, depth of ulceration, duration, and scarring after resolution, aphthous ulcers are classified into *minor, major,* and *herpetiform* types.

Minor

Minor aphthous ulcers are the most common clinical subtype representing approximately 80 to 85% of cases. Minor ulcers are more frequent in women and usually first appear between the age of 10 and 30.

Clinical features

Clinically, recurrent painful ulcers 3 to 7 mm in diameter, with a yellowish bottom and red areola are observed (**Figs. 22.1, 22.2**). There are one to six ulcers, lasting for 7 to 14 days and healing without leaving a scar. The ulcers are located in parts of the nonkeratinized oral mucosa, occur more often on the mucosa of the lips, tongue, and soft palate. Recurrences are common, with variable intervals of quiescence in between attacks. The diagnosis is based exclusively on clinical criteria.

Major

Major aphthous is a rare subtype of the disorder. It was previously known as recurrent periadenitis, or necrotizing disease of Sutton.

Clinical features

Clinically, it is characterized by large, circumscribed, and deep ulcers, 1 to 3 cm in diameter, with white-yellow surface and red inflammatory halo in the periphery (**Figs. 22.3, 22.4**). They are solitary or multiple (3–6), lasting 4 to 6 weeks. In cases where recurrent lesions develop often in the same site, after healing they may leave scarring and atrophy. The lesions are found, most often, in the mucosa of the lip, buccal mucosa, tongue, and soft palate. Recurring time ranges from 1 to 3 months. The diagnosis is based on the clinical criteria.

Herpetiform Ulcers

Herpetiform ulcers are a relatively rare clinical variety of aphthous ulcers.

The name derives from their clinical similarity with herpetic lesions in the mouth, although the two entities have distinct histopathologic, microbiological, and immunologic differences.

Clinical features

Clinically, the lesions appear as tiny ulcerations, which progressively grow and swarm in groups (**Fig. 22.5**). Ulcers are typically many (10–100); they have a diameter of 1 to 3 mm and are very painful. They are surrounded by erythematous halos and last for 1 to 2 weeks. The lesions recur frequently for period of 1 to 3 years. They may appear in any mobile area of the oral mucosa. The disease affects, most commonly, patients between ages 20 and 30. The diagnosis is based on the clinical characteristics.

Differential diagnosis

- Traumatic ulcer
- Chancre
- Herpetic stomatitis
- Herpangina
- Stomatitis due to drugs
- Erythema multiforme
- Adamantiades-Behçet disease
- Hand-foot-and-mouth disease
- Periodic fever, aphthous stomatitis, pharyngitis, cervical adenitis (PFAPA) syndrome
- Sweet's syndrome
- Cyclic neutropenia
- Leukemia
- Crohn's disease
- Ulcerative colitis
- Gluten enteropathy

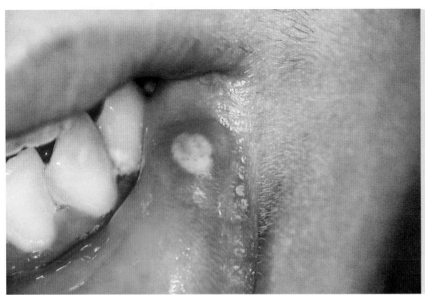

Fig. 22.1 Minor aphthous ulcer on the lower lip.

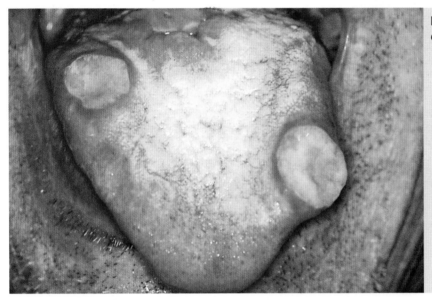

Fig. 22.2 Two minor aphthous ulcers on the tongue.

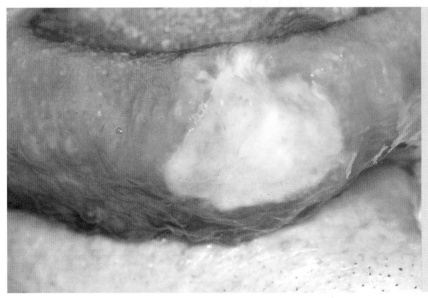

Fig. 22.3 Major aphthous ulcer on the tip of the tongue.

Pathology

There are no diagnostic laboratory tests. Histologically, non-specific ulceration, covered by a fibrin membrane is observed. The vessels of the lamina propria are dilated and a mixed-type inflammatory infiltrate consisting of lymphocytes, neutrophils, and histiocytes is present.

Treatment

There is no effective treatment for aphthae. Therapeutic interventions are aimed at reducing pain, shortening the duration of lesions, and if possible preventing recurrences. Treatment is local or systemic. Local treatment is palliative and is aimed at reducing pain and shortening the duration of lesions. Topical corticosteroids in the form of triamcinolone 0.1% in Orabase which is applied three times a day until the symptoms resolve is probably the most satisfactory treatment. Also, clobetasol propionate (Temovate gel 0.05%), fluocinonide (Lidex gel 0.5%), or tacrolimus (Protopic 0.03%) applied to the lesions three times a day for 4 to 6 days may be beneficial. Other anti-inflammatory ointments, i.e., amlexanox 5%, diclofenac 3% may also offer pain relief. For major aphthae and herpetiform ulcers, systemic administration of corticosteroids is recommended, e.g., prednisolone 20 to 30 mg for 7 to 10 days, followed by tapering and discontinuation within 5 to 10 days. Finally, in the case of major aphthae that are very large and recur frequently, satisfactory results have been achieved with the use of thalidomide at a dose of 100 to 200 mg/d for a period of 1 to 3 months. Administration of thalidomide requires careful monitoring and fertility planning, because of the well-known teratogenicity of the drug. Thalidomide is contraindicated in women of reproductive age and of course during pregnancy. Other systemic interventions include the use of azathioprine, dapsone, colchicine, or pentoxifylline, with uncertain results.

Adamantiades-Behçet's Disease

Key points

- A chronic multisystemic and polysymptomatic disease with strong evidence supporting autoimmune pathogenesis.
- The main features are oral ulcers, ocular lesions, ulcers on the genitals, and skin lesions.
- Positive pathergy test occurs in 50 to 60% of patients.
- Because of its systemic nature, any organ in the body may be affected. Therefore, diagnosis and treatment requires the contribution of many specialties.
- The diagnosis is based on clinical criteria.

Introduction

The Adamantiades-Behçet's disease is a chronic multisystem inflammatory disorder of uncertain cause and prognosis. The initial description of the disease was made by the Greek ophthalmologist Benedict Adamantiades in 1931 and was completed by the Turkish dermatologist Hulusi Behçet in 1937, who described the classical triad of the disease: mouth-eyes-genitals. Although the etiology and pathogenesis of the disease are not fully understood, there is evidence that autoimmune mechanisms including humoral- and cellular-

type responses against one or more endogenous antigens are possibly playing a major role in the pathogenetic mechanism. Along the same line of reasoning a relatively higher risk for developing the disease is observed in individuals bearing the histocompatibility antigens B5 and B51 (HLA-B5 and B51) immunogenetic haplotypes. This fact provides further evidence for a possible immunologic origin of the disease. Furthermore, bacteria (streptococci) and viruses (herpes simplex type 1 [HSV-1], Epstein-Barr, cytomegalovirus) may participate in the immunopathogenesis of the disease in genetically predisposed people. The end result is the development of vasculitis. The disease prevalence around the world varies. It is much more common in Japan and around the Mediterranean (Greece, Turkey, Italy, the Middle East). In Turkey, the frequency is 80 to 100 cases per 100,000 people, in Japan 10 cases per 100,000, in Greece the prevalence is estimated at 3 to 5 cases per 100,000, while in the United States it is 0.12 to 0.15 cases per 100,000. It affects men more often than women (5:1–10:1), usually between 20 and 30 years, but it may occur at any age. Almost all organs of the body may be affected. For this reason, the disease requires collective evaluation of the patients by many medical specialties.

Clinical features

The International Study Group for Adamantiades-Behçet's disease has established major diagnostic criteria (primary and secondary) of the syndrome which are as follows:

- Recurrent (three episodes per year) aphthous ulcers in the oral mucosa
- Recurrent ulcerations in the genitals
- Ocular lesions
- Dermal lesions
- Positive pathergy test, which is positive in 50 to 60% of cases

Furthermore, other lesions may occur less frequently (secondary criteria), such as the following:

- Arthralgias
- Arthritis
- Thrombophlebitis and phlebothrombosis
- Arterial occlusions and aneurysms
- Pericarditis
- Endocarditis
- Epididymitis
- Respiratory system manifestations and gastrointestinal and central nervous system (CNS) involvement

For the diagnosis of the syndrome, the required criteria are recurrent oral ulceration and two other main diagnostic criteria. However, the disease cannot be excluded when one of the main criteria and more than two of the secondary criteria are present.

The oral mucosa is almost always affected (95–100%). Frequently, the lesions precede other manifestations. Aphthous ulcers in the mouth may present in all clinical subtypes (minor, major, and herpetiform ulcers) (**Figs. 22.6, 22.7**).

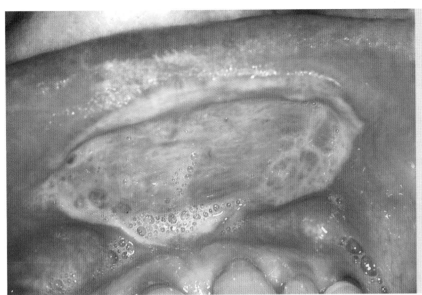

Fig. 22.4 Sizeable aphthous ulcer on the upper lip.

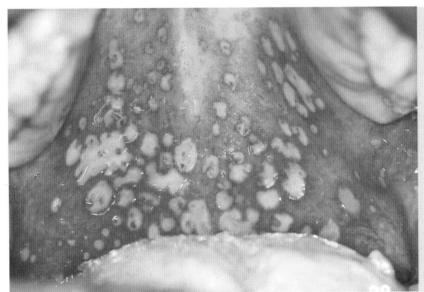

Fig. 22.5 Herpetiform ulcers, multiple lesions on the soft and hard palate.

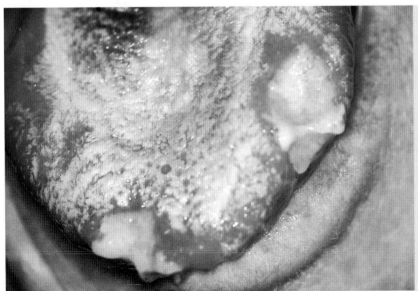

Fig. 22.6 Adamantiades-Behçet's disease, aphthous ulcers on the tongue.

In the genital area, deep, round, clearly circumscribed ulcers are observed, located mainly on the scrotum (**Figs. 22.8, 22.9**), penis, labia majora, vulva (**Fig. 22.10**), and the inner surface of the thighs (**Fig. 22.11**). Balanitis (**Fig. 22.12**) and perianal ulcers (**Fig. 22.13**) may also occur. Eye lesions are also frequent (80–90%) and may present as conjunctivitis (**Fig. 22.14**), iridocyclitis with hypopyon, uveitis, and retinitis which can cause blindness. Dermal lesions include papules, pustules, folliculitis, erythema nodosum, and more rarely necrotic lesions (**Figs. 22.15, 22.16**). The prognosis is usually good. However, severe cardiovascular, respiratory, and CNS complications can be fatal. The diagnosis of the disease is based almost exclusively on the history and clinical evaluation of the lesions.

Differential diagnosis

- Aphthous ulcers
- Herpetic stomatitis
- Erythema multiforme
- Mucous membrane pemphigoid
- Pemphigus
- PFAPA syndrome
- Sweet's syndrome
- Reiter's disease
- Pyostomatitis vegetans
- Pyoderma gangrenosum
- Crohn's disease
- Ulcerative colitis
- Systemic lupus erythematosus
- Other vasculopathies

Pathology

There are no pathognomonic diagnostic tests. Histologically, a neutrophilic angiocentric infiltrate with leukocytoclastic and lymphocytic vasculitis are the characteristic microscopic pattern. Fibrinoid necrosis may be present in involved veins and venules. The result is the destruction of the media and fibrous thickening of the intima and adventitia. Pseudoaneurysms of the aorta, femoral and pulmonary arteries may form and thrombosis is frequent. The presence of HLA-B5 and B51 is of limited diagnostic value.

Treatment

Treatment of the Adamantiades-Behçet's disease is difficult and complex because of the number of lesions, their unpredictable nature, and lack of evidence-based efficacy of the drugs currently used.

Various drugs have been used systemically or locally. It is highly desirable that prior to the initiation of treatment a multidisciplinary team of specialists determine the optimal individualized therapeutic strategy.

Systemic corticosteroids, immunosuppressants, colchicine, dapsone, thalidomide, and monoclonal antitumor necrosis factor α (TNF-α) antibodies (etanercept and infliximab) have been used either alone or in combination. The local symptomatic palliative treatment of oral lesions is the responsibility of stomatologist and is similar to aphthous ulcers treatment.

PFAPA Syndrome

Key points
- Defective overexpression of interleukin 1β (IL-1β).
- Clinically, it is characterized by periodic fever, aphthous ulcers, pharyngitis, and cervical lymphadenitis.
- Recurrences are common.
- Children under the age of 8 are most commonly affected.

Introduction

This is a rare disease reflecting excess release of IL-1β. Children under 8 years are most commonly affected. Occurrence in adolescents is uncommon.

Clinical features

Clinically, the disease is characterized by periodic fever (38–40°C) that lasts for 4 to 6 days and is accompanied by chills and fatigue. Aphthous-like ulcerations commonly appear in the mouth with a preference to the uvula and soft palate (**Figs. 22.17, 22.18**). Pharyngitis, tonsillitis, and bilateral lymphadenitis complete the clinical feature. Headache, abdominal pain, and arthralgia are less common symptoms. The disease usually recurs every 4 to 8 weeks for 1 to 2 years and then resolves spontaneously. The diagnosis is based solely on the history and clinical features as no specific laboratory tests are available.

Differential diagnosis

- Aphthous ulcers
- Adamantiades-Behçet's disease
- Hand-foot-and-mouth disease
- Herpetic gingivostomatitis
- Infectious mononucleosis
- Cyclic neutropenia
- Leukemia
- HIV infection
- Sweet's syndrome

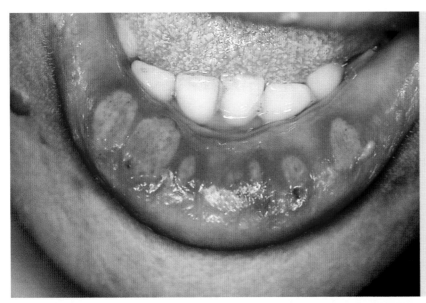

Fig. 22.7 Adamantiades-Behçet's disease, aphthous ulcer on the lower lip.

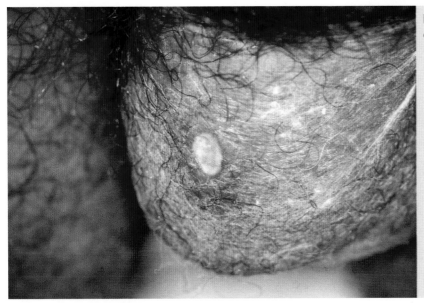

Fig. 22.8 Adamantiades-Behçet's disease, small ulcer on the scrotum.

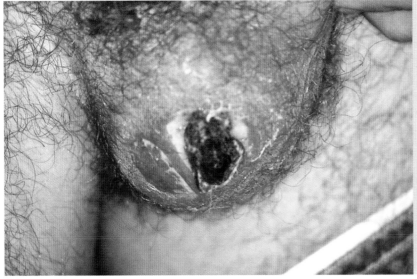

Fig. 22.9 Adamantiades-Behçet's disease, two necrotic lesions on the skin of the scrotum.

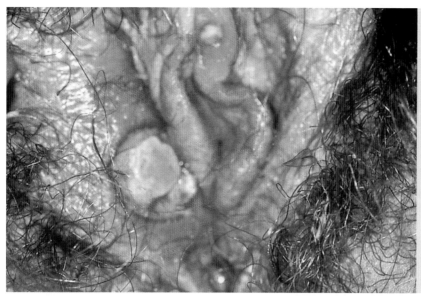

Fig. 22.10 Adamantiades-Behçet's disease, ulcers on the labia majora.

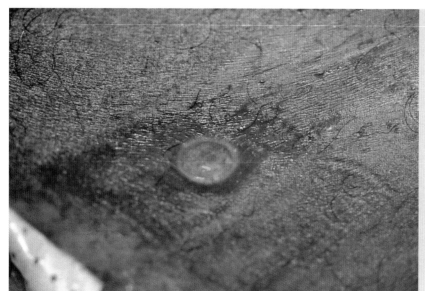

Fig. 22.11 Adamantiades-Behçet's disease, ulcer on the skin of the thigh.

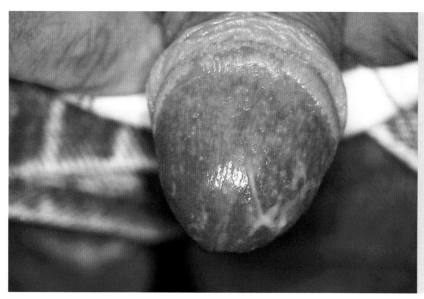

Fig. 22.12 Adamantiades-Behçet's disease, balanitis.

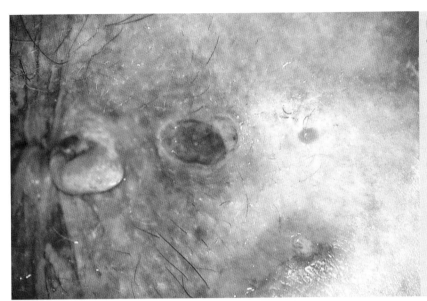

Fig. 22.13 Adamantiades-Behçet's disease, perianal ulcers.

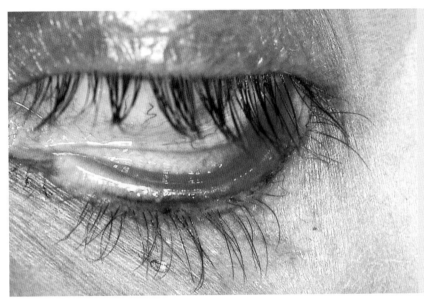

Fig. 22.14 Adamantiades-Behçet's disease, conjunctivitis.

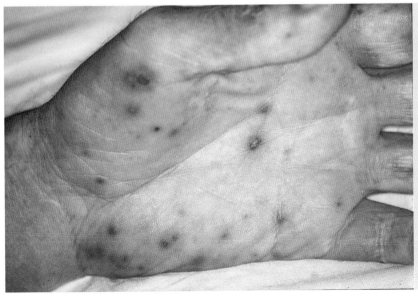

Fig. 22.15 Adamantiades-Behçet's disease, mild necrotic ulcers on the skin of the palm.

Pathology

This is of no diagnostic value.

Treatment

Treatment is symptomatic. Antipyretics are administered during the acute phase of fever. The drug of first choice is cimetidine, which is immunoregulatory, at a dose of 20 to 30 mg/kg/d for about a week. Anti-IL-1β causes resolution of disease.

The drug of second choice is systemic prednisolone, 10 to 15 mg daily for approximately 6 to 8 days.

Wegener's Granulomatosis

Key points

- A rare chronic granulomatous vasculitis.
- The disease is classified into *generalized* and *localized* forms.
- The classic triad is granulomatous inflammation of the upper and lower respiratory system, glomerulonephritis, and systemic vasculitis that affects the skin and mouth.
- The skin and oral mucosa are involved in 40% of patients.
- The detection of antineutrophil cytoplasmic antibodies (ANCAs) in the serum is crucial for diagnosis.

Introduction

Wegener's granulomatosis is a rare, chronic granulomatous vasculitis with questionable prognosis. Genetic and environmental factors may be involved in the pathogenesis. Some evidence exists for the pathogenetic role of a cell-mediated immune response to a microbial agent (e.g., *Staphylococcus aureus*) or aberrant hypersensitivity reaction to an unknown antigen. However, the exact etiology remains unknown. It affects equally both sexes of all ages, and the peak age is between 30 and 60 years.

Clinical features

The main diagnostic criteria of the disease are vascular granulomatous lesions in the upper and lower parts of the respiratory system with generalized necrotizing vasculitis of arteries and veins, necrotizing granulomatous glomerulonephritis, and necrotic lesions in the oral cavity and skin in approximately 40% of patients. The disease usually presents with respiratory symptoms and signs, such as cough, dyspnea, hemoptysis, and pleurisy. Then it extends quite often to the oral cavity and other organs. In rare cases, lesions can present exclusively in the oral cavity. Clinically, oral lesions present as multiple or solitary irregular ulcerations with inflammatory features, often located on the tongue, palate, buccal mucosa, and rarely in other areas (**Figs. 22.19–22.21**). Swelling and gingival red papillary granulomatous hyperplasia and prolonged healing time postextraction may also occur. Lesions of the skin include palpable purpura, nodules, ulcers, and necrotic papules. Other organs and systems that may be affected include the eyes, the gastrointestinal tract, CNS, and cardiac and musculoskeletal system. The clinical diagnosis should be documented histologically and immunologically.

Differential diagnosis

- Non-Hodgkin's lymphoma
- Nasal natural killer (NK)-T-cell lymphoma
- Tuberculosis
- Syphilis
- Necrotizing sialadenometaplasia
- Systemic mycoses
- Squamous cell carcinoma
- Aphthous ulcer

Pathology

Microscopically, vasculitis, with perivascular lymphocytic filtration and often frank leukocytoclastic vasculitis and granulomatous inflammation are observed. Lymphocytes, mast cells, eosinophils, and multinucleated giant cells are abundant in the areas of necrosis. Autoantibodies against neutrophil cytoplasm (c-ANCA) are positive in 80% of patients' serum with the systemic type of the disease and 60% with the localized type. Increase of erythrocyte sedimentation rate (ESR) and C-reactive protein (CRP) may also be present.

Treatment

The treatment of choice is the combination of corticosteroids (such as prednisolone 1 mg/kg/d) and cyclophosphamide 100 to 200 mg daily. Azathioprine and mycophenolate ester have been used in combination with prednisolone. These regimens have radically changed the prognosis for the better. In severe recurrent forms, trimethoprim-sulfamethoxazole can be administered simultaneously. Successful results have also been obtained with the biological agents, infliximab and rituximab.

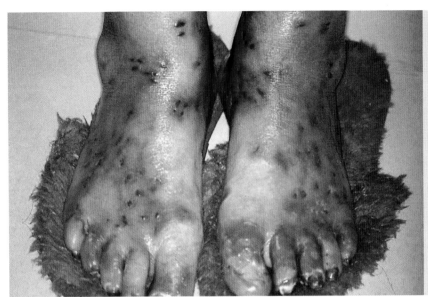

Fig. 22.16 Adamantiades-Behçet's disease, heavy necrotic lesions on the feet.

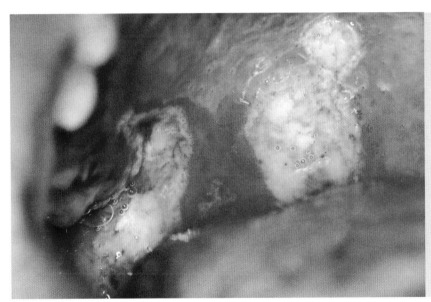

Fig. 22.17 PFAPA syndrome, two big ulcers on the soft palate and the uvula.

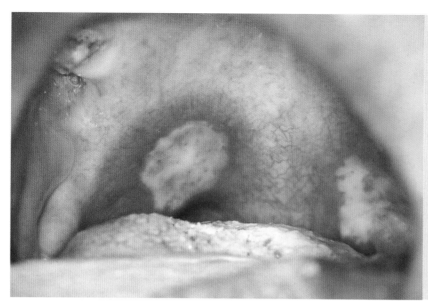

Fig. 22.18 PFAPA syndrome, ulcers on the soft palate close to the uvula.

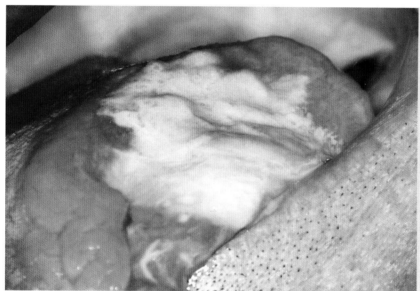

Fig. 22.19 Wegener's granulomatosis, large ulcer on the tongue.

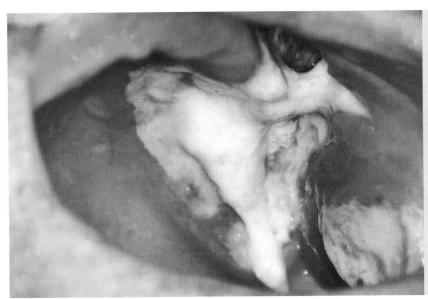

Fig. 22.20 Wegener's granulomatosis, large ulcers on the alveolar mucosa, palate, and buccal mucosa.

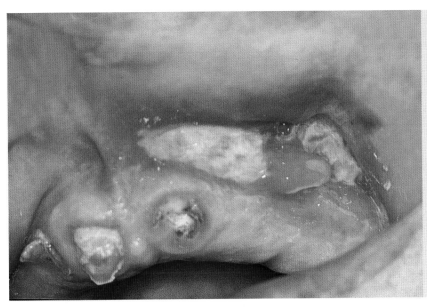

Fig. 22.21 Wegener's granulomatosis, early ulcer on the upper alveolar sulcus.

23 Autoimmune Diseases

Lupus Erythematosus

Key points

- An autoimmune disease that can have mucocutaneous, joint, and internal organ involvement.
- It can manifest as a skin condition or in a more systemic form.
- Cutaneous lupus is classified into *acute*, *subacute*, and *chronic*. The main representative of the chronic cutaneous form is discoid lupus erythematosus.
- Systemic lupus erythematosus is a common disease with significant morbidity and mortality.
- The oral mucosa is affected in 15 to 20% of the cases in discoid lupus and 20 to 40% of the cases in systemic lupus erythematosus.
- The clinical diagnosis of the oral lesions has to be confirmed by histology and immunology.

Introduction

Lupus erythematosus is an autoimmune disease affecting multiple systems. Genetic and environmental factors have been implicated in initiating and establishing the pathogenesis. It mostly affects females (ratio 6:1). Lupus has a very broad spectrum of clinical manifestations with the cutaneous form at one side and the systemic at the other and multiple variants between the two. Cutaneous lupus is classified into three major forms: *acute*, *subacute*, and *chronic*. The chronic type is the most common and includes discoid lupus erythematosus and four further subtypes: *lupus profundus* or *panniculitis*, *chilblain lupus*, *lupus tumidus*, and *neonatal lupus*. The mouth is involved mainly in the discoid and systemic forms.

Discoid Lupus Erythematosus

Discoid lupus erythematosus (DLE) is the more common form of the disease. It tends to be confined to the skin and oral mucosa and has a benign course in the vast majority of patients. In approximately 5 to 10% of the cases, the patients may progress to develop systemic lupus erythematosus. Using clinical criteria it can be classified into *localized* (which favors the head and neck region), *generalized*, and *hypertrophic*.

Clinical features

The skin lesions are characterized by violaceous papules and patches, scaling, and prominent follicular hyperkeratosis. The lesions are sharply demarcated from the surrounding healthy skin and progress to scarring with atrophy and telangiectasia. Progressively, the lesions have the potential for scarring demonstrating peripheral hyperpigmentation, central depigmentation, and disfiguring scarring. Discoid lupus lesions are very often located above the neck region (face, scalp, and ears). It is then characterized as localized and usually forms a characteristic "*butterfly-rash*" pattern on the face (**Fig. 23.1**). If the disease involves areas above and below the neck, it is characterized as generalized DLE, involving areas as the extensor forearms and hands. The cutaneous lesions persist for months to years. On occasion, discoid lesions occur on the oral mucosa, lips, nasal mucosa, conjunctivae, and genital mucosa.

The oral mucosa is involved in 15 to 25% of cases, usually in association with skin lesions. However, on rare occasions, oral lesions may occur alone. Clinically, the oral lesions appear as a well-defined erythematous central area surrounded by a sharp elevated border of irradiating whitish striae (**Fig. 23.2**). Telangiectasias and small, white dots may be present on the erythematous center. Ulcers, erosions, or white plaques may also present and progress to atrophic scarring (**Fig. 23.3**). The buccal mucosa is the most frequently affected site, followed by the lower lip, palate, gingiva, and tongue. The oral lesions may be associated with arthralgias. Rarely, squamous cell carcinoma develops in long-standing discoid oral lesions. In general, the clinical features of oral lesions are not pathognomonic and the clinical diagnosis has to be confirmed by further investigation.

Differential diagnosis

- Lichen planus
- Lichenoid reactions
- Leukoplakia
- Erythroplakia
- Mucous membrane pemphigoid
- Graft-versus-host disease (GVHD)
- Geographic tongue

Pathology

Histopathologic examination reveals hyperkeratosis, acanthosis, and vacuolar degeneration of the basal cell layer. Colloid bodies that represent apoptotic individual epithelial cells are occasionally observed. Edema in the papillary dermis or in the upper lamina propria along with vascular dilatation and extravasation of erythrocytes may also be noticed. Periadnexal and perivascular lymphocytic infiltrate are seen in papillary and reticular dermis. Direct immunofluorescence shows linear granular deposition of most commonly immunoglobulin G (IgG) and/or IgM and C3 antibodies at the basement membrane. Serology for anti-DNA, antinuclear antibody (ANA), Sjögren's syndrome A (SSA) (Ro), and SSB (La) antibodies is usually negative.

Treatment

The dermatologist usually manages DLE when the lesions are limited on the skin and the oral physician treats the oral disease when this is the only manifestation. Their collaboration is vital in the presence of mucocutaneous disease. Topical steroids are the first line of treatment in the more mild forms of the disease. That can be either the application topically of a steroid cream in Orabase, or intralesional injection of long-lasting steroids, such as Celestone Chronodose or

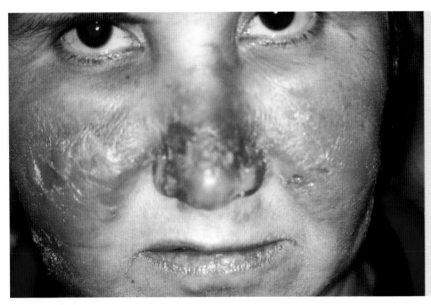

Fig. 23.1 Discoid lupus erythematosus, facial lesions forming the characteristic "butterfly rash."

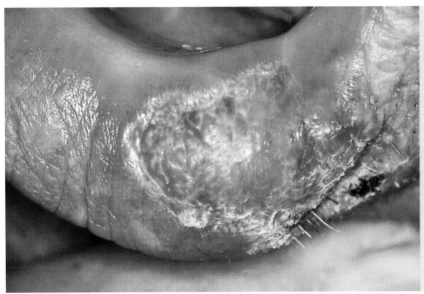

Fig. 23.2 Discoid lupus erythematosus on the lower lip. An atrophic, erythematous plaque is observed surrounded by telangiectasias and irradiating whitish striae peripherally.

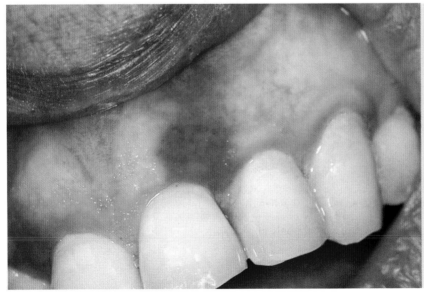

Fig. 23.3 Discoid lupus erythematosus, erythematous plaque on the maxillary gingiva and alveolar mucosa.

Propiochrone retard. Calcineurin inhibitors, such as tacrolimus have also been tried as an alternative. In the cases where topical steroids are not effective or the disease is more severe, the first line of treatment is systemic steroids (prednisolone 20–30 mg/d for 2–3 weeks with progressive decrease). Other systemic treatments include antimalarials, immunomodulators (such as dapsone), immunosuppressants (such as methotrexate and mycophenolate acid), oral retinoids and biological agents (rituximab, a chimeric monoclonal antibody for CD20, or belimumab, a B-lymphocyte stimulator-specific inhibitor).

Systemic Lupus Erythematosus

Systemic lupus erythematosus (SLE) is a serious multiorgan autoimmune disease although in some patients only one or a few organs are affected. The organ systems most frequently affected are the skin, mucosae, cardiovascular and gastrointestinal systems, lungs, kidneys, joints, and central nervous system (CNS).

Clinical features

SLE is accompanied by fever, fatigue, weight loss, myalgias, lymphadenopathy, and debilitation. These manifestations may be useful indicators of increased risk for SLE in patients who present with cutaneous or/and oral lesions. The Systemic Lupus Collaborating Clinics (SLICC) have revised and validated in 2012 the American College for Rheumatology (ACR) SLE classification criteria. They have come up with 17 criteria. The new SLE classification requires (a) fulfilment of at least four criteria with at least one clinical and one immunologic criterion or (b) biopsy-proven nephritis compatible with SLE as the sole clinical criterion in the presence of ANA or anti–double-stranded DNA (anti-dsDNA) antibodies.

The 11 clinical and 6 immunologic criteria are as follows:

Clinical criteria

1. Acute cutaneous lupus
2. Chronic cutaneous lupus
3. Oral ulcers
4. Nonscarring alopecia
5. Synovitis involving two or more joints
6. Serositis (pleurisy, pericarditis)
7. Renal findings (persistent proteinuria)
8. Neurologic disorders (seizures, psychosis, peripheral, or cranial neuropathy etc.)
9. Hemolytic anemia
10. Leukopenia (<4000/mm³ at least once) or lymphopenia (<1000/mm³ at least once)
11. Thrombocytopenia (<100,000/mm³ at least once)

Immunologic criteria

1. ANA above laboratory reference range
2. Anti-dsDNA above laboratory reference range except enzyme-linked immunosorbent assay (ELISA): twice above laboratory reference range
3. Anti-Sm: presence of antibody to Sm nuclear antigen
4. Positive finding of antiphospholipid antibody
5. Low complement
6. Direct Coombs' test in the absence of hemolytic anemia

The oral mucosa is involved in 20 to 40% of the cases and the oral manifestations are one of the basic clinical criteria toward diagnosis of the disease. Clinically, there are extensive painful erosions, or ulcers surrounded by a reddish or whitish zone (**Fig. 23.4**). Frequent findings include petechiae, edema, and hemorrhage. Xerostomia and parotid enlargement is observed in the cases of secondary Sjögren's syndrome. White hyperkeratotic lesions accompanied by erythema and edema are rarely observed (**Fig. 23.5**). The palate, lips, and buccal mucosa are the most frequently affected sites. Another common clinical finding is conjunctivitis (**Fig. 23.6**). On occasion, bullous eruption may develop on the skin and oral mucosa in patients with systemic disease. The oral manifestations of SLE are not pathognomonic and the diagnosis should be confirmed by further investigations.

Differential diagnosis

- Lichen planus
- Mucous membrane pemphigoid
- Bullous pemphigoid
- Pemphigus
- Drug-induced oral lesions
- Cinnamon contact stomatitis

Pathology

The same histologic findings of discoid lupus also apply in the systemic form. However, in contrast to discoid lesions, systemic lupus lesions tend to have little or no hyperkeratosis, basement membrane thickening, periadnexal infiltrate, and scarring. Direct immunofluorescence shows linear granular deposits of IgG, IgM, IgA, and C3 antibodies at the basement membrane and within the epidermis. Serology for anti-dsDNA, ANA, and anti-Sm antibodies usually reveals high titers, which are a strong indication of the disease. In addition, autoantibodies to Ro, La, U1 ribonucleoprotein (U1RNP), histones, and single-stranded DNA (ssDNA) are common in patients with SLE, but they are not disease-specific.

Treatment

Depending on the overall clinical severity of the disease, the therapy consists of systemic steroids, antimalarials, immunosuppressants, dapsone, thalidomide, use of monoclonal antibodies, and plasmapheresis if immune complexes are present. This should be led by appropriate specialists.

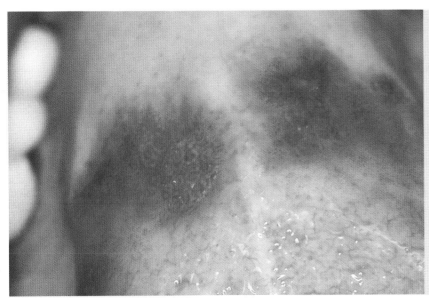

Fig. 23.4 Systemic lupus erythematosus, erythema, and ulceration on the palate.

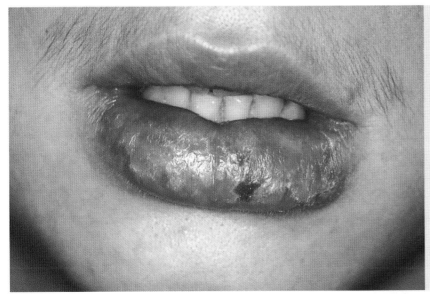

Fig. 23.5 Systemic lupus erythematosus, lower lip enlargement accompanied by red and white lesions.

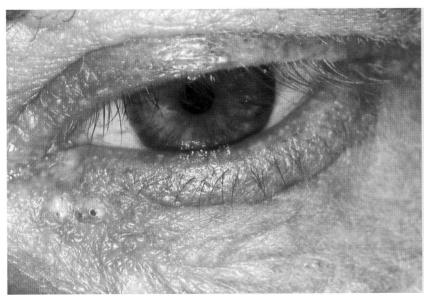

Fig. 23.6 Systemic lupus erythematosus, conjunctivitis, and edema of the eyelids.

Systemic Sclerosis

Key points

- An autoimmune connective tissue disease of unknown etiology.
- Classified into *localized* and *systemic* forms.
- Localized scleroderma affects only a few areas of skin and muscle while systemic affects multiple systems.
- It is characterized by symmetrical thickening of the skin of the fingers and the face that can then spread.
- Raynaud's phenomenon is common.
- The oral and perioral areas are commonly involved in the systemic form.

Introduction

Systemic scleroderma (SSc) is a chronic multisystem, connective tissue disorder that affects the skin, blood vessels, and internal organs. It primarily affects women (ratio 4:1) between 30 and 40 years. The etiology and pathogenesis remain unknown. Important pathogenic abnormalities in the skin and internal organs are vascular dysfunction, tissue fibrosis, and immune activation with autoantibody production. The increased fibroblast activity leads to excessive amounts of normal collagen. Vascular dysfunction in the form of impaired angiogenesis is an early event in the pathogenesis of SSc. Using clinical criteria, scleroderma is classified into *localized (morphea)* and *systemic sclerosis*. The localized form has a favorable prognosis and involves only the skin. The systemic form is characterized by multisystem involvement, including the skin and oral mucosa. Systemic sclerosis is further divided, based on the degree of skin involvement, into *diffuse* cutaneous scleroderma and *limited* cutaneous scleroderma (however, the two subtypes may commonly overlap). In limited form, the lesions are mainly confined to the fingers, hands, and face. In diffuse form, the fibrotic lesions usually begin in the fingers and hands and gradually spread to involve the arms, forearms, face, trunk, and lower extremities. Classically, diffuse form is associated with early internal organ involvement and has a worse prognosis. The limited disease tends to develop internal involvement later with better prognosis. It is important to remember that both subtypes are part of a systemic disease that also affects internal organs. Localized scleroderma has relatively good prognosis, while systemic sclerosis can have a poor prognosis.

Clinical features

Initially, the skin is edematous, but, as the disease progresses, it becomes thin, hard, and inelastic, with a pale appearance (**Fig. 23.7**). Involvement of the facial skin results in characteristic facies with a small, sharp nose, expressionless stare, and narrow oral aperture (microstomia) (**Fig. 23.8**). The oral mucosa is pale and thin with a smooth dorsal surface of the tongue due to papillary atrophy (**Fig. 23.9**). Frequent findings include smoothing out of the palatal folds, short and hard tongue frenum, which results in reduced mobility and can subsequently lead to dysarthria. As the disease progresses, there are limitations of mouth opening and difficulty in swallowing. Radiographic examination reveals characteristic widening of the periodontal ligament space and resorption of the mandibular condyle and coronoid processes. Finally, Raynaud's phenomenon can be quite common, while skin necrotic areas can be observed as a result of ischemia, progressive fibrosis, or trauma (**Fig. 23.10**). Secondary Sjögren's syndrome occurs in approximately 20% of the patients with systemic sclerosis.

In most patients with systemic sclerosis, internal organs are affected, causing multiple complications and increased disease morbidity. The most commonly affected organs are the heart, lungs, kidneys, and the gastrointestinal tract, resulting in relevant symptomatology. A clinical variant of limited scleroderma is the CREST syndrome, which is characterized by a combination of calcinosis cutis, Raynaud's phenomenon, esophageal dysfunction, sclerodactyly, and telangiectasia. Telangiectasia can occur on the face, the lips, and oral mucosa (**Fig. 23.11**). Diagnostic clinical criteria of SSc have been suggested by the American College of Rheumatology and include either one major criterion (symmetric cutaneous sclerosis proximal to the metacarpophalangeal or metatarsophalangeal joints) or two or more minor criteria (sclerodactyly, digital pitted scars or loss of substance from finger pads, bibasilar pulmonary fibrosis). The final diagnosis of systemic sclerosis is based on clinical and laboratory findings.

Differential diagnosis

- Oral submucous fibrosis
- Lipoid proteinosis
- GVHD, chronic
- Mixed connective tissue disease
- Epidermolysis bullosa
- Amyloidosis
- Werner's syndrome

Pathology

Histologic characteristics of scleroderma include atrophy of the epidermis, excessive accumulation of collagen in the extracellular matrix of the reticular dermis, leading to fibrous replacement of the subcutaneous fat. Lymphocytic perivascular infiltrate is also seen, along with small lymphocytic aggregates in the remaining subcutaneous fat. Autoantibody testing is useful for the diagnosis of SSc. Elevated titers of ANA, antibodies to topoisomerase and to RNA polymerase should be done. Finally, the modified Rodman skin score (MRSS) is widely used (17 different skin body areas are examined).

Treatment

The treatment of scleroderma is performed by the rheumatologist, dermatologist, and other specialists depending on the organs affected. Topical and systemic steroids, antimalarials, D-penicillamine, azathioprine, and other immunosuppressants, calcium channel blockers, prostaglandins, cyclophosphamide, interferon (α and γ) immunomodulatory agents, and some other have been tried with unsatisfactory results. Targeted molecular treatments give hope for better treatment of the disease.

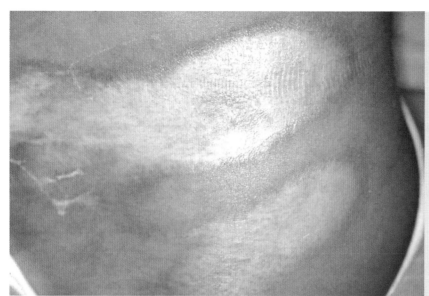

Fig. 23.7 Systemic sclerosis, characteristic white plaques on the skin.

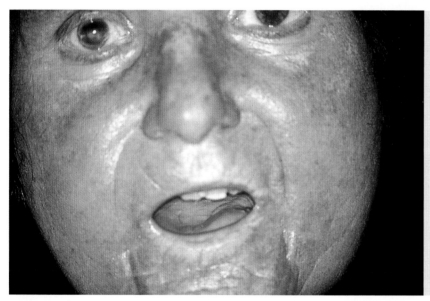

Fig. 23.8 Systemic sclerosis, characteristic facies and microstomia.

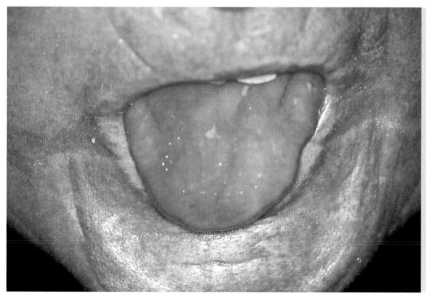

Fig. 23.9 Systemic sclerosis, pale and atrophic epithelium of the dorsum of the tongue.

Dermatomyositis

Key points

- Autoimmune connective tissue disease of unknown etiology.
- Classified into two main types: *adult* and *juvenile* based on the age of onset.
- Distinctive pink-violet poikiloderma favoring the scalp and periocular region and nailfold telangiectasias.
- The oral mucosa is rarely involved.
- The adult form is associated with malignancies (in 10–30% of the cases), but not the juvenile one.

Introduction

Dermatomyositis is a relatively rare inflammatory disease of the skin and underlying muscular tissue. The term polymyositis is used when there is no cutaneous involvement. While the exact etiology remains unknown, there are indications that genetic and immunologic factors (both humoral and cell-mediated), medication and viruses play a role in the pathogenesis. The disease most frequently affects women than men (ratio 2:1), over or 40 years and rarely children. The disease may be associated with an internal malignancy in 10 to 30% of cases, most commonly in elderly patients. The malignancies may precede or follow the disease. The most common neoplasias include ovarian and colon cancer, breast, lung, pancreatic, as well as non-Hodgkin's lymphomas, and female genital tract adenocarcinomas. Dermatomyositis and polymyositis can occur in association with other autoimmune connective tissue diseases (LE, SSc, Sjögren's syndrome, rheumatoid arthritis, and mixed connective tissue disease).

Clinical features

Clinically, progressive symmetrical muscle weakness is usually the first and most important clinical manifestation in the majority of patients with dermatomyositis. Myalgia and malaise accompanied by fever are also prominent early features. The most important diagnostic sign of cutaneous eruption of dermatomyositis is poikiloderma (hyperpigmentation, hypopigmentation, telangiectasias, and epidermal atrophy). It is characterized by a pink-violet color and the tendency of lesions to be distributed around the eyes (the *heliotrope sign*) and photodistribution and nailfold changes (telangiectasias). Characteristically, photodistributed poikiloderma involves the "V" of the chest and the upper back (*shawl sign*). *Gottron's sign* (violaceous erythema of the knuckles, elbows, and knees) is common. When lesions on the knuckles develop, secondary lichenoid lesions are termed *Gottron's papules*. Both sign and papules are diagnostic of dermatomyositis. In approximately 30% of cases, a purplish-red periorbital discoloration and a telangiectatic erythema at the nail margins are the initial manifestations (**Fig. 23.12**). During the course, the disease may be manifested by an erythematous, scaly maculopapular rash, skin discoloration, hyperpigmentation, and atrophy. The oral cavity is not commonly involved. The most frequent lesions are redness, painful edema, or ulcers on the tongue, soft palate, buccal mucosa, and uvula (**Fig. 23.13**). The diagnosis of dermatomyositis is based on clinical and laboratory evaluation.

Differential diagnosis

- Systemic lupus erythematosus
- Sarcoidosis
- Drug-induced oral manifestations
- Various atypical oral ulcers

Pathology

Histologically, the most common changes seen in skin biopsy are atrophy of the epidermis, vacuolar degeneration of the basal cells, basement membrane degeneration, mucin deposition in the lamina propria, and mild lymphocytic infiltration. Muscle specimens show muscle fiber atrophy, necrosis, degeneration and regeneration, perivascular and perifascicular lymphocytic infiltrate. Further investigations include serum enzyme determination (creatine phosphokinase, aspartate transaminase, alanine transaminase, aldolase), and other laboratory testing: ANA, anti-Ro/SSA, anti-La/SSB, anti-RNP, anti-Sm and anti-Jo-1. Imaging is also important (such as chest X-ray for the detection of interstitial lung disease). Pulmonary function tests and computed tomography (CT) can follow if the above is positive or in patients with pulmonary symptoms and signs. Electromyography and magnetic resonance imaging (MRI) may also be useful.

Treatment

The treatment of dermatomyositis can be complex, as the cutaneous and muscular lesions need to be precisely evaluated. First line of systemic treatment is steroids. Other drugs that have been tried include azathioprine, cyclophosphamide, mycophenolate acid, tacrolimus, methotrexate, thalidomide, rituximab, infliximab, and others.

Mixed Connective Tissue Disease

Key points

- A combination of clinical features similar to those observed in SLE, systemic sclerosis, polymyositis, and rheumatoid arthritis.
- Common clinical findings include arthritis, swollen hands or sclerodactyly, Raynaud's phenomenon, and pulmonary disorders associated with high-titers IgG anti-U1RNP antibodies.
- The oral mucosa is rarely involved.

Introduction

Mixed connective tissue disease (MCTD) is a relatively rare multisystemic disorder characterized by a combination of clinical features similar to those observed in SLE, scleroderma, polymyositis, and rheumatoid arthritis. The existence as a distinct entity is controversial, as patients often have overlapping clinical and serologic features of various combinations of other autoimmune connective tissue diseases. The etiology remains unknown, and the pathogenesis is unclear. An immune response to nuclear U1RNP antigens plays an essential role in the pathogenesis. Females are more commonly affected (ratio 9:1), with a mean age of onset in the second or third decade of life.

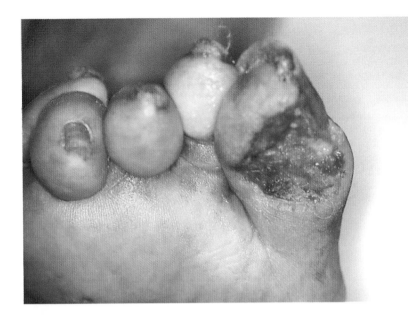

Fig. 23.10 Systemic sclerosis, necrosis of the great toe.

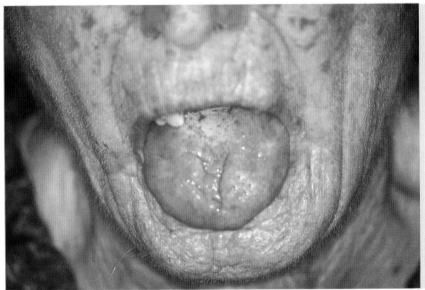

Fig. 23.11 CREST syndrome, facial and upper lip telangiectasia, and atrophy of the tongue.

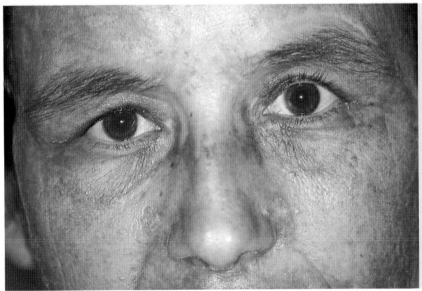

Fig. 23.12 Dermatomyositis, characteristic violaceous rash around the eyes and the nose.

Clinical features

Clinically, the disease is characterized by Raynaud's phenomenon, polyarthralgia or arthritis, sclerodactyly or swollen hands, inflammatory myopathy, pulmonary hypertension, esophageal dysmotility, and low-grade fever. There is also a plethora of other manifestations, such as cutaneous lesions resembling SLE, systemic sclerosis and also inflammatory myopathy, cardiac, renal, and neurologic abnormalities, lymphadenopathy, and Sjögren's syndrome, etc. Intraorally, erosions or ulcerations might be noticed that lack specific characteristics and can be localized or diffuse. The most commonly affected sites are the palate, buccal mucosa, and tongue (**Figs. 23.14, 23.15**). Other oral signs and symptoms may include telangiectasia, xerostomia, trigeminal nerve neuropathy, and facial nerve palsy.

Differential diagnosis

- SLE
- Systemic sclerosis
- Sjögren's syndrome
- Dermatomyositis-polymyositis
- Various vasculopathies
- Porphyria cutanea tarda

Pathology

There are no pathognomonic histopathologic findings for MCTD. The histopathologic features vary depending on the type of skin lesions examined (SLE, systemic sclerosis, and polymyositis). Of greater diagnostic value is the characteristically high titers of antibodies against nuclear U1RNP antigens. However, these antibodies can also be found in other connective tissue disorders, but in a lower scale.

Treatment

The treatment of MCTD is not simple and aims to cease the disease activity and control the manifestations from various organs and systems. It requires a multidisciplinary approach. The spectrum of medication used includes corticosteroids, immunosuppressants (azathioprine, cyclophosphamide, mycophenolic acid, methotrexate, tacrolimus, etc.). Plasmapheresis and autologous bone marrow transplantation have also been tried.

Sjögren's Syndrome

Key points

- A multiorgan autoimmune disorder that primarily affects secretory glands, predominantly the salivary and lacrimal ones.
- Xerostomia, xerophthalmia, and arthritis are the most common features.
- It is classified into *primary* and *secondary*.
- About 3 to 5% of the patients with primary Sjögren's syndrome develop a B-cell non-Hodgkin's lymphoma.

Introduction

Sjögren's syndrome is a chronic, multisystem, autoimmune exocrinopathy that predominantly involves lacrimal, salivary, and other exocrine glands, resulting in a decreased or eventually total absence of secretion. It is caused by a lymphocytic inflammatory infiltration of the exocrine glands. Women are more commonly affected (ratio 9:1) between 40 and 50 years. The most common features are xerostomia, keratoconjunctivitis sicca, and arthritis. Using clinical, serologic, and genetic criteria the disease is classified into *primary* and *secondary*. Sjögren's syndrome is primary when it is not accompanied by a collagen disease and secondary if it coexists with connecting tissue diseases, such as rheumatoid arthritis, SLE, systemic sclerosis, and more rarely, polymyositis, primary biliary cirrhosis, vasculitis, cryoglobulinemia, Hashimoto's thyroiditis, chronic active hepatitis, etc. The exact pathogenesis is unknown. However, genetic (increased HLA-B8, -DR3, -DQ2, -DRw52A) and immunologic (humoral and cellular) factors seem to play an important role in the pathogenesis.

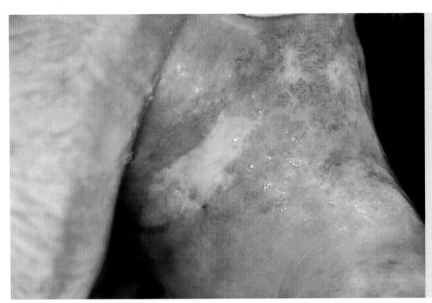

Fig. 23.13 Dermatomyositis, erythema, edema, and superficial ulceration on the buccal mucosa.

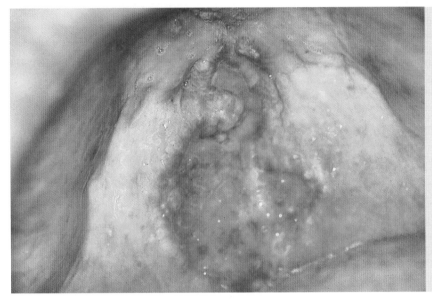

Fig. 23.14 Mixed connective tissue disease, ulceration on the palate.

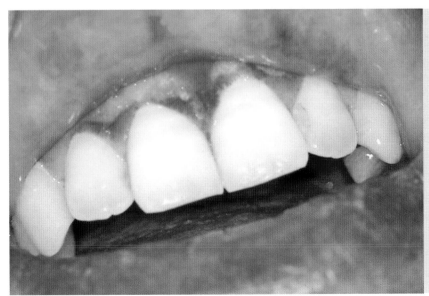

Fig. 23.15 Mixed connective tissue disease, ulceration on the upper gingiva.

Clinical features

The main clinical manifestations of Sjögren's syndrome are xerostomia, xerophthalmia, and vaginal dryness. The xerostomia is the classic symptom and sign due to destruction of the major and minor salivary glands. The oral mucosa appears erythematous, dry, glossy, shiny, and sometimes erosive (**Fig. 23.16**). The tongue is smooth and fissured and might appear lobulated (**Fig. 23.17**). Transient enlargement of the parotids and the other major and minor salivary glands may occur (**Fig. 23.18**). Purulent discharge from the major salivary gland ducts is not uncommon (**Fig. 23.19**). Other common clinical signs and symptoms include glossodynia, taste disturbances, dysphagia, difficulty in swallowing, extensive e caries, angular cheilitis, and candidiasis. Xerophthalmia is the second most common symptom of the disease and manifests as foreign body sensation and burning sensation, photophobia or pain, and reduction of tears. Complications following xerophthalmia include keratoconjunctivitis, corneal thinning, and ulceration and recurrent infection that can ultimately lead to perforation and blindness (**Fig. 23.20**). Ocular objective tests to verify decreased tear production and assess the integrity of the corneal surface e.g., Schirmer's test and Rose Bengal dye test should be performed by an ophthalmologist. Vaginal dryness, burning, and dyspareunia are common findings, while *Candida* and bacterial infections are common complications. The most common skin lesions are xeroderma accompanied by pruritus, purpura, vasculitis, porphyria cutanea tarda, erythema nodosum, and annular erythema. Extraglandular manifestations in primary Sjögren's are lymphadenopathy, arthritis, Raynaud's phenomenon, myositis, renal and pulmonary involvement, peripheral neuropathy, and hearing loss. There is an increased risk of B-cell non-Hodgkin's lymphoma development. These B-cell lymphomas are often extranodal and can originate from salivary and lacrimal glands.

New classification criteria for Sjögren's syndrome were defined in 2012 by the American College of Rheumatology. This was a data-driven expert consensus approach that suggested that target individuals with signs/symptoms suggestive of Sjögren's syndrome should present with at least two of the following three objective criteria:

1. Positive serum anti-SSA/Ro and/ or anti-SSB/La or positive rheumatoid factor (RF) and ANA titer greater than or equal to 1:320.
2. Presence of focal lymphocytic sialadenitis with a focus score greater than or equal to 1 focus/4 mm² in labial salivary gland biopsy samples.
3. Keratoconjunctivitis sicca with ocular staining score greater than or equal to 3.

The diagnosis and management of Sjögren's syndrome require three areas of specialty practice: oral medicine, rheumatology, and ophthalmology.

Differential diagnosis

- Xerostomia due to radiation
- HIV infection
- GVHD
- Mikulicz's syndrome
- Heerfordt's syndrome
- Sarcoidosis
- Mucous membrane pemphigoid
- Amyloidosis
- Xerostomia due to neurologic disorders
- IgG4-related disease
- Sialosis
- Diabetes mellitus

Pathology

Biopsy and histopathologic examination of minor salivary glands of the lower lip remains the most reliable diagnostic test. The presence of two or more aggregates of inflammatory cells (≥ 50 lymphocytes) in 4 mm² of salivary gland tissue is considered a reliable diagnostic marker. Additionally, the more focal points of lymphocytic infiltrate are observed, the stronger is the indication for the disease. Primary Sjögren's syndrome is associated with anti-SSA Ro (positive 60–80%) anti-SSB La (positive 30–50%). ANA test in titer greater than 1:320 and anti-α-fodrin is positive in 70% of the cases. Patients with secondary Sjögren's syndrome may have additional autoantibodies depending on the specific autoimmune connective tissue disease.

Treatment

Symptomatic treatment is suggested for most manifestations of Sjögren's syndrome. Artificial saliva, frequent ingestion of water, and chewing sugar-free gum may alleviate dryness of the mouth. Stimulation of the residual salivary and lacrimal glands can be achieved with systemic pilocarpine hydrochloride (Salagen tablet 5 mg three times daily). Cevimeline hydrochloride (Evoxac 30 mg caps three times daily) may also be used. Artificial tears and ophthalmic lubricants are indicated. Systemic treatment can include steroids, hydroxychloroquine, azathioprine, mycophenolic acid, and cyclophosphamide in different combinations and for different lengths of time depending on the disease activity. The new biological immunomodulating agents may also be used for the treatment of severe disease—and reverse non-Hodgkin's lymphoma.

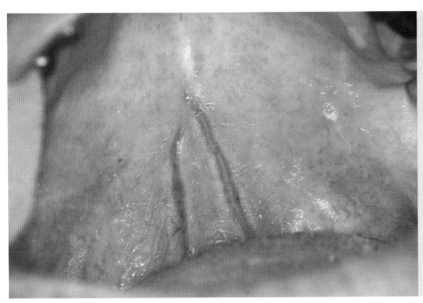

Fig. 23.16 Sjögren's syndrome, dry palate with presence of two linear erosive lesions.

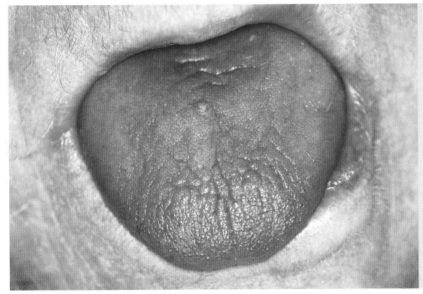

Fig. 23.17 Sjögren's syndrome, dry and lobulated tongue.

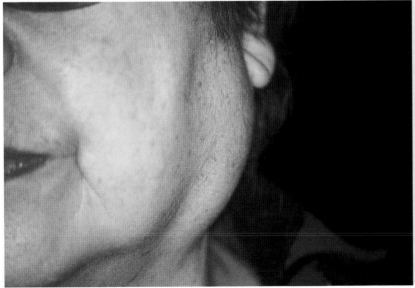

Fig. 23.18 Sjögren's syndrome, enlargement of the parotid.

Giant Cell Arteritis

Key points

- A vasculitis mainly involving the extracranial branches of the carotid artery and predominantly the temporal artery.
- Usually coexists with polymyalgia rheumatica.
- The hallmark of giant cell arthritis is fever, severe headache, visual disturbances, polymyalgia rheumatica, jaw claudication, and elevated erythrocyte sedimentation rate (ESR).
- Characteristic signs from the mouth are jaw and tongue claudication and ulceration on the tongue and buccal mucosa.

Introduction

Giant cell arteritis, also known as temporal or cranial arteritis is a granulomatous inflammation of medium- to large-size vessels. The extracranial branches of the carotid are mainly affected with predilection to the temporal artery. It mostly affects women than men (ratio [4:1]) over 60 years. The incidence is 20 to 30 new cases per 100,000 of population per year in the over 60s. The etiology remains unknown. However, immunologic mechanism, mainly of the cellular type, seems to be involved in the pathogenesis, leading to the ischemia in the areas supplied from the affected arteries.

Clinical features

The classic symptoms of giant cell arteritis are headache, loss of appetite, fatigue, scalp tenderness, visual symptoms, jaw claudication, and throat pain. The temporal artery is usually normal on physical examination but may be nodular, enlarged, and tender. About 50% of patients with giant cell arteritis also have polymyalgia rheumatica. Finally, unexplained head or neck pain and jaw claudication in an older patient may signal the presence of giant cell arteritis. The most common ocular manifestation include acute unilateral vision loss, episodes of amaurosis fugax, and in 30% of the cases permanent vision loss. Jaw claudication is common and has a high positive predictive value. Other oral manifestations include pain and claudication of the tongue and ulceration of the tongue and buccal mucosa as a result of ischemic necrosis (**Figs. 23.21, 23.22**).

The diagnosis is based on clinical features and the results of histologic examination and other tests.

Differential diagnosis

- Wegener's granulomatosis
- Takayasu arteritis
- Polyarteritis nodosa
- Other arteritis
- Amyloidosis
- Various oral ulceration

Pathology

Biopsy of the temporal artery is the most important diagnostic test. However, a negative biopsy does not confirm a negative diagnosis. Histology reveals inflammatory infiltrate in the media and adventitia of histiocytes, lymphocytes, plasma cells, and giant cells. The lumen of the artery is reduced and in some cases completely obliterated. Nearly 90% of patients with giant cell arteritis have raised ESRs (80–120 mm/h), C-reactive protein (CRP), and alkaline phosphatase.

Treatment

The first line of treatment with good results is systemic corticosteroids in high dose (prednisone 60–80 mg/d orally) for approximately 1 month before tapering, and a maintenance dose continues (5–10 mg/d) for up to 1 to 2 years. The concomitant administration of aspirin 60 to 80 mg/d orally may reduce the risk of complications.

Benign Lymphoepithelial Lesion

Key points

- A rare painless enlargement of the salivary and lacrimal glands.
- It may be a monosymptomatic form of Sjögren's syndrome.
- Histologically, there is a dense lymphocytic infiltrate.

Introduction

The term *benign lymphoepithelial lesion* is used to define a localized lymphocytic infiltration of the salivary or lacrimal glands of unknown etiology. Some investigators classify this lesion as a monosymptomatic form of Sjögren's syndrome. It mostly affects middle-aged women (ratio 5:1).

Clinical features

Clinically, there are small raised painless nodules of the minor salivary glands, usually on the posterior part of the hard or soft palate that might eventually ulcerate (**Fig. 23.23**). When the parotids are involved, there is a painless bilateral or unilateral enlargement that can cause mild xerostomia and an uncomfortable feeling. The duration of the disease may extend over months or years, with fluctuations in the size of the lesion. Patients that present with benign lymphoepithelial lesion have an increased risk of non-Hodgkin's lymphoma in the salivary glands or extraglandulary manifestations.

Differential diagnosis

- Non-Hodgkin's lymphoma
- Necrotizing sialadenometaplasia
- Mucocele
- Salivary gland tumors

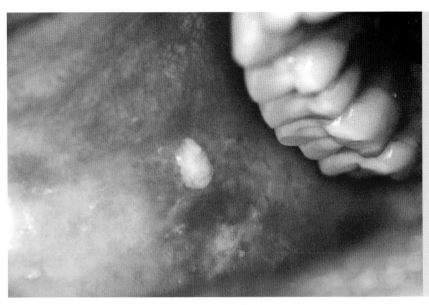

Fig. 23.19 Sjögren's syndrome, sero-purulent discharge from the parotid duct.

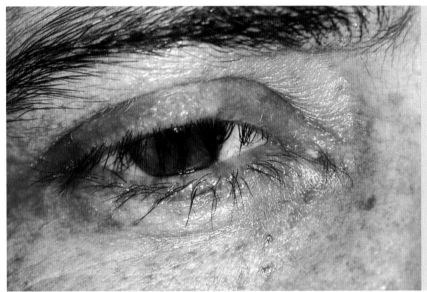

Fig. 23.20 Sjögren's syndrome, conjunctivitis, and edema of the eyelids.

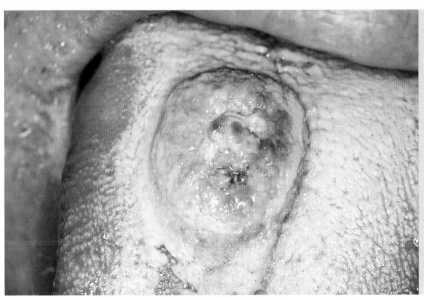

Fig. 23.21 Giant cell arteritis, necrosis on the dorsum of the tongue.

Pathology

Histologically, a dense lymphocytic infiltrate and destruction of the glandular parenchyma is seen along with the presence of epimyoepithelial islands among lymphocytes, which are the result of salivary gland ductal cells and myoepithelial cell proliferation.

Using special molecular techniques, it is important to diagnose the monoclonal or polyclonal nature of the lymphocytic infiltrate to exclude a progression to non-Hodgkin's lymphoma.

Treatment

The first line of treatment is the administration of systemic corticosteroids (i.e., prednisolone 30–40 mg/d for 3–4 weeks with gradual reduction for 2–3 months). Immunosuppressants can alternatively be used. Small enlargements of the minor salivary glands can be surgically removed.

Cryoglobulinemia

Key points

- It is characterized by the presence in serum or urine of globulins that have the property to sediment at a temperature of 4°C and redissolve at 37°C.
- Classified into three types: I, II, and III.
- Types II and II are mixed cryoglobulinemias.
- Palpable purpura, myalgias, arthralgias, peripheral neuropathy, and glomerulonephritis are common.
- Oral lesions are relatively rare and when present purpuric lesions and necrotic ulcers are observed.

Introduction

Cryoglobulinemia is characterized by the presence of globulins in serum or plasma that have the property to sediment at a temperature of 4°C and redissolve at 37°C. Serologically, the cryoglobulinemias are classified into three types. Type I cryoglobulinemia is caused by a monoclonal globulin (usually IgM or IgG) without RF activity and occurs usually in lymphoproliferative disorders and plasma cell dyscrasias. The RF component can be monoclonal—type II cryoglobulins or polyclonal—type III cryoglobulins. The polyclonal immunoglobulin is IgM. Mixed cryoglobulinemias are considered *idiopathic* if there is no underlying disease and *secondary* if they are associated with chronic infections, chronic hepatitis, hepatitis C, HIV infection, autoimmune, and malignant diseases.

Clinical features

Mixed cryoglobulinemias cause vasculitis of the small- and medium-size vessels. Clinically, they are characterized by recurrent palpable purpura of the lower extremities that might ulcerate and evolve to necrotic ulcerating lesions and peripheral neuropathy (**Figs. 23.24, 23.25**). Other signs and symptoms include polyarthralgias without arthritis and glomerulonephritis due to systemic vasculitis that is caused by the formation of immune complexes. Less frequently, purpuric lesions evolving to oral ulcers in the lips and the oral mucosa may occur (**Fig. 23.26**). Mixed cryoglobulinemias may be associated with malignancies such as non-Hodgkin's lymphomas, chronic lymphocytic leukemia, and Waldenström's macroglobulinemia. The diagnosis of cryoglobulinemias is based on a compatible clinical picture and a positive serum test for cryoglobulins.

Differential diagnosis

- Hypereosinophilic syndrome
- Waldenström's macroglobulinemia
- Thrombocytopenic purpura
- Leukemia
- Vasculitis

Pathology

Serologic identification and typing of cryoglobulins, serum protein electrophoresis, and ESR are all recommended toward diagnosis.

Histologically, papular lesions show amorphous eosinophilic, periodic acid–Schiff (PAS) positive, material due to cryoglobulin deposits on the wall and the lumen of the small vessels in the superficial dermis. There is also erythrocyte extravasation without inflammatory infiltrate with the exception of the mixed cryoglobulinemias where there is a picture of leukocytoclastic vasculitis. By direct immunofluorescence (DIF), granular deposits predominantly of IgM and C3 in a vascular pattern may be seen in the papillary dermis.

Treatment

The treatment of mixed cryoglobulinemia should be directed toward any underlying disease. Interferon-α plus ribavirin, aspirin, and corticosteroids are administered by the specialists. Plasma exchange or cyclophosphamide may also be used for neurologic or renal involvement. Rituximab followed by interferon-α and ribavirin have been suggested for severe cases.

Graft-versus-Host Disease

Key points

- A specific form of immune reaction caused by the immune cells in the graft against the host who lacks the donor's antigens.
- One of the most serious complications following allogeneic tissue transplant.
- Clinically, it is classified into *acute* and *chronic* depending on the time of onset.
- The main targets are the gastrointestinal tract and the skin.
- The oral mucosa is frequently affected in the chronic form.

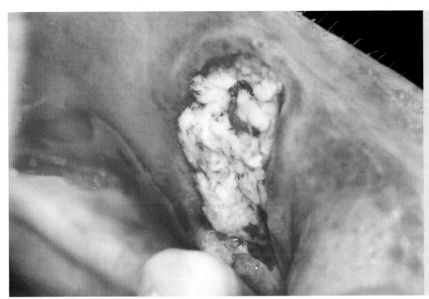

Fig. 23.22 Giant cell arteritis, necrotic ulcer on the buccal mucosa.

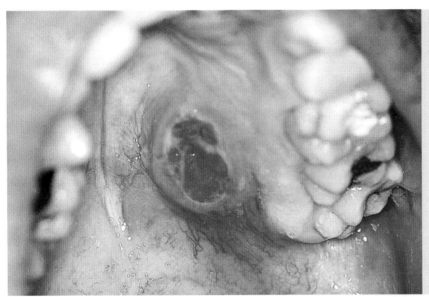

Fig. 23.23 Benign lymphoepithelial lesion, ulcerated nodules at the junction of the hard and soft palate.

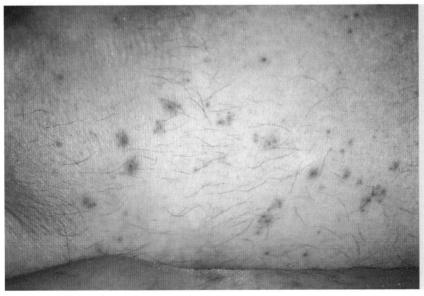

Fig. 23.24 Cryoglobulinemia, porphyric lesions on the skin of the lower extremities.

Introduction

GVHD is a complex multisystemic immune disorder that develops in patients who have undergone allogeneic bone marrow or stem cell transplantation to treat leukemias, myelodysplastic syndrome, myelin aplasia, immunodeficiency disorders, and solid tumors. The disorder is the result of the immune reaction caused by the allogeneic lymphoid cells of the donor against the host who lacks the donor's antigens. This reaction leads to GVHD that manifests with a plethora of signs and symptoms from multiple tissues and organs. Among the most affected systems are the gastrointestinal tract, liver, skin, nails, and oral and genital mucosa.

The disease is classified into *acute*, that occurs from the first week following the transplant and until 3 months after that and affects 20 to 40% of the patients and *chronic*, that starts 100 days after the transplantation and affects 40% of the patients. The risk of development of the chronic form is approximately 10 times greater in the patients who also presented the acute form of the disease. The pathogenetic mechanism is complex. CD8 T and natural killer (NK) lymphocytes seem to be implicated by releasing many cytotoxic cytokines. The most important predictor of GVHD remains human leukocyte antigen (HLA) compatibility between donor and recipient.

Clinical features

Clinically, the *acute* form is characterized by fever, diffuse erythematous, and maculopapular cutaneous rash with an initial predilection for acral areas. Gastrointestinal tract and liver are the two other primary organ systems affected. The mucosae are rarely affected with conjunctivitis dominating. Intraorally, erythema, atypical painful ulcerations, lichenoid lesions, and a burning sensation might be present.

The *chronic* form of the disease may manifest in nearly any organ system. Skin and mucosal involvement are common. Other sites of involvement include eyes, salivary glands, esophagus, liver, pancreas, and lungs. Early cutaneous changes include lichen planus–like lesions (reticulate pink to violet papules and plaques with overlying scale) (**Fig. 23.27**). Later involvement includes sclerotic changes and poikiloderma. When sclerotic changes occur, morphea-like sclerosis is initially observed that then spread in a diffuse pattern, similar to systemic scleroderma. In addition, poikiloderma, lupus erythematosus–like eruption, psoriasiform plaques, hyperpigmentation, scarring alopecia, myalgia, muscular weakness, and other symptoms are compatible with polymyositis. Oral manifestations are common in the chronic form (70–90%) and include erythema, lichenoid lesions, and painful ulceration that mainly affect the tongue, gingiva buccal mucosa and lips, and restriction of mouth opening (**Figs. 23.28, 23.29**). Superficial mucoceles, pyogenic granuloma, and verruciform xanthomas may occasionally occur. Because of the involvement of salivary glands and lacrimal glands, xerostomia and xerophthalmia are common mimicking Sjögren's syndrome (**Figs. 23.30, 23.31**). Genital involvement with pruritus burning, dyspareunia, and scarring are common. Nail changes are also common (thin, brittle nails). The morbidity and mortality are mostly associated with opportunistic infections (viral, bacterial, fungal) that are due to the immunosuppression from both the disease and the treatment. The diagnosis is mainly based on the history and the clinical features.

Pathology

Histopathologic examination of the skin reveals keratinocyte necrosis, hydropic degeneration of basal layer, and a band-like lymphocytic infiltrate in the upper dermis. In chronic scleroderma–like lesions, the histology is similar to scleroderma. The histologic features of minor salivary gland biopsy are similar to those of Sjögren's syndrome.

Treatment

The treatment of GVHD is not an easy task. First-line treatment consists of systemic corticosteroids. Immunosuppressants are administered such as azathioprine, mycophenolate mofetil, tacrolimus, rituximab, cyclosporine, depending on the gravity of the disease. Symptomatic therapy for oral, skin, eyes, and genital lesions is suggested. The management of the oral lesions includes saline rinses, topical anesthetics, antiseptic mouthwashes, topical steroid elixirs and gels, saliva substitutes, topical cyclosporine, and mouthwashes with granulocyte-macrophage colony-stimulating factor (GM-CSF). For persistent oral lesions, prednisolone per os 30 to 50 mg/d for 2 to 3 weeks and then gradually reduced in the period of 1 to 2 months gives very good results.

Chronic Viral Hepatitis

Introduction

Chronic viral hepatitis is a chronic disorder when the acute counterpart reaches 6 months. It is mainly caused by hepatitis B and C viruses.

Clinical features

The main clinical manifestations include jaundice, pruritus, diarrhea, and diffuse skin pigmentation and xanthomas. In later stages, when liver cirrhosis is established, portal hypertension, esophageal varices, hemorrhage, ascites, encephalopathy, and osteomalacia are observed among other signs. The disease may coexist with systemic sclerosis. In later stages of the disease, the oral mucosa becomes thin, erythematous, and atrophic and telangiectasia may develop, mainly on the lips (**Fig. 23.32**). The diagnosis is based on the clinical features and the results of further investigations.

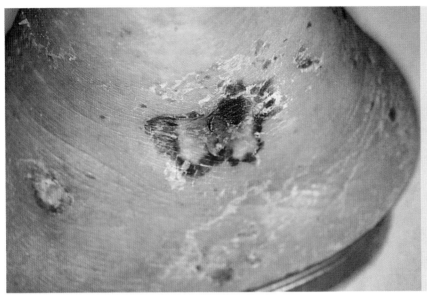

Fig. 23.25 Cryoglobulinemia, necrosis, and ulceration on the skin of the lower leg.

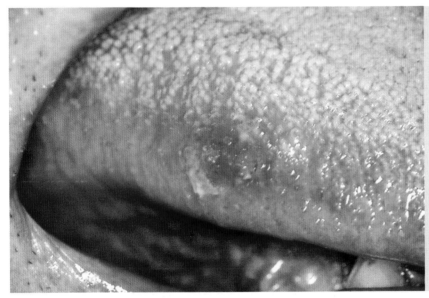

Fig. 23.26 Cryoglobulinemia, small ulceration on the lateral border of the tongue.

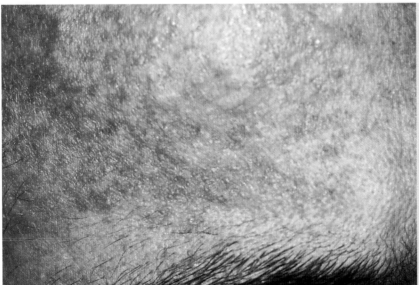

Fig. 23.27 Graft-versus-host disease, chronic form. Brown papules on the forehead.

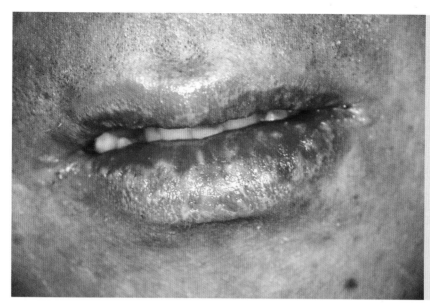

Fig. 23.28 Graft-versus-host disease, chronic form. Edema and lichenoid lesions on the lower lip.

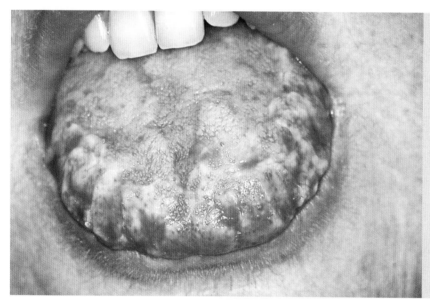

Fig. 23.29 Graft-versus-host disease, chronic form. Lichenoid lesions on the tongue.

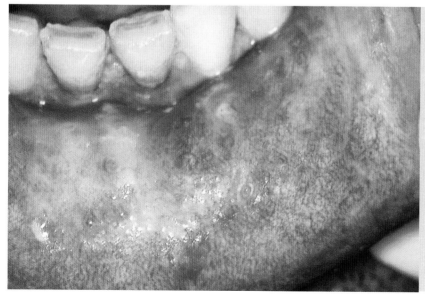

Fig. 23.30 Graft-versus-host disease, chronic form. Enlargement of the lower lip minor salivary glands.

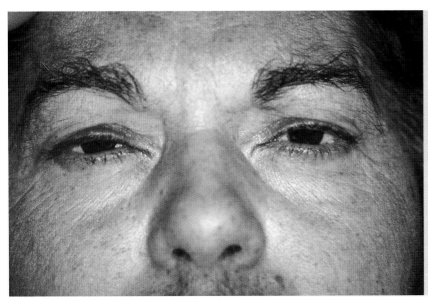

Fig. 23.31 Graft-versus-host disease, chronic form. Bilateral conjunctivitis and edema of the eyelids.

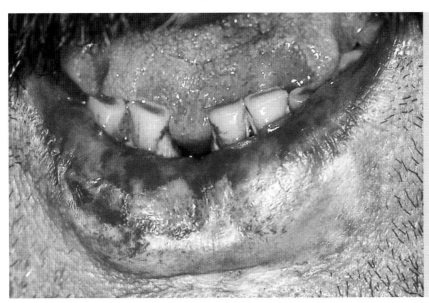

Fig. 23.32 Chronic virus hepatitis, telangiectasia, and erosion of the lower lip.

Differential diagnosis
- Systemic sclerosis
- CREST syndrome
- SLE

Laboratory tests

Special serologic, immunologic tests as well as liver biopsy are required.

Treatment

This is left to the specialist hepatologist.

Chronic Active Hepatitis

Key points
- An autoimmune hepatic disorder.
- Several manifestations from multiple organs.
- Oral mucosal lesions are rare.

Introduction

Chronic active hepatitis is a type of chronic virus hepatitis that gradually develops into hepatic cirrhosis.

Clinical features

Additionally, to the liver disease there are disorders occurring from the kidneys, lungs, joints, intestine, and hemolytic anemia and amenorrhea. The oral mucosa is rarely affected. The gingiva may appear erythematous, edematous, and painful on palpation (**Fig. 23.33**). However, rarely detach as in desquamative gingivitis. The diagnosis is based on the signs and symptoms present and the results of further investigations.

Differential diagnosis
- Plasma cell gingivitis
- Soft tissue plasmacytoma
- Granular gingivitis
- Desquamative gingivitis
- Psoriasis

Laboratory tests

Special serologic and immunologic tests as well as liver biopsy are required.

Treatment

This is left to the specialist hepatologist.

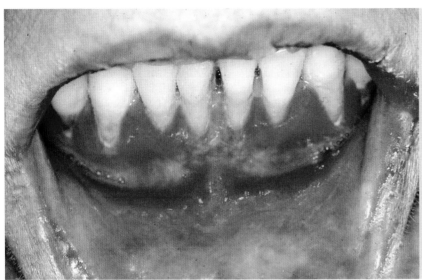

Fig. 23.33 Chronic active hepatitis, prominent erythema, and edema of the lower gingiva.

24 Immunodeficiencies

Immunodeficiencies are a large group of disorders whereby the body's immune system is either compromised or even absent. They are classified into (1) **primary** or **congenital** and (2) **secondary** or **acquired**. *Primary* immunodeficiencies are a genetically heterogeneous group of inherited disorders that can cause malfunction in different parts of the immune system. This results in individuals who are susceptible to topical and systemic opportunistic infections, malignancies, autoimmune disorders, and various allergic reactions. As a consequence, their life is in danger from infancy to adulthood. Using molecular criteria, the World Health Organization (WHO) recognized more than 150 primary immunodeficiencies in 2011. Following this, the International Union of Immunological Societies (IUIS) Expert Committee on Primary Immunodeficiency met in New York in April 2013 for an update. In this last report, more than 30 new gene defects were added that were subsequently identified. In general, primary immunodeficiencies can range from relatively common to very rare and affect humoral, or cell-mediated immunity, or both. A few selected types of primary immunodeficiency that present with oral manifestations are listed in **Table 24.1**.

Secondary immunodeficiencies are the result of acquired factors that suppress the immune system after birth. For those, see **Table 24.2**.

Immunosuppression caused by medication is a relatively recent problem. The most commonly used immunosuppressive medication, their indications, and oral side effects are presented in **Table 24.3**. The patients in this group often develop infections (*bacterial-fungal-viral*), neoplasias (mainly lymphomas and leukemias), and other disorders. In the following text, there is mention of the oral complications presented in patients with secondary immunodeficiency and their particular special features. For more details, please refer to the specific chapters of this book describing the various diseases.

Infections

Infections are the most common complication in immunosuppressed patients. These are facilitated by poor oral hygiene. The following infections belong to this group:

a. *Fungal infections* can be quite common. These are mainly candidiasis and rarely systemic fungal infections such as aspergillosis, mucormycosis, cryptococcosis, and histoplasmosis (see Chapter 19).

b. *Viral infections* are also common and are predominantly caused by the human herpes virus (HHV) group and the human papillomavirus (HPV) group. In **Table 24.4**, the herpes virus group is classified and the oral lesions that each virus causes, especially in transplant patients. HPV often cause condylomata acuminata in the mouth, verruca vulgaris, and focal epithelial hyperplasia.

c. *Bacterial infections* are often caused by anaerobic bacteria, *Staphylococcus aureus* and *Staphylococcus epidermidis*, and rarely by other bacteria (*Klebsiella*, *Pseudomonas* etc.). They can cause atypical ulceration, covered by a necrotic pseudomembrane and may be accompanied by fever and lymphadenopathy. Other common clinical manifestations in this group are necrotizing ulcerative gingivitis and necrotizing ulcerative periodontitis. Clinical features of oral infection in immunocompromised patients are: (1) the lesions are usually extensive, (2) they tend to recur, (3) they are more severe, (4) they can often evolve into systemic infection, (5) they can be resistant to treatment, and (6) they can be life threatening.

The treatment of oral infection in immunocompromised patients consists of antifungal, antiviral, and antibacterial medication used by nonimmunocompromised patients with the relevant infection. There are therapeutic protocols that apply to immunocompromised patients based on five parameters that are classified in **Table 24.5**.

Neoplasms

This group is classified into the following types:

a. Non-Hodgkin's lymphomas (see Chapter 40)
b. Kaposi's sarcoma (see Chapter 39)
c. Squamous cell carcinoma (see Chapter 39)

Non-Hodgkin's lymphomas and Kaposi's sarcoma are the most common, while squamous cell carcinoma is rare and occurs mostly on the lower lip of transplant patients. Their clinical features are the same as those of nonimmunocompromised patients and one can look in the relevant chapters of this book for more details. Finally, the various treatments are based on the same principles as in nonimmunocompromised patients.

Table 24.1 Primary immunodeficiencies with oral manifestations

Disorder	Main clinical manifestations	Oral manifestations
Severe combined immunodeficiency (SCI)	Recurrent infections (mucocutaneous candidiasis, pneumonia, viral gastroenteritis, cutaneous infections), chronic diarrhea, developmental delay	Mucocutaneous candidiasis, bacterial infections
Common variable immunodeficiency	Bacterial infections, cutaneous lesions, autoimmune disorders (hemolytic anemia, thrombocytopenic purpura, vasculitis), increased risk of neoplasias	Mucocutaneous candidiasis
Agammaglobulinemia	Recurrent bacterial infections, cutaneous infections, enteroviral infections, lymphomas	Staphylococcal and streptococcal infections
Selective IgA deficiency	Same as in common variable immunodeficiency	Mucocutaneous candidiasis
Hyper-IgM syndrome	Recurrent bacterial infections, autoimmune disorders, cutaneous lesions	Mucocutaneous candidiasis, ulceration, papillomas
Hyper-IgE syndrome	Cutaneous and respiratory bacterial infections, fungal infections, atopic dermatitis, papulovesicular dermatitis, osteopenia, skoliosis, CNS disorders	Chronic candidiasis, failure of deciduous teeth exfoliation, ectopic eruption/noneruption of permanent teeth
Hypohidrotic ectodermal dysplasia with immunodeficiency (see Chapter 25)	Opportunistic bacterial infections, pyodermatitis, hypohidrotic ectodermal dysplasia syndrome manifestations	Hypohidrotic ectodermal dysplasia features, infections
Complement deficiency (predominantly C2)	Bacterial infections, autoimmune disorders, Hodgkin's lymphoma	Bacterial infections, gingivitis, lupus
Ataxia-telangiectasia	Oculocutaneous telangiectasia, cerebellar ataxia, bacterial infections, lymphomas, leukemias, developmental delay	Palatal telangiectasia
DiGeorge syndrome	Chronic mucocutaneous candidiasis, eczematous dermatitis	Mucocutaneous candidiasis, labial anomalies
Various primary phagocytic disorders	Recurrent bacterial infections mainly of the skin and the respiratory system	Ulcerations, bacterial infections, gingivitis
Wiskott-Aldrich syndrome	Atopic dermatitis, bacterial infections, hemorrhage, "autoimmune disorders," lymphomas	Petechiae, ecchymoses, gingival hemorrhage
Chédiak-Higashi syndrome (see Chapter 25)	Skin hypopigmentation, silver-colored hair, photophobia, nystagmus, recurrent bacterial infections, hemorrhagic disposition, pancytopenia, hepatic, splenic, lymphatic lymphohistiocytic infiltration	Ulcerations, gingivitis, hemorrhage, periodontal destruction
Chronic granulomatous disease (see Chapter 25)	Recurrent bacterial infections and fungal infections of the skin and lungs, pulmonary, hepatic, splenic, and gastrointestinal granulomas	Ulceration mimicking aphthae, granulomatous cheilitis, perioral dermatitis
Chronic mucocutaneous candidiasis syndrome (see Chapter 19)	Serious, recurrent cutaneous, ungual, and mucosal infections by *Candida albicans*	Chronic mucocutaneous candidiasis
Good's syndrome (see Chapter 25)	Thymoma, serious myasthenia, infections, gastrointestinal disorders	Severe candidiasis
Leukocyte adhesion deficiency	Cutaneous, auricular, pulmonary infections, cutaneous ulcerations, mental and developmental delay, myelodysplastic syndromes	Gingivitis, severe periodontitis, early tooth loss

Abbreviation: CNS, central nervous system.

Table 24.2 Secondary immunodeficiencies, classification according to cause

- Immunosuppressive medication
- Organ transplant
- Human immunodeficiency virus infection
- Hematologic malignancy (lymphomas, leukemias)
- Bone marrow aplasia
- Neutropenias
- Solid neoplasms
- Nephrotic syndrome
- Uremia
- Second-degree burns and above
- Sickle cell anemia
- Splenectomy

Table 24.3 Common immunosuppressive medication and oral complications

Medication	Indications	Oral complications
• Corticosteroids	Autoimmune disorders, organ transplant, hematopoietic and lymphatic tissue malignancies	Candidiasis, viral infections
• Azathioprine	Autoimmune disorders, organ transplant, hematopoietic and lymphatic tissue malignancies	Ulceration, viral infections
• Mycophenolate mofetil	Autoimmune disorders, organ transplant, hematopoietic and lymphatic tissue malignancies	Infections
• Tacrolimus	Autoimmune disorders, organ transplant, hematopoietic and lymphatic tissue malignancies	Ulceration
• Cyclosporine	Autoimmune disorders, organ transplant, psoriasis	Gingival enlargement, infections
• Methotrexate	Autoimmune disorders, organ transplant, psoriasis	Ulceration, non-Hodgkin's lymphoma
Biological agents		
• Anti-TNF-α	Autoimmune disorders, inflammatory disorders, psoriasis	Infections
• Anti-IL2 antibody	Transplantation	Infections
• Antithymoglobulin	Transplantation	Infections

Table 24.4 Human herpes virus group and oral manifestations in immunosuppressed patients

Virus	Oral manifestations
• HHV1—herpes simplex virus 1	Extensive erosions and deep ulceration that mimic primary herpetic gingivostomatitis
• HHV2—herpes simplex virus 2	Extensive genital and oral erosions
• HHV3—varicella-zoster virus	Herpes zoster causing deep bilateral necrotic lesions and osteomyelitis that can be lethal in 18% of the cases
• HHV4—Epstein-Barr virus	Infectious mononucleosis, hairy leukoplakia. It predominantly affects kidney and other organ transplant patients and HIV patients
• HHV5—Cytomegalovirus (CMV)	Nonspecific ulcerations, erythema. They develop 1–3 mo posttransplant. It can be the main reason for transplant failure
• HHV6	CMV reactivation and increased severity of CMV disease
• HHV7	Greater risk of developing CMV disease
• HHV8	Kaposi's sarcoma

Table 24.5 Therapeutics of oral complications in immunosuppressed patients

1. Prophylactic medication
2. Increased dose of medication
3. Longer treatment
4. Combination of drugs
5. Collaboration of the oral medicine specialist with the consultant-in-charge (internal medicine, oncologist, hematologist, etc.)

25 Genetic Diseases

White Sponge Nevus

Key points

- An autosomal dominant disorder.
- Mutations in the genes encoding keratins 4 and 13 are the cause.
- The lesions commonly appear during the birth or early childhood.

Introduction

White sponge nevus, or Cannon's disease, is an uncommon autosomal dominant disorder. It may appear at birth or more commonly during childhood. It progresses until early adulthood, remaining stable thereafter.

Clinical features

Clinically, the affected oral mucosa is thick, white or gray-white with multiple furrows and a spongy texture (**Figs. 25.1, 25.2**). The lesions are benign, asymptomatic, and usually bilateral. The buccal mucosa, floor of the mouth, soft palate, alveolar mucosa, and labial mucosa are the most commonly affected sites. It can occasionally involve the nasal mucosa, esophagus, larynx, and vaginal or rectal mucosa. The extent of the lesions varies. The diagnosis is based on the history, the clinical features, and laboratory tests.

Differential diagnosis

- Leukoplakia
- Leukoedema
- Chronic biting
- Pachyonychia congenita
- Dyskeratosis congenita
- Hereditary benign intraepithelial dyskeratosis
- Focal palmoplantar and oral mucosa hyperkeratosis syndrome

Pathology

Histologic examination can be helpful in establishing the diagnosis, but it is not pathognomonic. The main features are hyperparakeratosis, marked acanthosis, and intracellular edema. Additionally, the cells of the prickle cell layer have abundant clear cytoplasm that gives the characteristics of large clear cells.

Treatment

No treatment is necessary.

Hereditary Benign Intraepithelial Dyskeratosis

Key points

- An autosomal dominant disorder.
- First described in North Carolina's inhabitants (USA).
- Primarily affects the mouth and the eyes.

Introduction

Hereditary benign intraepithelial dyskeratosis is a rare genetic disorder inherited in an autosomal dominant manner. It was first described after observation in North Carolina inhabitants where a mix of three different races had occurred (Indian, African-American, and Caucasian). The lesions usually appear during childhood.

Clinical features

Clinically, the oral lesions appear as thick, soft, corrugated white plaques (**Fig. 25.3**). The lesions are firm, asymptomatic, adherent, and benign in nature. The most commonly affected sites are the buccal and labial mucosa followed by other oral mucosal sites. The ocular lesions are early and common and present as a thick, opaque gelatinous plaque that covers the eyelid conjunctiva with extension to the cornea. The ocular lesions are more pronounced during spring time and tend to improve during the summer and autumn. The most common symptoms in the periods of exacerbation include lacrimation, pruritus, and photophobia, while blindness may occur in rare instances. The diagnosis is based on the history and the clinical features.

Differential diagnosis

- White sponge nevus
- Leukoedema
- Leukoplakia
- Dyskeratosis congenita
- Pachyonychia congenita
- Focal palmoplantar and oral mucosa hyperkeratosis syndrome

Pathology

Histologic examination of the oral mucosa lesions reveals hyperparakeratosis, marked acanthosis, and dyskeratosis similar to that of Darier's disease, throughout the prickle cell layer.

Treatment

There is no need for treatment of the oral lesions. The patients should be followed by an ophthalmologist for the ocular lesions.

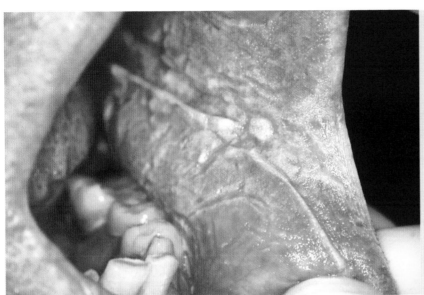

Fig. 25.1 White sponge nevus, lesions on the buccal mucosa.

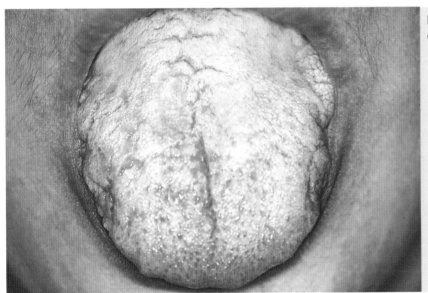

Fig. 25.2 White sponge nevus, lesions on the tongue.

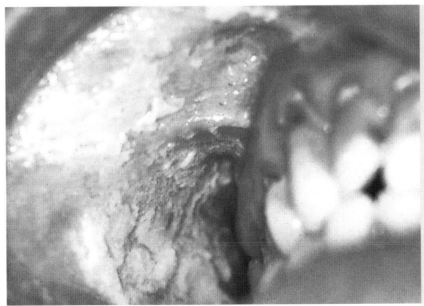

Fig. 25.3 Hereditary benign intraepithelial dyskeratosis, white plaques on the buccal mucosa.

Dyskeratosis Congenita

Key points

- A rare genodermatosis usually inherited in an X-linked recessive trait, therefore 90% of the patients are male.
- Main clinical characteristics are oral leukoplakia, skin hyperpigmentation, and nail dystrophy.
- Atresia of the lacrimal gland's duct leads to lacrimation.
- Bone marrow disorders (anemia, pancytopenia, thrombocytopenia).
- The disease predisposes to malignancies, mainly oral squamous cell carcinoma, Hodgkin's disease, acute myelogenic leukemia.

Introduction

Dyskeratosis congenita, or Zinsser-Engman-Cole syndrome, is a rare disorder with great genetic heterogeneity. It is usually transmitted via the X-linked trait and rarely via the autosomal dominant and autosomal recessive traits.

Clinical features

Clinically, the disorder is characterized by hyperpigmentation, telangiectasias, and atrophic areas of the skin during the first decade of life. This occurs primarily on the neck, chest, and the upper arms. Dystrophic nails, hyperhidrosis of palms and soles, and dermal and mucosal bullae may also occur (**Figs. 25.4, 25.5**). There is also increased lacrimation, chronic blepharitis, and ectropion (**Fig. 25.6**), ear anomalies, progressive bone marrow failure (anemia, leukopenia, thrombocytopenia, pancytopenia), gastrointestinal disorders, pulmonary fibrosis, liver cirrhosis, oral manifestations, and occasionally mental retardation. Oral lesions consist of recurrent blisters that rupture, leaving a raw ulcerated surface mainly on the tongue and less frequently on buccal mucosa and palate. Atrophy of the oral mucosa and the development of leukoplakia is the result of repeated episodes (**Fig. 25.7**). Malignant transformation of leukoplakia to squamous cell carcinoma may occur. Additionally, dental anomalies, usually regarding the teeth shape, hypodontia, and large interdental spaces may be observed. Increased risk for squamous cell carcinoma may develop in anus, vagina, cervix, esophagus, and skin, as well as Hodgkin's disease and acute myelogenous leukemia.

Differential diagnosis

- Pachyonychia congenita
- Fanconi's anemia
- Epidermolysis bullosa
- Goltz's syndrome
- Leukoplakia
- Lichen planus, hypertrophic type
- Graft-versus-host disease, chronic type

Pathology

Histopathologic examination of the oral lesions reveals hyperkeratosis, parakeratosis, acanthosis, but as the lesions progress to leukoplakia, epithelial dysplasia or carcinoma in situ or even squamous cell carcinoma can be developed.

Treatment

The management of dyskeratosis congenita requires multidisciplinary care. The oral lesions are managed symptomatically. However, periodic follow-up is necessary to check for malignant transformation.

Pachyonychia Congenita

Key points

- A disorder inherited in an autosomal dominant pattern.
- Two major types have been described: type 1 (Jadassohn-Lewandowsky) and type 2 (Jackson-Lawler).
- The main clinical characteristics are nail abnormalities, palmoplantar hyperkeratosis, and follicular hyperkeratosis.
- White lesions are observed on the oral mucosa.

Introduction

Pachyonychia congenita is classified into two major types: *type 1* (Jadassohn-Lewandowsky) and *type 2* (Jackson-Lawler). A considerable overlap exists between the two types and the classification is based on the affected gene. The disorder is inherited in an autosomal dominant pattern.

Clinical features

Clinically, the disorder is characterized by symmetrical thickening of the nails (**Fig. 25.8**), palmoplantar hyperkeratosis, hyperhidrosis, blister formation on the soles, especially during the warmer months, follicular keratosis, hoarseness, dyspnea, and hyperkeratosis of the oral mucosa (**Fig. 25.9**). The oral mucosa (tongue, palate, buccal mucosa gingiva) appears thick and white, or grayish-white. Angular cheilitis is also common. The oral lesions appear at birth or shortly thereafter and only in type 1 of the disorder. The diagnosis is based on the clinical features.

Differential diagnosis

- Dyskeratosis congenita
- Focal palmoplantar and oral mucosa hyperkeratosis syndrome
- Olmsted's syndrome
- Hereditary benign intraepithelial dyskeratosis
- White sponge nevus
- Leukoplakia

Pathology

Histopathologic examination of the oral lesions reveals hyperkeratosis, hyperparakeratosis, and acanthosis.

Treatment

The treatment is symptomatic. The oral lesions do not warrant any intervention as they are benign in nature and asymptomatic.

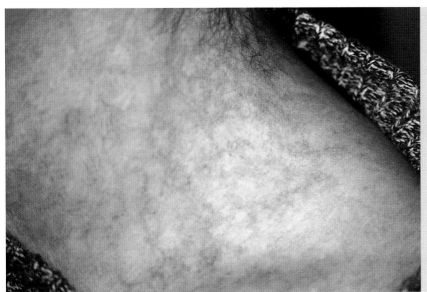

Fig. 25.4 Dyskeratosis congenita, pigmentation, and atrophy of the skin.

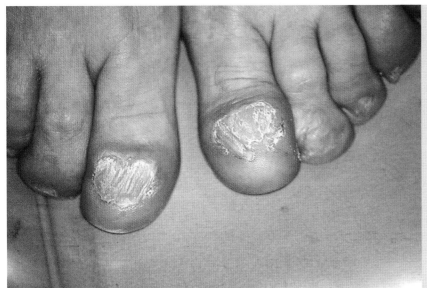

Fig. 25.5 Dyskeratosis congenita, nail dystrophy of the toes.

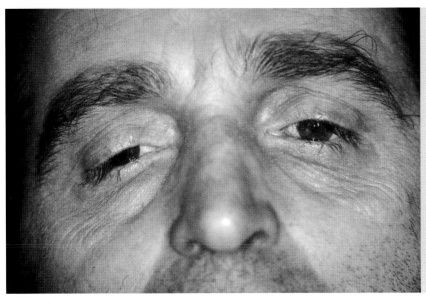

Fig. 25.6 Dyskeratosis congenita, blepharitis, and mild ectropion.

Hypohidrotic Ectodermal Dysplasia

Key points

- The most common disorder in the group of ectodermal dysplasias.
- Usually inherited in an X-linked pattern of inheritance.
- The main clinical features include anodontia or hypodontia, other dental anomalies, decreased ability to sweat, and hair and skin abnormalities.
- An early symptom is fever of unknown etiology during the summer months.

Introduction

Hypohidrotic ectodermal dysplasia is the most well-recognized genetic disease in the group of ectodermal dysplasias. It is characterized by dysplastic changes of tissues of ectodermal origin and is usually inherited as an X-linked recessive trait and less commonly as an autosomal dominant or autosomal recessive trait. The prevalence is approximately 1:10,000 live-born boys and may affect all racial and ethnic groups.

Clinical features

The main clinical manifestations include (1) characteristic faces (**Fig. 25.10**) (frontal bossing, saddle nose, large lips and ears); (2) thin, dry skin, and friable, sparse, blond, short hair; (3) decreased sweating or complete anhidrosis, due to the absence of sweat glands; (4) absence of eyebrows; and (5) oral lesions. The characteristic oral finding is hypodontia or anodontia, affecting both the deciduous and permanent dentition (**Fig. 25.11**). When teeth are present, they are hypoplastic and often have a conical shape. Xerostomia may occur because of salivary gland hypoplasia. The voice is frequently hoarse or raspy. The disease usually presents during the first year of life, with a fever of unknown cause (due to thermoregulation abnormalities caused by the absence of sweat glands) along with the retarded eruption or absence of the deciduous teeth.

Differential diagnosis

- Other forms of ectodermal dysplasias
- Idiopathic oligodontia
- Papillon-Lefèvre syndrome
- Chondroectodermal dysplasia
- Cleidocranial dysplasia
- Goltz's syndrome
- Incontinentia pigmenti

Pathology

Histopathologic examination of the skin reveals a thin and flat epidermis with reduction of the hair follicles and hair shaft abnormalities. There is a reduction in number of the sebaceous glands. The main finding, however, remains the great reduction or even total absence of the sweat glands.

Treatment

Multidisciplinary care is required for management of patients. There is no specific treatment. However, dental prosthetic rehabilitation should be applied from an early age. Sweat gland regulation is the work of the dermatologist.

Focal Palmoplantar and Oral Mucosa Hyperkeratosis Syndrome

Key points

- A rare genetic disorder inherited in an autosomal dominant trait.
- The oral characteristic is leukoplakia in areas of friction.
- Palmoplantar hyperkeratosis at the weight-bearing areas.

Introduction

Focal palmoplantar and oral mucosa hyperkeratosis syndrome is a rare genetic disorder inherited in an autosomal dominant pattern.

Clinical features

The disorder is characterized by (1) focal hyperkeratosis at the weight-bearing and pressure-related areas of the palms and soles (**Figs. 25.12, 25.13**) and (2) oral mucosal hyperkeratosis, mainly affecting the attached gingiva (**Fig. 25.14**). However, other areas bearing mechanical pressure or friction, such as the palate, alveolar mucosa, lateral border of the tongue, retromolar pad mucosa, and the buccal mucosa along the occlusal line, may manifest hyperkeratosis, presenting clinically as leukoplakia. Rarely, hyperhidrosis, hyperkeratosis, and thickening of the nails may be observed. The lesions appear early in puberty and their severity increases with age. The diagnosis is based on the clinical features.

Differential diagnosis

- Pachyonychia congenita
- Dyskeratosis congenita
- Hyperkeratosis and esophageal carcinoma syndrome
- White sponge nevus
- Papillon-Lefèvre syndrome
- Oral leukoplakia
- Focal palmoplantar hyperkeratosis

Pathology

Histopathologic examination of the oral mucosa reveals hyperorthokeratosis, hyperparakeratosis, and acanthosis.

Treatment

The treatment is symptomatic. Systemic retinoids may occasionally be helpful for the skin lesions.

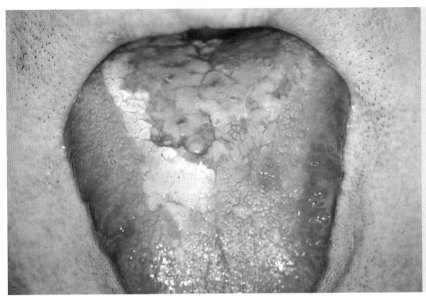

Fig. 25.7 Dyskeratosis congenita, leukoplakia on the dorsum of the tongue.

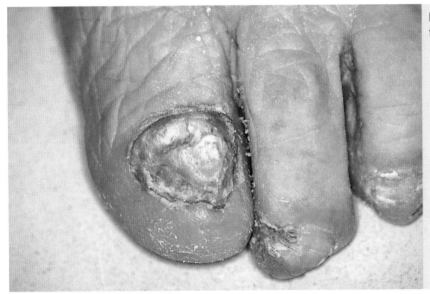

Fig. 25.8 Pachyonychia congenita, thickening of the toe nails.

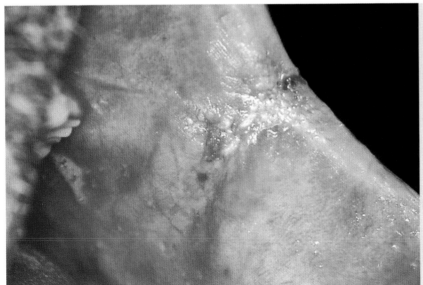

Fig. 25.9 Pachyonychia congenita, hyperkeratosis of the buccal mucosa.

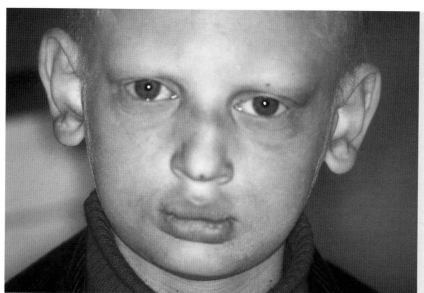

Fig. 25.10 Hypohidrotic ectodermal dysplasia, characteristic face.

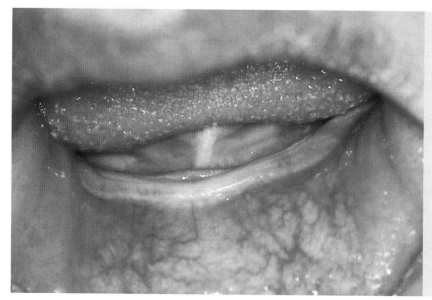

Fig. 25.11 Hypohidrotic ectodermal dysplasia, anodontia.

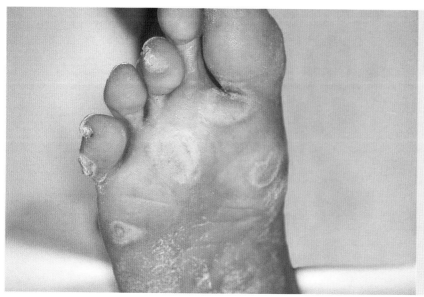

Fig. 25.12 Focal palmoplantar and oral mucosa hyperkeratosis syndrome, hyperkeratosis of the sole.

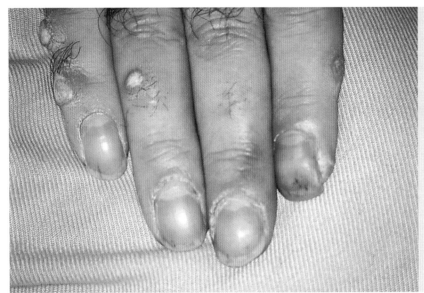

Fig. 25.13 Focal palmoplantar and oral mucosa hyperkeratosis syndrome, hyperkeratosis of the fingers, and thickening of the nails.

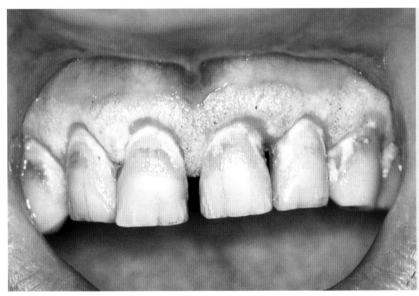

Fig. 25.14 Focal palmoplantar and oral mucosa hyperkeratosis syndrome, leukoplakia of the maxillary attached gingiva.

Papillon-Lefèvre Syndrome

Key points

- A genetic disorder inherited in an autosomal recessive fashion.
- A main characteristic is rapidly progressing periodontitis, affecting both deciduous and permanent dentition, leading to rapid loss of teeth.
- Other features include palmoplantar hyperkeratosis and other cutaneous lesions.

Introduction

Papillon-Lefèvre syndrome is a rare genetic disorder, inherited in an autosomal recessive fashion. Loss of function mutations in the cathepsin C gene are responsible for the syndrome. Its incidence is one to four cases per million of population.

Clinical features

Clinically, Papillon-Lefèvre is characterized by (1) hyperkeratosis of the palms and soles, as well as elbows and knees (**Figs. 25.15, 25.16**), psoriasiform lesions, follicular hyperkeratosis, nail dystrophy, and hyperhidrosis; (2) severe destruction of periodontal tissues of both deciduous and permanent dentitions; and (3) meningeal calcifications, recurrent pyoderma, and susceptibility to infections that are rare. Eruption of the deciduous teeth proceeds normally, but inflammation of the periodontal tissues, with periodontal pocket formation and bone destruction, ensues. The severity of the destruction of the periodontal tissues results in premature loss of all the deciduous teeth at about the fourth year of life (**Fig. 25.17**). The inflammatory response subsides at this stage, and the gingiva resumes its normal appearance. The periodontitis again develops with the eruption of the permanent teeth and results in a new cycle of periodontal destruction. The responsible cathepsin C gene is also expressed in various inflammatory cells that are vital to the body's immune defenses. This possibly leads to the impaired chemotactic and phagocytic function of polymorphonuclear leukocytes and the impaired reactivity to T- and B-cell mitogens, described in many reports. The periodontal lesions and the cutaneous manifestations usually appear between the second and fourth year of life. The diagnosis is mainly based on clinical criteria.

Differential diagnosis

- Aggressive periodontitis
- Haim-Munk syndrome
- Acatalasia
- Hypophosphatasia
- Langerhans' cell histiocytosis
- Hypohidrotic ectodermal dysplasia
- Chédiak-Higashi syndrome
- Congenital neutropenia
- Cyclic neutropenia

Pathology

Histopathologic examination of the periodontal tissues is nonspecific. A dense inflammatory infiltrate in the lamina propria with polymorphonuclear neutrophils, lymphocytes, plasmocytes, and histiocytes is seen. The epithelium appears normal or mildly hyperplastic. Dental panoramic tomography reveals severe periodontal destruction and bone loss.

Treatment

Therapy of the periodontal disease has not proved to prevent teeth loss. However, plaque control, scaling, and oral hygiene instructions are to be recommended. The treatment of any cutaneous lesions is overseen by a dermatologist.

Olmsted's Syndrome

Key points

- An extremely rare genetic disorder with an unclear pattern of inheritance.
- Predominantly affects males with a ratio 3:1.
- The lesions appear during the first year of life.
- The main clinical characteristics are palmoplantar hyperkeratosis and hyperkeratotic plaques in the perioral, genital, inguinal, and intergluteal areas.

Introduction

Olmsted's syndrome, or congenital palmoplantar and perioral keratoderma, is a rare genetic disorder first described by Olmsted in 1927 in a 5-year-old boy. About 73 cases have been reported so far. The pattern of inheritance has not been established and most cases are sporadic. There are, however, reports of possible autosomal dominant trait (mutations in *TRPV3*—transient receptor potential vanilloid 3) and X-linked recessive trait (mutations in *MBTPS2*—membrane-bound transcription factor protease, site 2). Additional genes remain to be identified.

Clinical features

Clinically, the first lesions become obvious immediately after the birth or during the first months of life. The main clinical characteristics are severe symmetrical palmoplantar

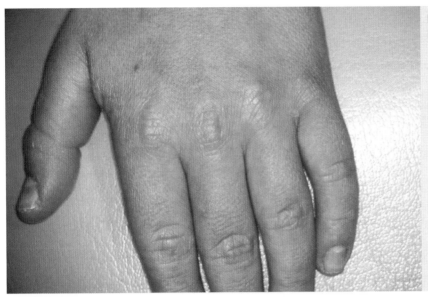

Fig. 25.15 Papillon-Lefèvre syndrome, hyperkeratosis of the hand.

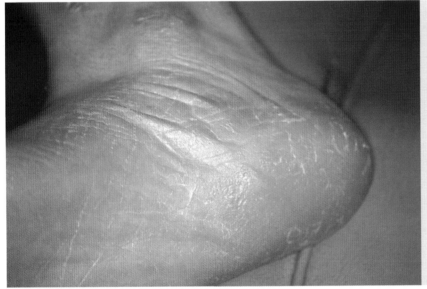

Fig. 25.16 Papillon-Lefèvre syndrome, hyperkeratosis of the sole.

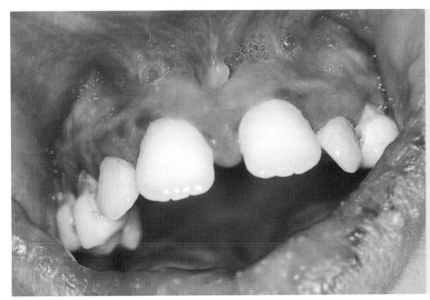

Fig. 25.17 Papillon-Lefèvre syndrome, periodontitis, and teeth displacement.

hyperkeratosis (**Figs. 25.18, 25.19**) and perioral hyperkeratosis. Periorificial lesions are common around the commissures as irregular, elevated hyperkeratotic plaques (**Fig. 25.20**). Similar lesions can be observed in the anal, inguinal, genital, and natal areas. The keratoderma is severe and progressive and may lead to dysmorphies and autoamputation of the digits. Nail dystrophy, alopecia, palmoplantar hyperhidrosis, mental retardation, failure to thrive, and oral mucosal leukoplakia may also occur. The diagnosis is based on the clinical features.

Differential diagnosis

- Mal de Meleda disease
- Vohwinkel's syndrome
- Clouston's syndrome
- Papillon-Lefévre syndrome
- Pachyonychia congenita
- Focal palmoplantar and oral mucosa hyperkeratosis syndrome

Pathology

When differential diagnosis from other severe forms of palmoplantar keratosis is difficult, genetic studies are essential to search for *TRPV3* or *MBTPS2* mutation.

Treatment

The treatment is symptomatic. Topical and systemic treatment of hyperkeratosis can provide some relief and includes corticosteroids, retinoids, and keratolytics. Surgical treatment may be offered for the milder perioral lesions.

Benign Acanthosis Nigricans

Key points

- A group of mucocutaneous disorders.
- Traditionally, it is classified into benign and malignant forms.
- The malignant form is associated with internal malignancy.
- The benign forms include hereditary and secondary (obesity-related, endocrine forms) subtypes.
- Acanthosis nigricans can also be divided according to the cause.

Introduction

Acanthosis nigricans is a rare group of mucocutaneous disorders, characterized by dark discoloration and papillary lesions. Using clinical criteria, the disorder is classified into two major types: *benign* and *malignant*. The benign variety is subdivided into (1) *familial*, which is a genodermatosis, inherited in an autosomal dominant pattern and rarely involves the oral cavity, (2) *secondary* acanthosis nigricans that occurs as part of other syndromes, such as Prader-Willi, Crouzon, Lawrence and Bloom, and various endocrinopathies such as insulin-resistant diabetes mellitus (hypothyroidism, Addison's disease, acromegaly); this subtype is manifested during childhood and does not involve the oral mucosa, and (3) *pseudoacanthosis*, which is an acquired, secondary form that affects obese and dark-skinned people 25 to 60 years and involves the skin only.

Clinical features

The familial (genetic) type of acanthosis nigricans involves the oral mucosa in approximately 10 to 15% of cases. Clinically, there is hypertrophy and elongation of the filiform papillae resulting in a shaggy appearance of the tongue (**Fig. 25.21**), while the lips and the gingiva may be covered by papillomatous growths giving them a papillary appearance (**Figs. 25.22, 25.23**). The oral lesions are characteristically of normal color without any pigmentation. The tongue and lips, and less frequently gingiva, buccal mucosa, and palate, are most frequently affected. The skin is thick with small, velvety papillary nodules and dark pigmentation. The axillae, neck, groin, umbilicus, perianal area, and the genitalia are the most common sites of involvement (**Fig. 25.24**). The diagnosis is based on clinical criteria.

Differential diagnosis

- Malignant acanthosis nigricans
- Cowden's syndrome
- Ichthyosis hystrix

Pathology

Histopathologic examination of the oral mucosa exhibits papillomatosis, hyperorthokeratosis, marked acanthosis and elongation of the rete ridges, and usually minimal increased melanin deposition.

Treatment

There is not an effective treatment. Keratolytic agents or electrosurgery is sometimes applied with partial success.

Darier's Disease

Key points

- An uncommon autosomal dominant disorder.
- Cutaneous hyperkeratotic macules and plaques favor seborrheic areas. The palms and soles are also affected.
- Oral mucosal lesions occur in approximately 20 to 40% of the cases with whitish papules.
- Microscopically, acantholytic dyskeratosis with "corps ronds" and "grains" formation.

Introduction

Darier's disease or dyskeratosis follicularis is an uncommon autosomal dominant genodermatosis. Several pathogenic mechanisms have been proposed. Recently, the abnormal gene in Darier's disease has been identified as *ATP2A2*, found on chromosome 12q23–24.1. This gene codes for the SERCA2b enzyme that is required to transport calcium within the cell and finally cause both acanthosis and apoptosis. More than

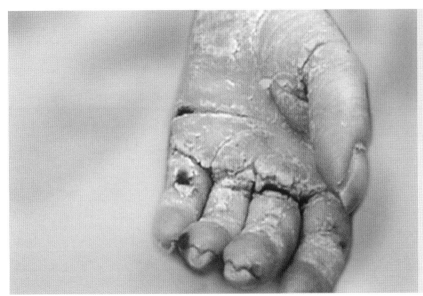

Fig. 25.18 Olmsted's syndrome, palmar hyperkeratosis, and nail dystrophy.

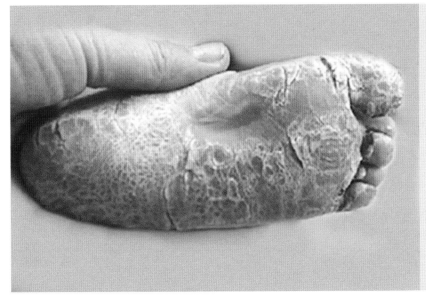

Fig. 25.19 Olmsted's syndrome, hyperkeratosis of the sole.

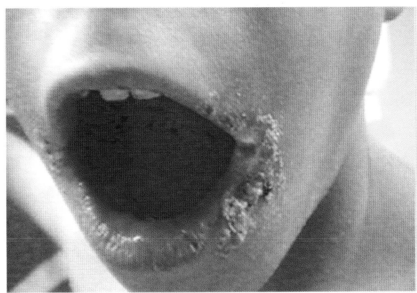

Fig. 25.20 Olmsted's syndrome, hyperkeratosis of the commissures.

120 ATP2A2 mutation have been identified. Darier's disease equally affects males and females. In 70% of the cases, the disease starts between 6 and 20 years with a peak around 10 to 15 years. The disease affects mainly skin and nails, but the mucosae may also be involved (mouth, rectum, genitalia).

Clinical features

Clinically, multiple skin keratotic papules of a few millimeters in diameter, which occasionally may coalesce into large plaques, are seen (**Fig. 25.25**). They are brownish-red in color and are covered by a yellowish to tan scaly *seborrheic crust*. The lesions tend to become confluent and may form papillomatous masses. Small hypomelanotic macules may develop and intermix with the keratotic papules. Rarely, vesicles or bullae may form. The most common affected sites are the scalp, neck, breast, back ear, nasolabial fold, dorsal aspect of the hands and feet. The nails present with subungual keratosis and longitudinal, white or red ridges and lines. The cutaneous lesions usually deteriorate during the summer months and may be then accompanied by pruritus and odor.

The oral mucosa is affected in 20 to 40% of the cases. The severity of oral lesions is following the pattern of activity of the disease on the skin. The typical oral lesions are small whitish confluent papules that may subsequently coalesce, giving a micropapillomatous appearance, or form into plaques and become hypertrophic, assuming a cobblestone appearance. The

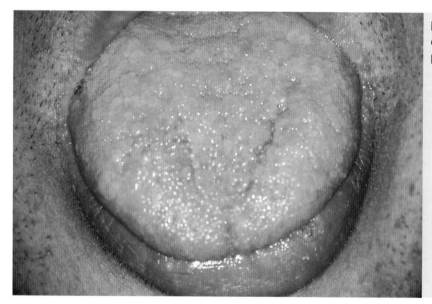

Fig. 25.21 Benign acanthosis nigricans, elongation of the papillae, and papillomatous elevations of the tongue.

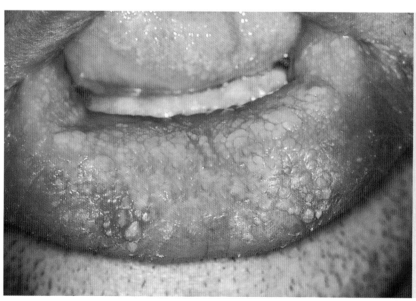

Fig. 25.22 Benign acanthosis nigricans, multiple papillary nodules of the lower lip mucosa.

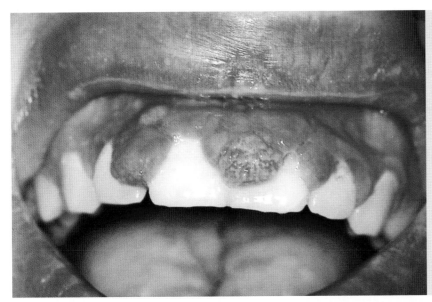

Fig. 25.23 Benign acanthosis nigricans, papillomatous enlargement of the interdental papillae.

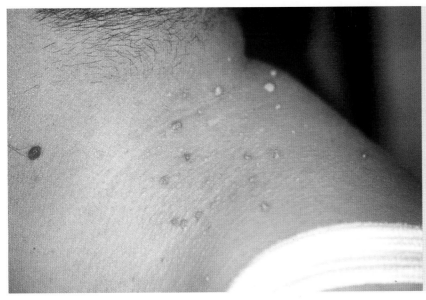

Fig. 25.24 Benign acanthosis nigricans, small cutaneous nodules.

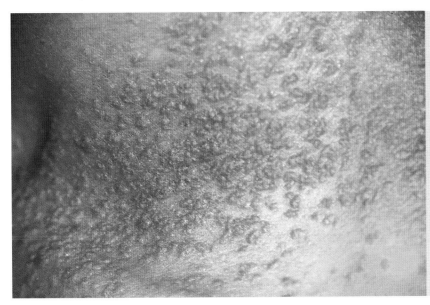

Fig. 25.25 Darier's disease, coalescing cutaneous papules.

most common sites of involvement are the palate, followed by the gingiva, buccal mucosa, and tongue (**Figs. 25.26, 25.27**). Salivary gland obstruction and painful swelling may occasionally occur.

The ocular, rectal, vaginal, vulval, and pharyngeal mucosae may also be involved. The disease has a chronic course with periods of exacerbation and regression, but with no spontaneous remission. The diagnosis is mainly based on clinical criteria, but should be confirmed by a biopsy.

Differential diagnosis

- Acanthosis nigricans
- Papillary hyperplasia of the palate
- Nicotinic stomatitis
- Warty dyskeratoma
- Pemphigus vegetans
- Grover's disease
- Acrokeratosis verruciformis of Hopf
- Seborrheic dermatitis
- Hailey-Hailey disease

Pathology

Histopathologic examination reveals acantholysis at all levels and dyskeratosis. Dyskeratosis is due to apoptosis of premature keratinocytes and has two distinct features: *corps ronds*, which are acantholytic cells with small pyknotic nuclei, a perinuclear clear halo, and eosinophilic cytoplasm and *grains* which are small oval cells with an intensely eosinophilic cytoplasm composed of keratin bundles containing parakeratotic nuclear remnants mainly seen in the stratum corneum and the granular layer. Acantholysis is caused by suprabasal disruption of the desmosomes.

Treatment

The treatment of the oral lesions is symptomatic. The treatment of the cutaneous lesions is performed by the dermatologist and can be local, systemic, and surgical, depending on the extent

of the disease, its severity, and the affected sites. Moisturizers, dermabrasion, systemic retinoids, cyclosporine, and methotrexate among others have been tried with variable results.

Hailey-Hailey Disease

Key points

- A rare autosomal dominant genodermatosis.
- Clinically, it is characterized by flaccid vesicles and erosions on the axillae, groin, perianal region and the neck.
- The oral mucosa is rarely involved.
- Characteristic histologic feature is acantholysis.

Introduction

Hailey-Hailey disease or familial benign chronic pemphigus is a rare genodermatosis inherited in an autosomal dominant pattern. The defect responsible has been identified on gene *ATP2C1* found on chromosome 3q21–24. This gene codes for the protein SPCA1 (secretory pathway calcium/manganese-ATPase), a calcium and manganese pump. That subsequently has an effect on desmosomes. The exact prevalence is not known, and the disease affects both sexes around the second and third decades of life.

Clinical features

Clinically, it is characterized by a recurrent group of small flaccid vesicles arising on an erythematous or normal skin base. The vesicles rapidly rupture, leaving erosions covered with crusts. The skin lesions are usually localized, with a tendency to spread peripherally, although the center heals with pigmentation or exhibits granular vegetations (**Fig. 25.28**). Widespread lesions are unusual. The cutaneous lesions often exhibit secondary infection by bacteria, fungi, or viruses.

The lesions regress during the winter and are exacerbated during the summer. The most frequently affected sites are those under mechanical friction such as the axillae, groin, neck, and perianal region. Nail changes may rarely occur. The

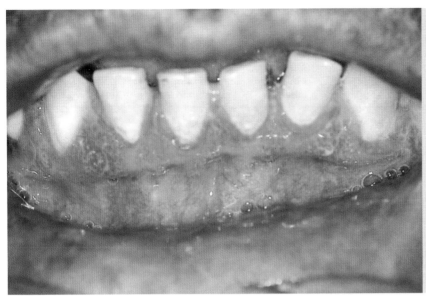

Fig. 25.26 Darier's disease, coalescing hypertrophic papules of the gingiva.

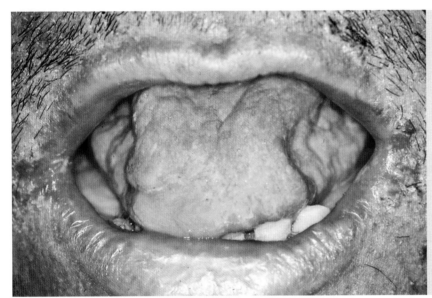

Fig. 25.27 Darier's disease, coalescing papules of the tongue that give a micropapillomatous appearance.

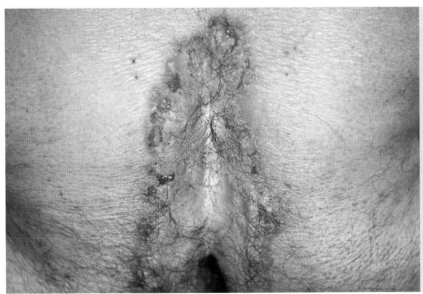

Fig. 25.28 Hailey-Hailey disease, erosions and vegetative hyperplasia of the natal grove.

oral mucosa is rarely affected and always after the skin involvement. The oral lesions consist of small, painful erosions (**Figs. 25.29, 25.30**). Very rarely, the conjunctivae and vaginal mucosa may be affected. The disease has a good prognosis, although the clinical course is characterized by remissions and exacerbations and shows little tendency for complete remission. The patients are usually in remission after the 50th year of life. The diagnosis is based on clinical and histopathologic criteria.

Differential diagnosis

- Darier's disease
- Pemphigus
- Mucous membrane pemphigoid
- Bullous pemphigoid
- Linear immunoglobulin A (IgA) disease
- Grover's disease

Pathology

Histopathologic examination is indispensable for definite diagnosis. Characteristically, prominent, generalized acantholysis is observed throughout the epidermis. A moderate perivascular lymphocytic infiltration is found in the lamina propria. Direct immunofluorescence is negative.

Treatment

Topical applications of steroids or tacrolimus are effective treatment and are often associated with topical antimicrobials and cleanses. Systemic steroids and immunosuppressants are used only in severe cases. The treatment is performed by the dermatologists.

Epidermolysis Bullosa

Key points

- Epidermolysis bullosa is referred to a group of distinctive disorders with numerous clinical characteristics that share three major features: (1) genetic inheritance, (2) bullae formation, and (3) cutaneous and mucosal fragility even under minor pressure.
- Using genetic, histopathologic, immunohistochemical, and clinical criteria, three major types are identified: simplex, junctional, and dystrophic. There are at least 30 clinical phenotypes between the three major groups.
- The oral mucosa is involved in all the three groups.
- There is no effective treatment.

Introduction

Epidermolysis bullosa is a heterogeneous group of inherited disorders characterized by bullae formation on the skin and mucous membranes spontaneously or after mechanical friction. The incidence in United States is 8.2 per 1 million population and 19.6 per million live births. However, the incidence varies greatly worldwide. Over 300 mutations have been implicated so far, involving at least 18 genes that encode structural proteins that reside within the epidermis (EB-simplex), dermoepidermal junction (EB-junctional), and the upper papillary dermis (EB-dystrophic). Based on the anatomical level of the skin where the bullae formation occurs, also the pattern of inheritance and the clinical characteristics, the group is classified into three main types and over 30 clinical phenotypes.

Epidermolysis bullosa *simplex* is a nonscarring intraepidermal skin separation. It is usually inherited in an autosomal dominant pattern and rarely via the X-linked recessive pattern.

Epidermolysis bullosa *junctional* shows skin separation at the basement membrane zone. It is inherited in an autosomal recessive pattern.

Epidermolysis bullosa *dystrophic* shows sublamina densa basement membrane zone separation. Clinically, it manifests with bullae formation, atrophy, and scarring. It is inherited in an autosomal dominant or autosomal recessive patterns. Epidermolysis bullosa may begin from birth and up until the 10th year of life, depending on the type.

Clinical features

Cutaneous findings of epidermolysis bullosa are classified according to the ultrastuctural level of bulla formation, antigenic alterations in the skin, the mode of inheritance, and the clinical phenotype. The cutaneous lesions occur in areas of mechanical friction and pressure, such as the digits, knees, elbows, intertriginous areas, etc., followed by the oral mucosa lesions (mainly in the junctional and dystrophic types) and less frequently by other mucosae. In all types, there is skin friability under even mild mechanical pressure. This leads to bullae formation and subsequently erosions, ulcers, scarring, or disfigurement depending on the type (**Figs. 25.31–25.36**). Intraorally, bullae occur which rupture leaving erosions or ulcers leading to atrophic scarring, tongue dyskinesia, symphises, microstomia, and dystrophic lesions of the dental tissues depending on the type of the disease (**Figs. 25.37–25.41**). The severity of the lesions greatly depends on the type of the disease. Occasionally, leukoplakia and even squamous cell carcinoma may occur on the atrophic lesions, mainly in the dystrophic type.

Other involved mucosae include the conjunctivae that lesions may lead to neoangionesesis and blindness, the esophagus that lesions may lead to scarring and stricture, the small intestine, and the genitourinary system. Rarely, pseudosyndactyly, chronic renal failure, and osteoporosis may occur. The most serious complication, mainly in the dystrophic form, is the development of multiple squamous cell carcinomas of the skin and melanomas.

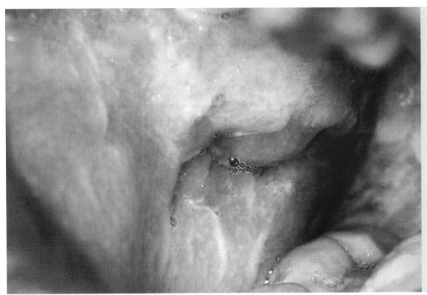

Fig. 25.29 Hailey-Hailey disease, erosion of the buccal mucosa surrounded by leukoedema.

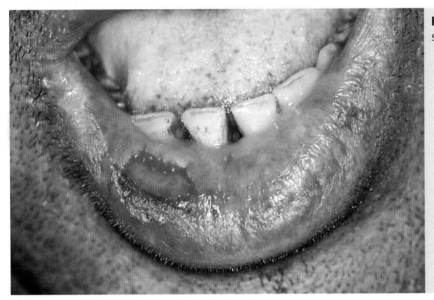

Fig. 25.30 Hailey-Hailey disease, erosion of the lower lip.

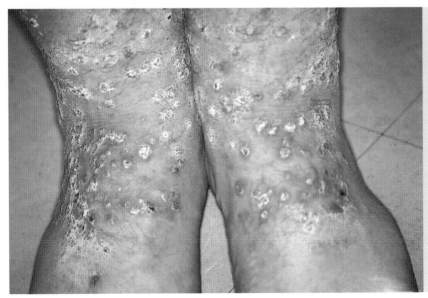

Fig. 25.31 Epidermolysis bullosa simplex, coalescing lesions of the skin.

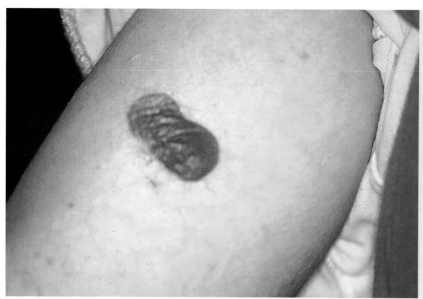

Fig. 25.32 Epidermolysis bullosa simplex, hemorrhagic bulla of the skin.

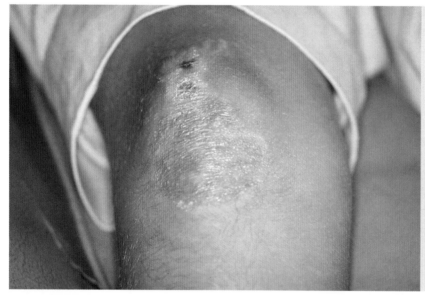

Fig. 25.33 Junctional epidermolysis bullosa, scars on the knee.

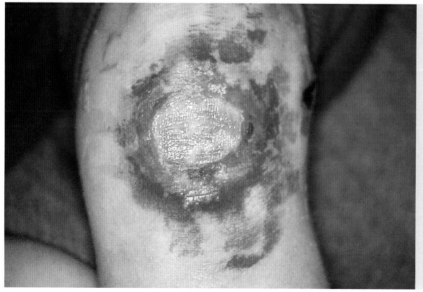

Fig. 25.34 Dystrophic epidermolysis bullosa, severe scars on the knee.

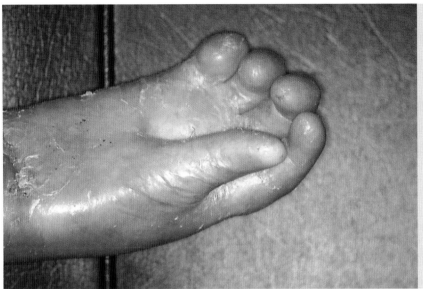

Fig. 25.35 Dystrophic epidermolysis bullosa, severe lesions with deformity of the palm and fingers.

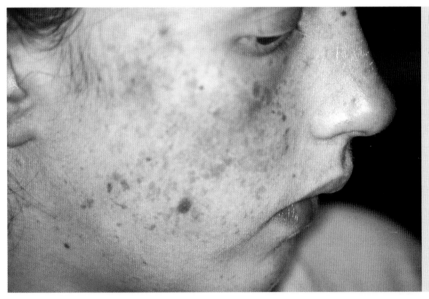

Fig. 25.36 Dystrophic epidermolysis bullosa, mottled pigmentation, nevi, and dryness of the face.

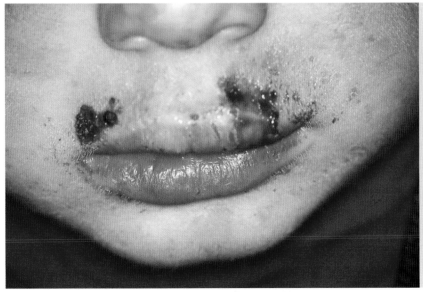

Fig. 25.37 Epidermolysis bullosa simplex, labial and perioral lesions.

Differential diagnosis

- Hailey–Hailey disease
- Pemphigus
- Mucous membrane pemphigoid
- Bullous pemphigoid
- Acrodermatitis enteropathica
- Incontinentia pigmenti
- Pachyonychia congenita
- Other rare genodermatoses

Pathology

The classical histopathologic examination offers little diagnostic help between the different types of epidermolysis bullosa, as it is difficult to determine the exact level of bulla formation. More reliable techniques are electron microscopy examination, immunofluorescent antigen mapping, mutation analysis, and molecular genetics for the determination of the specific subtypes.

Treatment

There is no effective treatment for any of the types of epidermolysis bullosa. Any treatment is aimed to prevent complications and address the symptoms, such as prevention of mechanical trauma and prevention and treatment of any infection. There are several approaches for the cutaneous lesions. Systemic corticosteroids, phenytoin, thalidomide, and retinoids have been tried but with not very encouraging results. For the oral lesions, oral or systemic corticosteroids have been used in combination with good oral hygiene and crowns treatment for the hypoplastic teeth.

Promises in treatment include the use of inducible pluripotent stem cells, revertant mosaicism, bone marrow stem cell therapy, intradermal injection of mesenchymal stromal cells, intradermal injection of allogeneic fibroblasts, recombinant protein therapy, and gene therapy.

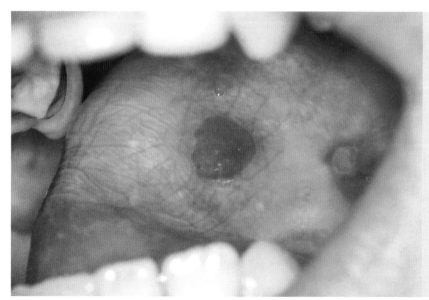

Fig. 25.38 Dystrophic epidermolysis bullosa, atrophy and bulla formation on the tongue.

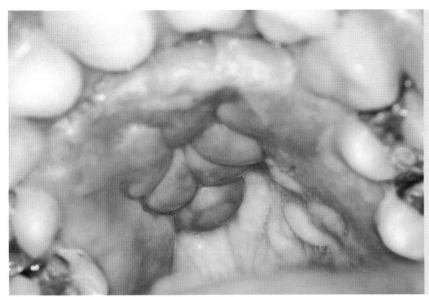

Fig. 25.39 Dystrophic epidermolysis bullosa, multiple nodules on the hard palate.

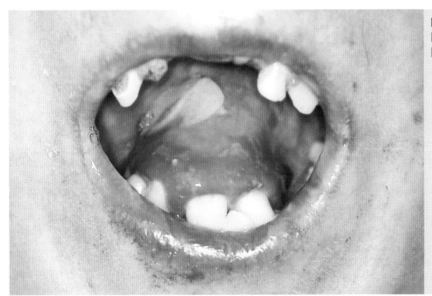

Fig. 25.40 Dystrophic epidermolysis bullosa, scarring on the tongue and lips, and microstomia.

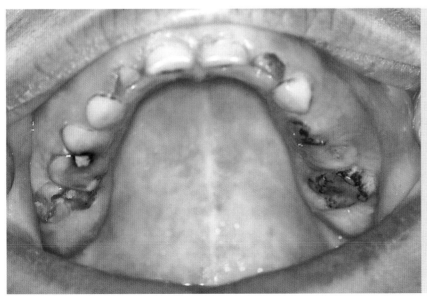

Fig. 25.41 Dystrophic epidermolysis bullosa, dystrophy, and premature damage of the teeth.

Neurofibromatosis type 1

Key points

- Neurofibromatosis refers to a heterogeneous group of neurocutaneous disorders.
- Two distinct types are recognized: neurofibromatosis type 1 (NF1), which affects 85% of the patients and neurofibromatosis type 2 (NF2) which affects 10% of the cases.
- NF1 is an autosomal dominant disorder.
- In over 50% of the cases, there are mutations of the NF1 gene, coding for the tumor suppressor neurofibromin on chromosome 17q11.2.
- Clinically, it is characterized by café au lait spots, multiple neurofibromas, clusters of freckles in unusual areas such as the axillae and the inguinal area, osseous lesions, and ocular lesions.
- The mouth is involved in more than 70 to 80% of the cases with the development of neurofibromas.

Introduction

The term neurofibromatosis represents a group of etiologically heterogeneous multisystemic neurocutaneous disorders involving both neuroectodermal and mesenchymal derivatives. Riccardi's classification of neurofibromatosis, on molecular basis, includes eight subtypes. Among these, *NF1 or von Recklinghausen's disease* is the most common and accounts for 80 to 90% of cases. This type is inherited in an autosomal dominant pattern. Its incidence is about 1 case per 3,000 live births.

Clinical features

Seven diagnostic criteria have been suggested for NF1. Two or more of the following clinical signs must be present: (1) café au lait macules (six or more macules over of 5 mm in diameter in prepubertal children and over of 15 mm in postpubertal individuals), (2) two or more neurofibromas of any type or one plexiform neurofibroma, (3) multiple freckles in the axillary or inguinal areas, (4) two or more iris hamartomas (Lisch nodules), (5) optic gliomas, (6) osseous lesions (such as sphenoid wing dysplasia or thinning of long bone cortex, with or without pseudarthrosis), and (7) first-degree relative with NF1 by the above criteria. Other symptoms and signs may include cardiovascular manifestations, neurologic disorders, and malignancies such as neurosarcomas, rhabdomyosarcoma, central nervous system (CNS) malignancies, myelomonocytic leukemia, and some others.

Although almost every organ system may be involved, the cutaneous manifestations represent the most important clinical features.

The main clinical features of the disease are the café au lait macules that are tan to dark-brown, uniformly pigmented macules and patches, which may appear during the first year of life or later during the childhood, and the multiple neurofibromas. The neurofibromas are nodules of varying sizes that may occur on the skin (**Fig. 25.42**), mouth (**Figs. 25.43, 25.44**), and internal organs such as the stomach, heart, intestine, kidneys, bladder, etc.

The mouth is affected in more than 70 to 80% of the cases with neurofibromas mainly on the tongue and less commonly on the jaws. Malocclusions and disorders in teeth positions may also be observed. Enlargement of the fungiform papillae of the tongue can also be seen. Finally, osseous lesions may occur in the jaws that can be detected radiographically. These may include an enlarged mandibular canal, mandibular foramen, and mental foramen as well as increased bone density.

Differential diagnosis

- Other types of neurofibromatosis
- Multiple endocrine neoplasia syndrome, types 1 and 2B (MEN1 and MEN2B)
- Cowden's syndrome
- Tuberous sclerosis
- McCune-Albright syndrome
- Gardner's syndrome

Pathology

Histopathologic examination of the oral neurofibromas reveals well-circumscribed, small neural bundles, and loosely arranged spindle cells containing scant cytoplasm and large elongate nucleus. The underlying connective tissue demonstrates mucoid degeneration. The spindle cells represent fibroblasts, Schwann cells, and perineural cells in a collagenous stroma with varying amounts of mucin and scattered mast cells. The tumor cells, immunohistochemically, exhibit positive reaction for S-100 protein.

Additionally, neurofibromas can develop intraosseously producing a well-demarcated, unilocular, or rarely multilocular, radioluscent lesion. Routine radiographic, or computed tomography (CT) scan monitoring of patients with neurofibromatosis is recommended.

Treatment

The treatment of neurofibromatosis requires a multidisciplinary approach. It is focused on the prevention and treatment of complications. Surgical excision of oral neurofibromas is recommended for preventive or esthetic reasons.

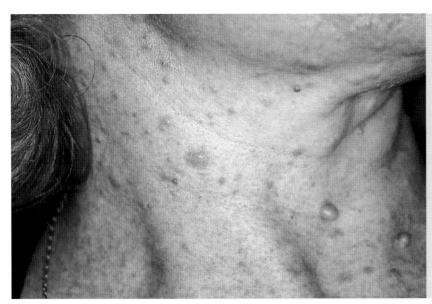

Fig. 25.42 Neurofibromatosis type 1, multiple cutaneous neurofibromas, and café au lait macules.

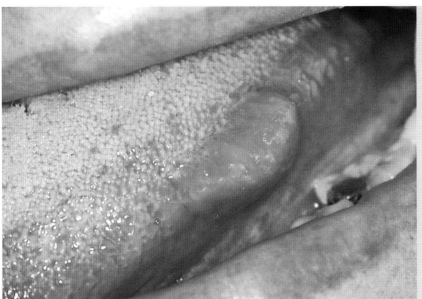

Fig. 25.43 Neurofibromatosis type 1, neurofibroma on the lateral border of the tongue.

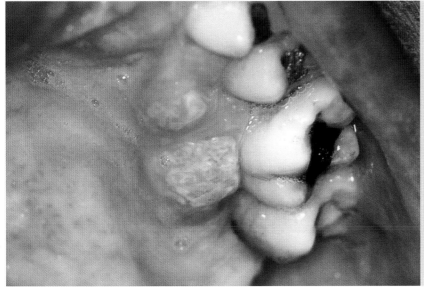

Fig. 25.44 Neurofibromatosis type 1, two neurofibromas on the palate.

Multiple Endocrine Neoplasia Syndrome, Type 2B

Key points

- A group of disorders characterized by hyperplasia or neoplasia of endocrine glands.
- Autosomal dominant disorder, with high penetrance but variable expressivity.
- About 50% of the cases are caused by spontaneous new mutations.
- Often coexists with pheochromocytoma and thyroid gland carcinoma.
- Multiple mucosal neuromas are observed on the oral mucosa and conjunctivae.

Introduction

MEN2B is a rare autosomal dominant genetic disorder with incidence of 1 in 10 million births. It affects both sexes. The cause is mutation in the RET proto-oncogene on chromosome 10, which encodes a tyrosine kinase receptor. About half of all cases are caused by spontaneous new mutations.

Clinical features

The most distinct and characteristic constant clinical feature is the presence of multiple, asymptomatic mucosal neuromas. The lesions appear as small and soft and painless papules or nodules and start to appear during the first decade of life. The tongue and lips are more frequently affected followed by buccal mucosa, palate, and gingiva (**Fig. 25.45**). Multiple neuromas are also observed on the eyelid ridge, conjunctivae, laryngeal, and nasal mucosa. The face is narrow with osseous anomalies and the palate is arched. A characteristic clinical sign is the development of medullary thyroid carcinoma (90%) and usually bilateral pheochromocytoma (50%), usually during the second or third decade of life.

Differential diagnosis

- MEN2A
- Werner's syndrome
- Neurofibromatosis

Pathology

Histologically, oral neuromas reveal hyperplastic neural bundles, surrounded by a thick perineurium in a background of loose endoneurium-like fibrous stroma.

Analysis of the *PET* gene is the currently preferred method for establishing the diagnosis of MEN2B. It is almost 100% sensitive and specific. Measurement of serum and urinary calcitonin should be done as it is elevated if a medullary thyroid carcinoma is developed. If a pheochromocytoma is present, it results in increased level of furinary vanillylmandelic acid.

Treatment

Early diagnosis is important especially regarding prophylaxis against the thyroid and adrenal gland carcinomas. Prophylactic thyroidectomy is recommended together with close monitoring of the adrenal glands. The oral lesions do not require any treatment unless they cause a functional or esthetic problem when a conservative surgical excision of neuromas is indicated. In those cases, surgery can take place.

Chondroectodermal Dysplasia

Key points

- A rare genetic disorder, inherited via an autosomal recessive pattern.
- Main characteristic include postaxial polydactyly, finger nail dysplasia, short limbs, dwarfism, congenital heart defects, cleft palate, and disorders of the number, shape, and size of the teeth.

Introduction

Chondroectodermal dysplasia or Ellis-van Creveld syndrome is inherited as an autosomal recessive trait. The incidence is approximately 7 cases per 1 million births.

Clinical features

The main clinical characteristics of the disease are: (1) bilateral polydactyly, (2) chondrodysplasia of long bones leading to short-limbed dwarfism, (3) involvement of ectodermal tissues (hair, nails, teeth), and (4) congenital heart disease and CNS involvement. The most constant oral finding is fusion of the upper or lower lip to the gingiva, resulting in the disappearance of the mucolabial fold or the formation of multiple fibrous bands (**Fig. 25.46**). There can also be teeth present at birth, oligodontia, small conical teeth with enamel hypoplasia, and cleft palate. The diagnosis is based on clinical criteria.

Differential diagnosis

- Orofacial–digital syndrome
- Acrofacial dysostosis of Weyers
- Achondroplasia

Treatment

There is no effective treatment. The treatment is supportive and largely depends on the case.

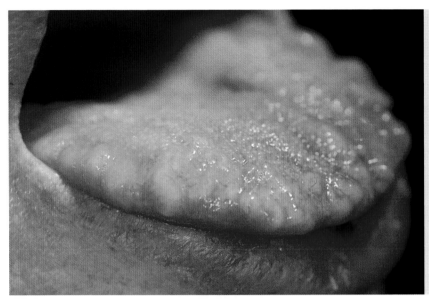

Fig. 25.45 Multiple endocrine neoplasia syndrome type 2B, multiple neuromas on the lateral borders of the tongue.

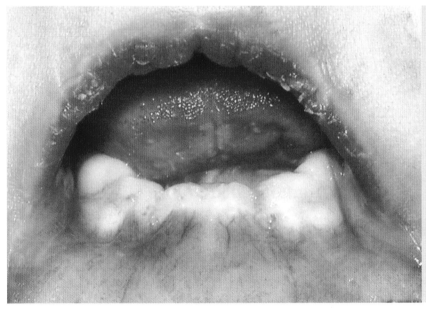

Fig. 25.46 Ellis-van Creveld syndrome, fusion of the lower lip with the gingiva, and subsequent disappearance of the mucolabial sulcus.

Gardner's Syndrome

Key points

- A rare autosomal dominant disorder, caused by a mutation in the *APC* gene, located in chromosome 5q21.
- It is considered to be a phenotypic variant of familial adenomatous polyposis.
- Characterized by colorectal premalignant polyps, multiple osteomas, cutaneous fibromas, epidermoid cysts, and desmoid tumors.
- Congenital hyperpigmentation of the retinal pigment epithelium is an early sign.
- Oral manifestations are common.

Introduction

Gardner's syndrome is a rare genetic disorder, inherited in an autosomal dominant pattern. About 30% of the cases represent spontaneous, new gene mutations. All mutations occur in the *APC* gene, on chromosome 5q21, a tumor suppressor gene which controls proliferation of colon epithelial cells. The incidence is approximately 1 case per 8,000 to 16,000 births. The syndrome is considered to represent a phenotypic variant of the familial adenomatous polyposis syndrome.

Clinical features

Clinically, the oral manifestations are common and important for early diagnosis. These include multiple impacted teeth, supernumerary teeth (20%) and multiple odontomas, benign soft tissue tumors, and jaw osteomas (80%) with a characteristic *cotton-wool* radiographic appearance. Occasionally, the latter protrude externally, giving the appearance of an exostosis (**Fig. 25.47**). Multiple osteomas are a common finding usually located at the facial bones and the calvaria.

Epidermoid cysts occur in 40 to 50% of the cases and usually become obvious after puberty. Other cutaneous lesions include sebaceous cysts, subcutaneous fibromas, and rarely increased skin pigmentation (**Fig. 25.48**). In approximately 3 to 15% of the cases, soft tissue desmoid tumors occur. They are benign in nature, but locally aggressive and with a tendency to recur. A main feature remains the presence of multiple intestinal tumors (colon and rectum) that usually appear before puberty. They have a high rate of malignant transformation into adenocarcinomas that increases with age to reach 100%. Rarely, benign or malignant neoplasms occur in other organs. Finally, congenital hyperpigmentation of the retinal pigment epithelium is one of the most important and early diagnostic sign. For final diagnosis, the presence of four or more lesions are necessary.

Differential diagnosis

- Jaw and other bone exostoses
- Peutz-Jeghers syndrome
- Juvenile polyposis syndromes
- Cowden's syndrome
- Cleidocranial dysplasia

Pathology

Histopathologic examination of the jaw osteomas shows features of compact osteomas without any additional findings. The intestinal polyps exhibit epithelial adenomatous hyperplasia, or a histologic picture of adenocarcinoma if they have undergone malignant transformation.

Treatment

The treatment of osteomas, fibromas, other soft tissue tumors and cysts is surgical excision if they cause a functional or esthetic problem. Prophylactic removal of the intestinal polyps is of great importance to prevent malignant transformation. It is crucial that the patients are closely monitored by a gastroenterologist.

Gorlin's Syndrome

Key points

- A rare genetic disorder inherited in an autosomal dominant pattern.
- It is due to *PTCH* gene mutation, located on 9q22.3–q31 chromosome.
- The main clinical features are odontogenic keratocysts in the jaws, cutaneous basal cell carcinomas, and other skin abnormalities and CNS disorders.
- Regular follow-up of the patients is highly recommended to prevent cutaneous carcinomas and monitor the odontogenic cysts.

Introduction

Gorlin's syndrome, or nevoid basal cell carcinoma syndrome is a rare genetic disorder. It is inherited in an autosomal dominant pattern, with a very high penetrance and extremely variable expressivity. Over 50% of the cases represent new, spontaneous mutations. The responsible gene is the tumor suppressor *PTCH* gene, located on 9q22.3–q31 chromosome. The incidence of the disease ranges from 1 in 50,000 to 150,000 individuals with higher incidence in Australia. The signs and symptoms start to appear usually between 20 and 40 years.

Clinical features

The clinical spectrum of signs and symptoms of Gorlin's syndrome is very wide. However, the hallmark of the syndrome is the early presence of numerous nevoid basal cell carcinomas of the skin, which exhibit some special features such as multiple, early onset (during childhood), frequently may occur in sun-protected areas, are usually pigmented, and most cases are of good prognosis (**Fig. 25.49**). Palmoplantar pits

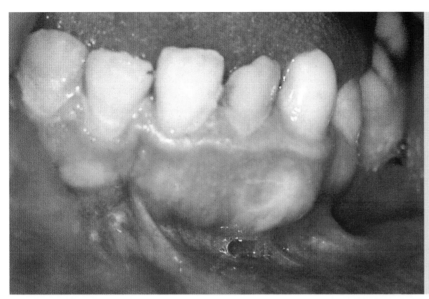

Fig. 25.47 Gardner's syndrome, multiple osteomas of the mandible.

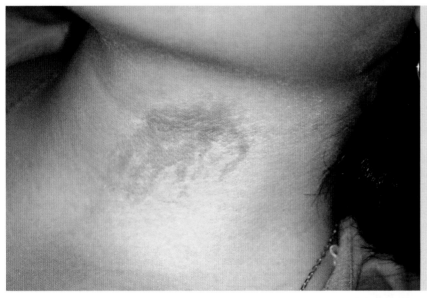

Fig. 25.48 Gardner's syndrome, pigmentation of the neck.

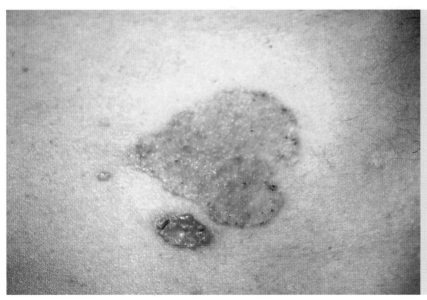

Fig. 25.49 Gorlin's syndrome, cutaneous basal cell carcinomas.

and epidermoid cysts and facial milia are common features (**Fig. 25.50**). Craniofacial anomalies are frequent with characteristic facies with frontal and temporoparietal bossing, resulting in an increased head circumference. Additionally, there is a broadened nasal bridge, hypertelorism and mild mandibular prognathism. A constant finding (in ~70–80% of the cases) is the presence of multiple odontogenic keratocysts of the jaws that develop between the ages of 10 and 30. Displacement or even teeth loss and malocclusion may occur (**Fig. 25.51**).

Other features that may be present include rib anomalies (absence, bifid, splayed, fused, missing), spina bifida occulta, short metacarpals, kyphoscoliosis, lumbarization of the sacrum, calcifications of the falx cerebri, osseous pseudocysts, CNS disorders, mental retardation, genetic anomalies, clefts, etc. The diagnosis is mainly based on the major diagnostic criteria: more than two BCCs or one before the age of 20, odontogenic keratocysts of the jaw, three or more palmar or plantar pits, calcification of falx cerebri, bifid-fused ribs, and first-degree relatives with the syndrome. The diagnosis needs two major or one major and two minor criteria.

Differential diagnosis

- Solitary dentigerous cysts
- Bazex's syndrome
- Pseudohypoparathyroidism
- Multiple hamartomas on a background of severe myasthenia

Pathology

Histologically, the odontogenic keratocysts and the cutaneous basal cell carcinomas exhibit the same characteristics as their solitary counterparts. Radiographic examination and CT scans are required for the determination of jaws, osseous and other lesions.

Treatment

As the disorder has a very broad spectrum of manifestations, therapeutics depend on the complications and malfunctions caused by the disease. The cutaneous basal cell carcinomas are treated either with surgical excision, radiation, or photodynamic therapy. The odontogenic keratocysts should be surgically enucleated.

Tuberous Sclerosis

Key points

- An autosomal dominant disorder.
- Up to 75% of cases are caused by spontaneous, new mutations.
- The genes responsible are *TSC1* on chromosome 9q34, encoding hamartin and TSC2 on chromosome 16p13.3, encoding tuberin.
- The main clinical feature is the presence of hamartomas predominantly affecting the skin, eyes, brain, heart, and kidneys.
- Gingival fibromas and tooth enamel pits are common oral findings.

Introduction

Tuberous sclerosis, or Bourneville-Pringle syndrome, is a rare genetic disorder inherited in an autosomal dominant pattern. In 50% of the cases, the disease is caused by new, spontaneous mutations. Mutations have been identified in two genes: *TSC1* on chromosome 9q34, encoding hamartin and *TSC2* on chromosome 16p13.3, encoding tuberin. The disease is usually manifested between the ages of 2 and 6. Many patients die by the age of 20, but some may survive longer.

Clinical features

Tuberous sclerosis is clinically characterized by epilepsy, mental retardation, mucocutaneous lesions and rarely tumors affecting the heart, kidneys, and eyes and also skeletal anomalies. Cutaneous lesions are often the first clinical features. The most characteristic lesions, starting the first 2 years of life, occur on the face, particularly along the nasolabial fold, cheeks, and chin. These are numerous small nodules that can be flat or raised, red to brown in color. They are *angiofibromas*, formed by connective tissue and vascular tissue hyperplasia (**Fig. 25.52**). Other characteristic features are the presence of hypomelanotic and cafe au lait macules, shagreen patch, periungual fibromas, and nail dysplasia (**Fig. 25.53**). The oral mucosa may be involved in 10 to 56% of cases. Usually, the gingiva or less frequently other parts of the oral mucosa may exhibit multiple confluent fibrous nodules, usually 1 to 6 mm in diameter. They are whitish or normal in color and are caused

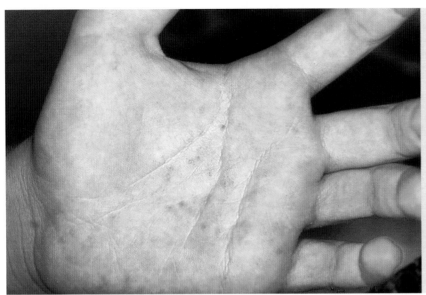

Fig. 25.50 Gorlin's syndrome, very small palmar pits.

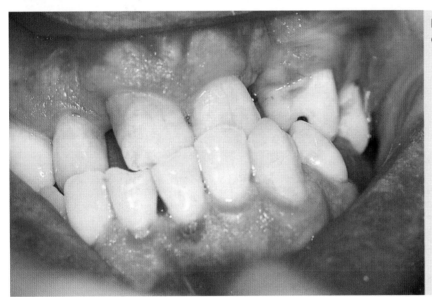

Fig. 25.51 Gorlin's syndrome, teeth displacement and malocclusion.

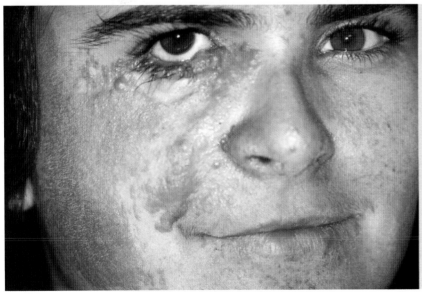

Fig. 25.52 Tuberous sclerosis, multiple facial angiofibromas.

by hyperplasia of the connective tissue (**Fig. 25.54**). Erythema on the tongue with absence of the fungiform papillae and hypertrophy of the filiform papillae may also occur (**Fig. 25.55**). Enamel pits may also be present on the facial aspect of the anterior permanent dentition. The diagnosis is mainly based on the clinical features.

Differential diagnosis

- Cowden's syndrome
- Neurofibromatosis
- Multiple fibromas
- Focal epithelial hyperplasia
- MEN1

Pathology

Histopathologic examination of oral mucosa lesions reveals fibrous hyperplasia without any special features. The skin angiofibromas consist of an irregular proliferation of fibrous tissue and blood vessels. Genetic testing for the affected genes can be performed.

Treatment

The treatment is symptomatic. As nearly every organ can be affected, the management should be performed by specialists. The oral lesions can be surgically removed. A high level of oral hygiene is recommended.

Cowden's Disease

Key points

- A rare autosomal dominant disorder.
- Mutations in the *PTEN* gene has been implicated in the pathogenesis.
- Main clinical manifestations include hamartomas and carcinoma of breast, colon, thyroid, multiple trichilemmomas, palmoplantar keratoses, and oral mucosa lesions.
- It is associated with certain types of malignancy.
- Oral mucosal lesions are common.

Introduction

Cowden's disease or multiple hamartoma syndrome is a rare genetic disorder inherited in an autosomal dominant pattern showing a high degree of expression and a range of expressivity. Mutation of the *PTEN* gene, located on chromosome 10, is responsible for the disease. The prevalence of the disease is approximately 1:200,000 individuals.

Clinical features

Cowden's disease is characterized by multiple hamartomas and malignant neoplasms such as breast, thyroid, colon, and kidney cancers. The main cutaneous manifestations are hamartomas that appear as multiple small papules that represent hair follicle hamartomas (trichilemmomas), primarily on the face, usually around the mouth (nasolabial folds) and ears. Less frequently, palmoplantar punctate keratoses are present

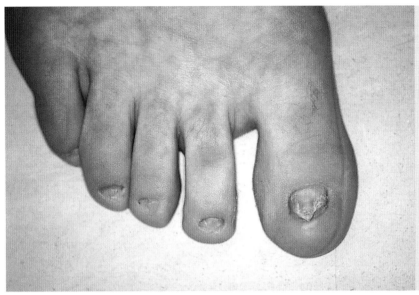

Fig. 25.53 Tuberous sclerosis, dysplasia of the nails.

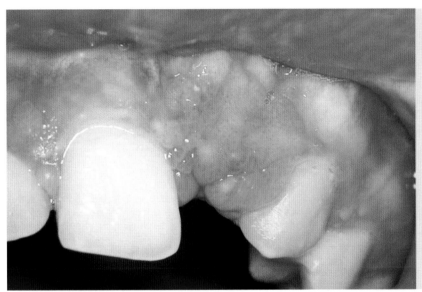

Fig. 25.54 Tuberous sclerosis, multiple nodules on the gingiva, and the alveolar mucosa.

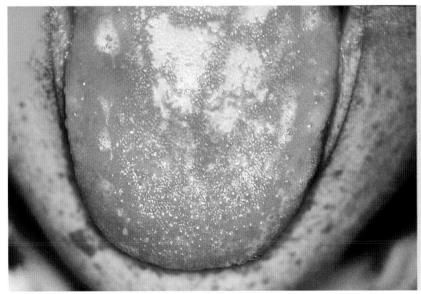

Fig. 25.55 Tuberous sclerosis, absence of the fungiform papillae, and hypertrophy of the filiform papilla of the tongue.

(**Fig. 25.56**). Cutaneous benign tumors, hemangiomas, lipomas, xanthomas, and neuromas have been described. The oral lesions consist of multiple, small, asymptomatic papules or nodules of white or normal color that may be isolated or coalesce in a cobblestone pattern, usually on the gingiva and alveolar mucosa, and less frequently on buccal mucosa, tongue, and lips (**Fig. 25.57**). The diagnosis is based on the clinical criteria.

Differential diagnosis

- Tuberous sclerosis
- Benign acanthosis nigricans
- Focal epithelial hyperplasia
- MEN3

Pathology

Histopathologic examination of the oral lesions reveals hyperplasia of the connective tissue with some contribution by the epithelium, with no other special feature. Genetic testing for mutation of the *PTEN* gene is sometimes useful.

Treatment

There is no specific treatment. The patient is followed by a team of specialists. It is of great importance to identify the individuals early in life for monitoring against the potential malignancies.

Hereditary Hemorrhagic Telangiectasia

Key points

- An autosomal dominant disorder.
- Mutations in two different genes are responsible for the disorder: *ENG* (endoglin, HHT1) and *ALK1* (activin receptor–like kinase 1).
- In rare cases, it can occur as the result of new, spontaneous mutation.
- Clinically, it is characterized by the development of telangiectasias on the mucosae, skin, and viscera.
- The oral mucosa is very commonly affected with characteristic signs and symptoms.
- In most cases, the first symptom is epistaxis.

Introduction

Hereditary hemorrhagic telangiectasia or Osler-Rendu-Weber disease is inherited in an autosomal dominant pattern. Mutations in two different genes are responsible for the disorder. Mutation of the *ENG* gene, encoding the cell surface coreceptor endoglin is associated with type 1 (HHT1). Mutation of the *ACVRL1 gene*, also encoding a cell surface receptor, previously known as *ALK1*, is associated with type 2 (HHT2). The above encoding proteins seem to play a role in blood vessel maturation and vascular smooth muscle development. While no absolute genotype–phenotype correlation exists between clinical phenotypes and specific mutations, certain clinical features are more common in particular types, for example, in type 1 there is more frequent pulmonary involvement.

The prevalence is estimated at 1:10,000 individuals, but this is likely to be an underestimate. The age of onset of vascular malformation usually develops during adolescence and affects both sexes.

Clinical features

The cardinal manifestations are cutaneous, mucosal, and visceral (liver, spleen, brain, lungs, etc.) telangiectasias. Clinically, three varieties of telangiectasias have been described: (1) *microscopic lesions* of less than 1 mL in diameter, (2) *nodules*, and (3) *spider-like lesions*. These round or slightly elevated lesions have a bright red, purple, or violet color and disappear on pressure with a glass slide and reappear straight after. The oral mucosa is frequently involved with multiple lesions usually on the tip and dorsum of the tongue and lips (**Fig. 25.58**). Rarely, the palate, buccal mucosa, and gingiva are involved

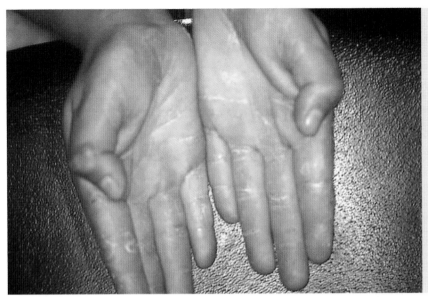

Fig. 25.56 Cowden's syndrome, palmar hyperkeratosis.

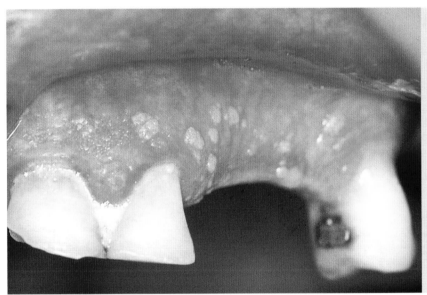

Fig. 25.57 Cowden's syndrome, multiple small nodules on the gingiva and alveolar mucosa.

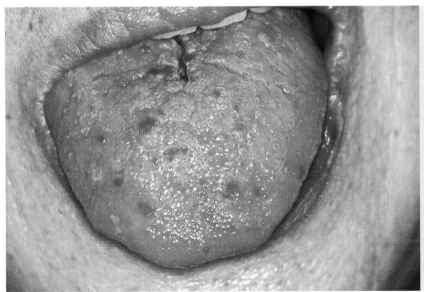

Fig. 25.58 Hereditary hemorrhagic telangiectasia, multiple telangiectasias on the tongue.

(**Fig. 25.59**). Hemorrhage from oral lesions may be spontaneous or caused by minimal mechanical friction and can be vigorous. Epistaxis and gastrointestinal bleeding are early and occasionally serious complications and may lead to iron deficiency anemia. Cutaneous telangiectasias are more common on the face and less frequent on the fingers and toes, as well as the periungual areas. Arteriovenous malformations and fistulas may develop in the lungs, liver, and brain. The most important diagnostic criteria are recurrent epistaxis, cutaneous and mucosal telangiectasias, arteriovenous malformations in the lung, liver, or brain and a family history of the disorder. The diagnosis is based on the clinical features.

Differential diagnosis

- Varicosities of the tongue and other anatomical areas
- Fabry's disease
- Calcinosis, Raynaud phenomenon, esophageal dysmotility, sclerodactyly, and telangiectasia (CREST) syndrome
- Maffucci's syndrome
- Sturge-Weber syndrome
- Klippel-Trénaunay-Weber syndrome

Pathology

The histologic examination is not pathognomonic. Superficial vascular spaces with thin walls, filled with red blood cells, are observed. Genetic testing may establish the diagnosis of the disorder particularly in individuals who do not yet fulfill the diagnostic clinical criteria.

Treatment

There is no specific treatment. Control of spontaneous hemorrhage is important. The angiomatous lesions that pose a risk of bleeding can be cauterized, or treated with the cryoprobe.

Maffucci's Syndrome

Key points

- A rare sporadic disease with less than 200 cases described worldwide.
- Multiple, enchondromas, hemangiomas, and occasionally lymphangiomas of the skin and mucosa.

Introduction

Maffucci's syndrome is a very rare disorder of unknown cause with sporadic appearance and no sexual or racial predilection. It manifests early in life (around 4–5 years) and 25% of the cases are congenital.

Clinical features

Clinically, it is characterized by: (1) multiple enchondromas, principally in the small bones of the hands and feet, (2) bone abnormalities, (3) multiple mucocutaneous hemangiomas, and (4) phleboliths. The oral mucosa is affected by multiple hemangiomas in approximately 10 to 20% of all cases, most commonly on the tongue and less frequently in other anatomical areas (**Fig. 25.60**). Fractures are a common complication of the disease. Additionally, the risk of malignant transformation of the enchondromas, hemangiomas, or lymphangiomas is approximately 15 to 30%. The disease is also associated with a higher risk of pancreatic, ovarian, and CNS malignancies.

Differential diagnosis

- Solitary vascular malformation
- Ollier's disease
- Klippel-Trénaunay-Weber syndrome
- The blue rubber bleb nevus syndrome
- Proteus syndrome

Pathology

Histopathologic examination of the enchondromas and hemangiomas exhibits the same features as in their isolated counterparts.

Treatment

Surgical excision of the enchondromas and hemangiomas may be attempted if they are symptomatic.

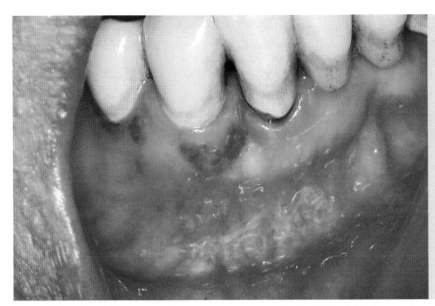

Fig. 25.59 Hereditary hemorrhagic telangiectasia, multiple telangiectasias on the gingiva.

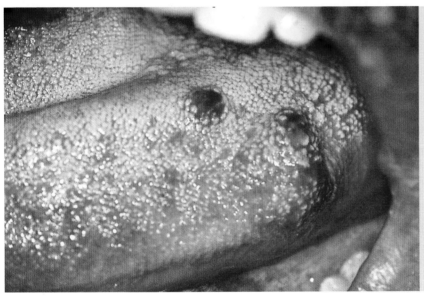

Fig. 25.60 Maffucci's syndrome, hemangiomas on the tongue.

Sturge-Weber Angiomatosis

Key points

- A sporadic disorder in which the facial capillaries malformation is associated with ipsilateral ocular and leptomeningeal or brain anomalies.
- The facial port-wine stain typically involves the trigeminal nerve distribution.
- The lesions are usually unilateral and rarely bilateral.
- Oral lesions are common and are characterized by great vascular hyperplasia.

Introduction

Sturge-Weber angiomatosis or encephalotrigeminal angiomatosis is a sporadic congenital, neurologic, and skin capillaries malformation. Both sexes may be affected.

Clinical features

Sturge-Weber angiomatosis is characterized by: (1) great hyperplasia of the capillaries of the face and oral mucosa; (2) hemangiomas of the leptomeninges; (3) calcification of the brain; (4) ocular dysplasias (angiomas, glaucoma, hemianopsia); and (5) neurologic disorders (epilepsy, seizures, migraine headaches, contralateral hemiparesis, developmental motor delays, and mild mental retardation). The facial hemangioma is the most constant clinical manifestation and is apparent at birth. It is usually unilateral, has a bright red or purple color, and typically involves the trigeminal nerve region (**Fig. 25.61**). Hemangiomas of the oral mucosa are common and occur on the ipsilateral side with the skin lesions. They mainly affect the gingiva, buccal mucosa, lips, and tongue. These lesions have a bright red or purple color and are usually flat (**Fig. 25.62**), but may also have a raised irregular surface that causes gingival enlargement, macroglossia, and macrocheilia. The gingival enlargement may cause early or delayed teeth eruption, teeth displacement, and malocclusion. Care must be taken during any surgical, or blood-borne, intervention and tooth extractions as hemorrhage may be severe. When the classic signs and symptoms are present, the diagnosis of Sturge-Weber syndrome is apparent, otherwise laboratory confirmation is necessary.

Differential diagnosis

- Klippel-Trénaunay-Weber syndrome
- Proteus syndrome
- Telangiectasias
- Hereditary hemorrhagic telangiectasia
- Angiokeratoma

Pathology

Histopathologic examination of the oral lesions reveals multiple, enlarged vessels in the lamina propria that lack any special characteristics. In early atypical cases, magnetic resonance imaging (MRI), magnetic resonance arteriography (MRA), single-photon emission computed tomography (SPECT), and positron emission tomography (PET) are important diagnostic tools.

Treatment

There is no specific treatment. Improvement of the mucocutaneous lesions can be achieved with the use of laser. Great care should be taken for all oral interventions.

Klippel-Trénaunay-Weber Syndrome

Key points

- Most cases are sporadic, although few cases are inherited in an autosomal dominant pattern.
- Common angiogenic factor gene, *AGGF1* variants may confer a risk of the disease.
- Clinically, it is characterized by capillary-venous and capillary-lymphatic-venous malformations and limb hypertrophy.
- Vascular malformations are observed of the gastrointestinal and urinary systems.
- Oral involvement is common.

Introduction

Klippel-Trénaunay-Weber syndrome or angio-osteohypertrophy syndrome is a rare congenital, dysplastic vascular disorder.

Clinical features

Clinically, the disorder is characterized by: (1) vascular malformations of the face and brain that may cause neurologic abnormalities (**Fig. 25.63**); (2) vascular masses that can involve the soft tissues and bone and are accompanied by asymmetric

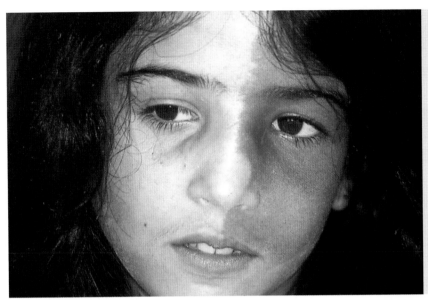

Fig. 25.61 Sturge-Weber angiomatosis, unilateral facial hemangioma.

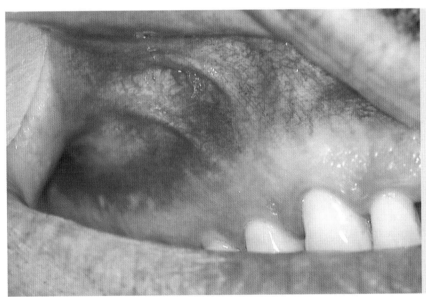

Fig. 25.62 Sturge-Weber angiomatosis, hemangioma affecting the labial and buccal sulcus.

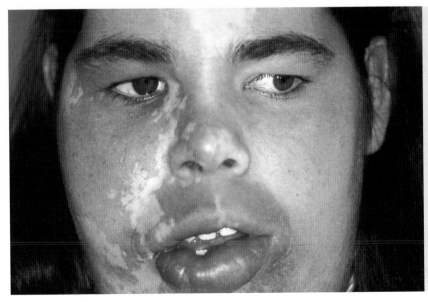

Fig. 25.63 Klippel-Trénaunay-Weber syndrome, multiple hemangiomas on the face and lips.

enlargement of the extremities (**Fig. 25.64**); (3) vascular cutaneous lesions that can affect various areas and occasionally pigmentation; (4) ocular abnormalities such as scleral pigmentation (**Fig. 25.65**), glaucoma, cataract, iris heterochromia; etc.; (5) vascular lesions of the viscera; and (6) oral vascular malformations. The latter most commonly affect the palate and upper gingival and less frequently the tongue (**Fig. 25.66**). They clinically appear as vascular masses that can cause premature tooth eruption and malocclusion. The cutaneous lesions present either as a pink-to-red blotchy stain or a red-to-purple, well-demarcated stain that tend to involve the lateral aspects of the thigh, knee, and leg.

Differential diagnosis

- Sturge-Weber angiomatosis
- Proteus syndrome

Pathology

Histopathologic examination of the oral lesions reveals multiple enlarged vessels (capillaries and veins) that lack any special features. Duplex ultrasonography and lymphoscintigraphy are useful in investigating the vascular malformations.

Treatment

There is no specific treatment. Some improvement of the oral and facial lesions can be achieved with the use of laser.

Cleidocranial Dysplasia

Key points

- Usually, inherited in an autosomal dominant pattern.
- In 30 to 40% of the cases, new spontaneous mutations occur.
- Genetic mutations occur on the *CBFA1* gene (also known as Runx2) on chromosome 6p21.
- Predominantly, affected sites are the clavicles and jaws.

Introduction

Cleidocranial dysplasia is a rare genetic autosomal dominant disorder. In 30 to 40% of the cases, new spontaneous mutations occur. The genetic mutations occur on the *CBFA1* gene (also known as Runx2) on chromosome 6p21. The gene plays an important role in the differentiation from stem cells to osteoblasts, resulting in problematic ossification. The prevalence is approximately 1:1,000,000 individuals.

Clinical features

Clinically, cleidocranial dysplasia is characterized by: (1) unilateral or bilateral hypoplasia or complete absence of the clavicles; thus, the patient has the capability of approximating of shoulders (**Fig. 25.67**); (2) skull abnormalities such as delayed closure or open fontanelles, open sutures, large skull, frontal bossing, broad flat nose; (3) exophthalmos, hypertelorism, deafness, and other osseous dysplasias; (4) short stature; and (5) oral lesions. The oral manifestations include high-arched

and narrow palate, delayed eruption or noneruption of deciduous and permanent teeth, supernumerary ectopic permanent teeth, and cleft palate. Malformation of the maxilla results in apparent mandibular prognathism of the normally developed mandible (**Fig. 25.68**).

The diagnosis is based on the clinical features and is confirmed by the radiographic imaging of the jaws and the skeleton.

Differential diagnosis

- Craniofrontonasal dysplasia
- Hypohidrotic ectodermal dysplasia
- Osteogenesis imperfecta
- Apert's syndrome

Laboratory tests

Radiographic examination, CT scan, and dental scan tomography help toward the diagnosis.

Treatment

There is no specific treatment. Dental care is essential (management of the unerupted teeth, surgical excisions where required, orthodontic treatment, prosthetic rehabilitation, etc.).

Orofacial–Digital Syndrome

Key points

- A group of related disorders that affect the face, mouth, digits, and the brain.
- At least 13 different forms have now been identified.
- Mutations in the *OFD1* gene have been associated with orofacial–digital syndrome, type 1.
- Orofacial–digital syndrome type 1 is inherited in an X-linked dominant fashion, while most of the other types are inherited in an autosomal recessive fashion.

Introduction

Orofacial–digital syndrome refers to a group of related conditions that affect the face, mouth, digits, and the brain. Mutations in the *OFD1* gene at chromosome 22.3–P.22.2 have been associated with orofacial–digital syndrome type 1. This mutation is believed to cause cilia defects that can affect numerous developmental signaling pathways that are critical to cellular development. As type 1 is inherited in an X-linked dominant pattern, females present with the disorder, but male embryos rarely survive. Most of the other types are inherited in an autosomal recessive pattern.

Clinical features

Clinically, orofacial–digital syndrome type 1 is characterized by: (1) digital malformations (brachydactyly, syndactyly, clinodactyly, polydactyly) (**Figs. 25.69, 25.70**); (2) skeletal abnormalities (kyphoscoliosis, zygomatic arch hypoplasia, osteoporosis, etc.); (3). cutaneous lesions (milia, xeroderma, alopecia, sparse hair, dermatoglyphic abnormalities); (4) mental retardation, ocular hypertelorism (**Fig. 25.71**); and (5) oral lesions, which

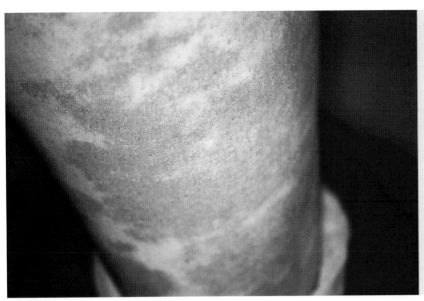

Fig. 25.64 Klippel-Trénaunay-Weber syndrome, extensive hemangiomas on the shin.

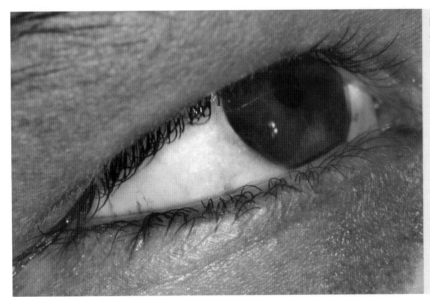

Fig. 25.65 Klippel-Trénaunay-Weber syndrome, scleral pigmentation, and periocular hemangioma.

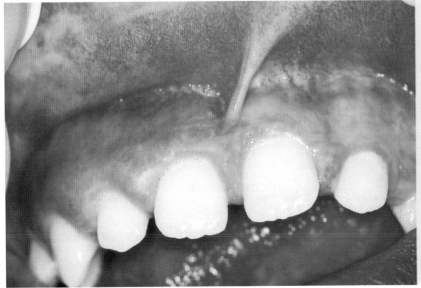

Fig. 25.66 Klippel-Trénaunay-Weber syndrome, hemangiomas on the upper gingiva and alveolar mucosa.

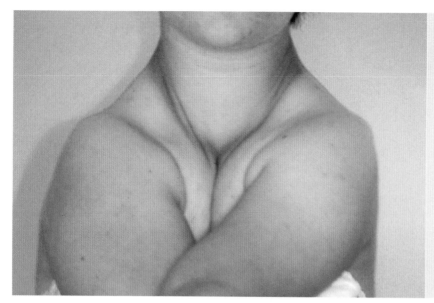

Fig. 25.67 Cleidocranial dysplasia, absence of the clavicles, and approximation of the shoulders in the midline.

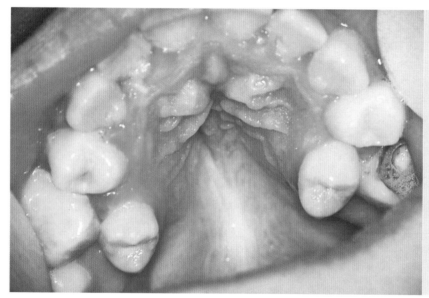

Fig. 25.68 Cleidocranial dysplasia, high-arched palate and ectopic teeth.

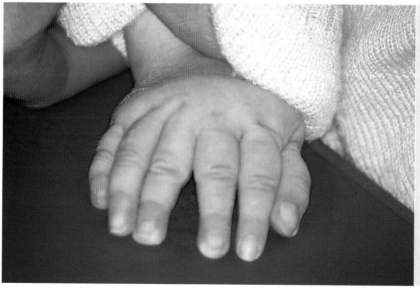

Fig. 25.69 Orofacial–digital syndrome, exadactyly, and brachydactyly on the hand.

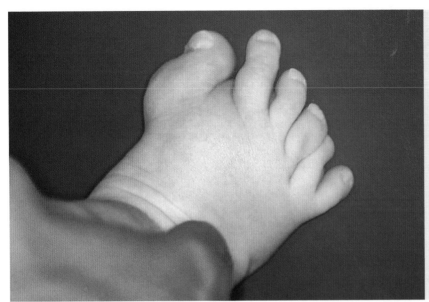

Fig. 25.70 Orofacial–digital syndrome, exadactyly, brachydactyly, clinodactyly on the foot.

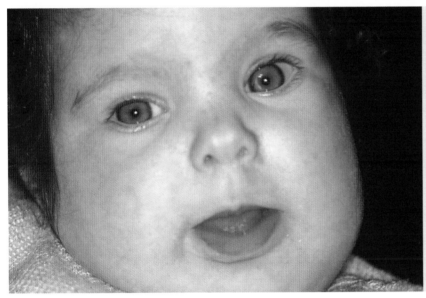

Fig. 25.71 Orofacial–digital syndrome, ocular hypertelorism, and characteristic facial appearance.

are numerous and variable. Constant oral mucosal findings are multiple hyperplastic frenula on the upper and lower vestibular sulci (**Fig. 25.72**). There is also hypertrophy and shortening of the lingual frenulum, nodules, and fissures on the tongue that divide it into two or more lobes. Clefts of the lips and palate are common. Finally, teeth abnormalities regarding the shape, position, and number of teeth are observed (**Fig. 25.73**). The diagnosis is based on clinical features.

Differential diagnosis

- All other types of orofacial–digital syndrome
- Chondroectodermal dysplasia
- Oculodentodigital syndrome

Laboratory tests

Radiographic examination, CT scan, and dental scan tomography may be helpful.

Treatment

There is no specific treatment, but the oral problems require the appropriate management.

Focal Dermal Hypoplasia

Key points

- A rare genetic disorder, inherited in an X-linked dominant pattern.
- Caused by mutations in the *PORCN* gene.
- The disorder affects the endoderm, mesoderm, and ectoderm, so that it can involve almost any organ in the body, resulting in a wide range of clinical manifestations.
- The cutaneous lesions follow Blaschko's lines, consist of dermal atrophy associated with telangiectasias, hypopigmentation, and/or hyperpigmentation.
- Papillomatous lesions intraorally and periorally are a common finding.

Introduction

Focal dermal hypoplasia or Goltz's syndrome is a rare genetic disorder inherited in an X-linked dominant pattern. Most male embryos do not survive. It is caused by mutations of the *PORCN* gene. This is a gene required ultimately for the formation of proteins that participate in chemical signaling pathways and are crucial for normal development. It involves all three embryonic layers (endoderm, mesoderm, and ectoderm). Approximately 95% of all cases are sporadic.

Clinical features

Clinically, cutaneous manifestations of the disorder include linear hypoplastic streaks which follow the Blaschko's lines, atrophy, telangiectasias, multiple soft raspberry-like

papillomas, and hypo- and hyperpigmentation. The papillomas may develop at any location. However, they are more common at the anogenital region, lips, larynx, and acral sites (**Fig. 25.74**). Other features include nail dystrophy, brittle and sparse hair, syndactyly, polydactyly or oligodactyly, brachydactyly, microcephaly and other skeletal anomalies, ocular abnormalities (displaced lens, chorioretinal atrophy, blocked lacrimal duct, microphthalmia, and anophthalmia), mental retardation, and oral lesions. The oral manifestations are multiple papillomas (40–50%) on the tongue, buccal mucosa, palate, gingiva, and lips (**Fig. 25.75**). Oligodontia, small teeth, enamel hypoplasia, delayed eruption, malocclusion, and more rarely cleft lip or palate can also be observed (**Fig. 25.76**). The diagnosis is based on the clinical criteria.

Differential diagnosis

- Multiple papillomas
- Multiple condyloma acuminatum
- Focal epithelial hyperplasia
- Orofacial–digital syndrome
- Rothmund-Thomson syndrome
- Incontinentia pigmenti
- Conradi-Hünermann-Happle syndrome

Pathology

Histopathologic examination of the oral papillomas reveals epithelial hyperplasia around a fibrovascular stalk, composed of loose connective tissue and dilated vessels.

Treatment

There is no specific treatment. The treatment is symptomatic and depends on the case. Surgical excision or electrosurgery of oral papillomas can be of help if they cause problems.

Incontinentia Pigmenti

Key points

- A rare disorder inherited via the X-linked dominant pattern.
- Some cases represent new, spontaneous mutations.
- Caused by mutation in the *NEMO* gene.
- Linear skin lesions that follow Blaschko's lines.
- Oral manifestations include dental anomalies.

Introduction

Incontinentia pigmenti is a rare genetic disorder that affects multiple body systems, inherited in an X-linked dominant pattern. As a result, it is prevalent to females and lethal to most males. It has been associated with a deletion of the *NEMO* (also known as *IKBKG*) gene that encodes a protein that ultimately protects from cellular apoptosis, rendering the individuals affected susceptible to unregulated cellular apoptosis.

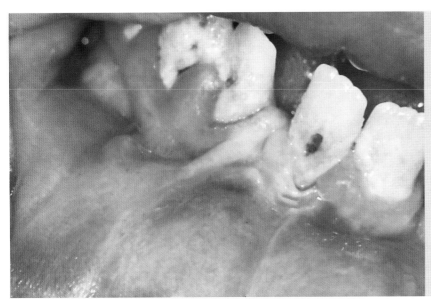

Fig. 25.72 Orofacial–digital syndrome, multiple frenula on the lower vestibule.

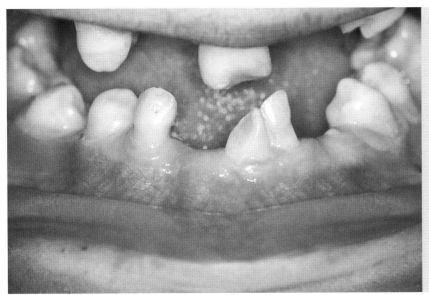

Fig. 25.73 Orofacial–digital syndrome, hypodontia, ectopic teeth, and shape abnormalities.

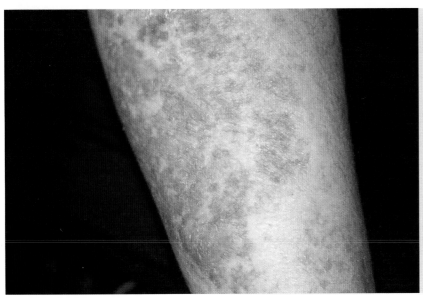

Fig. 25.74 Focal dermal hypoplasia, multiple nodules, and macules on the forearm.

Clinical features

Clinically, cutaneous manifestations of incontinentia pigmenti are the most common ones and evolve in four stages: (1) *blistering*: a blistering rash appears at birth and in early infancy and follows Blaschko's lines, or coalesces on the limbs, the trunk, and the scalp, (2) *verrucous linear plaques*: the development of wart-like lesions follows the healing of the blistering rash, (3) *hyperpigmentation*: gray-to-brown patches develop in a swirled pattern (**Fig. 25.77**), and (4) *hypopigmentation*: linear hyperpigmented bands fade with time leaving lines of light-colored skin and occasionally atrophy on the posterior aspects of the limbs and may be the only stigmata of the disease during adulthood.

The oral manifestations include dental anomalies presenting with small, conical, sharp teeth, hypodontia, delayed eruption, large interdental spaces, and enamel hypoplasia (**Fig. 25.78**).

Other rarer clinical features include alopecia, dystrophic nails, ocular defects, mental retardation, epilepsy, skeletal defects, and pulmonary hypertension.

The diagnosis is mainly based on the medical history and the clinical features.

Differential diagnosis

- Hypomelanosis of Ito
- Epidermolysis bullosa
- Goltz's syndrome
- Hypohidrotic ectodermal dysplasia
- Infections (chicken pox, herpes zoster, congenital syphilis)

Pathology

Histopathologic examination of the skin can be useful if genetic testing is inconclusive. Microscopically, in stage 1, eosinophilic spongiosis, a dyskeratotic keratinocytes are present; in stage 2, acanthosis, hyperkeratosis, and foci of dyskeratosis are present; in stage 3, pigmentary incontinence and vacuolization of basal cells; and in stage 4, thinned epidermis and dermis devoid of adnexa are seen.

Treatment

There is no specific treatment. The treatment is symptomatic and tailored to each case.

Ehlers-Danlos Syndrome

Key points

- A heterogeneous group of connective tissue disorders with an autosomal dominant and autosomal recessive inheritance patterns.
- Caused by a defective function of the collagen meshwork.
- From 1997, it is classified into six major types and several other novel subtypes.
- Oral and joint symptoms and signs are common.
- The hallmark of clinical features include hyperextensible fragile skin and joint hypermobility.
- The oral lesions are common.

Introduction

Ehlers-Danlos syndrome is a heterogeneous group of genetic collagen disorders inherited in an autosomal dominant or autosomal recessive patterns. The pathogenesis of the disorder may involve mutations in genes for collagen-processing enzymes and those encoding collagen α-chains. Some of the cases are caused by new, spontaneous mutations. The genes involved are multiple (*ADAMTS2, COL1A1, COL1A2, COL3A1, COL5A1, COL5A2, PLOD1,* and *TNXB*) and encode proteins required for collagen formation or proteins that interact with

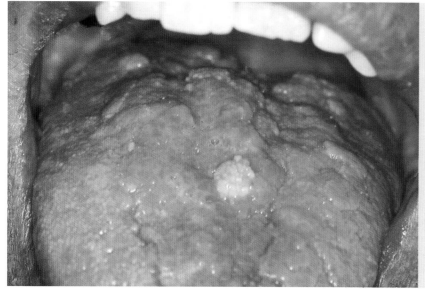

Fig. 25.75 Focal dermal hypoplasia, multiple papillomas on the tongue.

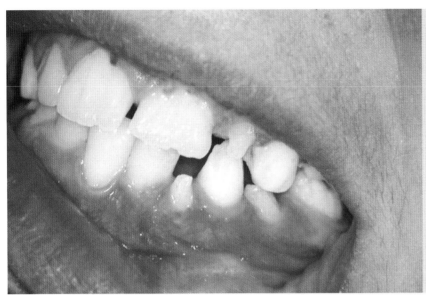

Fig. 25.76 Focal dermal hypoplasia, hypodontia, and small teeth.

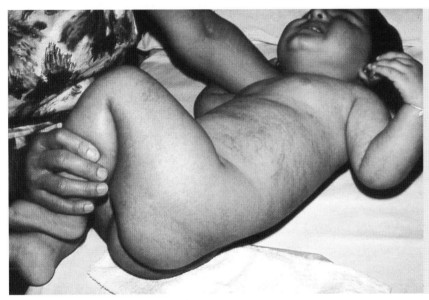

Fig. 25.77 Incontinentia pigmenti, black-brown linear hyperpigmentation of the trunk and extremities.

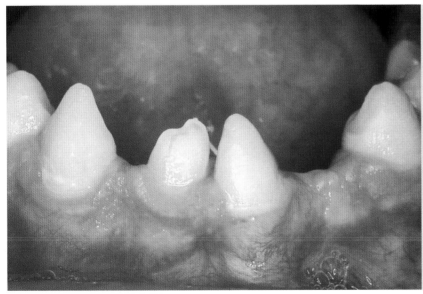

Fig. 25.78 Incontinentia pigmenti, hypodontia, and conical teeth.

collagen. The result is disruption of the structure, production or processing of collagen. Ultimately, this leads to weakened connective tissues in the multiple parts of the body, causing several characteristic symptoms and signs.

Previously more than 10 recognized types of Ehlers-Danlos syndrome existed. In 1997, a new classification was introduced into six major categories and named them by description: *classic type*, *hypermobility type*, *vascular type*, *kyphoscoliosis type*, *arthrochalasia type*, and *dermatosparaxis type*. Several other minor novel forms have also been reported in single families but are not well characterized.

Clinical features

The cardinal clinical features of the syndrome include extensibility and fragile skin, joints hypermobility (**Fig. 25.79**), bruisability, varicose veins, molluscoid pseudotumors, subcutaneous spheroids, fragility of blood vessels and delayed wound healing, atrophic scars, ocular abnormalities, oral manifestations, and several others. About 80% of patients have the classic type that is inherited as an autosomal dominant pattern.

The oral mucosa is excessively fragile and subject to bruising and subsequent hematomas formation and gingival bleeding, reflecting the fragility of small blood vessels. Delayed wound healing may be observed as well as hypermobility of the temporomandibular joint. A characteristic clinical sign is the ability, of approximately 50% of the patients, to touch the tip of their nose with their tongue tip (*Gorlin's sign*) compared with 10% of the general population (**Fig. 25.80**). Common oral radiographic findings include the presence of multiple pulp stones and abnormal and short roots. Dental abnormalities, such as enamel, dentine, and cementum defects may also be observed. The signs and symptoms usually become apparent after the first year, but some patients, depending on the type, may be undiagnosed for many years. The diagnosis is based on clinical criteria but may be supported by laboratory tests.

Differential diagnosis
- Differentiation between different types of the syndrome
- Marfan's syndrome
- Other causes of hyperelastic skin
- Osteogenesis imperfecta

Pathology

Histopathologic skin examination may support the diagnosis of connective tissue disorder when reduced and disorganized collagen fibrils are present. However, the histologic findings are not specific and diagnostic. Alternatively, genetic testing, electron microscopy examination, immunohistochemical analysis, protein electrophoresis of collagen from cultured dermal fibroblasts may be diagnostically helpful.

Treatment

There is no specific treatment available. The treatment is symptomatic and tailored to each case.

Marfan's Syndrome

Key points
- An autosomal dominant disorder with variable connective tissue weakness.
- It is caused by mutations of the *FBN1* gene on chromosome 15 which encodes fibrillin 1.
- The clinical characteristics include anomalies of the skin, ocular, skeletal, and cardiovascular systems.
- The patients have a characteristic appearance, being very tall, with long limbs and long, thin digits.
- Oral abnormalities are few and not pathognomonic.

Introduction

Marfan's syndrome is a rare genetic disorder of the connective tissue. The disorder is inherited in an autosomal dominant pattern, with at least 25% of the cases being caused by new, spontaneous mutations. Mutations of the *FBN1* gene on chromosome 15 ultimately result in the misfolding of fibrillin 1. That is a glycoprotein which forms elastic fibers in connective tissue and plays a role to cell signaling by binding to and sequestering transforming growth factor β (TGF-β). The altered fibrillin binds poorly to TGF-β, which results in its accumulation in various organs and systems causing more than 30 different symptoms and signs.

Clinical features

The most serious changes occur in the musculoskeletal and cardiovascular systems, the eyes, and skin. Characteristically, the patients are very tall with long and slender fingers and toes (arachnodactyly), long arms and legs, chest deformities, scoliosis, and less often kyphosis. Hyperextensibility of joints is also present. Cardiovascular anomalies are common and include mitral valve prolapse, aortic dilatation, and aneurysms that can be life threatening. Ocular abnormalities include myopia, glaucoma, and retinal detachment. The cutaneous manifestations may include striae and decrease of subcutaneous fat. The more common oral manifestation is a narrow, high-arched palate and, less commonly, cleft palate, bifid uvula, teeth anomalies of shape, mandibular prognathism, and malocclusion (**Fig. 25.81**). The symptoms can appear straight after birth, or later during childhood, or even puberty. The diagnosis is mainly based on clinical criteria.

Differential diagnosis
- Marfan's syndrome–like condition
- Ehlers-Danlos syndrome
- Loeys-Dietz syndrome

Pathology

There is no specific laboratory tests. In 2010, the Ghent Nosology was revised to suggest seven new criteria for the syndrome's diagnosis.

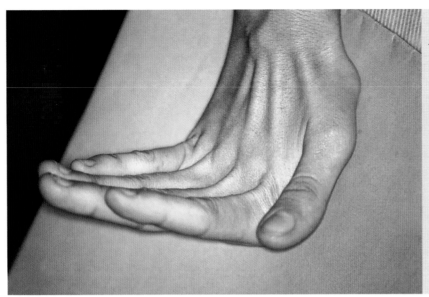

Fig. 25.79 Ehlers-Danlos syndrome, joint hyperextensibility of the fingers.

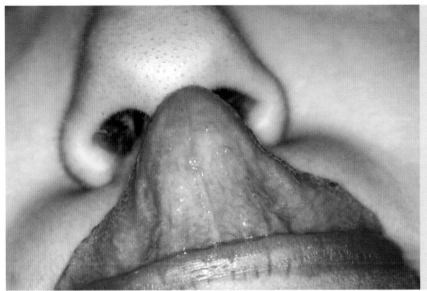

Fig. 25.80 Ehlers-Danlos syndrome, ability to touch the tip of the nose with the tongue tip.

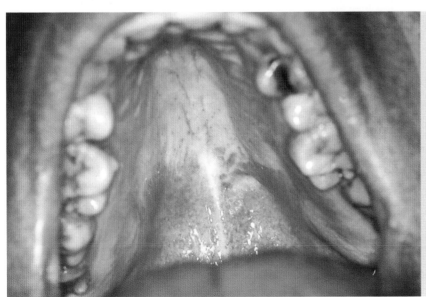

Fig. 25.81 Marfan's syndrome, narrow and arched palate.

Treatment

The treatment is symptomatic. Because these patients tend to develop dissecting aneurysms, control of blood pressure is mandatory. Life expectancy has increased significantly over the past decades, to reach similar levels to that of the average person.

Hypomelanosis of Ito

Key points

- A disorder characterized by hypopigmentation along the Blaschko's lines.
- No clear genetic causative picture.
- May arise as a result of chromosomal mosaicism.
- The disorder involves mainly the skin, but also may cause ocular, CNS, musculoskeletal, and dental abnormalities.

Introduction

Hypomelanosis of Ito is a description term rather than a diagnosis. The disorder is characterized by hypopigmented areas of skin and variable extracutaneous abnormalities. It was first described by Ito in 1952 who only reported cutaneous changes. A directly causative mutation remains unclear and it is believed that chromosomal mosaicism gives rise to the disorder.

Clinical features

Hypomelanosis of Ito can first appear straight after birth, or during infancy and early childhood. Clinically, the characteristic cutaneous lesions consist of hypopigmented whorls, or lines, or even plaques that follow the Blaschko's lines (**Fig. 25.82**). These lesions can be unilateral or bilateral and usually affect the trunk and extremities. Less frequently, hypertrichosis, alopecia, lentigines, nail and hair abnormalities may be observed. In approximately 30 to 40% of the patients, extracutaneous abnormalities such as musculoskeletal, CNS, cardiac, and ocular may be present (**Fig. 25.83**). Intraorally, dental anomalies such as enamel and dentin hypoplasia, conical and pitted anterior deciduous teeth, teeth with multiple cusps, brown-yellow–colored crowns, and gingivitis may occur (**Fig. 25.84**). The diagnosis is based on clinical criteria.

Differential diagnosis

- Leukoderma
- Achromic nevus
- Goltz's syndrome
- McCune-Albright syndrome
- Vitiligo
- Other genetic forms of hypomelanosis

Pathology

The histopathologic examination of the cutaneous lesions with dihydroxyphenylalanine (DOPA) staining reveals decreased size and number of melanosomes and smaller and fewer melanocytes. However, in some cases there are no pathologic findings. A blood karyotype can be performed to confirm the diagnosis.

Treatment

The treatment is symptomatic.

Hypophosphatasia

Key points

- A rare metabolic bone disease that is characterized by a deficiency of tissue alkaline phosphatase.
- The perinatal and infantile types are inherited in an autosomal recessive pattern. The milder forms are inherited in an autosomal recessive or autosomal dominant pattern.
- At least six types of the disease are recognized.
- The earlier forms of the disease have the most serious signs and symptoms.
- Early loss of the deciduous teeth is one of the early signs of the disease.

Introduction

Hypophosphatasia is a rare (1:100,000 births) enzyme, inherited disorder that affects the development of bones and teeth. The early forms of the disease are inherited in an autosomal recessive fashion, while the milder (later) forms are inherited in an autosomal recessive or autosomal dominant fashion. The disorder is caused by mutation of the *ALPL* gene, encoding the tissue nonspecific isoenzyme of alkaline phosphatase. This results in reduced serum and tissue levels of alkaline phosphatase that ultimately leads to problems in mineralization.

Clinical features

There is a great spectrum of clinical presentations with the most severe forms of the disorder developing early in life (perinatally and infantile) and the milder forms developing even in adult life, going undetected for several years.

Depending on the severity and the age of onset of the signs and symptoms, four major forms are recognized: *perinatal*, *infantile*, *childhood*, and *adult*. Two other forms include *odontohypophosphatasia* with only biochemical and dental manifestations and *pseudohypophosphatasia* with normal or elevated alkaline phosphatase activity levels.

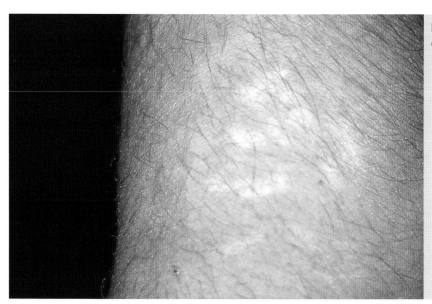

Fig. 25.82 Hypomelanosis of Ito, cutaneous hypopigmentation.

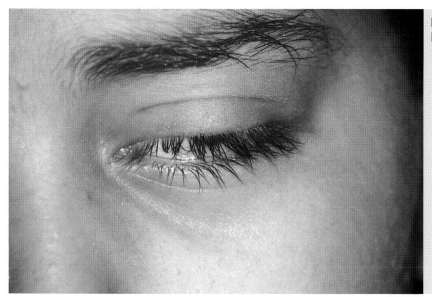

Fig. 25.83 Hypomelanosis of Ito, blepharoptosis, and photophobia.

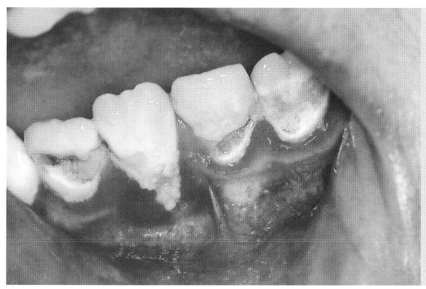

Fig. 25.84 Hypomelanosis of Ito, enamel hypoplasia, multiple cusps, dental caries, and gingivitis.

Systems, organs, and tissues commonly affected include the skeleton, pulmonary system, kidneys, eyes, and the periodontium. The childhood form affects mainly the periodontium and occurs usually during the second to third year of life, but periodontal lesions may less frequently occur in the adult form. Clinically, early loss of deciduous teeth is observed, during the second or third year of life. This involves the lower anterior teeth that lack any signs of periodontal disease. The same can be observed in the permanent teeth (**Fig. 25.85**). Teeth loss might be the first and only sign of the disease. In addition, other features may include alveolar bone loss and enlarged pulp chambers and root canals.

In the more serious forms of the disease, scull deformities and intracranial hypertension, failure to thrive and skeletal abnormalities (shortened, bowed limbs, ribs deformities), nephrolithiasis, respiratory failure, and ocular disorders may be observed.

Perinatal and infantile forms have the more severe manifestations with high mortality. The infantile and adult types are of better prognosis. The diagnosis is based on the clinical manifestations and the appropriate laboratory tests.

Differential diagnosis

- Acatalasia
- Papillon-Lefèvre syndrome
- Langerhans' cell histiocytosis
- Cyclic neutropenia
- Aggressive periodontitis
- Osteogenesis imperfecta
- Rickets

Laboratory tests

Laboratory tests to confirm the clinical diagnosis are the low levels of serum alkaline phosphatase and the increased levels of phosphoethanolamine in both blood and urine. Radiographic examination of the jaws, skull, and skeleton reveals radiolucencies.

Histopathologically, the teeth present with reduction or absence of cementum.

Treatment

The treatment is symptomatic. Alkaline phosphatase infusion, phosphorus, vitamin D, and parathormone have been used but without very promising results. It is important to prevent the built-up of intracranial pressure and bone fractures.

Odonto-Onychodermal Dysplasia

Key points

- A rare type of ectodermal dysplasia, inherited in an autosomal recessive pattern.
- Mutations occur on the *WNT10A* gene on chromosome 2q35.
- Mainly is characterized by cutaneous and dental abnormalities.

Introduction

Odonto-onychodermal dysplasia is a rare type of ectodermal dysplasia inherited in an autosomal recessive pattern. Mutations occur on the *WNT10A* gene which encodes a protein involved in signaling and plays a role in early development. The result of the mutation is a truncated protein which leads to impaired signal transduction during early development.

Clinical features

A main clinical feature is the presence of dental abnormalities which include oligodontia, microdontia, macrodontia, peg-shaped mandibular incisors, conical incisors, large interdental spaces, and overbite (**Fig. 25.86**). Macrocheilia may also be observed (**Fig. 25.87**). Cutaneous abnormalities include partial or total alopecia of the scalp, folliculitis, scarring, erythematous atrophic patches, cysts, mainly on the cheeks, nose, neck, and extremities, and also nail dystrophy (**Fig. 25.88**). Hyperkeratosis of the palms and soles, and hyperhidrosis of the palms can also occur. Ocular abnormalities include photophobia, blepharitis, and tearing. The diagnosis is based on clinical criteria.

Differential diagnosis

- Other types of ectodermal dysplasias
- Witkop's tooth–nail syndrome
- Goltz's syndrome

Laboratory tests

Genetic testing can be used; affected children are often born in consanguineous families.

Treatment

The treatment is symptomatic.

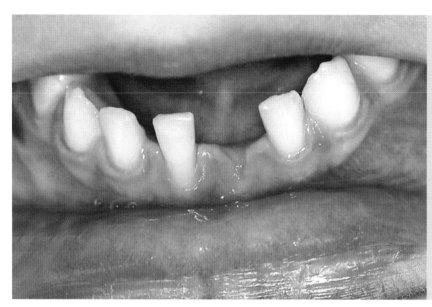

Fig. 25.85 Hypophosphatasia, premature loss of the lower incisors in a 10-year-old boy.

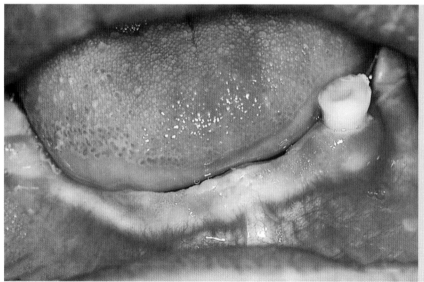

Fig. 25.86 Odonto-onychodermal dysplasia, oligodontia.

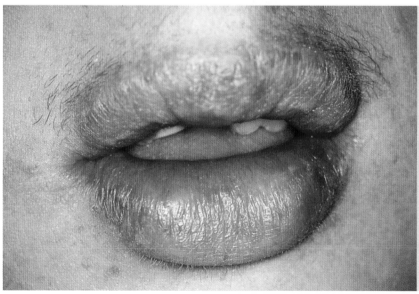

Fig. 25.87 Odonto-onychodermal dysplasia, macrocheilia.

Werner's Syndrome

Key points

- A rare genetic disorder inherited in an autosomal recessive pattern.
- It is due to mutations in the *RECOL2* gene, which encodes a helicase.
- The disease becomes apparent in the second and third decades of life.
- The disorder involves the skeletal system, skin, nails, eyes, and mouth.
- Premature aging is associated with the development of malignancies.

Introduction

Werner's syndrome is a rare genetic disorder inherited in an autosomal recessive pattern. It was first described in 1904 by the German Ophthalmologist Otto Werner who observed progeria-like features and juvenile cataracts in his patients. The disorder is caused by mutation of the *RECOL2* gene, which encodes a helicase. This protein thought to perform functions related to the maintenance and repair of DNA and DNA replication prior to cell division. The protein encoded by the mutated gene is a short, nonfunctional protein. It is speculated that cells with the altered protein divide more slowly, or stop dividing earlier, causing growth problems. Additionally, DNA damage may accumulate causing health problems associated with the condition.

Clinical features

The signs and symptoms of the disorder usually appear during the second and third decades of life. Until then, the patients develop normally. The clinical spectrum is variable depending on which the potentially affected organ presents changes at the time of diagnosis. The typical presentation involves short stature with short limbs, thin face, and obvious signs of premature aging. The skin lesions are prominent and are characterized by thin and atrophic skin, particularly over areas depleted of fat and connective tissue, and musculature. This leads in shiny smooth, inelastic, and dry skin giving a scleroderma-like pattern. Other cutaneous changes include hyperpigmentation, hypopigmentation, telangiectasias, hyperkeratosis, loss of subcutaneous fat, and ankle ulcerations. The main areas of skin involvement are the face and extremities. Microstomia and micrognathia may also be observed (**Fig. 25.89**). The oral mucosa is thin and atrophic, the nose is thin and the ears are also thin and inelastic. There is also a plethora of skeletal, ocular, cardiovascular, hormonal, and neurologic abnormalities. The patients are at risk of developing malignancies such as basal cell and squamous cell carcinomas, melanoma, thyroid carcinoma, sarcoma, etc. (**Fig. 25.90**). Malignancies or myocardial infarctions are usually responsible for death by the fifth decade. The diagnosis is based on the clinical criteria.

Differential diagnosis

- Progeria
- Systemic sclerosis
- Rothmund-Thomson syndrome
- Ataxia-telangiectasia

Laboratory tests

There is no diagnostic laboratory test. Genetic testing is only used for research purposes.

Treatment

There is no specific treatment. The treatment is symptomatic, aiming at the problems caused by the disease.

Chédiak-Higashi Syndrome

Key points

- An uncommon genetic disorder inherited in an autosomal recessive pattern.
- It is caused by mutations in the lysosomal trafficking regulator gene (*LYST*).
- Silver hair, diffuse pigmentary dilution, photophobia, nystagmus, recurrent infections, bleeding diathesis, and periodontal disease are the most common manifestations.
- The prognosis is poor and if bone marrow transplantation is not performed, most patients die.
- Gingivitis, hemorrhage, and oral ulceration can be observed.

Introduction

Chédiak-Higashi syndrome is a rare genetic disorder that causes primary immunodeficiency. It is inherited in an autosomal recessive pattern. It has been associated with mutations of the *CHS1* gene (also known as *LYST*). This gene encodes the lysosomal trafficking regulator that is believed to play a role in the transport of materials into lysosomes. As a result, they lose their ability to break down toxic substances, digest bacteria, and carry out general recycling. This ultimately leads to the development of large intracellular vesicles that impair the function of melanosomes, white blood cells, and platelets. The immune system is also affected.

Clinical features

Clinically, the syndrome manifests during early infancy and is characterized by mild diffuse pigmentary dilution of the skin, hair, and eyes. Cutaneous areas of bronze to slate-gray hyperpigmentation often admixed with guttate hypopigmented macules in sun-exposed areas may occur. Silvery hair is

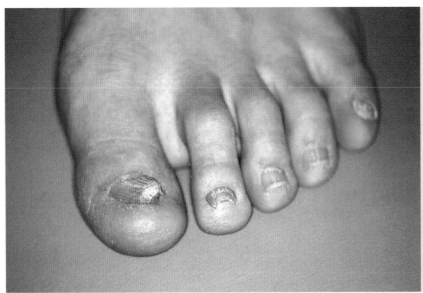

Fig. 25.88 Odonto-onychodermal dysplasia, nail dystrophy.

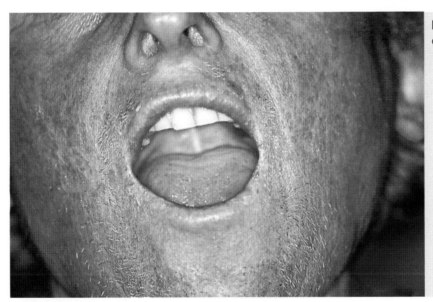

Fig. 25.89 Werner's syndrome, thin, dry, and inelastic skin and microstomia.

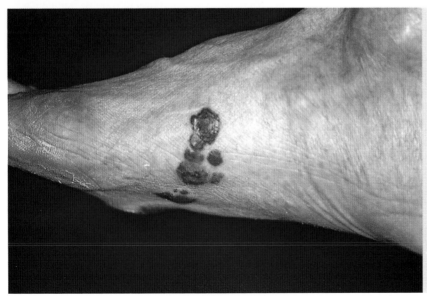

Fig. 25.90 Werner's syndrome, malignant melanoma on the foot.

characteristic feature (**Fig. 25.91**). Decreased ocular pigment usually results in photophobia, nystagmus, and strabismus. Patients are also prone to gram-positive and gram-negative bacterial infections classically caused by *Staphylococcus aureus* and *Streptococcus pyogenes* that primarily affect the skin and lungs. Other common findings are epistaxis, petechiae, and ecchymoses. Intraorally, dental caries, gingivitis, hemorrhage, and ulceration have been described (**Fig. 25.92**).

Most of the children affected (80%) reach a stage known as the *accelerated phase*, or *lymphoma-like syndrome*. In that stage, defective white blood cells divide uncontrollably and invade many organs, which can be life threatening.

Differential diagnosis
- Griscelli's syndrome
- Hermansky-Pudlak syndrome
- Other primary immunodeficiencies
- Hypomelanosis of Ito
- Neutropenia
- Leukemia

Pathology

Blood smears demonstrate characteristic abnormal giant granules in the neutrophils, eosinophils, and granulocytes. Bone marrow cytology reveals giant inclusion bodies in the leukocyte precursor cells. Histologically, the silver hair is characterized by clumps of melanin and giant melanosomes within melanocytes. With the use of polarized light microscopy, a bright and polychromatic refringence pattern can be seen on the hair.

Treatment

Hematopoietic stem cell allogeneic transplantation from a human leukocyte antigen (HLA)-matched sibling or unrelated donor is the treatment of choice. Therefore, it is crucial to recognize the disease early to prevent the onset of the accelerated phase. Prophylactic antibiotics to prevent recurrent infections are recommended.

Zimmermann-Laband Syndrome

Key points
- A very rare genetic disorder inherited in an autosomal dominant pattern.
- One of the main clinical characteristics is great gingival enlargement.

Introduction

Zimmermann-Laband syndrome is a very rare genetic disorder that is inherited in an autosomal dominant pattern. It has been recently reported that the cause is mutations of the *KCNH1* gene, on chromosome 1q32, which encodes the voltage-gated K$^+$ channel EAG1. A change in the *ATP6V1B2* gene, on chromosome 8p21, is also noted.

Clinical features

Clinically, Zimmermann-Laband syndrome is characterized by hypertrichosis, facial dysmorphism, gingival enlargement, nail and distal phalanges, joint hyperextensibility, macrosomia at birth, hepatosplenomegaly, and mental retardation. Gingival enlargement is one of the prominent features. It is usually observed during the second or third month of life. Clinically, the gingiva appear lobular and enlarged and if teeth are present, they are fully or partially covered (**Fig. 25.93**). Rarely, macroglossia and macrocheilia may also be observed. The diagnosis is based on the history and clinical features.

Differential diagnosis
- Hereditary gingival fibromatosis
- Murray-Puretic-Drescher syndrome
- Rutherford's syndrome
- Cross and Rammon syndromes
- Drug-induced gingival enlargement

Pathology

Histologic examination of the gingiva exhibits dense collagenous tissue, which forms multiple interlacing bundles which run in all directions. The surface epithelium exhibits long and thin rete ridges that extend into the fibrous connective tissue.

Treatment

There is no specific treatment. Gingivectomy of enlarged gingiva along with a program of high levels of oral hygiene are suggested.

Chronic Granulomatous Disease

Key points
- A genetic group of immunodeficiencies.
- The disorder is inherited in an X-linked recessive or autosomal recessive pattern.
- Recurrent bacterial and fungal infections, granulomas, lymphadenopathy, and hepatosplenomegaly.
- Atypical oral ulceration and granulomatous cheilitis.

Introduction

Chronic granulomatous disease is a rare group of life-threatening, congenital disorders classified under primary immunodeficiencies. It is caused by the inability of phagocytes to produce the superofide radical that is used to kill ingested pathogens, due to defects in the nicotinamide adenine dinucleotide phosphate (NADPH) oxidase enzyme complex. This results in severe, recurrent, bacterial and fungal infections. Subsequently, the intracellular survival of the ingested microorganisms leads to granulomas formation in the lymph nodes, skin, lungs, liver, and gastrointestinal tract.

Approximately, 80% of cases are inherited as an X-linked recessive pattern, while the rest are autosomal recessive. The incidence of the disorder is approximately 1:200,000 per live births.

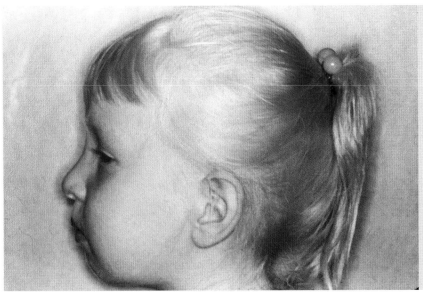

Fig. 25.91 Chédiak-Higashi syndrome, thin light skin and thin silver hair.

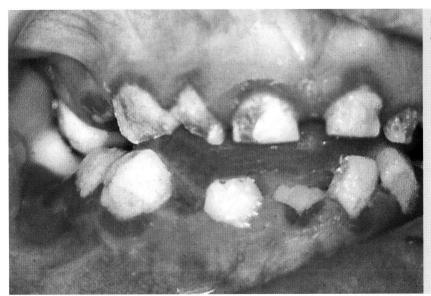

Fig. 25.92 Chédiak-Higashi syndrome, gingivitis, and dental caries.

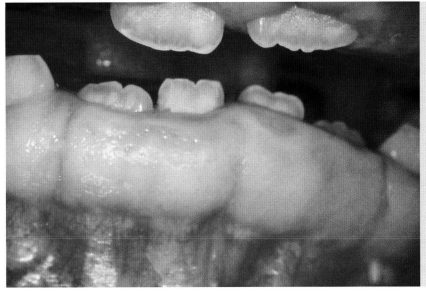

Fig. 25.93 Zimmermann-Laband syndrome, great gingival enlargement with a lobular pattern.

Clinical features

Clinically, chronic granulomatous disease is characterized by recurrent serious bacterial and fungal infections of the lungs, lymph nodes, liver and spleen, bones, and subcutaneous tissue. The most common pathogens are *S. aureus* and *Serratia marcescens*, causing infections and abscesses around the nose and the ears that usually start during the neonatal stage. Cutaneous lesions include seborrheic dermatitis, scalp folliculitis, lupus erythematosus–like lesions, erythema, ulceration, and granulomas formation. Other findings include lymphadenopathy, hepatosplenomegaly, pneumonia, gastrointestinal disorders (diarrhea, abdominal pain), conjunctivitis and choroiditis, osteomyelitis, etc. Granulomas and abscesses in internal organs, e.g., lungs, liver, spleen, gastrointestinal and urinary tracts occur more frequently than those of the skin. The oral manifestations are oral infections with nonspecific, irregular ulcerations resembling aphthous ulcers (**Fig. 25.94**). Rarely, gingivitis, salivary gland swelling, granulomatous cheilitis, and perioral dermatitis may occur. Fungal infections involving the mouth are candidiasis and aspergillosis.

The clinical diagnosis should be confirmed by laboratory tests.

Differential diagnosis
- Other primary immunodeficiencies disorders
- Neutropenia
- Cyclic neutropenia
- Other inherited phagocytic deficiencies

Pathology

Histopathologic examination from cutaneous granulomas demonstrates histiocytic infiltrates associated with foreign body giant cells and accumulation of neutrophils. Peripheral blood examination reveals leukocytosis, anemia, reduction of the T lymphocytes, elevated erythrocyte sedimentation rate (ESR), and hypergammaglobulinemia.

Nitroblue tetrazolium slide test remains the simplest and most reliable diagnostic test. It is also very fast, but it does not quantify the enzymes. A similar test is dihydrorhodamine, where the whole blood is stimulated to produce superoxide radicals. A more advanced test, the cytochrome C reduction assay, can determine the amount of superoxide the phagocytes can produce. A genetic analysis can be used to determine the mutation responsible.

Treatment

The use of antibiotics and antifungal drugs both prophylactically and therapeutically has improved the outcome. Short courses of systemic corticosteroids are also used to improve the granulomas. Other medications used include sulfasalazine, azathioprine, tumor necrosis factor α (TNF-α), and interferon γ (INF-γ). Additional therapies include granulocyte transfusion, hematopoietic stem cell transplantation, and bone marrow transplantation.

Good's Syndrome

Key points
- The disorder is classified under primary immunodeficiencies.
- Coexists with thymoma and hypogammaglobulinemia.
- Common findings are recurrent opportunistic infections.
- A frequent oral feature is severe *Candida* infection.

Introduction

Good's syndrome was first described by Good in 1954. It is classified under primary immunodeficiencies and usually coexists with thymoma. The immunodeficiency might precede or follow the thymoma diagnosis.

The etiology and pathogenesis remain unclear, but there is some evidence to suggest that a bone marrow defect is involved, combined with a B- and T-cell deficiency. The disease is usually detected during the fourth or fifth decade of life. It is common for the thymoma to be detected during testing performed for severe myasthenia in patients greater than 40 years. Other autoimmune conditions may coexist, including severe myasthenia, pernicious anemia, diabetes mellitus, and idiopathic thrombocytopenia.

Clinical features

Clinically, the first symptoms are persistent cough, dysphagia, dyspnea, hoarseness, and retrosternal pain. Recurrent opportunistic infections are frequent (bacterial, viral, and candidal). Common targets of the infections are the respiratory and gastrointestinal systems, the sinuses, and the skin. Intraorally, severe *Candida* infection can occur, extending throughout the oral cavity and to the upper parts of the respiratory and digestive systems (**Figs. 25.95, 25.96**). Candidiasis can also affect the nails and skin.

Good's syndrome should be suspected in patients more than 40 years that present with immunodeficiency, thymoma, and all the relevant symptoms and signs. The diagnosis is based on clinical features and immunologic investigations.

Pathology

An assessment of quantitative immunoglobulins can be performed as part of an immunologic evaluation. B- and T-lymphocyte subsets should also be looked at. The humoral response may also be impaired.

Treatment

Surgical removal of the thymoma and intravenous immunoglobulin are widely suggested. Prophylactic antibiotics and treatment of any infections are very important.

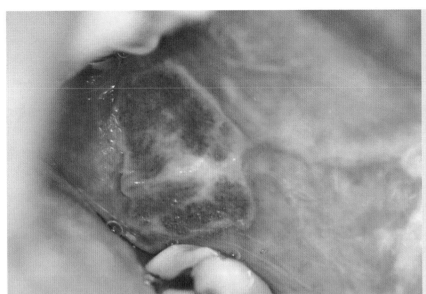

Fig. 25.94 Chronic granulomatous disease, large ulcer of the buccal mucosa.

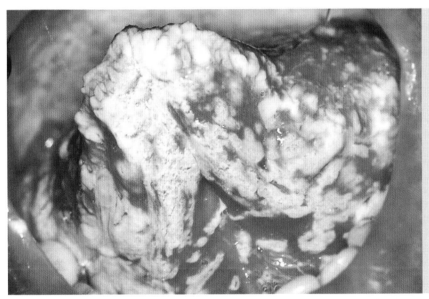

Fig. 25.95 Good's syndrome, severe candidiasis extending to the whole tongue.

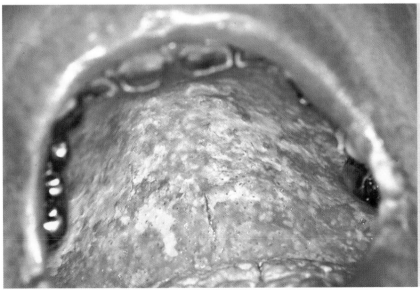

Fig. 25.96 Good's syndrome, severe candidiasis on the palate.

26 Skin Diseases

Erythema Multiforme

Key points

- An acute condition that tends to recur.
- The most important factors implicated in the pathogenesis are herpes simplex 1 and 2 and less frequently other infections or drugs.
- Two types are recognized: minor and major.
- The oral mucosa is mainly involved in the major type of the disease.
- "Target lesions" are the characteristic cutaneous lesions of erythema multiforme.

Introduction

Erythema multiforme is an acute or subacute self-limited disease that mainly involves the skin and mucous membranes. It tends to recur, especially during autumn and spring. The exact etiology remains unknown. It is considered as a distinct skin or/and mucous membrane–directed reaction associated with certain recognized triggers in predisposed individuals. Herpes simplex virus (HSV1, HSV2) seems to trigger erythema multiforme minor in almost all cases and erythema multiforme major in approximately 55% of the cases. Other infectious agents triggering the disease include *Mycoplasma pneumoniae*, *Epstein-Barr virus*, and *Histoplasma capsulatum*. Other triggers include other viruses, fungi, and more rarely medication (< 10%) including nonsteroidal anti-inflammatory drugs, sulphonamides, antibiotics, antiepileptics, and systemic diseases. Erythema multiforme predominantly affects young adults between 20 and 40 years, with a slight male preponderance.

Stevens-Johnson syndrome was separated from the major erythema multiforme as they are distinct clinical disorders.

Clinical features

Clinically, erythema multiforme is divided into two forms: *minor* with typical and/or atypical papular target lesions and minimal or no mucosal involvement and no systemic symptoms and *major* that is more severe, with typical and/or atypical papular target lesions with severe mucosal involvement and systemic features.

Erythema multiforme does not carry the risk of progressing to toxic epidermal necrolysis (TEN).

The clinical presentation has a sudden onset with the occurrence of a red maculopapular exanthema that may be small or increase in size centrifugally, reaching a diameter of 1 to 2 cm. Almost all the lesions appear within 24 to 48 hours and full development by 72 hours. Characteristically, the periphery remains erythematous, but the center becomes cyanotic or even purpuric, forming the characteristic "target" or "iris" lesions (**Fig. 26.1**). Two types of *target* lesions are recognized: (1) the *typical*, with at least three different zones and (2) the *atypical papular*, with two different zones and/or a poorly defined border. Less frequently, vesicles and bullae may develop.

The oral mucosa is affected in 25 to 50% of the cases, mainly in the major type and rarely in the minor. Clinically, the primary lesion is erythema and multiple small vesicles, or bullae that coalesce and then rupture, leaving painful, extensive erosions or ulcerations covered by a necrotic pseudomembrane. Any oral area can be affected with a predilection toward the lips, soft palate, tongue, and buccal mucosa (**Figs. 26.2, 26.3**). Rarely, conjunctivitis, balanitis, and vaginitis may be observed (**Fig. 26.4**). Fever, coughing, difficulty in swallowing, arthralgias, atypical pneumonia, and malaise occur in the major type, but are absent in the minor form of the disease. The diagnosis is primarily based on clinical criteria, but should be confirmed by a biopsy and histologic examination.

Differential diagnosis

- Fixed drug eruption
- Stevens-Johnson syndrome
- Toxic epidermal necrolysis
- Primary herpetic gingivostomatitis
- Systemic lupus erythematosus
- Pemphigus
- Mucous membrane pemphigoid
- Kawasaki's disease
- Recurrent aphthous ulcers

Pathology

Histopathologic examination of the lesions is indicative of the condition, but not diagnostic. The features observed are keratinocyte apoptosis, throughout all layers of the epidermis, and marked basal cell hydropic degeneration. Superficial dermal edema and a perivascular infiltrate of mononuclear cells and exocytosis of T lymphocytes into the epidermis are common. At an early stage, there might be intra- or subepithelial vesicles.

Using direct immunofluorescence granular deposit of immunoglobulin M (IgM) and C3 can be seen around the vessels and focally at the epidermodermal junction, but these findings are nonspecific.

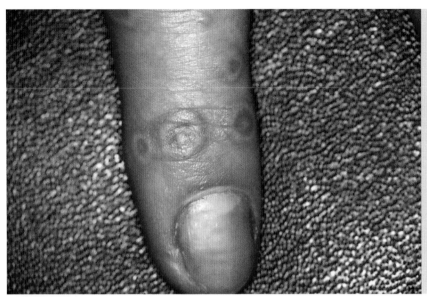

Fig. 26.1 Erythema multiforme, typical target lesions on the finger.

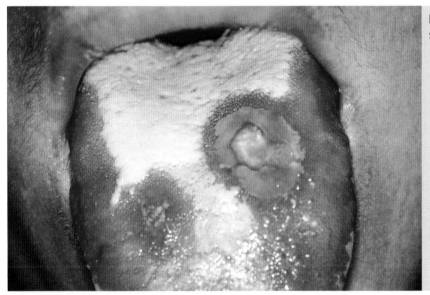

Fig. 26.2 Erythema multiforme, erosions on the dorsum of the tongue.

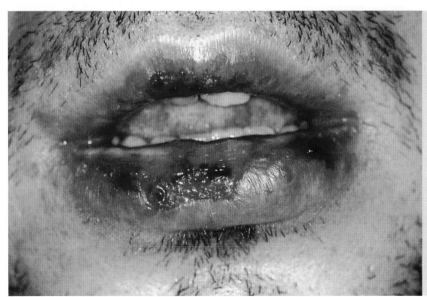

Fig. 26.3 Erythema multiforme, erosions on the lips covered by hemorrhagic crusts.

Treatment

The treatment includes topical and systemic therapy. The topical treatment includes oral antihistamines, analgesics, antiseptic mouthwashes, local skin care. If an underlying cause is identified, treatment toward it should be administered. If medication is implicated, it should be withdrawn. In severe major forms, early therapy with systemic corticosteroids, e.g., prednisolone 0.5 to 1 mg/kg/d in divided doses should be considered. In patients with HSV-associated disease with frequent recurrences, prophylactic use for 4 to 6 months with valacyclovir (500–1000 mg/d) or famciclovir (500 mg/d) or acyclovir (10 mg/kg/d) for 4 to 6 months should be used.

Other treatments which may help patients with recurrent disease are dapsone, antimalarials, azathioprine, mycophenolate mofetil, cyclosporine, thalidomide, and psoralens plus ultraviolet light A (PUVA).

Stevens-Johnson Syndrome

Key points

- An acute mucocutaneous disease with general signs and symptoms that can initially resemble these of upper respiratory tract infection.
- Most commonly represents adverse drug reaction.
- Extensive lesions mainly in the oral and other mucosae and skin.
- Exfoliation of the skin is due to extensive death of keratinocytes via apoptosis.
- Early diagnosis, cessation of the causative drug, and rapid start of supportive and specific treatment are recommended.

Introduction

Stevens-Johnson syndrome is a relatively rare, acute, life-threatening mucocutaneous disease of an immune complex–mediated hypersensitivity, which is nearly always drug-related. The disease is unrelated to erythema multiforme and is considered as a milder form of TEN. It presents with less than 10% of body surface area detachment, with a considerable overlap with TEN. The medications most frequently associated with Stevens-Johnson syndrome include antiepileptics, sulfasalazine, trimethoprim-sulfamethoxazole, nonsteroidal anti-inflammatory drugs (NSAIDs), allopurinol, antibiotics, barbiturates, and others.

Genetic susceptibility and immune response play a role in the pathogenesis of the disease, which leads to epidermal and mucosal necrosis and detachment. Stevens-Johnson syndrome has an annual incidence of 1.2 to 6 per million while is slightly more common in women than men (1.5:1).

Clinical features

Prodromal symptoms include fever, cough, fatigue, malaise, sore throat, arthralgia, myalgias, diarrhea, photophobia, etc. usually precede by 1 to 3 days the development of mucosal and skin manifestations.

The oral mucosa is almost always involved, with extensive formation of vesicles or bullae that rupture quickly to leave extensive and painful erosions that are covered by grayish-white or hemorrhagic pseudomembranes/crusts (**Fig. 26.5**). The lesions usually extend to the pharynx, larynx, esophagus, and respiratory system. The ocular lesions follow in frequency and consist of severe conjunctivitis and more rarely chorioretinitis, corneal ulceration, and ocular pain (**Fig. 26.6**). The genital involvement manifests as balanitis and vulvovaginitis (**Fig. 26.7**). The oral, ocular, and genital mucosa lesions are present in more than 90 to 95% of patients. The skin lesions are variable in both gravity and extent. They start as erythematous, dusky red, or purpuric macules of irregular shape and size that tend to coalesce. As the epidermal lesions progress toward full-thickness necrosis of the epidermis, the dusky red macular lesions take a gray hue and soon detach from the dermis giving rise to bullae. Finally, the skin assembles *wet cigarette paper* "*scalding*" as it is pulled away after mechanical trauma. The Nikolsky's sign might be positive in certain areas. The exanthema starts from the trunk and neck, face,

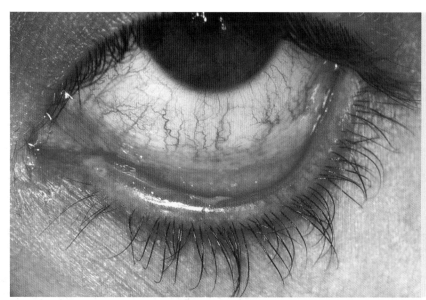

Fig. 26.4 Erythema multiforme, conjunctivitis.

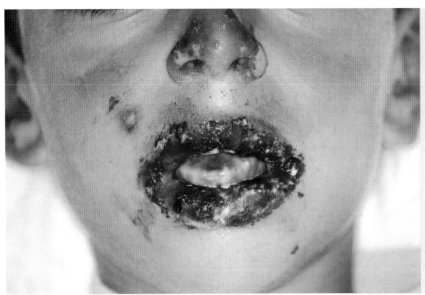

Fig. 26.5 Stevens-Johnson syndrome, severe lesions on the lips.

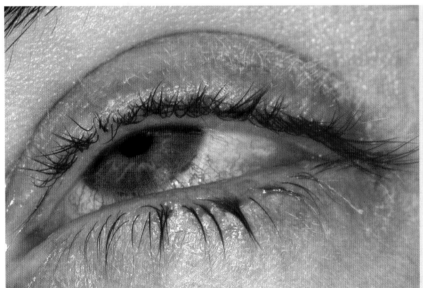

Fig. 26.6 Stevens-Johnson syndrome, conjunctivitis, and edema of the eyelids.

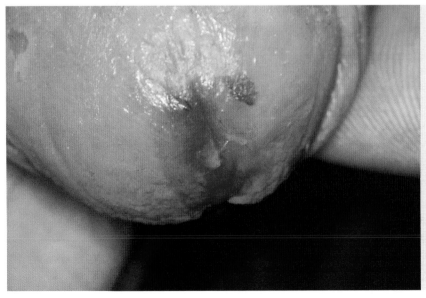

Fig. 26.7 Stevens-Johnson syndrome, erosions on the glans penis.

and upper extremities (**Fig. 26.8**). Occasionally, the cutaneous and other manifestations resemble TEN, making their distinction challenging. The extent of epidermal detachment is the criterion of classification of the patients into three groups: (1) Stevens-Johnson syndrome detachment less than 10% of body surface area, (2) Stevens-Johnson syndrome and TEN overlap: 10 to 30%, and (3) TEN greater than 30%. In severe cases, there can be renal and hepatic involvement and also pneumonia. The mortality rate ranges between 1 and 3%. The diagnosis is based on the history and the clinical features. Skin biopsy may be helpful, but is not routinely performed in the acute setting.

Differential diagnosis

- Toxic epidermal necrolysis
- Erythema multiforme
- Generalized fixed bullous drug eruption
- Staphylococcal scalded skin syndrome
- Paraneoplastic pemphigus
- Graft-versus-host disease, acute
- Sweet's syndrome

Pathology

Histopathologic examination of skin biopsy is useful for confirming the diagnosis. It reveals subepidermal bullae with epidermal cell necrosis. Apoptotic keratinocytes can be seen scattered throughout the basal and suprabasal layers. There is also perivascular lymphocytic infiltrate in the lamina propria.

Treatment

The treatment of patients with Stevens-Johnson is performed in intensive care units or burn units, by a team of specialists. If the responsible agent is identified and withdrawn quickly, the outcome is more favorable in most of the cases. Supportive treatment is indicated with emphasis on airway maintenance and hemodynamic stability, fluid replacement, and electrolyte correction. Prevention and treatment of any secondary infection is important. Agents that have been tried include systemic corticosteroids, immunosuppressants, thalidomide, tumor necrosis factor α (TNF-α) antagonistic, e.g., infliximab, etanercept. Additionally, plasmapheresis, hemodialysis, and parenteral administration of Ig have also been reported. Recently, a treatment regimen of 1 g/kg/d of intravenous immunoglobulin (IVIg) for 3 consecutive days (total dose 3 g/kg) or total dose of 4 g/kg over 4 days is currently recommended treatment.

Toxic Epidermal Necrolysis

Key points

- A rare, acute mucocutaneous disorder associated with drug reactions.
- It is characterized by detachment of the epidermis in over 30% of the whole body surface.
- The oral and other mucosae are always involved.

Introduction

Toxic epidermal necrolysis (TEN), also known as Lyell's disease, is a rare acute and life-threatening mucocutaneous disease characterized by extensive (> 30% of the whole body surface) detachment of the epidermis. In more than 95% of the cases it represents a form of severe drug reaction. More than a hundred different medications have been associated with TEN such as antibiotics, sulphonamides, trimethoprim-sulfamethoxazole, analgesics, nonsteroidal anti-inflammatory drugs, antiepileptics etc. It has also been associated with human immunodeficiency virus (HIV) infection, autoimmune disease, and malignancies.

The pathogenesis is similar with that of Stevens-Johnson syndrome. The annual incidence of TEN is 0.4 to 1.2 per million and are slightly more common in women than men (ratio 1.5:1).

Clinical features

Clinically, toxic epidermal necrolysis presents with prodromal symptoms such as malaise, low-grade fever, burning sensation of the conjunctivae, and coughing that precede the mucocutaneous manifestations by 1 to 3 days. Following the above, a painful rash appears that begins on the face and extremities in a symmetrical fashion and within 1 to 2 days it coalesces, forming flaccid bullae and eventually causing the characteristic *sheet-like epidermal detachment resembling "scalding."* As the very thin skin detaches, with even the mildest form of friction and trauma it leaves extensive, raw, painful, uncovered areas that can bleed (**Fig. 26.9**). The Nikolsky's sign is usually positive.

The mouth is involved in 85 to 95% of the cases with severe inflammation and painful erosions that predominantly affect the lips, tongue, palate, buccal mucosa, and gingiva (**Fig. 26.10**). Similar lesions may be seen on the pharyngeal mucosa, conjunctivae, genitals, and anus (**Fig. 26.11**). The prognosis is poor with mortality rates range from 25 to 35%. If the disease is the result of a drug reaction, the quickest the responsible medication is identified and withdrawn, the better the prognosis.

The diagnosis is based on the history, clinical features, and histologic examination.

Differential diagnosis

- Stevens-Johnson syndrome
- Staphylococcal scalded skin syndrome
- Generalized bullous fixed drug eruption
- Systemic lupus erythematosus
- Pemphigus
- Bullous pemphigoid
- Sweet's syndrome
- Graft-versus-host disease

Pathology

The histopathologic picture of affected skin lesions is similar to the one of Stevens-Johnson syndrome.

Treatment

Admission to intensive care units or burn units in hospital is mandatory for most of the cases. The same therapeutic principles apply as in the Stevens-Johnson syndrome.

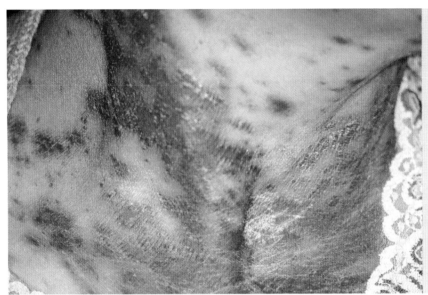

Fig. 26.8 Stevens-Johnson syndrome, macular rash, and erosions covered by hemorrhagic crust.

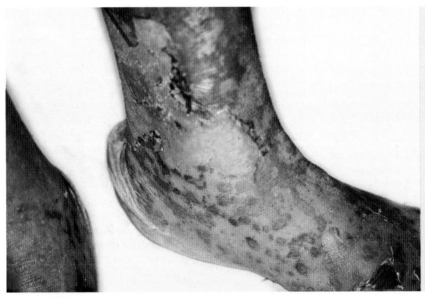

Fig. 26.9 Toxic epidermal necrolysis, characteristic detachment of the epidermis.

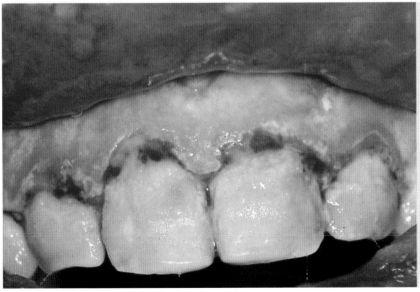

Fig. 26.10 Toxic epidermal necrolysis, erosions on the gingiva.

Pemphigus

Key points

- A group of chronic autoimmune mucocutaneous diseases.
- Pemphigus is classified into three major types: pemphigus vulgaris, pemphigus foliaceus, and paraneoplastic pemphigus and several subtypes.
- Oral involvement (> 95%) is observed in pemphigus vulgaris and paraneoplastic pemphigus and less frequently in the other types.
- The main pathogenic mechanism is the functional inhibition of desmogleins 1 and 3 which play an important role in cell–cell adhesion of keratinocytes, by IgG autoantibodies resulting in bullous formation.
- Desmoglein 3 autoantibodies are responsible for the oral lesions while desmoglein 1 autoantibodies for the cutaneous lesions.
- Over the past 20 years, advances in treatment have improved the outcome of the disease.

Introduction

The term *pemphigus* refers to a group of chronic blistering autoimmune diseases affecting the skin and mucosae. It is caused by autoantibodies directed against desmogleins 3 and 1. These are cadherin-type epithelial cell adhesion molecules of the keratinocyte cells. When this phenomenon occurs, the keratinocyte cells loose adhesion resulting in to cell–cell adhesion acantholysis. Ultimately, intraepithelial bullae formation in several layers of the epithelium and the epidermis occurs. When the autoantibodies target desmoglein 3 lesions present in the oral mucosa, while when the target is desmoglein 1 lesions that occur on the skin. When the autoantibodies target both types of desmogleins, mucocutaneous manifestations occur. The disease shows a high prevalence in Mediterranean races (Jewish, Greeks, Italians, Tunisians, and Balkans in general) without any familial distribution. The incidence is be-

tween 1 and 7 new cases/annum per 1,000,000 per year of the population. Females are more frequently affected (1.6:1) with the mean age of onset being between 50 and 60 years. It can, however, affect any age group, including children. Using clinical, histopathologic, and immunologic criteria, pemphigus is classified into three major types: *pemphigus vulgaris, pemphigus foliaceus, paraneoplastic pemphigus,* and several subtypes: *pemphigus vegetans, pemphigus erythematosus, IgA pemphigus, drug-induced pemphigus.* The oral mucosa is affected in over 95% of the cases in pemphigus vulgaris and paraneoplastic pemphigus and less frequently in the other types. **Table 26.1** includes the different types of pemphigus with the target antigens and autoantibodies responsible for each type.

Pemphigus Vulgaris

Pemphigus vulgaris is the most common and severe form of the disease representing 90 to 95% of all cases. In approximately 60 to 70% of the cases, the oral mucosa is the region of onset, but finally, almost all patients develop oral lesion. The lesions may remain in the oral mucosa for weeks, months, or even years before spreading to the skin or other mucosa, while many times the disease is confined in the oral cavity. Using clinical criteria pemphigus vulgaris is classified into three types: (1) the mucosal-dominant type, with mucosal lesions but minimal or no skin lesions, (2) the mucocutaneous type, with extensive skin lesions besides the mucosal involvement, and (3) cutaneous type, with only skin lesions that is rare (1–2%).

Clinically, oral mucosal lesions present as painful erosions. Intact bullae are rare, because they are fragile and break easily. These spread with time to ultimately occupy large areas, resulting in dysphagia and difficulty swallowing. A characteristic feature of the oral lesions is the presence of small linear discontinuities of the epithelium surrounding active erosions, resulting in epithelial disintegration. Any site of the mouth may be affected, but the soft palate, buccal mucosa, lower lip, tongue, gingiva, and floor of the mouth predominate (**Figs. 26.12–26.14**). Lesions can affect other mucosal surfaces such as the pharynx, larynx, esophagus, nose,

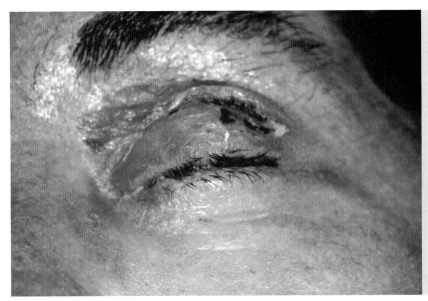

Fig. 26.11 Toxic epidermal necrolysis, severe lesions on the eye and the eyelids.

Table. 26.1 Clinical manifestations and target antigens in pemphigus

Pemphigus type	Skin	Oral	Other mucous membranes	Antigens	Autoantibodies
Pemphigus vulgaris					
• *Mucosal type*	Rare	100%	Frequently	Desmoglein 3	IgG
• *Mucocutaneous type*	100%	90%	Frequently	Desmoglein 1, 3	IgG
• *Cutaneous type*	100%	0	0	Desmoglein 1 mainly	IgG
Foliaceus	100%	Rarely	Very rarely	Desmoglein 1	IgG
Paraneoplastic	Frequently	100%	Frequently	Desmogleins 1, 3 Envoplakin Periplakin BP 180 Desmoplakins I, II α_2-microglobulin–like-1 protease inhibitor (A$_2$ML1)	IgG, IgA
Vegetans	Frequently	Up to 88%	Rarely	Desmogleins 1, 3	IgG
Drug-induced	Frequently	Frequently	Rarely	Desmogleins 3, 1	IgG
IgA-pemphigus	100%	Rarely	Rarely	Desmocollin 1	IgA

Abbreviation: Ig, immunoglobulin.

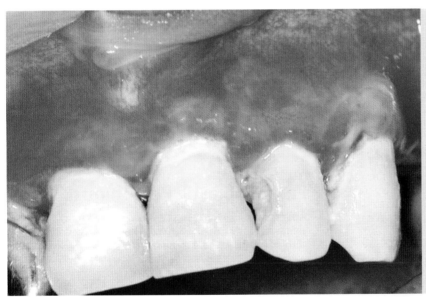

Fig. 26.12 Pemphigus vulgaris, erythema, and erosions on the gingiva in the form of desquamative gingivitis.

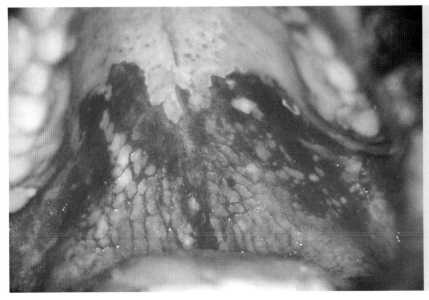

Fig. 26.13 Pemphigus vulgaris, extensive erosions on the palate.

conjunctivae, genitals, and anus (**Fig. 26.15**). On the skin, wrinkled thin-walled bullae are seen that rupture easily, leaving eroded areas, with a tendency to enlarge centrifugally as the epidermis strips off at the edges (**Fig. 26.16**). The erosions soon become partially covered with crusts, without tendency to heal. Eventually, after healing, pigmentation remains on the skin, but not scarring. The most commonly affected areas of the skin are the trunk, axillae, genital areas, umbilicus, scalp, periocular areas, and the ears.

A characteristic clinical sign of pemphigus is the Nikolsky's sign, where detachment of clinically healthy epidermis following slight pressure or rubbing may occur. This sign is due to the absence of cohesion of cells within the epidermis. The course of pemphigus vulgaris is chronic and the prognosis has improved greatly throughout the past three decades. Without appropriate treatment, pemphigus vulgaris can be fatal.

Pemphigus Vegetans

Pemphigus vegetans is a rare variant of pemphigus vulgaris.

Clinical features

The skin eruption consists of bullae and erosions identical to those of pemphigus vulgaris. Following that is the development of vegetating plaques, or papillomatous-like areas. The lesions most commonly occur on the crurogenital area, genitalia, axillae, face, and scalp (**Fig. 26.17**). Lesions are rare in the mouth and vegetating lesions may form at the commissures and the lower lip and rarely on the tongue and gingiva (**Fig. 26.18**). There are two subtypes of pemphigus vegetans: (1) pemphigus vegetans of *Hallopeau*, a milder form and (2) pemphigus vegetans of *Neumann*, a more severe form of the disease. The course and prognosis of pemphigus vegetans are similar to those of pemphigus vulgaris.

Pemphigus Foliaceus

Pemphigus foliaceus is a rare, benign form of pemphigus. It predominantly affects the skin while the oral and other mucosae are rarely involved. *Fogo selvage*, is an endemic variety in certain region of Brazil which has clinical, histologic, and immunologic features similar to pemphigus foliaceus. This form of pemphigus is caused by environmental factors.

Clinical features

The onset of the disease is usually mild with a few scattered lesions that are transient and are frequently resemble impetigo. Following this stage the skin lesions present as flaccid bullae that are fragile resulting to crusts and scales that resemble seborrheic dermatitis. The lesions usually develop on the scalp, face, and trunk (**Fig. 26.19**). The disease may be limited for months or even years or it may rapidly progress to generalized involvement resembling an exfoliative erythroderma. The Nikolsky's sign is positive. In contrast to pemphigus vulgaris the oral mucosa is rarely affected with limited superficial erosions that can cause a diagnostic problem (**Fig. 26.20**).

Pemphigus Erythematosus

Pemphigus erythematosus, also known as Senear-Usher syndrome, is a rare, localized variety of pemphigus foliaceus, with a mild course and usually a good prognosis. The disease may have clinical and immunologic features similar to lupus erythematosus, while rarely the two diseases coexist.

Clinical features

The disease affects the malar region of the face and other seborrheic areas, similar to systemic lupus erythematosus. Clinically, typical scaly and crusted lesions develop associated with superficial erosions, resembling seborrheic dermatitis (**Fig. 26.21**). The oral mucosa is rarely affected with mild superficial erosions (**Fig. 26.22**).

Paraneoplastic Pemphigus

Paraneoplastic pemphigus is a rare variant of pemphigus most commonly associated with non-Hodgkin's lymphoma and chronic lymphocytic leukemia in 80% of the cases and rarely with Castleman's disease, Waldenström's macroglobulinemia, sarcomas, and thymomas. In up to one-third of cases, the underlying malignancy has not been diagnosed at the time of diagnosis. It equally affects both sexes, with mean age of onset around 60 years. The paraneoplastic pemphigus has specific clinical, histopathologic, and immunologic characteristics that differ from those of pemphigus vulgaris.

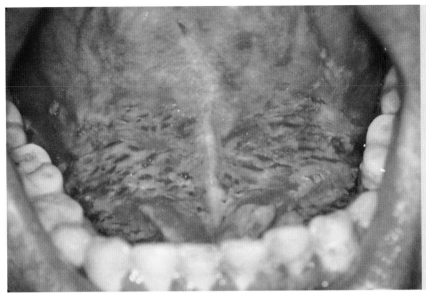

Fig. 26.14 Pemphigus vulgaris, erosions and disruption of the epithelium of the floor of the mouth.

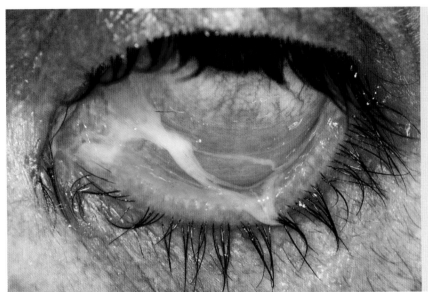

Fig. 26.15 Pemphigus vulgaris, erosions of the conjunctiva.

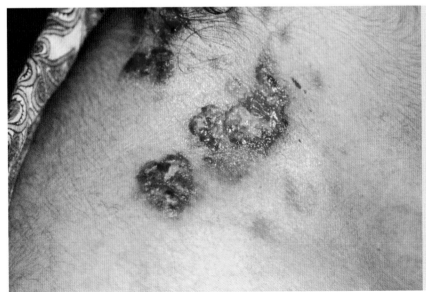

Fig. 26.16 Pemphigus vulgaris, multiple, crust-covered, erosions on the skin.

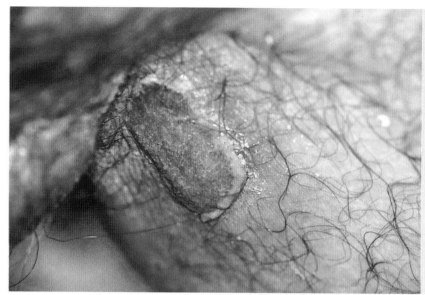

Fig. 26.17 Pemphigus vegetans, vegetating, erosive plaque on the crurogenital area.

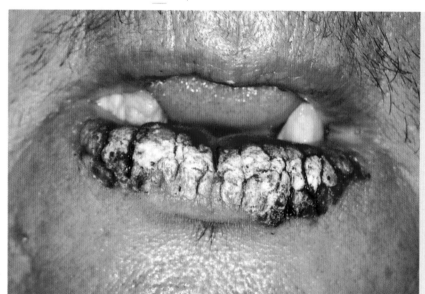

Fig. 26.18 Pemphigus vegetans, vegetating, papillomatous lesions on the lower lip.

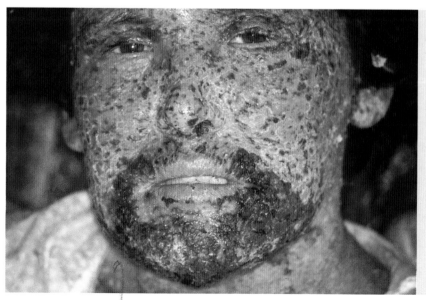

Fig. 26.19 Pemphigus foliaceus, generalized lesions on the face.

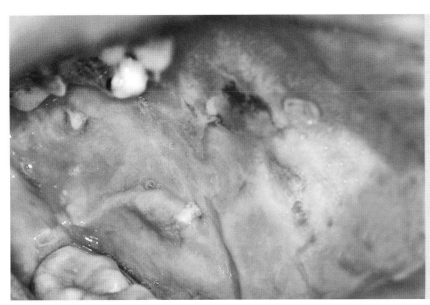

Fig. 26.20 Pemphigus foliaceus, erosion on buccal mucosa.

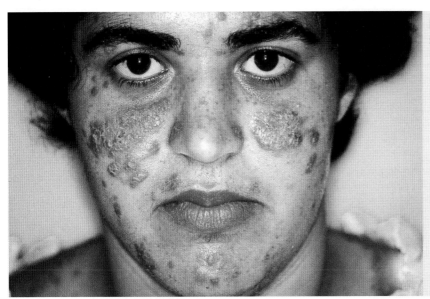

Fig. 26.21 Pemphigus erythematosus, characteristic lesions on the face like lupus erythematosus.

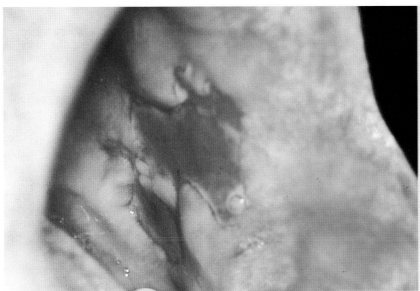

Fig. 26.22 Pemphigus erythematosus, erosions on buccal mucosa.

Clinical features

The clinical features of the disease are characterized by early, generalized, persistent, and severe erosions of the oral mucosa that often extend to the vermilion border of lips, pharynx, and the upper part of esophagus (**Fig. 26.23**). The severe oral lesions is usually the first presenting sign and after treatment, the one that persists as it is resistant to therapy. The mucosa of the genitals is also affected. Severe and persistent pseudomembranous conjunctivitis with erosions and edema which may progress to scarring and adhesions may occur (**Fig. 26.24**). Finally, polymorphous skin lesions with flaccid blisters and erosions, erythematous macules and plaques that mimic erythema multiforme, bullous pemphigoid, and lichenoid eruptions are observed. The clinical manifestations may precede the neoplasia or follow it.

Drug-Induced Pemphigus

This is a special form of pemphigus associated with the use of certain medication. The medication implicated is divided into two groups: *thiol* (such as penicillamine, captopril, and enalapril) and *nonthiol* (penicillins, cephalosporins). The thiol medication is predominantly associated with drug-induced pemphigus, contain sulfhydryl groups (-SH) that are speculated to interact with the sulfhydryl groups in desmogleins 1 and 3. This interaction modifies the antigenicity of desmoglein 1 or 3, which may lead to autoantibody production.

Clinical features

The clinical manifestations of drug-induced pemphigus are similar to those of pemphigus vulgaris, or pemphigus foliaceus. An eruption usually occurs within weeks from the beginning of treatment with the responsible medication. In the case of penicillamine, the onset of pemphigus can take up to 6 months after the beginning of treatment. Bullae and erosions appear that are clinically and histologically similar to pemphigus vulgaris or to pemphigus foliaceus (**Fig. 26.25**). The oral mucosa is frequently involved and sometimes can be the site of onset. Most patients with drug-induced pemphigus go into remission after the discontinuation of the responsible drug. However, in some cases it persists for a long time.

IgA Pemphigus

Immunoglobulin A (IgA) pemphigus is a recently recognized type of the disease, first described in 1982. It is characterized by vesiculopustular eruption, neutrophilic infiltration of the skin, and in vivo–bound and circulating IgA autoantibodies instead of IgG autoantibodies. Two types of IgA pemphigus exist: (1) the *subcorneal pustular dermatosis* type and (2) *intraepidermal neutrophilic* type.

Clinical features

IgA pemphigus mostly affects patients between 60 and 70 years of both sexes. Clinically, flaccid vesicles or pustules are observed, on an erythematous or normal base, that tend to coalesce. They subsequently rupture to leave erosions that are covered by crusts. They develop in a circinate or "*sunflower-like*" pattern and are accompanied by pruritus. The most common areas of involvement are the axilla and groin, following by trunk, extremities, and face (**Fig. 26.26**). The oral and other mucosa membranes are rarely involved. Intraorally, erosive areas that are limited and lack any special characteristics are seen. Clinically, the lesions resemble other forms of pemphigus (**Fig. 26.27**) and distinction and definite diagnosis is based on immunologic findings.

Differential diagnosis of all types

- Differentiation among the different types of pemphigus
- Bullous pemphigoid
- Mucous membrane pemphigoid
- Dermatitis herpetiformis
- Pemphigoid gestationis
- Erythema multiforme
- Stevens-Johnson syndrome
- Toxic epidermal necrolysis
- Drug-induced oral ulcerations
- Erosive lichen planus
- Recurrent aphthous ulceration
- Adamantiades-Behçet's disease
- Acute herpetic gingivostomatitis
- Sneddon-Wilkinson disease
- Hailey-Hailey disease
- Grover disease

Pathology

The definite diagnosis of pemphigus should be confirmed by histopathologic examination and direct and indirect immunofluorescence. As there are both immunologic and histologic differences between the different types of pemphigus, they will be discussed separately. A common histologic characteristic shared by all types is *acantholysis*.

Pemphigus vulgaris. Suprabasilar acantholysis is observed in the epithelium or the epidermis. However, intraepithelial separation may occasionally be higher in the stratum spinosum. The basal cells may maintain their attachment to the basal membrane via hemidesmosomes giving at the characteristic "*row of tombstones*" pattern. Frequently, the dermal papillae protrude into the blister cavity giving a "*villi-like*" appearance. The blister cavity may contain a few inflammatory cells. Cleftin and blister formation may also be seen. The hallmark of pemphigus is the finding of IgG autoantibodies against the cell surface of epithelial or epidermal cells. Direct immunofluorescence is positive (almost 100%) for IgG, IgA, and C3 in an intercellular, mesh-like pattern. Indirect immunofluorescence reveals circulating IgG autoantibodies directed against epithelial cell surfaces. Usually, the circulating autoantibody titer reflects the disease activity. However, in cases where only limited oral lesions are present indirect immunofluorescence may be negative. Detection of antidesmogleins 1 and 3 IgG autoantibodies by enzyme-linked immunosorbent assay (ELISA) is available. Immunoprecipitation and immunoblot may be used to demonstrate pemphigus

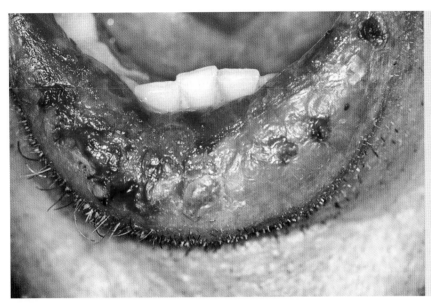

Fig. 26.23 Paraneoplastic pemphigus, severe erosions of the lower lip in a patient associated with chronic lymphocytic leukemia.

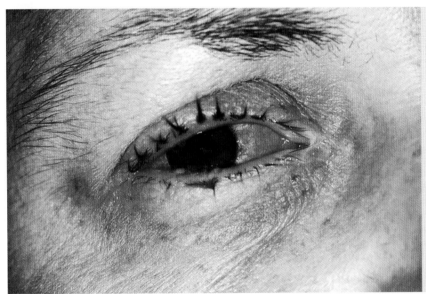

Fig. 26.24 Paraneoplastic pemphigus, conjunctival erosions, and edema of the eyelid in a patient with chronic lymphocytic leukemia.

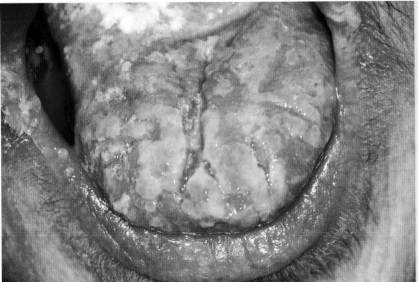

Fig. 26.25 Drug-induced pemphigus, erosions on the tongue.

autoantibodies against desmogleins 1 and 3, envoplakin, periplakin, and other pemphigus antigens.

Pemphigus vegetans. The histologic and immunologic findings are similar to those of pemphigus vulgaris. However, the suprabasal acantholysis may be masked by proliferation of the epithelium that may show pseudoepitheliomatous hyperplasia associated with papillomatosis. Additionally, there are intraepithelial microabscesses with numerous eosinophils and occasionally acantholytic keratinocytes.

Pemphigus foliaceus and erythematosus. The histologic findings of pemphigus foliaceus and pemphigus erythematosus are similar. Acantholysis in the upper epithelial, or epidermal layers, mainly of the granular cell layer is present. Occasionally, superficial blisters contain numerous neutrophils. Eosinophilic spongiosis can also occur in early lesions. Direct and indirect immunofluorescence findings are identical with those of pemphigus vulgaris. However, different antigenic targets are identified with specific techniques. ELISA testing for desmogleins 1 and 3 reveals desmoglein 1 in pemphigus foliaceus and desmoglein 3 in pemphigus vulgaris.

Paraneoplastic pemphigus. The histologic pattern of paraneoplastic pemphigus exhibits considerable variability. The findings show a combination of pemphigus vulgaris, erythema multiforme–like and lichen–like features. The direct and indirect immunofluorescent pattern of paraneoplastic pemphigus differ from the other types of pemphigus. Direct immunofluorescence exhibits deposition of IgG and C3 on epithelial cell surfaces and along the basement membrane region. Indirect immunofluorescence autoantibodies also react with simple or transitional epithelia. Characteristically, IgG autoantibodies react against multiple antigenic targets (desmoglein 1 and 3, desmoplakins I and II, envoplakin, periplakin, plectin, BPAG1).

Drug-induced pemphigus. The histologic findings that resemble pemphigus foliaceus show superficial acantholysis, while lesions that resemble pemphigus vulgaris reveal suprabasal acantholysis. Eosinophilic spongiosis may be observed. The findings of direct immunofluorescence are the same as in pemphigus vulgaris.

IgA pemphigus. The classic histologic pattern in IgA pemphigus is the intraepidermal blister or pustule formation with the characteristic neutrophil infiltration that tends to form neutrophilic microabscesses. IgA deposition is detected on keratinocyte cell surfaces. In conclusion, histology and direct immunofluorescence are the most reliable and sensitive diagnostic tests for all types of pemphigus.

Treatment

Systemic corticosteroids (prednisone or prednisolone) are the drugs of choice in patients with pemphigus. There are several strategies regarding the initial dose of treatment which may range between 0.5 and 3 mg/kg/d. In our experience, the initial dose of prednisone or prednisolone should be flexible and should be customized to the individual needs of each patient depending on the severity of the disease. For example, patients with mild lesions may be treated initially with 50 mg/d for 2 to 3 weeks. Patients who do not respond to this treatment regimen or those who present initially with severe or rapidly progressive lesions should be treated with 80 to 120 mg/d or more until disease activity is controlled. The disease is thought to be clinically controlled when old lesions have healed and new lesions are absent. The dose that achieves clinical control of the disease is maintained for 2 to 3 weeks and then gradually tapered by 30% every 2 weeks until the dose of 20 mg/d is reached while maintaining clinical disease control. The dosage may subsequently be continued alternate days and lowered by 5 mg every month until the dose of 5 to 10 mg every other day is achieved over a long period of time (1–3 years). Cessation of all treatment remains a judgment call for every physician.

Adjuvant Therapies

As a rule, adjuvant therapies should be used almost exclusively in combination with corticosteroids and rarely, if ever, as monotherapy for controlled cases of pemphigus. The reasons for using adjuvant therapies in pemphigus are (1) to reduce the need for corticosteroids and hence their side effects, and (2) to achieve better control of the disease. Depending on the mechanism of action, adjuvant therapies of pemphigus can be classified into the following three categories:

- Immunosuppressive drugs (azathioprine, mycophenolate mofetil or acid, cyclophosphamide, cyclosporine, and methotrexate)
- Immunomodulatory procedures (plasmapheresis, extracorporeal photochemotherapy)
- Azathioprine in a dose of 100 to 200 mg/d and mycophenolate mofetil in a dose of 2 to 3 g/d are the major immunosuppressive agents currently used more frequently. Plasmapheresis is indicated in very severe cases or cases resistant to corticosteroids.

Recently, rituximab, a potent B-cell–depleting chimeric anti-CD20 monoclonal antibody is used to treat pemphigus. When rituximab is used as adjuvant therapy in severe resistant cases, it led to a full remission of the disease. The suggested dose is 375 mg/m² once weekly for 4 weeks. The most common side effects of the drug is infections and leukoencephalopathy. High-dose of IVIg (400 mg/kg/d for 5 days) is an additional option for steroid-resistant pemphigus.

Pulse Therapy

Pulse therapy refers to the intermittent IV infusion of very high doses (megadoses) of corticosteroids (dexamethasone or methylprednisolone) and cyclophosphamide over a short period. This regimen must be used only in very severe cases and only in a hospital setting because it is associated with high morbidity and mortality.

Topical Treatment

Painful, resistant, localized oral lesions may require the use of topical corticosteroids either in the form of a paste (0.1% triamcinolone acetonide in Orabase or 0.05% clobetasol propionate gel) or in the form of intralesional injection every 2 weeks until the lesions heal. Topical corticosteroids alone is insufficient for sustained control of the disease, as pemphigus is a systemic autoimmune disease and lesions will develop as long as there are adequate amounts of circulating pemphigus antibodies. Topical cyclosporine has also been used for oral lesions of pemphigus with partial success.

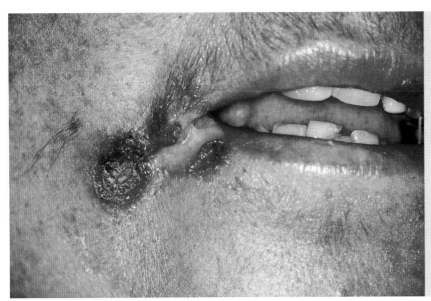

Fig. 26.26 IgA pemphigus, crust-covered erosions on commissure and the skin.

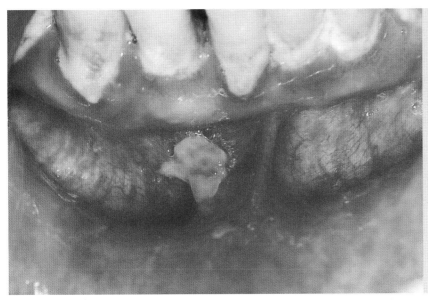

Fig. 26.27 IgA pemphigus, small erosion on the lower vestibule.

Mucous Membrane Pemphigoid

Key points

- A chronic, autoimmune, blistering disorder that primarily affects the mucous membranes and rarely the skin.
- The disorder should not be regarded as a single clinical entity, but rather a "disease phenotype" with clinical and antigenic heterogeneity.
- Based on the clinical type and the antigenic target, four variants are recognized.
- The oral mucosa is involved in over 95% of the cases and is usually the first manifestation of the disease.
- A common oral sign is desquamative gingivitis.

Introduction

Mucous membrane pemphigoid, or cicatricial pemphigoid, is a chronic bullous disease of autoimmune origin. The disorder represents a heterogeneous group of diseases (disease phenotype) with respect to disease severity, clinical site of involvement, and the isotype of the associated autoantibodies. It primarily affects the mucous membranes and rarely the skin with the tendency for scarring. It is histologically characterized by the development of subepithelial blistering and autoantibodies fixation to the basement membrane zone. The variants of the disease differ in the hemidesmosomal structural components or components of the epithelial basement membrane that are targeted (e.g., laminin 5, laminin 6, type XVII collagen, bullous pemphigoid antigen 180, b4 integrin subunit, and antigens with unknown identities: a 45-kd protein, uncein, a 168-kd epithelial protein, and a 120-kd epithelial protein). Four variants are currently recognized based on the clinical expression of the disease and the antigenic target (**Table 26.2**).

Clinical features

Mucous membrane pemphigoid predominantly affects females with a ratio of 1.5 to 2:1. The mean age of onset is around 66 years (~10 years later than pemphigus). It very rarely affects children and is then confined to the mouth. The oral mucosa is approximately affected in 90 to 95% of the cases and may be the only site of disease activity.

The oral mucosal lesions are recurrent vesicles or small bullae that quickly rupture leaving painful, erosions with smooth surface and irregular shape (**Figs. 26.28, 26.29**). These lesions recur for a long time and finally heal with scarring. They are usually localized, but widespread involvement may be seen. The most commonly affected sites are the gingiva, buccal mucosa, palate, alveolar mucosa, tongue, and more rarely lower lip. The gingiva is involved in more than 60% of the cases in the form of *desquamative gingivitis* (**Fig. 26.30**). Occasionally, the gingival involvement is the only clinical manifestation of the disease. The ocular lesions are second in frequency (30–45%) and consist of conjunctivitis, symblepharon, fibrotic sequels, trichiasis, entropion, dryness, and corneal perforation that may result in blindness (**Fig. 26.31**). Less commonly, other mucosae (genitals, anus, nose, pharynx, esophagus, larynx) are involved (**Fig. 26.32**). Skin lesions occur in approximately 5 to 10% of all cases and consist of bullae, which usually appear on the scalp and neck and may heal with scarring (**Fig. 26.33**).

Differential diagnosis

- Linear IgA disease
- Bullous pemphigoid
- Pemphigus
- Pemphigoid gestationis
- Epidermolysis bullosa acquisita
- Dermatitis herpetiformis
- Angina bullosa hemorrhagica
- Chronic ulcerative stomatitis
- Bullous and erosive lichen planus
- Erythema multiforme
- Systemic lupus erythematosus

Pathology

Histologically, there is detachment of the whole epithelium at the basement membrane zone and development of subepithelial blistering, similar to that of bullous pemphigoid. Electron microscopy shows dermal–epidermal cleavage develops within the lamina lucida. Direct immunofluorescence reveals linear autoantibody fixation (mainly IgG and C3) at the basement membrane zone of mucosa and skin in 80 to 95% of the cases, also similar to that of bullous pemphigoid. Indirect immunofluorescence reveals mainly IgG

Table 26.2 Mucous membrane pemphigoid

Phenotype	Clinical expression	Main antigens	IgG, C3 antibodies	
			Perilesional	Circulating
Oral pemphigoid	Oral mucosa only	C-terminal of BPAG-2, integrin β_4 subunit, integrin α_6 subunit	Positive 60–95%	Positive in 30–40%
Ocular pemphigoid	Always ocular lesions with or without oral lesions	Integrin β_4 subunit	Yes	Rare
Antilaminin pemphigoid	Mucosae and rarely skin	Laminin 5	Yes	Yes
Mucous membrane pemphigoid with BP antigen	Oral mucosa and skin with or without other mucosae	BP2, Laminin 5 (332), integrin $\alpha_6\beta_4$	Yes	Yes

Abbreviations: IgG, immunoglobulin G; BP, bullous pemphigoid.

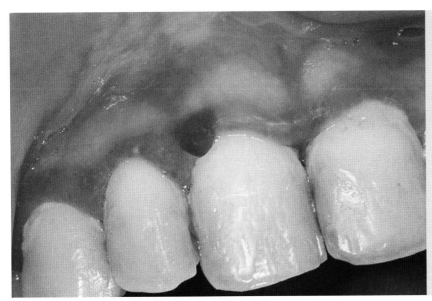

Fig. 26.28 Mucous membrane pemphigoid, hemorrhagic bulla on the gingiva, and desquamative gingivitis.

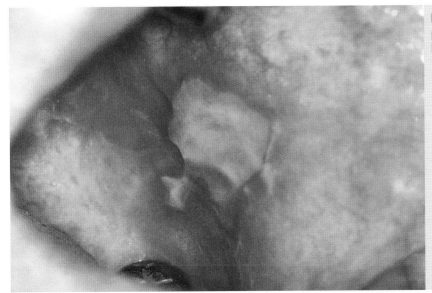

Fig. 26.29 Mucous membrane pemphigoid, superficial ulceration on the buccal mucosa.

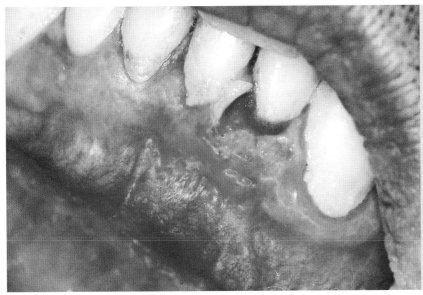

Fig. 26.30 Mucous membrane pemphigoid, epithelial detachment on desquamative gingivitis, following friction.

and more rarely IgA and IgM serum autoantibodies against the basement membrane in approximately 20 to 30% of the cases. Antibody titers are usually low (1:10, 1:20, 1:40). The sensitivity of indirect immunofluorescence can be increased by the use of normal oral mucosa as substrate. Other tests include immunoblotting (Western blot), immunoprecipitation, and immunoelectron microscopy, which can define the target antigens.

Treatment

Oral corticosteroids (prednisone or prednisolone) are the cornerstone of therapy for cicatricial pemphigoid. The initial dose varies from 30 mg/d to 60 mg/d depending on the severity of the disease. It usually takes 2 to 3 weeks to stop new bullae formation and for old ones to heal. The dose is subsequently tapered by 20% every 2 to 3 weeks until the dose of 10 mg/d is reached. This dose is subsequently maintained on alternate days and reduced by 5 mg every 2 weeks until cessation. Recurrence of oral lesions is not uncommon and may be treated with local corticosteroids or low doses of systemic corticosteroids. Corticosteroid-sparing immunosuppressants are usually required only in severe cases that present with ocular, laryngeal, or esophageal involvement. Azathioprine 100 mg/d and cyclophosphamide 100 to 200 mg/d are most frequently used. Mycophenolate mofetil 2 g/d may also be used in some cases.

Dapsone: 50 to 100 mg/d is beneficial in mild-to-moderate diseases, particularly for patients with oral lesions alone. Localized, mild, oral lesions or recurrences may be treated with topical corticosteroids alone; 0.1% triamcinolone acetonide in an oral adhesive base (Orabase) or 0.5% fluocinonide gel, or 0.05% clobetasol propionate gel applied to the lesions 2 to 3 times a day for 2 to 6 months or more is particularly effective for gingival lesions. Recently, 0.05% clobetasol mouthwash in aqueous solution has been shown to be effective for localized oral lesions. Intralesional injection of triamcinolone acetonide retard or betamethasone dipropionate and sodium phosphate retard may be beneficial for localized resistant oral lesions. New immunomodulators for topical use, with anti-inflammatory action, such as tacrolimus and 0.1% pimecrolimus ointment, have been used with promising results in the treatment of oral lesions of autoimmune disease. Combination therapy with tetracyclines (minocycline or doxycycline) 1 to 2 g/d and nicotinamide 1 to 2 g/d may be effective.

Bullous Pemphigoid

Key points

- It is the most common chronic autoimmune skin bullous disease that predominantly affects the elderly.
- It is characterized by tissue-bound and circulating autoantibodies directed against bullous pemphigoid antigens (BP 180, BP 230).
- The oral mucosa is affected in 30 to 40% of the cases.
- Clinical diagnosis should be confirmed by histopathologic examination and direct and indirect immunofluorescence.

Introduction

Bullous pemphigoid is the most common chronic autoimmune bullous disease, mainly affecting the skin, and, less often, the mucous membranes. It is characterized by tissue-bound and circulating autoantibodies directed against bullous pemphigoid antigens (BP 180, BP 230), components of hemidesmosomes of the epidermal and/or epithelial basal cells that promote dermoepidermal cohesion. Bullous pemphigoid is a disease of the elderly with a mean onset at approximately 65 years. Men are more commonly affected than women (ratio 1.7:1). The disease may rarely occur in children. Occasionally, it is drug-induced, with diuretics, analgesics, D-penicillamine, antibiotics, and captopril being most often incriminated.

Clinical features

The cutaneous lesions are multiform. During the nonbullous stage, they appear as intensely pruritic, erythematous, urticarial-like plaques. Later, tense bullae develop (bullous stage) on normal or erythematous base, 0.5 to 4 cm in diameter, usually containing clear or serosanguineous fluid. The bullae rupture leaving superficial ulcerations covered by hemorrhagic crusts. The eruption is most commonly located on the extremities and the trunk in a symmetrical

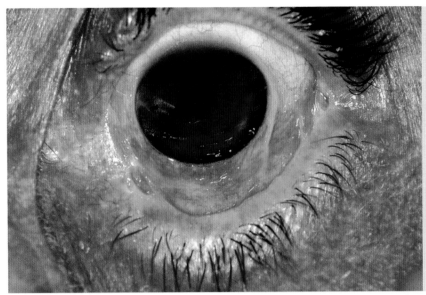

Fig. 26.31 Mucous membrane pemphigoid, symblepharon, fibrotic sequels, and the beginning of corneal opacity.

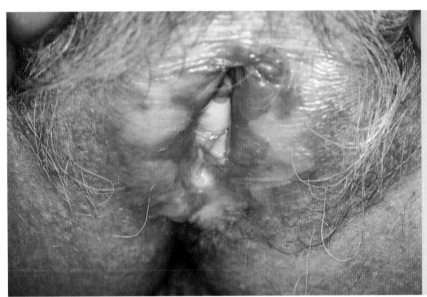

Fig. 26.32 Mucous membrane pemphigoid, scarring atrophy of the vulva and labia majora.

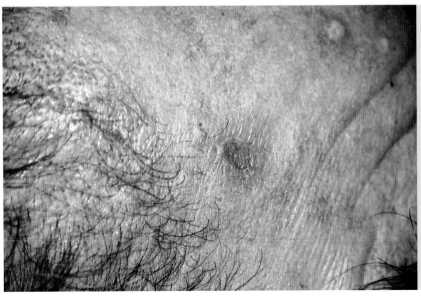

Fig. 26.33 Mucous membrane pemphigoid, localized scarring atrophy on the forehead.

distribution. It may be localized or generalized (**Fig. 26.34**). The oral mucosa is affected in 30 to 40% of the cases. In 6% of the cases, oral mucosa is the first site of involvement. Clinically, oral lesions are bullae that rupture in 2 to 4 days leaving painful superficial erosions (**Figs. 26.35, 26.36**). The buccal mucosa, palate, tongue, and lower lip are more frequently affected. Gingival involvement is seen in 16% of the cases, most often appearing as desquamative gingivitis. Less frequently, conjunctivae, esophagus, vagina, and anus may also be affected. The course is chronic with exacerbations and remissions. The prognosis is usually good. Most of the patients get full clinical remission after treatment. Rarely, bullous pemphigoid may be associated with internal malignancies (paraneoplastic manifestations), inflammatory bowel disease, or other autoimmune disorders. The clinical diagnosis should be confirmed by histopathologic examination and direct and indirect immunofluorescence.

Differential diagnosis

- Pemphigus
- Mucous membrane pemphigoid
- Dermatitis herpetiformis
- Linear IgA disease
- Pemphigoid gestationis
- Epidermolysis bullosa acquisita
- Lichen planus, erosive type
- Lupus erythematosus
- Bullous drug eruptions

Pathology

On histologic examination, a subepithelial bulla is observed, accompanied by a dermal inflammatory infiltrate of eosinophils and neutrophils. Direct immunofluorescence shows linear deposition in the form of a continuous fine line of immunoreactants, mostly IgG and C3, along the basal membrane. Salt-split-skin method reveals that the deposition of autoantibodies is on the epidermal side (roof) and/or the dermal side (base) of the blister. Circulating autoantibodies directed against basal membrane are detected by indirect immunofluorescence in 60 to 80% of the cases in high titers. Immunohistochemistry and ELISA method detect the antigenic target (BP 180, BP 230).

Treatment

Patients with mild localized lesions should be treated with topical ointment and/or intralesional corticosteroids. Those with severe generalized lesions must be treated with systemic prednisolone, 0.5 to 1 mg/kg/d and usually controls the disease within 2 to 3 weeks. Second-line therapy includes azathioprine, cyclophosphamide, mycophenolate acid (Myfortic 360 mg four times a day), and cyclosporine. They can be usually used in combination with systemic corticosteroids. In addition, tetracycline in combination with nicotinamide and dapsone, are another alternative second-line therapeutic regimen. In cases of recalcitrant to treatment, plasmapheresis, high-dose IVIg, and, most recently, monoclonal antibody to CD20 (rituximab) have been tried.

Linear IgA Disease

Key points

- An autoimmune subepidermal–subepithelial disease.
- It is characterized by linear IgA deposits along the basement membrane zone of the epidermis/epithelium.
- Depending on the age group, two types are recognized: *adult linear IgA disease* (usually in the age group of > 60) and *childhood linear IgA disease* (usually in the age group of < 6 years).
- The disease predominantly affects the skin, while the oral mucosa is involved in approximately 25 to 30% of the cases.

Introduction

Linear IgA disease or linear IgA bullous dermatosis is a rare, chronic, autoimmune subepithelial blistering disease. It is mostly idiopathic, but can also be triggered by medication, with vancomycin, being one of the more common inducers. In addition, other agents have also been reported (phenytoin, amiodarone, captopril, and NSAIDs). Association of linear IgA disease with inflammatory gastrointestinal diseases, infections, malignancies, and autoimmune diseases have been reported. The disease is classified into two groups, based on the age of onset: *adult linear IgA disease* (usually at ages > 60) and *childhood linear IgA disease* (usually age < 6). The adult form of the disease affects almost equally to both sexes. The average age of onset is after 60, while in childhood occurs around 4 to 5 years. The disease has many clinical and laboratory similarities to other bullous conditions such as dermatitis herpetiformis and bullous pemphigoid. Several different antigens have been identified at the basement membrane of epidermis in patients with linear IgA disease. Immunologically, disease is characterized by the linear deposition of IgA along the basement membrane of the epithelium as well as circulating antibodies against the basement membrane zone antigens. Based on the region of IgA deposition, the disease is classified into two types: (1) a *lamina lucida type* and (2) a *sublamina densa type*. In the lamina lucida type the IgA antibody reacts against a 97-kDa antigen, while in the sublamina densa type IgA binds VII collagen in anchoring fibrils.

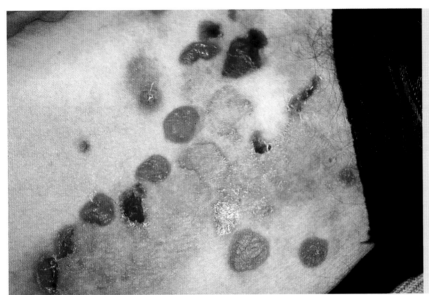

Fig. 26.34 Bullous pemphigoid, skin blisters of different stage of evolution.

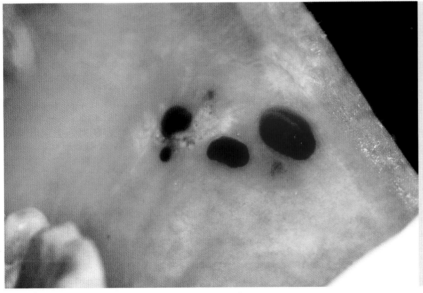

Fig. 26.35 Bullous pemphigoid, hemorrhagic blisters on the buccal mucosa.

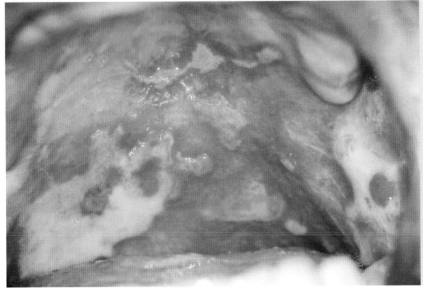

Fig. 26.36 Bullous pemphigoid, extensive erosions on the soft palate.

Clinical features

Clinically, linear IgA disease is characterized by a sudden onset of vesicles and bullae, which affect, in a symmetrical pattern, the face, trunk, and extremities. They tend to have a herpetiform or annular pattern and a normal, or erythematous base (**Fig. 26.37**). The bullae rupture leaving superficial ulcerations that usually heal without scarring. The oral mucosa is involved in approximately 25 to 30% of the cases with vesicles that rapidly evolve into painful superficial ulceration without any special characteristics (**Fig. 26.38**). More rarely, the gingiva, the conjunctival, nasal, pharyngeal, and esophageal mucosae may be affected (**Fig. 26.39**). The clinical features of the disease have many similarities with bullous pemphigoid, mucous membrane pemphigoid, and dermatitis herpetiformis. The diagnosis is therefore mainly based on the histologic and immunologic findings.

Differential diagnosis

- Dermatitis herpetiformis
- Bullous pemphigoid
- Mucous membrane pemphigoid
- Epidermolysis bullosa acquisita
- Erythema multiforme
- Stevens-Johnson syndrome

Pathology

Histopathologic examination, direct and indirect immunofluorescence are essential for the diagnosis. Histologically, in fully developed lesions there is subepithelial blistering accompanied by very prominent neutrophilic infiltrate along the basement membrane zone. Some eosinophils may also be observed. Neutrophilic microabscesses can be seen in the dermal papillae. There are a lot of histologic similarities with dermatitis herpetiformis. Linear fixation of IgA antibodies along the basement membrane zone is revealed with direct immunofluorescence. Circulating antibasement membrane zone autoantibodies are detected through indirect immunofluorescence in up to 50% of the cases.

Treatment

The treatment of choice is dapsone100 to 200 mg/d for adults and 1 to 2 mg/kg/d for children. Occasionally, it may be necessary to add prednisolone 40 to 60 mg/d for better results.

Other alternative treatments include sulfapyridine and antibiotics (e.g., tetracycline, erythromycin). Mycophenolate mofetil, azathioprine, methotrexate, cyclophosphamide, rituximab, IVIgs, colchicine, and thalidomide may be used as second-line treatment in patients who do not respond to a combination of dapsone and prednisolone.

Pemphigoid Gestationis

Key points

- A rare, autoimmune bullous dermatosis of pregnancy.
- It occurs usually during the last trimester of pregnancy, or shortly after.
- Clinically, it is characterized by a pruritic vesiculobullous eruption.
- The oral mucosa is rarely involved with bullae and erosion.
- Linear C3 deposition along the basement membrane zone of the epidermis by direct immunofluorescence.

Introduction

Pemphigoid gestationis, formerly known as herpes gestationis, is a rare, distinctive, self-limited autoimmune bullous dermatosis that usually appears during the second or third trimester of pregnancy, as well as in the immediate postpartum period, and usually resolves within 3 to 4 months after delivery. The incidence has been estimated at approximately 1:1,700 to 1:50,000 pregnancies, to connect with the prevalence of HLA-DR3 and -DR4 in different populations.

In pemphigoid gestationis the circulating antibodies trigger an immune response when they bind to the basement membrane. These antibodies target usually two hemidesmosomal proteins, BPAG2 and collagen XVII and less frequently BP230. That leads to the formation of subepidermal blistering. It is believed that cross-reactivity between placental tissue and skin plays a role in the pathogenesis.

Clinical features

Clinically, the cutaneous manifestations present as intensely pruritic, urticarial plaques with an abrupt onset that then evolve into vesicles and small tense bullae that coalesce to occupy extensive areas on the trunk, abdomen, axillae,

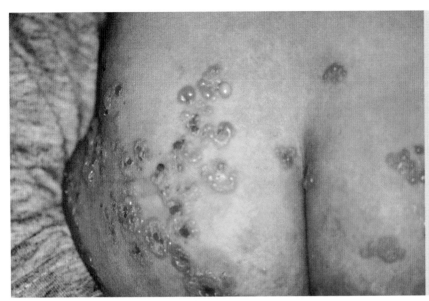

Fig. 26.37 Linear IgA disease, small bullae in an herpetiform pattern on the buttock area.

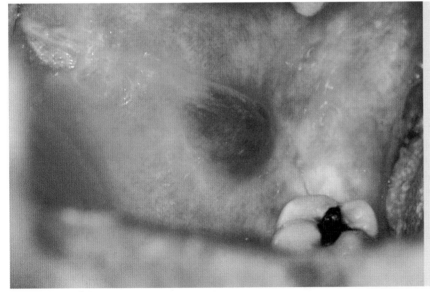

Fig. 26.38 Linear IgA disease, hemorrhagic bulla on the buccal mucosa.

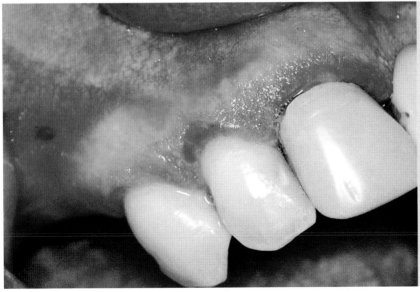

Fig. 26.39 Linear IgA disease, mild desquamative gingivitis, and erosion of the gingiva.

extremities, and face (**Figs. 26.40, 26.41**). Rapid progression to a generalized pemphigoid-like eruption usually occurs. The lesions may involve the entire body. The oral mucosa is rarely involved with hemorrhagic bullae that rupture leaving superficial, painful ulceration (**Fig. 26.42**). The most commonly affected sites are the buccal mucosa, palate, tongue, and gingiva. The oral lesions follow the cutaneous manifestations and quickly respond to treatment. The clinical manifestations and progress of the disease presents in a wide spectrum. Most disease activity spontaneously remits during weeks or months following delivery. Fewer than 10% of newborns present with mild, self-limiting disease due to passive transfer of maternal antibodies and the disease severity.

The clinical diagnosis should be confirmed by the histologic and immunologic findings.

Differential diagnosis

- Bullous pemphigoid
- Linear IgA disease
- Mucous membrane pemphigoid
- Dermatitis herpetiformis
- Pemphigus
- Drug eruptions
- Allergic contact dermatitis

Pathology

Histopathologic examination reveals subepithelial bulla and a nonspecific mixed cellular infiltrate with a variable number of eosinophils. Direct immunofluorescence of perilesional skin and oral mucosa frequently demonstrates C3 with or without IgG, in a linear band along the basement membrane zone. Indirect immunofluorescence reveals circulating IgG antibodies against the basement membrane zone. Immunoblotting and ELISA testing can detect autoantibodies to BP 180 antigen. Additionally, ELISA can be useful for monitoring autoantibody levels in serum.

Treatment

Systemic corticosteroids are the cornerstone of therapy. Depending on the gravity of the disease, 0.5 mg/kg/d of prednisolone can be administered initially. The dose is tapered as soon as blister formation is suppressed. As adjuvant therapies azathioprine, dapsone, methotrexate, IVIg, cyclosporine, pyridoxine, and others have been used.

Dermatitis Herpetiformis

Key points

- A chronic, autoimmune vesiculopapular dermatosis.
- It is a cutaneous manifestation of celiac disease and is associated with gluten sensitivity in almost all cases.
- Histologically, it is characterized by papillary neutrophilic microabscesses.
- The disease is a genetic disorder associated with the HLA-DQ2 genotype in which IgA antiendomysial antibodies are directed against epidermal transglutaminase.
- The oral mucosa can be involved in approximately 5 to 10% of the cases.

Introduction

Dermatitis herpetiformis, or Duhring's disease is a chronic autoimmune dermatosis associated with a gluten-sensitive enteropathy. Patients with gluten-sensitive enteropathy develop dermatitis herpetiformis in approximately 15 to 25% of the cases. However, even if patients with dermatitis herpetiformis are asymptomatic, in more than 90% of the cases there is gluten-sensitive enteropathy upon endoscopic examination. Additionally, both dermatitis herpetiformis and celiac disease demonstrate increased expression of HLA-A1, HLA-B8, HLA-DR3, and strongly HLA-DQ2 genotypes. That implies an underlying genetic predisposition for gluten sensitivity. The former together with a diet high in gluten leads to IgA antibody formation against intestinal gluten-tissue transglutaminase. These also cross-react with the highly homologous epidermal transglutaminase. The deposition of IgA and epidermal transglutaminase complexes in the dermal papillae is the cause of dermatitis herpetiformis.

Clinical features

The disease occurs at any age, but is more common between ages 15 and 50, and males are more frequently affected than females with a ratio of 1.5 to 2:1.

The prevalence is reported to be 10 to 11.2 cases per 100,000 of general population. Clinically, the dermatitis herpetiformis is characterized initially by very pruritic, erythematous papules or plaques, and vesicles that coalesce in a herpetiform pattern. They symmetrically affect the extensor surfaces of the skin: the elbows, knees, scapular region,

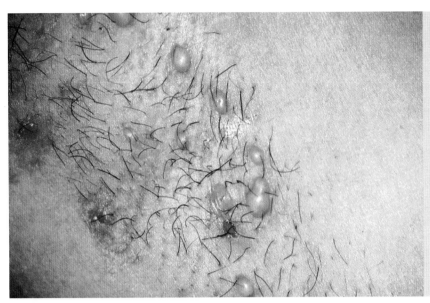

Fig. 26.40 Pemphigoid gestationis, coalescent vesicles on the axilla.

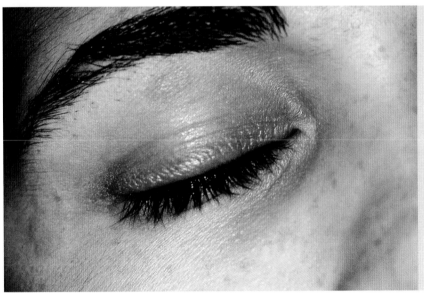

Fig. 26.41 Pemphigoid gestationis, edema of the eyelid.

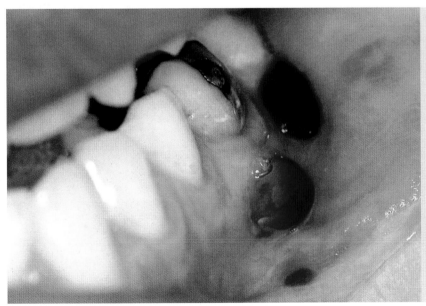

Fig. 26.42 Pemphigoid gestationis, hemorrhagic bullae on the alveolar mucosa.

glutes, neck, trunk, and scalp (**Fig. 26.43**). Following that crust-covered superficial ulceration occur. The oral mucosa is affected in 5 to 10% of cases. Oral lesions follow the skin eruption and very rarely precede skin involvement. Clinically, erythema, maculopapular lesions, and vesicles are observed in a centrifugal or hemicircular pattern (**Fig. 26.44**). The vesicles rupture leaving superficial painful erosions resembling small aphthous ulcers. The most frequently affected sites are the palate, tongue, and buccal mucosa and more rarely the gingiva, lips, and tonsils.

The disease runs a very prolonged course with remissions and exacerbations. Dermatitis herpetiformis may be associated with Hashimoto's thyroiditis, insulin-dependent diabetes mellitus, and rarely with other autoimmune diseases and T-cell lymphoma.

The clinical diagnosis needs to be confirmed histologically and immunologically.

Differential diagnosis

- Linear IgA disease
- Bullous pemphigoid
- Mucous membrane pemphigoid
- Systemic lupus erythematosus
- Erythema multiforme
- Aphthous ulcers
- Primary herpetic gingivostomatitis

Pathology

Histopathologically, dermatitis herpetiformis is characterized by papillary neutrophilic microabscesses and subepithelial vesicle formation associated with prominent perivascular, lymphocytic infiltrates. When an intact vesicle is biopsied, a subepidermal/subepithelial blister containing predominantly neutrophils are seen. Direct immunofluorescence reveals granular IgA deposits in the dermal papillae of perilesional skin. IgA antiendomysial antibodies and antibodies–epidermal transglutaminase complexes can also be found in the serum and are specific for dermatitis herpetiformis and celiac disease.

Treatment

Long-term adherence to a gluten-free diet is recommended. Dapsone is the first-line treatment with initial dose of 25 to 50 mg in adults and 0.5 mg/kg in children daily. Follow-up of the patients receiving dapsone is crucial due to the side effects. Nevertheless, the drug is usually well tolerated. Sulfapyridine 500 to 1,000 mg three times a day is a second-line choice.

Epidermolysis Bullosa Acquisita

Key points

- A rare chronic, autoimmune, subepidermal blistering disease.
- The responsible antigen is type VII collagen, the major component of anchoring fibrils of the dermal–epidermal junction.
- Mild friction can be responsible for the development of lesions.
- It mainly affects the skin and less commonly mucosae.
- The oral mucosa is involved in approximately 30 to 50% of the cases.

Introduction

Epidermolysis bullosa acquisita is a rare, noninherited, chronic, autoimmune blistering disease. Immunologically, it is characterized by autoantibodies, mostly IgG, against the noncollagenous domain of type VII collagen. The latter is the major component of anchoring fibrils that connect the basement membrane to the dermal structures. Patients may present either with a mechanobullous lesion mimicking dystrophic epidermolysis bullosa or with clinical features indistinguishable to those found in mucous membrane pemphigoid or bullous pemphigoid. The disease may occur at any age in both sexes.

Clinical features

Clinically, the disease is characterized by the formation of tense, recurrent bullae, mainly on the skin areas that can be the subject of friction, such as the knees, elbows, joints, dorsal aspect of the hands, feet, toes, and scalp. The bullae then rupture to leave ulceration that heal with scarring (**Fig. 26.45**). Other common findings include atrophic areas, milia hyper- or hypopigmentation, and dystrophic nails (**Fig. 26.46**). The clinical features may mimic a bullous pemphigoid-like or mucous membrane pemphigoid. The oral mucosa is involved in approximately 30 to 50% of the cases. Clinically, a few hemorrhagic bullae may appear, usually following mild trauma (**Fig. 26.47**). These rupture, leaving ulcers that may heal with scarring. The oral lesions are limited and mainly affect the buccal mucosa, palate, tongue, and gingiva. Other mucosae may be involved, including the larynx, esophagus, and conjunctiva which may lead to laryngeal stenosis, dysphagia, and blindness. The age of onset is usually after 20. The diagnosis is based on the history and clinical features, but mostly on the immunologic findings.

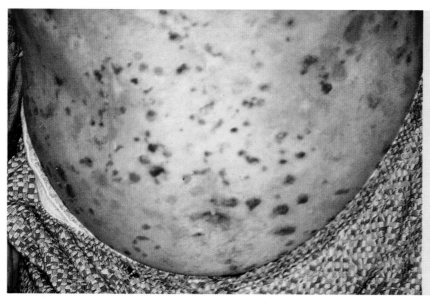

Fig. 26.43 Dermatitis herpetiformis, multiple vesicles, and crusting on the trunk.

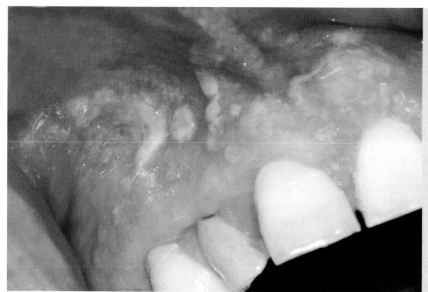

Fig. 26.44 Dermatitis herpetiformis, vesicles in a hemicircular pattern on the alveolar mucosa.

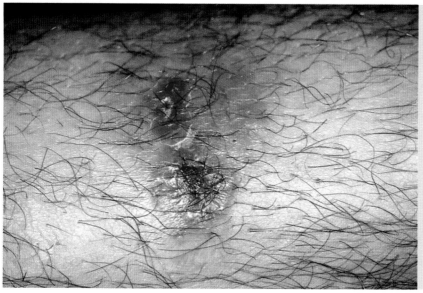

Fig. 26.45 Epidermolysis bullosa acquisita, erythema, and scarring on the skin.

Differential diagnosis

- Inherited dystrophic epidermolysis bullosa
- Bullous pemphigoid
- Mucous membrane pemphigoid
- Porphyria cutanea tarda
- Linear IgA disease
- Pemphigus
- Systemic lupus erythematosus
- Angina bullosa hemorrhagica

Pathology

Histopathologic examination reveals the presence of sub-epithelial bulla without acantholysis, accompanied by mild, mixed, inflammatory infiltrate in the lamina propria. It is not a pathognomonic picture, as it is shared by other subepithelial blistering diseases. Direct immunofluorescence reveals IgG deposits and more rarely IgA, IgM, and C3, along the basement membrane zone of the epithelium or/and epidermis, appearing as a continuous broad linear pattern.

In indirect immunofluorescence, circulating antibasement membrane autoantibodies usually of the IgG, IgA, and collagen VII type can be detected. On salt-split-skin circulating antibodies bind to the dermal side of the bulla.

Immunoelectron microscopy reveals autoantibodies specifically bind to the anchoring fibrils and the lamina densa.

Treatment

Systemic corticosteroid is the first line of treatment, i.e., 30 to 50 mg of prednisolone, depending on the disease activity. Immunosuppressive agents can also be used either alone or together with steroid treatment such as azathioprine, methotrexate, mycophenolate mofetil, and cyclophosphamide. Colchicine and dapsone have also be used. Newer treatments include IVIgs and intravenous infusion of anti-CD20 antibodies (rituximab).

It is important that the patient should avoid trauma and other friction on the skin and in the mouth.

Lichen Planus

Key points

- A relatively common, chronic, inflammatory disease.
- It is characterized by T-cell–mediated immune reaction damage to basal epithelial cells that express altered self-antigens on their surface.
- It affects the oral and genital mucosae, skin, nails. and hair.
- The oral mucosa is commonly involved.
- Six clinical oral variants are recognized: *reticular*, *atrophic*, *erosive* or *ulcerative*, *plaque-like*, *bullous*, and *pigmented*.
- Topical or systemic corticosteroids are the first line of treatment.

Introduction

Oral lichen planus represents a T-cell–mediated immune reaction of unknown etiology. Clinical observation and evidence have suggested that an autoimmune reaction against antigenic targets of the epithelial basal cells that might have been modified by viruses (e.g., hepatitis C virus, human herpes virus 6), bacteria, contact allergens, drugs, or chemical antigens are responsible for the development of the disease. About 1 to 2% of all populations is affected with a female-to-male ratio of 2:1 and a middle-to-late life onset. Oral manifestations occur in more than 70% of the patients with cutaneous lichen planus, while commonly the mouth is the only affected site.

Clinical features

Clinically, the cutaneous lesions appear as small, flat, polygonal, shiny papules (**Fig. 26.48**). Early papules are red, whereas older lesions display the characteristic violaceous color. Several variants of lichen planus of the skin have been described according to clinical pattern and configuration of lesions. They are distributed in a symmetrical pattern, more frequently over the flexor surfaces of the forearms

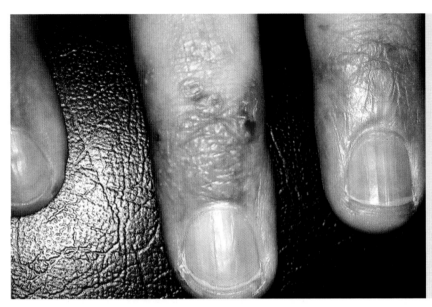

Fig. 26.46 Epidermolysis bullosa acquisita, milia, and scarring on the fingers.

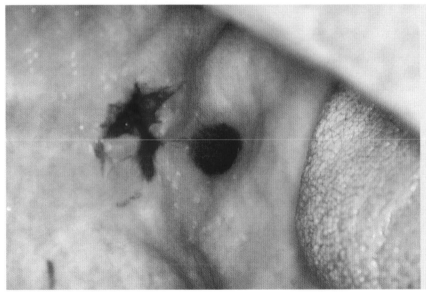

Fig. 26.47 Epidermolysis bullosa acquisita, bulla, and erosion on the buccal mucosa.

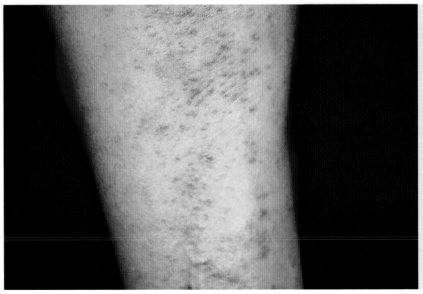

Fig. 26.48 Lichen planus, typical lesions on the forearm.

and wrists, the sacral area, the back, and the lateral sides of the neck, and they are usually accompanied by pruritus. Linear lesions may develop after scratching (*Koebner's phenomenon*). Nails are also involved (**Fig. 26.49**). The oral mucosa may be affected without skin manifestations.

Clinically, six forms of oral lichen planus have been described. The *reticular form* is the most common variant and is characterized by small white papules, which may be discrete but more often coalesce and form lines (*Wickham's striae*) and networks of line (**Figs. 26.50, 26.51**). Linear and annular distribution of the papules may be seen. The *erosive or ulcerative form* is the second most frequent variant and is characterized by small or extensive painful erosions with isolated papules or lines at the periphery (**Fig. 26.52**). The *atrophic form* is less common and usually the result of the erosive forms and is characterized by epithelial atrophy. The lesions have a smooth red surface and poorly defined borders and at the periphery papules or lines may be seen (**Fig. 26.53**). The *hypertrophic form* is rare and appears as a well-circumscribed elevated white plaque resembling homogeneous leukoplakia and is the result of coalescing hypertrophic papules (**Fig. 26.54**). The *bullous form* is rare and is characterized by formation of bullae of varying sizes, which rupture rapidly leaving painful ulcerations (**Fig. 26.55**). The bullae usually arise on a background of papules or striae. The *pigmented form* is uncommon variant and is characterized by pigmented papules arranged in a reticular pattern interspersed with whitish lesions (**Figs. 26.56, 26.57**). This form is due to local melanin overproduction and dermal melanophages during the acute phase of the disease. It is most common on the skin and should not be confused with pigmentation that may develop after healing of lichen planus lesions. Frequently, the erosive and atrophic forms of lichen planus, when located on the gingiva may manifests as *desquamative gingivitis* (**Fig. 26.58**). Lesions are also commonly seen on the glans penis (**Fig. 26.59**) and the vagina usually in the erosive and annular forms.

Oral lichen planus may follow a course of remissions and exacerbations. The disease most frequently affects the buccal mucosa, tongue, gingiva, and rarely the lips, palate, and floor of the mouth. The lesions are usually symmetri-cal and asymptomatic or cause mild discomfort, such as a burning sensation, irritation after contact with certain foods, and an unpleasant feeling of roughness in the mouth. However, erosive and bullous forms tend to be painful. The oral lesions of lichen planus may be associated with *Candida* infections. The prognosis is good, although it has been suggested that there is a possibility of malignant transformation in the erosive and atrophic forms, but this topic is still subject to some controversy. The diagnosis is mainly based on the clinical features but occasionally should be confirmed by histology.

Differential diagnosis

- Lichenoid reaction to dental materials
- Lichenoid drug eruption
- Cinnamon contact stomatitis
- Discoid lupus erythematosus
- Secondary syphilis
- Candidiasis
- Graft-versus-host disease
- Leukoplakia
- Erythroplakia
- Mucous membrane pemphigoid
- Bullous pemphigoid
- Pemphigus
- Other chronic bullous diseases
- Chronic ulcerative stomatitis

Pathology

Histologically, oral lichen planus is characterized by parakeratosis, acanthosis, "*saw-tooth*" rete ridges, liquefaction degeneration of the basal cell layer, and a band-like lymphocytic infiltration mainly CD3—T cells of the connective tissue at the epithelial–lamina propria junction. *Civatte's or colloid*

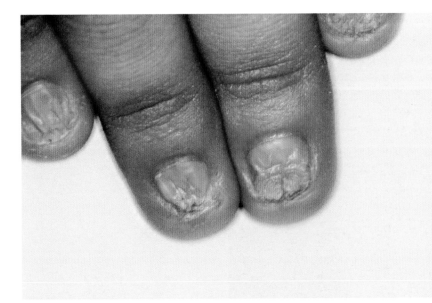

Fig. 26.49 Lichen planus, onycholysis.

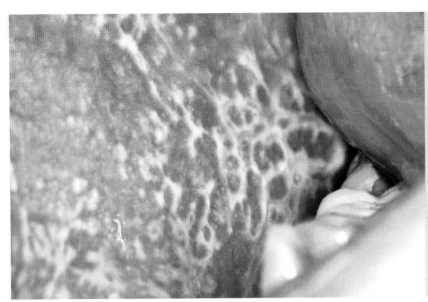

Fig. 26.50 Lichen planus, reticular type on the buccal mucosa.

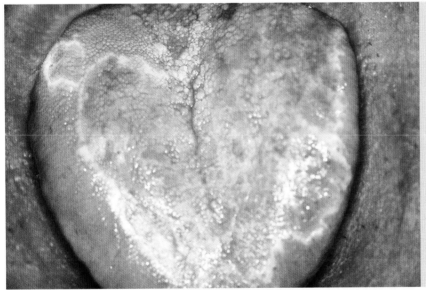

Fig. 26.51 Lichen planus, reticular type on the dorsum of the tongue.

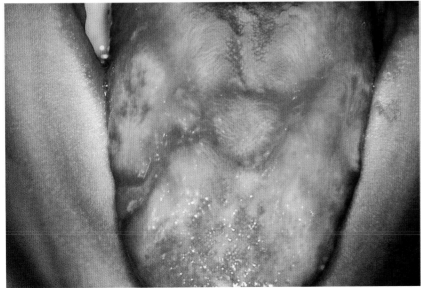

Fig. 26.52 Lichen planus, erosive type on the dorsum of the tongue.

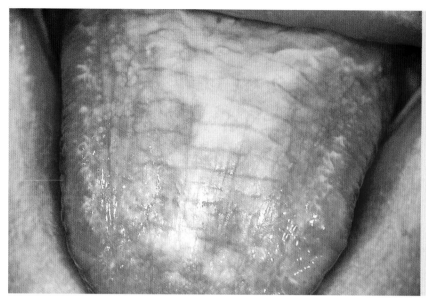

Fig. 26.53 Lichen planus, atrophic type on the dorsum of the tongue.

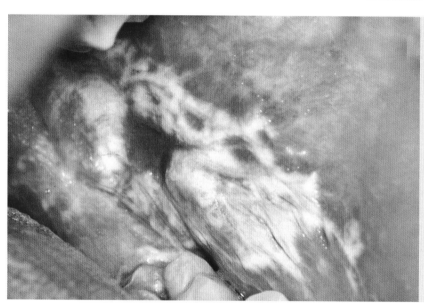

Fig. 26.54 Lichen planus, hypertrophic lesions with a central erosion on the buccal mucosa.

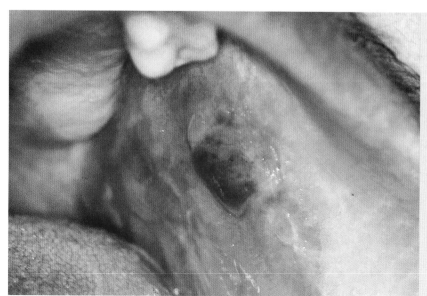

Fig. 26.55 Lichen planus, bullous type on the buccal mucosa.

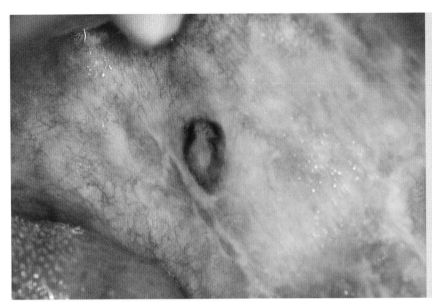

Fig. 26.56 Lichen planus, pigmented lesion on the buccal mucosa.

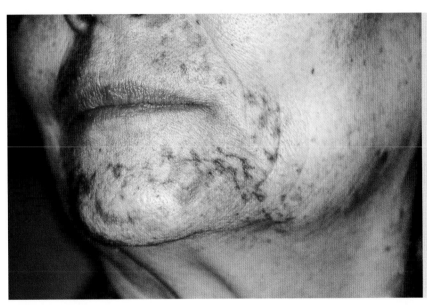

Fig. 26.57 Lichen planus pigmentosus on the face.

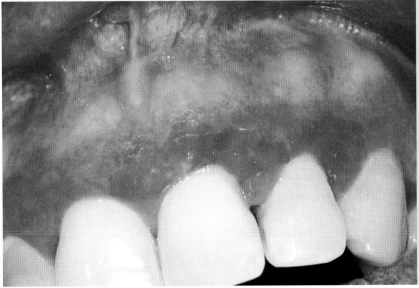

Fig. 26.58 Lichen planus, desquamative gingivitis.

bodies representing apoptotic basal cell layer keratinocytes are observed. They are usually present in the lower epithelial layers or the superficial lamina propria.

Direct immunofluorescent reveals mainly fibrin and to a lesser extend IgG and C3 along the basement membrane and the upper lamina propria. Colloid bodies often stain with fibrin and IgG, IgA, IgM, C3 are representative findings of lichen planus.

Treatment

Asymptomatic forms of oral lichen planus do not need therapy. Dental restorative materials such as amalgam and gold near the oral lesions should be replaced by other materials as they may produce lichenoid reactions or aggravate the lichen planus lesions.

Systemic oral corticosteroids (prednisone or prednisolone) 20 to 40 mg/d are the mainstay of treatment in severe, symptomatic oral lichen planus, particularly the erosive form. The lesions usually respond well in approximately 2 to 3 weeks and then the dose can be tapered to 5 mg every week and finally stopped not later than 4 to 6 weeks. Azathioprine 50 to 100 mg/d and cyclosporine 3 to 5 mg/kg/d have been used with partial success as corticosteroid-sparing adjuncts to systemic corticosteroid therapy or as single-modality treatment if corticosteroid use is contraindicated. However, both immunosuppressive agents should be avoided in the treatment of oral lichen planus and used only in exceptional cases. Systemic retinoids have no place in the treatment of oral lichen planus as complete remission is difficult to achieve and there is the possibility of severe adverse effects. Dapsone, levamisole, hydroxychloroquine sulfate, thalidomide, and pentoxifylline have been used but with doubtful results. Topical corticosteroids applied in an adhesive paste (triamcinolone acetonide, fluocinolone acetonide, fluocinonide, clobetasol propionate) are usually effective and control the disease. They are particularly useful in maintaining the therapeutic result after systemic corticosteroid therapy. Intralesional injection of triamcinolone acetonide or betamethasone dipropionate and sodium phosphate in resistant localized erosions is effective. Topical tacrolimus in a 0.5% adhesive ointment form appears to be effective in controlling erosive oral lichen planus.

Chronic Ulcerative Stomatitis

Key points

- An inflammatory, chronic autoimmune disease with characteristic immunofluorescent findings.
- Clinically, manifests as desquamative gingivitis and erosions on the tongue and buccal mucosa.
- Circulating and tissue-bound autoantibodies against DeltaNp63α protein are the prominent diagnostic features.

Introduction

Chronic ulcerative stomatitis is a rare, chronic, autoimmune oral disease characterized by a unique immunofluorescent pattern. It was first described in 1989. The prevalence cannot be easily estimated as there is a lack of awareness among clinicians and specific tests are required for its diagnosis. Specific autoantibodies cause a change to the cell-binding proteins that allow the epithelial cells to attach the underlying connective tissue. These antibodies target DeltaNp63α protein which is a 70-kDa epithelial nuclear protein. Women, usually older than 40 years are more frequently affected.

Clinical features

Clinically, the oral lesions present as erythema and painful erosions of the gingiva, usually localized, in the form of desquamative gingivitis (**Fig. 26.60**). Painful erosions, associated with white striation, similar to those seen in oral lichen planus and discoid lupus erythematosus, mainly on the tongue and buccal mucosa may also occur (**Fig. 26.61**). Rarely, skin lesions similar to lichen planus may be seen. The clinical diagnosis should be confirmed by immunofluorescent tests and histologic examination.

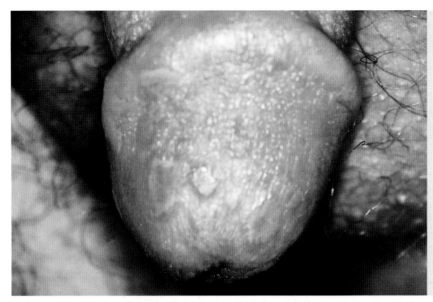

Fig. 26.59 Lichen planus, papules on the glans penis.

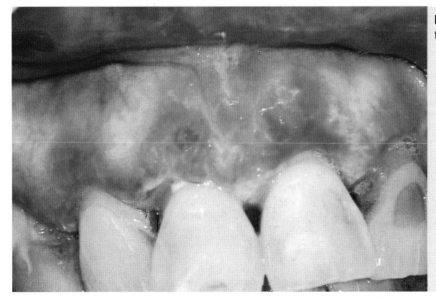

Fig. 26.60 Chronic ulcerative stomatitis, desquamative gingivitis.

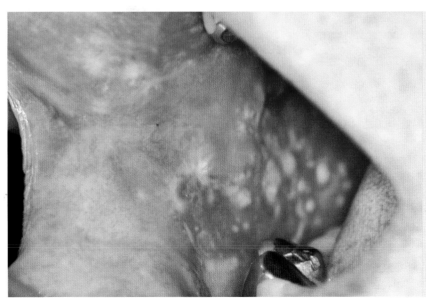

Fig. 26.61 Chronic ulcerative stomatitis, erosions interspersed with white striated lesions on the buccal mucosa.

Differential diagnosis

- Lichen planus
- Discoid lupus erythematosus
- Mucous membrane pemphigoid
- Linear IgA disease
- Epidermolysis bullosa acquisita
- Bullous pemphigoid
- Pemphigus
- Oral psoriasis

Pathology

The histologic features from oral mucosal biopsies are nonspecific, resembling those of lichen planus. Direct immunofluorescence reveals a unique speckled pattern of antinuclear IgG antibodies on the basal and parabasal cell of stratified epithelium.

Indirect immunofluorescence reveals IgG and/or IgA autoantibodies against keratinocyte nuclei in high titer. An ELISA test assay has recently been developed to detect these specific antibodies, called stratified epithelium–specific antinuclear antibody (SES-ANA) in quite high titers.

Treatment

Hydroxychloroquine 200 to 300 mg/d is the treatment of choice. The lesions usually respond to treatment in 1 to 2 weeks and may disappear in about a month. Systemic corticosteroids, e.g., prednisolone 20 to 40 mg/d reduce the symptoms and signs in approximately 2 to 4 weeks. Then the dose is tapered slowly and stops in approximately 1 to 2 months. Topical treatment with 0.1% triamcinolone acetonide in an oral adhesive base or 0.05% clobetasol propionate gel either alone in mild lesions or in association with systemic treatment may be used. The patient should also avoid inducing trauma to the gingiva with hard toothbrush as it may cause gingival relapse.

Sweet's Syndrome

Key points

- A rare disease classified in the group of noninfectious neutrophilic dermatoses.
- Clinically, it is characterized by constitutional signs and symptoms, cutaneous lesions, conjunctivitis, and oral lesions.
- The association with underlying diseases suggests a hypersensitivity reaction.
- Associated disorders include infections, malignancies, inflammatory bowel disease, drugs, and pregnancy.
- Neutrophilia is observed both in the peripheral blood and skin lesions.

Introduction

Sweet's syndrome or acute febrile neutrophilic dermatosis is an uncommon acute condition that was first described in 1964 by Robert Sweet. The classic or idiopathic form accounts for more than 50% of all cases. It has been associated with malignancies (11–54%), mostly hematopoietic (acute myeloid leukemia, chronic myelogenous leukemia, myelodysplastic syndrome, Hodgkin's disease) but also some solid tumors (breast, genitourinary, gastrointestinal). Sweet's syndrome may frequently follow an upper respiratory tract infection. It has also been associated with drugs such as granulocyte-colony stimulating factor (G-CSF), trimethoprim-sulfamethoxazole, minocycline. Less common associations are inflammatory and autoimmune diseases such as Crohn's disease, ulcerative colitis, and less frequently Sjögren's syndrome, Adamantiades-Behçet's disease, lupus erythematosus, and rheumatoid arthritis. The disease is more common in female (ratio 4:1) usually between 30 and 60 years.

Clinical features

Clinically, Sweet's syndrome presents with constitutional signs and symptoms such as high fever (38–39°C) of sudden onset, arthralgias, myalgias, malaise, skin rash, ocular lesions, and oral ulceration. The cutaneous lesions first appear as nonpruritic edematous and erythematous papules or plaques that coalesce and have a tendency to spread. Subepidermal edema can give a pseudovesicular appearance. The vesiculobullous lesions can progress to ulceration (**Figs. 26.62, 26.63**). The cutaneous lesions favor the head and neck and upper extremities. The pathergy test, injury-induced, is usually positive. Ocular lesions include conjunctivitis, episcleritis, scleritis, periorbital and orbital inflammation. Oral lesions are rare and present as deep, large ulcers, similar to major aphthous ulcers with size from 1 to 5 cm or more (**Fig. 26.64**). The lip, tongue, buccal mucosa, and palate are more frequently affected. The lip lesions present with great edema and ulceration covered by hemorrhagic crusts (**Fig. 26.65**). The cutaneous manifestations of Sweet's syndrome may spontaneously resolve in 1 to 3 months and recur in 30% of the cases. The diagnostic criteria of Sweet's syndrome are classified into *major* (abrupt onset of cutaneous lesions, characteristic histopathologic pattern) and *minor* (fever and constitutional signs and symptoms, one of the associated disorders, leukocytosis, and excellent response to systemic corticosteroids). For final diagnosis, both the major and two minor criteria are necessary.

Differential diagnosis

- Aphthous ulcers
- Adamantiades-Behçet's disease
- Periodic fevers with aphthous stomatitis, pharyngitis, and adenitis (PFAPA) syndrome
- Autoimmune collagen diseases
- Erythema multiforme
- Pyostomatitis vegetans
- Pyoderma gangrenosum
- Other neutrophilic dermatoses
- Acute leukemias
- Non-Hodgkin's lymphoma
- Wegener's granulomatosis

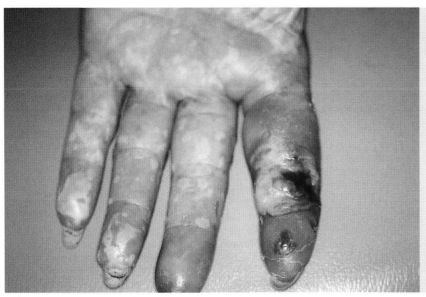

Fig. 26.62 Sweet's syndrome, edema, pustules, and ulceration on the fingers.

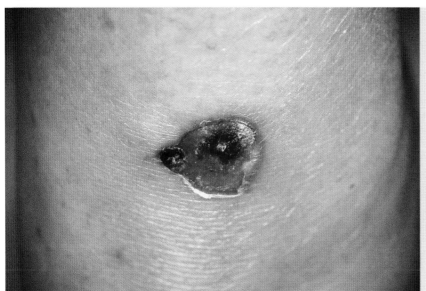

Fig. 26.63 Sweet's syndrome, ulceration on the knee.

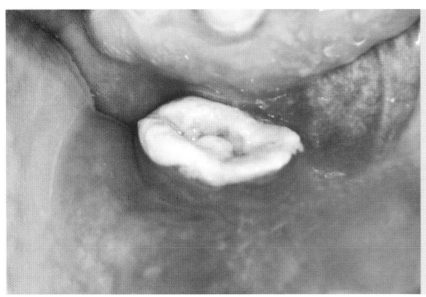

Fig. 26.64 Sweet's syndrome, deep ulceration on the lower labial mucosa.

Pathology

In the peripheral blood, leukocytosis is observed with characteristic neutrophilic domination (60–80%), however, the absence of this does not rule out the syndrome. Erythrocyte sedimentation rate (ESR) and C-reactive protein (CRP) are elevated in more than 90% of the cases. Histopathologic examination reveals a dense and diffuse neutrophilic infiltrate in the dermis. The neutrophils can migrate into the epidermis causing subcorneal pustules. A characteristic finding is the presence of perivascular neutrophilic infiltrates without vasculitis.

Treatment

Corticosteroids are the drugs of choice for the treatment of Sweet's syndrome. Prednisone 50 to 60 mg/d for 3 to 6 weeks is usually enough to control the disease. In resistant cases, low-dose prednisone, 20 to 30 mg/d for an additional 1 to 3 months may be necessary to prevent recurrence. When the disease is associated with a recognized infection (e.g., *Streptococcus*, *Staphylococcus*), antibiotics may be helpful. Dapsone 100 to 200 mg/d or colchicine 1 to 2 mg/d or potassium iodine 900 mg/d are the main alternative drugs. NSAIDs, thalidomide, cyclosporine, tacrolimus, and interferon-α have been reported to be useful. Topical treatment of oral lesions is necessary to reduce the pain and the duration of the ulcers. Triamcinolone acetonide in Orabase or 0.05% clobetasol propionate gel is applied to the ulcer three to six times a day for 1 to 2 weeks. Amlexanox 5% oral paste and topical anesthetics such as 2% viscous lidocaine may improve the symptoms. Intralesional injection of corticosteroids may be helpful.

Kawasaki's Disease

Key points
- An acute febrile multisystem disease affecting young children.
- The main symptoms and signs include fever, ocular and oral involvement, cervical lymphadenopathy, polymorphous skin rash, and acral swelling.
- Represents the most common cause of acquired cardiovascular disorders in children.

Introduction

Kawasaki's disease or mucocutaneous lymph node syndrome, is an acute, multisystem, febrile vasculitis, primarily affects children of usually less than 5 years. It was first described in Japan in 1967 by Tomisaku Kawasaki. It has a predilection for people of Asian origin (especially Japanese and Korean) but also of Afro-Caribbean descent. However, it may occur in Caucasians but the incidence varies from country to country. Boys are most commonly affected (1.5:1). The cause remains unknown, but an infectious etiology, by an agent with tropism for vascular tissues, is possible. Genetic predisposition and gene associations may also play a role.

Clinical features

There is a great range of signs and symptoms associated with Kawasaki disease. It has been suggested that diagnosis can be based on the presence of sudden onset, high-grade fever (3840°C) lasting at least 5 days plus four of the following five criteria: (1) erythema, edema, and fissuring of the lips or the oral mucosa, strawberry tongue, crusting of the lips, erythema and enlargement of the lingual papilla (**Fig. 26.66**); (2) polymorphous, maculopapular, cutaneous rash; (3) cervical lymphadenopathy, (4) bilateral nonpurulent conjunctivitis, or choroiditis, (**Fig. 26.67**); and (5) swelling or erythema of the hands or feet followed by characteristic peeling (**Fig. 26.68**).

The disease runs a course that is usually divided into three stages: *acute*, *subacute*, and *convalescent* with some authors adding a fourth, *chronic stage*. Other symptoms and signs observed throughout those stages include coughing, vomiting, diarrhea, arthralgias, arthritis, cardiovascular disorders, thrombocytosis, urethritis, aseptic meningoencephalitis, hepatitis, myocarditis, pericarditis, and renal involvement. The mortality rate is 0.1 to 2% and predominantly occurs because of cardiac complications. Early detection and treatment lead to good prognosis. The diagnosis is mainly based on the clinical features.

Differential diagnosis
- Measles
- Scarlet fever
- Staphylococcal scalded skin syndrome
- Erythema multiforme
- Drug eruption
- Childhood polyarteritis nodosa
- Periodic fever syndromes
- Acute herpetic gingivostomatitis

Pathology

There are no specific investigations for the detection of the disease. However, ESR, CRP, and α_1-antitrypsin levels are elevated initially. Mild-to-moderate normochromic anemia is observed during the acute phase along with a moderate-to-high white cell count with neutrophilia. During the subacute phase, there is thrombocytosis, while thrombocytopenia is associated with severe cardiovascular disease.

Echocardiography has to be performed in both diagnosed and suspected cases in a serial manner for evaluation and diagnosis of possible cardiovascular complications.

Biopsy is not routinely performed for the diagnosis of Kawasaki's disease. The findings are nonspecific, characterized by edema in the lamina propria and perivascular inflammatory infiltrates.

Treatment

Intravenous administration of Ig in a single infusion of 2 g/kg over 10 to 12 hours is the first line of treatment. Hospital admission and observation until the fever is resolved is recommended. Monitoring for cardiovascular disease should

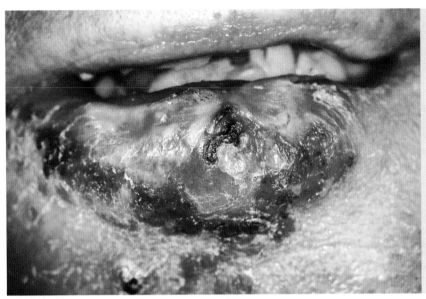

Fig. 26.65 Sweet's syndrome, edema, and ulceration on the lower lip and the perioral area.

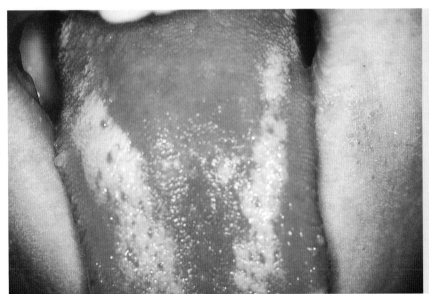

Fig. 26.66 Kawasaki's disease, erythema, and enlargement of the fungiform papillae of the tongue.

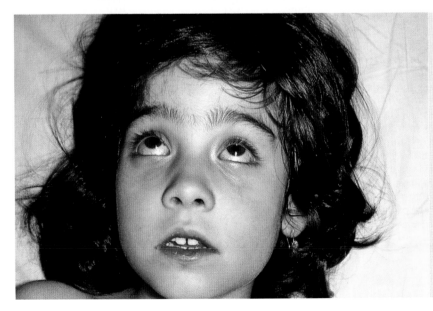

Fig. 26.67 Kawasaki's disease, bilateral conjunctivitis, blepharitis, and erythema of the lower lip.

take place. Aspirin has also been part of the treatment during the acute phase, 80 to 100 mg/kg/d for approximately 14 days, followed by a maintenance dose for 4 to 6 weeks.

Psoriasis

Key points

- A chronic, multifactorial, immune-mediated dermatosis combined with genetic, environmental, and drugs' predisposing factors.
- The disease can first appear at any age with two peaks: one at 20 to 30 years and second at 50 to 60 years.
- Predominantly affects the skin (scalp, elbows, knees, hands, nails, feet, trunk).
- The oral mucosa is rarely involved, mainly in the pustular type.

Introduction

Psoriasis is a chronic, inflammatory dermatosis of multifactorial etiology with genetic, environmental, and immunologic factors playing an important role. Contributing and triggering factors include trauma, sunburn, stress, infections, endocrine disorders, several medications (β- blockers, antimalarials, NSAIDs, calcium channel blockers, captopril, G-CSF), and others. It affects both sexes and can occur at any age with the onset of the disease before the age of 40 in 75 to 80% of patients, while 10 to 15% of new cases occur in children of less than 10 years. The prevalence is estimated to be 2 to 4% of the world's population making it one of the most common cutaneous diseases.

Clinical features

Clinically, the lesions are usually located on the extensor surfaces of the extremities, particularly the elbows and knees, lumbar area, scalp, and nails. Psoriasis presents with great polymorphism, but certain types have been described according to the presentation: *chronic plaque* or *psoriasis vulgaris* which is the most common, making approximately 90% of the cases, *guttate*, *inverse*, *pustular*, and *erythrodermic*. About 10 to 20% of patients develop psoriatic arthritis and approximately 10% present with ocular lesions (conjunctivitis, blepharitis). Clinically, the most common type, chronic plaque psoriasis is characterized by a symmetric distribution of well-circumscribed, erythematous, thickening and scaly plaques (**Fig. 26.69**). The lesions are arranged in a circular, oval, or polycircular pattern. *Koebner's phenomenon* is positive. Psoriatic lesions are occasionally surrounded by a pale branching ring (*Worong of ring*). The oral mucosa is affected in approximately 2 to 4% of the cases following the skin lesions, mainly in the pustular form of the disease and the acrodermatitis continua of Hallopeau (**Fig. 26.70**).

Clinically, oral lesions are characterized by erythema, white plaques, and circular or semicircular white, raised lesions similar to geographic tongue (**Fig. 26.71**). Rarely, when xerostomia coexists, erythematous and scaly lesions may appear on the dorsal surface of the tongue. The most commonly affected site is the tongue, followed by the gingiva, buccal mucosa, palate, floor of the mouth, and lips (**Fig. 26.72**). Generally, oral manifestations are not pathognomonic and pose diagnostic problems that may be solved with histologic examination and the diagnosis of cutaneous psoriasis.

Differential diagnosis

- Geographic tongue
- Geographic stomatitis
- Candidiasis
- Cinnamon contact stomatitis
- Lichen planus
- Desquamative gingivitis
- Linear gingival erythema
- Reactive arthritis
- Leukoplakia

Pathology

Histopathologic examination reveals mild parakeratosis, acanthosis, and orthokeratosis. The rete ridges are broader at the base. A superficial perivascular infiltrate of lymphocytes and macrophages is seen in the dermis along with papillary edema and a dilatation of capillaries. Similar histologic findings are also observed in cinnamon contact stomatitis and geographic tongue.

The accumulation of neutrophils within a spongiotic pustule is characterized as "spongiform pustule of Kogoj" while the accumulation of neutrophil remnants in the stratum corneum as "microabscess of Munro."

Treatment

Numerous topical and systemic agents and other therapies have been tried in the treatment of psoriasis. In 2013 dermatologists from 33 different countries contributed to the transitioning therapies program that aimed to provide guidance on treatment optimization and transitioning for moderate-to-severe plaque psoriasis. The American Academy of Dermatology is developing a series of recommendations and has published guidelines on treatment.

The topical treatments include the use of daily moisturizers, daily sun exposure, ultraviolet A irradiation, sea bathing, and relaxation if possible. Topical corticosteroids and retinoids, anthralin, salicylic acid, phenolic compounds, and calcipotriene can be administered. Combination therapy with a vitamin D analogue or a retinoid and a topical corticosteroid seems to be more effective than momotherapies. In severe cases, systemic retinoids, methotrexate, cyclosporine, azathioprine, "biological" therapies or hydroxyurea, or photochemotherapy can be used.

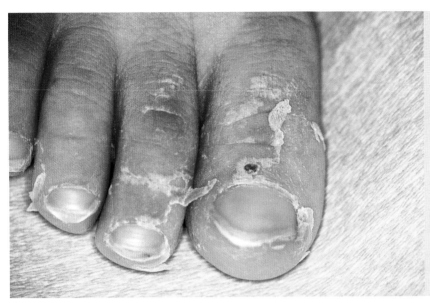

Fig. 26.68 Kawasaki's disease, characteristic peeling of the skin of the toes.

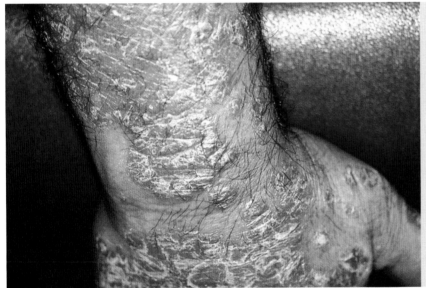

Fig. 26.69 Psoriasis, plaque-like type, cutaneous lesions.

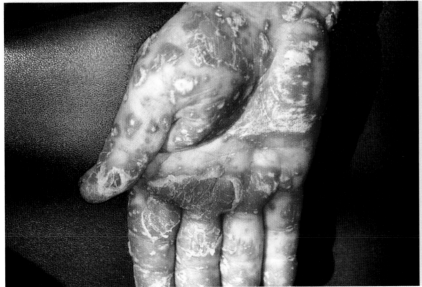

Fig. 26.70 Psoriasis, pustular type, lesions on the palm.

Reactive Arthritis

Key points

- A condition that usually affects young males.
- The main features are arthritis, urethritis, ocular, oral, and skin lesions.
- Clinically and histologically, it can resemble psoriasis.
- The oral mucosa is affected in approximately 20 to 30% of the cases.

Introduction

Reactive arthritis or Reiter's syndrome is a rare condition in response to infection. Before its manifestation, the infection that may proceed can include nongonococcal urethritis by *Chlamydia trachomatis* or *Ureaplasma urealyticum*, or intestinal infection from *Salmonella, Shigella, Campylobacter,* or *Yersinia* species. HIV-infected patients may develop the disease more commonly in the severe form. The disorder primarily affects men of 20 to 30 years and is uncommon in children. Reactive arthritis has a strong association with HLA-B27.

Clinical features

Clinically, the classical triad of nongonococcal urethritis, arthritis, and conjunctivitis is observed in about one-third of the patients in addition to mucocutaneous lesions. Oral lesions occur in 20 to 30% of the patients. They appear as diffuse erythema and painful superficial erosions. Red and slightly elevated painless plaques, occasionally surrounded by a thin, whitish line in a circular pattern are common. The gingiva, tongue, buccal mucosa, palate, and lips are the most frequently affected sites. On the tongue, there is prominent erythema and apoptosis of the filiform papillae, giving an appearance similar to that of geographic tongue (**Fig. 26.73**). Conjunctivitis is common (30%) although iritis, uveitis, and keratitis may also occur. The genital lesions include balanitis circinata, urethritis, and prostatitis. The cutaneous lesions start as vesicles and pustules to evolve in scales and hyperkeratosis (keratoderma blennorrhagicum) and most commonly affect the palms, soles, and other areas (**Fig. 26.74**). Papules and plaques that are covered by scales resembling psoriasis are common. Onychodystrophy is also observed. Asymmetrical arthritis of the large joints is the most important and early manifestation that occasionally may produce disability. Other rare manifestations include cardiac, renal, and neurologic disorders. The diagnosis is based on the clinical features as there are no specific diagnostic tests.

Differential diagnosis

- Psoriasis
- Geographic tongue
- Geographic stomatitis
- Adamantiades-Behçet's disease
- Erythema multiforme
- Sneddon-Wilkinson Disease

Pathology

Histologic examination of the mucocutaneous lesions reveals features similar to psoriasis. The epithelium and epidermis present with parakeratosis, acanthosis, spongiosis, and microabscess formation by neutrophils and lymphocytes (*Munro's microabscesses*) in the parakeratotic areas. Elongation of the rete ridges is observed and a mixed inflammatory perivascular infiltrate in the underlying lamina propria, predominantly consisting of lymphocytes, neutrophils, and macrophages. A blood test for HLA-B27 may also be helpful.

Treatment

Treatment is symptomatic. Potent nonsteroidal anti-inflammatory medications are used for the treatment of arthritis. Sulfasalazine, corticosteroids, and immunosuppressants may also be used in more severe, or nonresponsive cases.

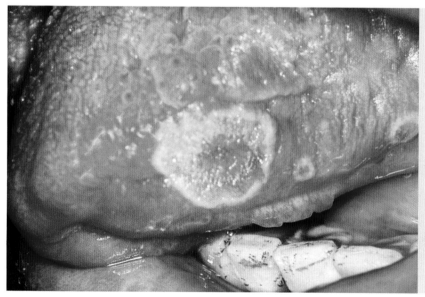

Fig. 26.71 Psoriasis, white lesions on the tongue similar to geographic tongue.

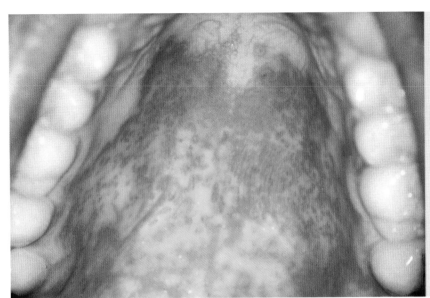

Fig. 26.72 Psoriasis, erythematous lesions on the palate.

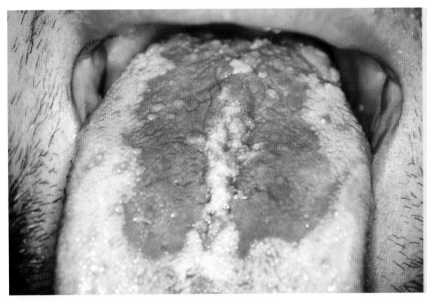

Fig. 26.73 Reactive arthritis, erythema, and apoptosis of the filiform papillae.

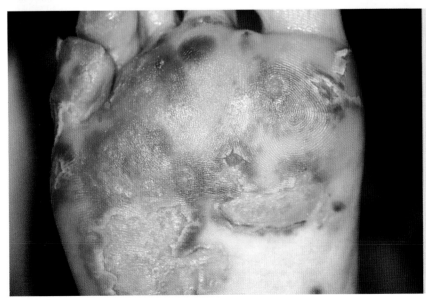

Fig. 26.74 Reactive arthritis, hyperkeratotic plaques on the sole.

Ichthyosis Hystrix

Key points

- The ichthyosis family is a large, heterogeneous group of skin disorders.
- Ichthyosis vulgaris is the most common type.
- Ichthyosis hystrix is very rare.
- The mouth is rarely involved.

Introduction

The ichthyosis family is comprised of various skin disorders with different etiology, genetics, and clinical manifestations, making it a large heterogeneous group. At least 28 different types have been described. Ichthyosis hystrix is a very rare variant that is inherited as an autosomal dominant pattern. Curth-Macklin type ichthyosis hystrix can be caused by mutation in the *KRT1* gene. The disease has many clinical phenotypes.

Clinical features

Clinically, ichthyosis hystrix is characterized by massive hyperkeratosis with an appearance like spiny scales (in the past the term "*Porcupine man*" was used) (**Fig. 26.75**). There can also be hearing problems, nail dystrophy, predisposition to infections, and skin neoplasias. The oral mucosa is not affected. However, there can be microerosions on the lips and angular cheilitis with hyperkeratosis (**Fig. 26.76**). The diagnosis is mostly based on the clinical findings and also on electron microscopy. The prognosis is poor.

Differential diagnosis

- Different types of ichthyosis
- Angular cheilitis of other etiology
- Leukoplakia of the lips

Treatment

The dermatologist is in charge of the therapeutic regime. Systemic retinoids have been tried with varied response.

Perioral Dermatitis

Key points

- It is thought to be a rosacea-like disorder.
- The patients may or may not have a history of topical steroid usage.
- The lesions characteristically have a perioral, perinasal, and periorbital distribution pattern.

Introduction

Perioral dermatitis or periorificial dermatitis has a resemblance to rosacea. It is mainly characterized by persistent eruption that affects the area around the mouth. It most commonly occurs in young adult females, especially if they are using topical corticosteroid in the area. Some cases have been associated with cosmetic creams, fluorinated toothpaste, and contraceptives. The exact cause is not well understood.

Clinical features

Clinically, perioral dermatitis is characterized by an erythematous area with small papules and vesicles or pustules in clusters, intermixed with thin crust-covered plaques around the mouth (**Fig. 26.77**). There is a typical clear zone between the affected skin and the vermilion border of the lips that appears pale. The lesions may extend to the sides of the chin, the upper lip, and the cheeks. The term periorificial dermatitis is used for the same condition when it spreads around the nose and eyes. Pruritus and a burning sensation may accompany the lesions. The diagnosis is based on clinical criteria.

Differential diagnosis

- Contact dermatitis
- Lip-licking dermatitis
- Seborrheic dermatitis
- Rosacea

Laboratory tests

No laboratory tests are required.

Treatment

If topical corticosteroids are used, their discontinuation is recommended. In mild cases, topical erythromycin, metronidazole gel, pimecrolimus cream, and azelaic acid preparations may be used. In severe cases, systemic oral antibiotics are recommended (tetracycline, minocycline, erythromycin, azithromycin).

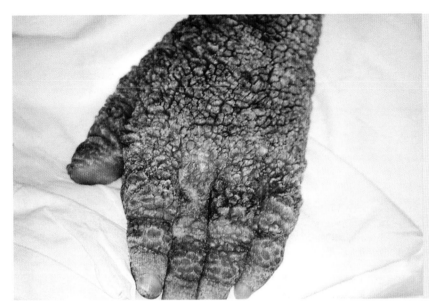

Fig. 26.75 Ichthyosis hystrix, very prominent hyperkeratotic lesions with a papillomatous appearance of the skin.

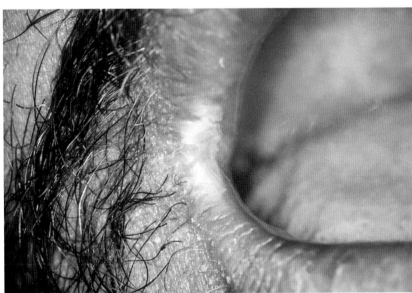

Fig. 26.76 Ichthyosis hystrix, hyperkeratosis (leukoplakia) on the commissure.

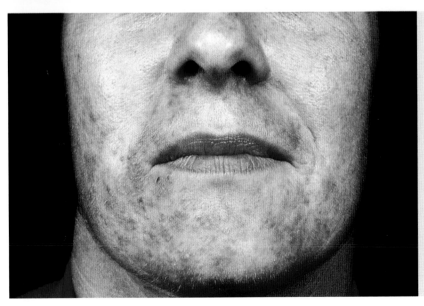

Fig. 26.77 Perioral dermatitis.

Warty Dyskeratoma

Key points

- A rare solitary lesion that affects the skin and rarely the oral mucosa.
- Histologically, similar with keratosis follicularis (Darier's disease).
- The palate is the most common site of oral involvement.

Introduction

Warty dyskeratoma is an uncommon, rare, solitary, cutaneous lesion that is histologically similar to Darier's disease. An acquired genetic mutation in *ATP2A2* has been shown to play a role in its development.

Clinical features

Warty dyskeratoma has a moderate male predilection with a median age of appearance around 52 years. The oral lesion occurs in keratinized oral sites such as the hard palate, alveolar mucosa, and gingiva. Clinically, it appears as a painless papule or small nodule with a central crater and smooth or papillomatous surface (**Fig. 26.78**). The lesion is sessile with whitish or normal color and a diameter ranging from a few millimeters to 1 cm. As the clinical features are nonpathognomonic, biopsy and histopathologic examination confirm the diagnosis.

Differential diagnosis

- Keratosis follicularis
- Necrotizing sialadenometaplasia
- Foreign body reaction
- Benign lymphoepithelial lesion
- Trauma
- Pyogenic granuloma
- Squamous cell carcinoma
- Minor salivary gland adenocarcinoma

Pathology

Histologic examination reveals epithelial suprabasal acantholysis and dyskeratosis. The epithelium overlying shows acantholytic and dyskeratotic foci and hyperkeratosis and papillomatosis. Sporadic *corps ronds* and *grains* are observed as in Darier's disease. A central keratin-filled invagination may be observed.

Treatment

Surgical excision is the treatment of choice.

Vitiligo

Key points

- An acquired disorder characterized by depigmented macules and patches.
- The precise cause remains unknown.
- Its global incidence is 0.5 to 2%.
- The oral mucosa is spared, but the lips and perioral area can be affected.

Introduction

Vitiligo is a multifactorial disorder of unknown cause related to both genetic and nongenetic factors. Factors believed to play a role include an autoimmune mechanism, cytotoxic mechanisms, oxidant–antioxidant mechanisms, neural mechanisms, and an intrinsic defect of melanocytes. Vitiligo can appear at any age with mean age of onset around 20 to 25 years.

Clinical features

Because of the lack of melanin production, amelanotic, asymptomatic macules or plaques appear that are well demarcated and are of chalk, or milk-white color. They are surrounded by a zone of normal skin. Characteristically, the lesions have discrete margin and are round, oval, linear, or irregular in shape. The size varies from several millimeters to several centimeters in diameter. Progressively, the lesions increase in size centrifugally and might extend to very large areas. The most commonly affected sites are the dorsal aspect of the hands, neck, nipples, umbilicus, and genital area. Facial vitiligo typically occurs around the eyes and mouth. The lips can also be affected, while the oral mucosa usually remains unaffected (**Figs. 26.79, 26.80**).

The diagnosis of vitiligo is predominantly based on clinical criteria.

Differential diagnosis

- Skin disorder of a different etiology
- Leukoderma
- Hypomelanosis of Ito
- Nevi
- Scars

Pathology

Histopathologic examination of the affected skin reveals partial or total absence of melanocytes and absence of melanin. The Langerhans cell density of vitiligo skin have been reported as normal, decreased, or increased.

Treatment

Topical and systemic treatments have been tried to stop the progression of the depigmentation process and to stimulate repigmentation. The management is undertaken by dermatologists.

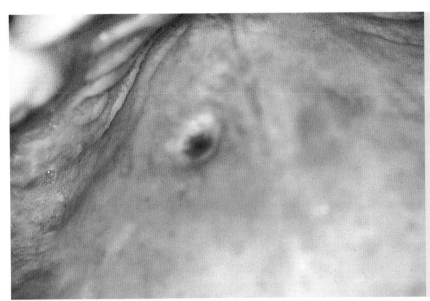

Fig. 26.78 Warty dyskeratoma, small nodule with a central crater on the palate.

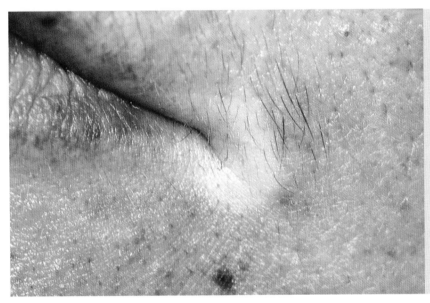

Fig. 26.79 Vitiligo of the skin on the commissure.

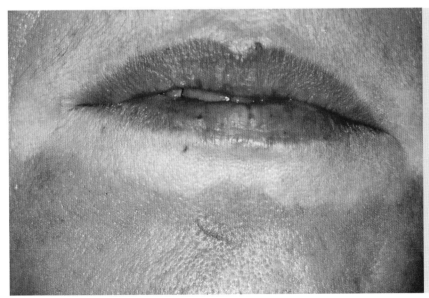

Fig. 26.80 Vitiligo periorally.

27 Blood Diseases

Iron Deficiency Anemia

Key points

- It is mainly caused by blood loss and less frequently by insufficient iron intake, decreased absorption, increased requirements, or hemoglobinopathy.
- Reliable markers are serum ferritin, less than 12 µg/L and serum iron, less than 30 µg/dL.
- Oral manifestations are common.

Introduction

Iron deficiency anemia is the most common form of anemia. It is caused by blood loss, decreased iron intake from foods, decreased iron absorption, disorders in the iron incorporation into the hemoglobin molecule, increased iron demand (pregnancy, breast-feeding), or hemolysis. The disease is more common in children with restrictive diets, women with heavy menstruation, patients with gastrointestinal tract disorders and malignancies.

Clinical features

The spectrum of clinical manifestations is very wide and depends on the degree of the anemia. Fatigue, loss of appetite, headaches, arrhythmias, pallor of the skin and mucosae, koilonychia, and neurologic disorders are the symptoms and signs. The oral mucosa appears pale and the tongue appears smooth and shiny due to atrophy of the filiform and fungiform papillae (**Fig. 27.1**). The atrophy can initially be patchy and then extend throughout the dorsum of the tongue. Rarely, leukoplakia and erosions might develop. Angular cheilitis, glossodynia, and candidiasis are not uncommon (**Fig. 27.2**). The clinical diagnosis should be confirmed by laboratory investigations.

Differential diagnosis

- Other types of anemia
- Myelodysplastic syndromes
- Lichen planus, atrophic type
- Mucous membrane pemphigoid
- Geographic tongue
- Avitaminoses
- Syphilitic tertiary glossitis
- Malnutrition disorders

Laboratory tests

Full blood count will reveal reduced red blood cells, changes in their morphology and a drop of the hematocrit. The serum ferritin may become low. A ferritin value less than 12 µg/L is a highly reliable marker of iron deficiency. Serum iron values decline to less than 30 µg/dL and transferrin levels rise, leading to transferring saturation of less than 15%.

Treatment

The first step of treatment is identification of the cause, particularly a source of occult blood loss. Ferrous sulfate per os 325 mg three times daily or ferrous fumarate together with vitamin C 250 to 500 mg/d are the first line of treatment. Alternatively, parenteral iron therapy with sodium ferric gluconate is available. Referral to a hematologist should be considered.

Plummer-Vinson Syndrome

Key points

- A form of iron deficiency anemia.
- Clinically, characterized by anemia, dysphagia, difficulty in swallowing, and atrophy of the dorsum of the tongue.
- The atrophic epithelium may predispose to the development of squamous cell carcinoma.
- The findings of the peripheral blood tests are the same as those in iron deficiency anemia.

Introduction

Plummer-Vinson syndrome or sideropenic dysphagia occurs mostly in the middle-aged women and is characterized by iron deficiency anemia, dysphagia, difficulty in swallowing, and oral lesions. Plummer-Vinson syndrome is classified into the precancerous conditions of the oral mucosa.

Clinical features

Clinically, the oral mucosa, particularly the dorsum of the tongue, appears smooth and atrophic that might also be mildly erythematous and occasionally with erosions (**Fig. 27.3**). Angular cheilitis, lip atrophy, xerostomia, glossodynia, dysphagia, and difficulty in swallowing, because of the formation of esophageal webs, may occur. The oral lesions predispose to the development of leukoplakia and oral squamous cell carcinoma.

Differential diagnosis

- Iron deficiency anemia
- Megaloblastic anemia
- Avitaminoses
- Protein and mineral deficiency

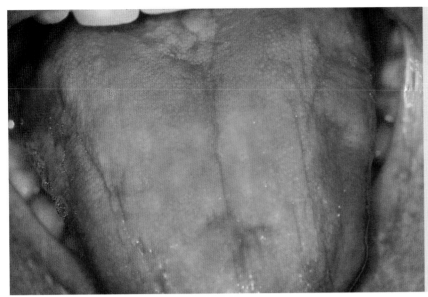

Fig. 27.1 Iron deficiency anemia, atrophy on the dorsum of the tongue.

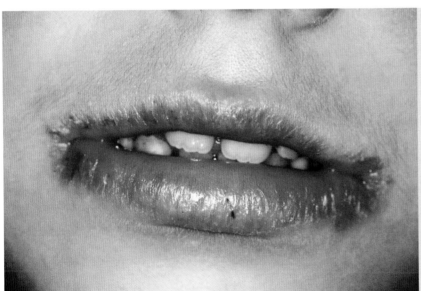

Fig. 27.2 Iron deficiency anemia, angular cheilitis.

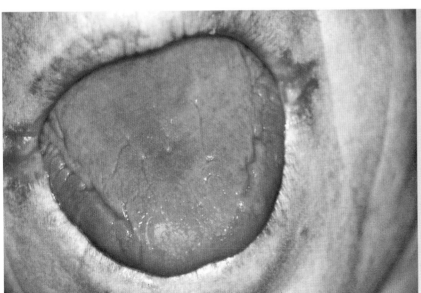

Fig. 27.3 Plummer-Vinson syndrome, erythematous and smooth tongue, and angular cheilitis.

Laboratory tests

The same as in iron deficiency anemia.

Treatment

The treatment is the same as in iron deficiency anemia.

Megaloblastic Anemia

Key points

- A macrocytic anemia caused by vitamin B_{12} deficiency.
- Decreased production of intrinsic factor and abdominal surgery may lead to vitamin B_{12} deficiency in several ways.
- Oral lesions are common and early.
- Serum vitamin B_{12} level less than 170 pg/mL.

Introduction

Megaloblastic or pernicious anemia is caused by deficiency of vitamin B_{12}, mainly due to decreased production of *intrinsic factor* (which is required for vitamin B_{12} absorption) by the gastric mucosa parietal cells. Reduced production of intrinsic factor is usually the result of an autoimmune reaction to the stomach lining. Other causes of vitamin B_{12} deficiency are dietary deficiency, gastrectomy, *Helicobacter pylori* infection, B_{12} malabsorption as the result of competitive neutralization by other factors, reduced absorption due to surgical resection, Crohn's disease, and pancreatic insufficiency. Vitamin B_{12} belongs to the cobalamin family that plays an important role in hematopoiesis and the deficiency leading to ineffective hematopoiesis affects all cell lines. All vitamin B_{12} comes from the diet and is present in all animal foods. The daily absorption is 5 µg.

Clinical features

Megaloblastic anemia affects both sexes, usually older than 30 years of age. Clinically, the patients present with anemia, pallor, weakness, fatigue, anorexia, diarrhea, weight loss, gastrointestinal and neurologic disorders (mainly of the peripheral nerves/paresthesia). The oral signs and symptoms are early and common. Clinically, there is atrophy of the lingual papillae which appears smooth, shiny, and red (**Figs. 27.4, 27.5**). The rest of the oral mucosa may be pale, with or without superficial erosions. The patients complain of burning mouth, taste disturbance, and xerostomia. The clinical diagnosis should be confirmed by the necessary investigations.

Differential diagnosis

- Iron deficiency anemia
- Folic acid deficiency
- Myelodysplastic syndromes
- Pellagra
- Malnutrition disorders

Laboratory tests

The serum vitamin B_{12} level remains the most reliable finding. Values less than 170 pg/mL are considered pathognomonic. A level of 170 to 240 pg/mL is considered borderline. Elevated levels of serum methylmalonic acid (> 1,000 nmol/L) are also diagnostic of the disease. Because vitamin B_{12} deficiency affects all hematopoietic cell lines, in severe cases the white blood cell count and the platelet count are reduced and pancytopenia is present. Bone marrow morphology is abnormal.

Treatment

The treatment is arranged by the physician or the hematologist. Intramuscular injections of 100 to 250 µg/d of vitamin B_{12} or oral cobalamin in a dose of 100 to 200 µg/d are the drugs of choice.

Thalassemia

Key points

- Classified into *α-thalassemia* and *β-thalassemia*.
- β-Thalassemia is the most common form of the disease. Elevated levels of hemoglobin A_2 or F.
- β-Thalassemia is classified into *major* and *minor*.
- Oral lesions occur in the major type and include disorders of the jaws' occlusion and teeth.

Introduction

Thalassemias are a heterogeneous group of hereditary disorders characterized by reduction in the synthesis of globin chains (α or β). They are classified into several types (α, β, δβ, δ, and γδβ) according to which globin chain or chains are affected. The gene for β-globin is located in chromosome 11 while that for α-globin on chromosome 16. The thalassemias are described as *"trait"* when there are laboratory findings without clinical features, *"intermedia"* when there is a red blood transfusion requirement and *"major"* when the disease is life threatening. α-Thalassemia is primarily due to gene deletion causing reduced α-globin chain synthesis. β-Thalassemia are usually caused by point mutations rather than deletions. These mutations result in reduced or absence of β-globin chain synthesis. The most common form is β-thalassemia or Mediterranean anemia that is classified into *heterozygous/minor* and *homozygous/major*. The disease primarily affects Greeks, Italians, and other Mediterranean populations.

Clinical features

The signs and symptoms of the disease (thalassemia major, homozygous type) usually develop after 6 months of life and become progressively more severe. The course of the disease depends on whether the child is maintained on an adequate transfusion program. The inadequately transfused patient has the typical clinical features, such as skin pallor, low fever, malaise, weakness, growth failure, hepatosplenomegaly, and bony deformities. Gradually, the face assumes mongoloid appearance. There is protrusion of the upper anterior teeth, delayed eruption, and disorders of the teeth position and occlusion caused by craniofacial abnormalities (**Fig. 27.6**).

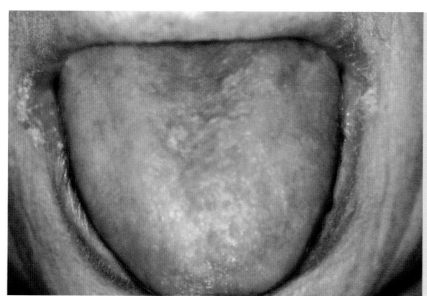

Fig. 27.4 Megaloblastic anemia, smooth and atrophic dorsal aspect of the tongue, and angular cheilitis.

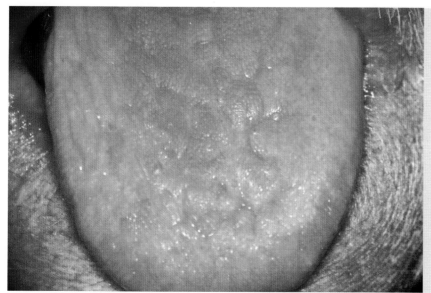

Fig. 27.5 Megaloblastic anemia, papillary atrophy of the tongue.

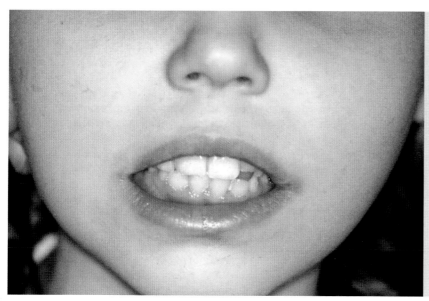

Fig. 27.6 β-Thalassemia major, pallor of the skin, anomalies of the teeth position, and malocclusion.

The oral mucosa presents with pallor, the tongue papillae are atrophic while swelling of parotid glands may occur. Quite often the patients complain of glossodynia.

Differential diagnosis

- Other forms of thalassemia
- Iron deficiency anemia
- Various hemoglobinopathies

Laboratory tests

Anemia is detected through the full blood count and the hematocrit may fall to less than 10%. There are also alterations of the shape and size of the red blood cells. Electrophoresis of hemoglobin is also useful.

Treatment

The pediatrician decides upon a transfusion program for support. Allogeneic bone marrow transplantation is the treatment of choice for β-thalassemia major.

Neutropenia

Key points

- A hematologic disease characterized as neutropenia when the peripheral blood neutrophils is less than 1,800/μL.
- The causes of neutropenia may be *hereditary* or *acquired*.
- Acquired causes may include bone marrow disorders or peripheral disorders.
- Patients with neutropenia are susceptible to infections.
- The oral cavity can be a target of infections and other lesions.

Introduction

Neutropenia is hematologic disorder characterized by a low neutrophil count (< 1,800/μL). Patients are susceptible to infections, mainly by gram-positive and gram-negative bacteria and by fungi. The risk of infection is related to the severity of neutropenia. It is high when the neutrophil count is less than 500/μL and very high when the count is less than 100/μL. In contrast, patients with *chronic benign neutropenia* are not susceptible to infections.

The causes of neutropenia are divided into *bone marrow* disorders: congenital neutropenia, cyclic neutropenia, aplastic anemia, chronic benign neutropenia, drugs reaction, e.g., sulphonamides, chlorpromazine, phenytoin, cimetidine, penicillin, cephalosporins, chemotherapeutic agents, radiotherapy, T-cell large granular lymphocytic leukemia, etc., and *bone marrow* conditions (splenomegaly, HIV infection and other viral infections, Felty's syndrome, systemic lupus erythematosus, and other autoimmune diseases).

Clinical features

Regardless of the cause and the type of neutropenia, the clinical signs and symptoms are similar and their gravity is directly related to the degree of neutrophil reduction. The patients are susceptible to infections due to gram-positive or gram-negative aerobic bacteria. Systemic symptoms include high fever, malaise, loss of appetite, and other signs and symptoms mainly from the respiratory and uropoietic systems, the inner ear, the skin etc. They may progress to develop septicemia. Systemic fungal infections may be developed, such as candidiasis, aspergillosis, mucormycosis, cryptococcosis, with all the relevant signs and symptoms. Oral manifestations are common and include multiple ulcers, primarily on the gingiva, palate, tongue, and lips. Soft tissue abscesses, advanced periodontal disease, and bacterial and fungal infections may also occur (**Figs. 27.7, 27.8**). In severe neutropenia, the usual signs of inflammatory response to infection may be reduced or absent. The clinical diagnosis should be confirmed by hematologic investigations.

Differential diagnosis

- Different specific forms of neutropenia
- Leukemia
- Myelodysplastic syndromes
- Agranulocytosis
- Aplastic anemia

Laboratory tests

The examination of the peripheral blood reveals a reduction in neutrophils with values usually less than 500 to 1,000/μL depending on the severity of the disease.

Treatment

The responsibility for the treatment falls on the hematologist and is usually taking place in hospital. Systemic antibiotics are administered for the different bacterial infections and antifungal medication for the systemic mycoses. Granulocyte colony-stimulating factor (G-CSF), once or twice weekly will often be sufficient to increase neutrophil count.

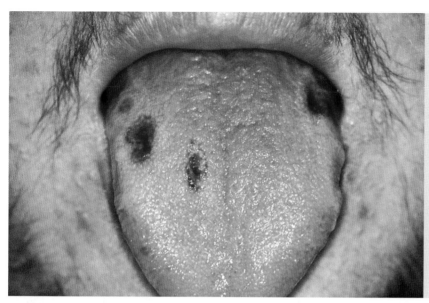

Fig. 27.7 Neutropenia, multiple ulcers on the tongue.

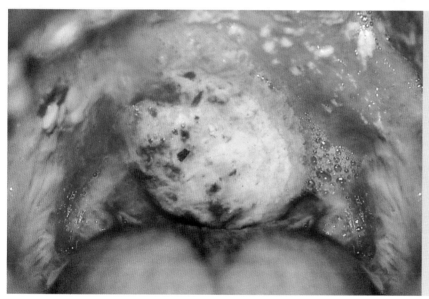

Fig. 27.8 Neutropenia, ulceration on the soft palate.

415

Congenital Neutropenia

Key points

- A genetic disease inherited by an autosomal dominant or autosomal recessive pattern.
- It manifests in early childhood with recurrent infections.
- Oral manifestations are common and are mainly characterized by atypical ulceration and periodontal disease.

Introduction

Congenital neutropenia or infantile genetic agranulocytosis is a rare form of neutropenia transmitted with the autosomal dominant or the autosomal recessive pattern of inheritance. It is characterized by a marked persistent decrease in circulating neutrophils. The disease becomes apparent during early childhood with recurrent infections. The severity of clinical manifestations is related to the degree of neutropenia.

Clinical features

Multiple bacterial infections characterize the clinical picture of the disease. The most common infections involve the skin, lungs, middle ear, and urinary tract and may be life threatening. Oral manifestations are common and include persistent and recurrent ulcerations, gingivitis and periodontal disease, bacterial infections, and candidiasis (**Figs. 27.9–27.11**). Periodontal disease is very common and is characterized by extensive bone destruction and tooth mobility and loss. The marginal and attached gingiva are fiery red and edematous and the interdental papillae are hyperplastic. The disease is gradually improving with age. The diagnosis is based on the history, the clinical features, and the hematologic investigations.

Differential diagnosis

- Shwachman-Diamond syndrome
- Papillon-Lefèvre syndrome
- Dyskeratosis congenita
- Cyclic neutropenia
- Agranulocytosis
- Aplastic anemia
- Acute leukemia
- Glycogen storage disease type 1b
- Acatalasia
- Hypophosphatasia

Laboratory tests

Peripheral blood test and myelogram are diagnostic of neutropenia. Remarkably decreased neutrophils or absence of neutrophils are common findings. Radiographic examination of the jaws may show severe alveolar bone loss.

Treatment

High level of oral hygiene is required regarding the periodontal disease. Systemic treatment is the responsibility of the pediatrician or hematologist and follows the guidelines of neutropenia treatments.

Cyclic Neutropenia

Key points

- A rare form of neutropenia with a genetic background.
- Mutations of *ELA2* gene for neutrophil elastase is linked to the disease.
- Characteristically, in the peripheral blood cyclic reduction in the number of circulating neutrophil is observed.
- There is a risk of infection when the neutrophils are at the lower levels.
- Oral lesions are common.

Introduction

Cyclic neutropenia is a rare form of neutropenia with a genetic pattern that is characterized by a cyclic, repeated reduction in the number of circulating neutrophil leukocytes. In many of the cases, the disease is transmitted as an autosomal dominant trait with variable expression, but there are also many isolated cases. The reduction in neutrophils occurs regularly at 3-week intervals and may last for 1 to 3 days. A recovery phase of 5 to 8 days follows when the number of neutrophils returns to normal. The disease is usually manifested in infancy or childhood, but it may occur at any age.

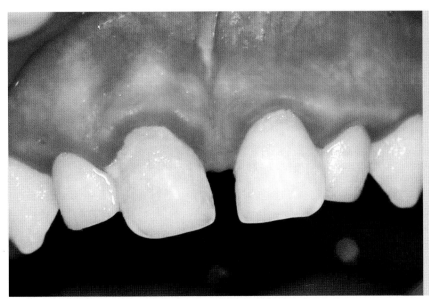

Fig. 27.9 Congenital neutropenia, gingivitis, and early periodontitis in the maxilla of a 6-year-old child.

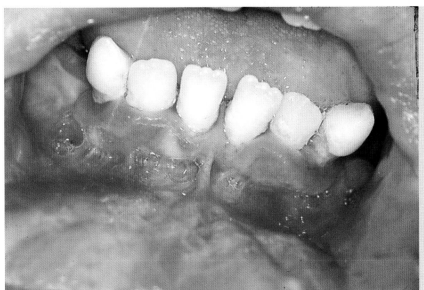

Fig. 27.10 Congenital neutropenia, advanced periodontitis with tooth mobility in a 6-year-old child.

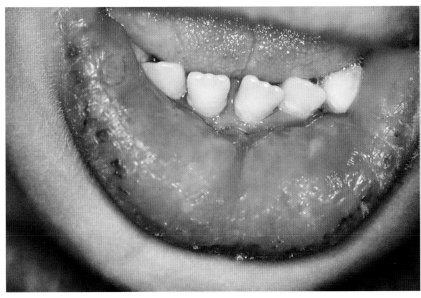

Fig. 27.11 Congenital neutropenia, scars from recurrent ulceration, and edema of the lower lip.

Clinical features

During an episode of profound neutropenia, the signs and symptoms include low-grade fever, malaise, headache, loss of appetite, oral lesions, less frequently dysphagia, arthralgias, cervical adenitis, skin infections, and rarely intestinal ulceration. Painful oral ulcers, covered by a whitish membrane and surrounded by slight erythema, are usually seen (**Fig. 27.12**). The size of ulcers varies from a few millimeters to 1 cm, and they may appear at any area of the oral mucosa for 1 to 2 weeks. The most commonly affected sites are the lower lip, tongue, buccal mucosa, and soft palate. Gingivitis, also a common finding, deteriorates during the phase of neutropenia (**Fig. 27.13**). A characteristic feature of the oral lesions is the cyclic recurrence which coincides with the phase of neutrophil drop.

Differential diagnosis
- Congenital neutropenia
- Agranulocytosis
- Leukemias
- Aphthous ulceration
- Oral herpetic lesions

Laboratory tests

Hematologic test that determines the neutrophil number is performed three times per week for 6 to 8 weeks. The neutrophil count is usually varied, however, during the phase of greatest risk of neutropenia (third to sixth day), the number can be less than 600/mm³.

Treatment

The systemic treatment is performed by the pediatrician or the hematologist. It includes corticosteroids, splenectomy, administration of G-CSF growth factor, and treatment of infections. Local oral measures should include high level of oral hygiene. For the ulceration, topical application of steroid ointments or tacrolimus and the use of antiseptic mouthwashes are recommended.

Agranulocytosis

Key points
- A severe reduction or even complete absence of all granulocytes in the peripheral blood and the bone marrow.
- It can be caused by either a reduction in production or increase in destruction of granulocytes.
- Classified into *idiopathic*, *secondary*, and *genetic*.
- Clinically, it is characterized by signs and symptoms of acute infection.
- The mouth is often affected at early stages with necrotic lesions of the mucosa and the periodontal tissues.

Introduction

Agranulocytosis is an acute hematologic disorder characterized by a severe reduction or complete absence of all granulocytes, especially neutrophils, both in the peripheral blood and the bone marrow. It is classified into *idiopathic* (of unknown etiology), *secondary* (usually caused by medication, infections, etc.), and *genetic* (congenital agranulocytosis, Kostmann's syndrome) that is caused by cytokine G-CSF insufficiency.

Clinical features

The disease may affect both sexes of any age. The onset is sudden and is characterized by chills, fever, malaise, dysphagia, and arthralgias. Within 12 to 24 hours, evidence of oral, pharyngeal, respiratory, skin, and gastrointestinal infections usually appear. Pneumonia related to death may occur within a few days in serious cases. Oral mucosal lesions are common and occur early. Clinically, multiple necrotic ulcers appear covered by gray-white or dark "dirty" pseudomembranes without an inflammatory red halo (**Fig. 27.14**). The palate, gingiva, tongue, and tonsils are the most common sites of involvement. Severe necrotizing gingivitis with destruction of

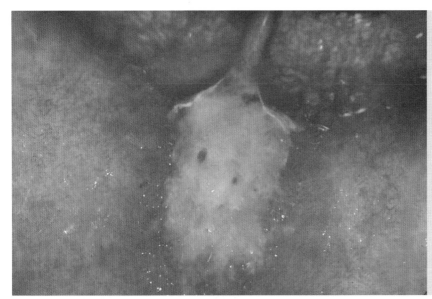

Fig. 27.12 Cyclic neutropenia, atypical ulceration of the lower lip mucosa.

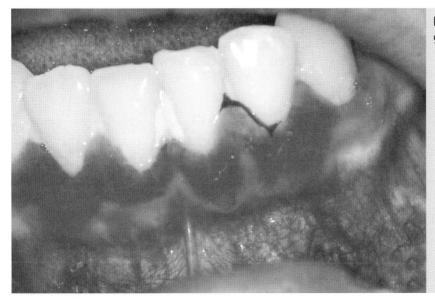

Fig. 27.13 Cyclic neutropenia, gingivitis.

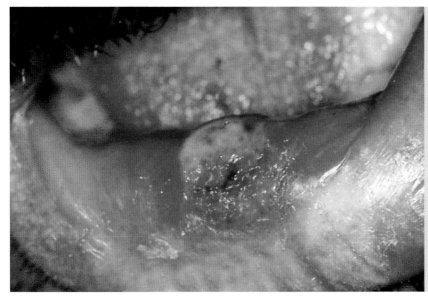

Fig. 27.14 Agranulocytosis, early ulceration on the mucosa of the lower lip.

periodontal tissues may occur (**Figs. 27.15–27.17**). The oral lesions are frequently accompanied by increased salivation, painful mastication, and difficulty in swallowing. The diagnosis is based on the history, the clinical features, and mainly the hematologic investigations.

Differential diagnosis

- Aplastic anemia
- Neutropenias
- Acute leukemia
- Infectious mononucleosis
- Wegener's granulomatosis
- Acute necrotizing ulcerative gingivitis and periodontitis

Laboratory tests

Hematologic examination of the peripheral blood and the bone marrow reveals a great reduction or even absence of granulocytes and the relevant stem cells.

Treatment

If medication is responsible for the agranulocytosis, it should be discontinued immediately. Hematopoiesis growth factors such as G-CSF, or granulocyte-macrophage colony-stimulating factor (GM-CSF) are administered. Antibiotics and cytokines can also be useful. The treatment is the responsibility of the hematologist and requires hospital admission.

Aplastic Anemia

Key points

- A life-threatening hematologic disease, caused by inability of the bone marrow to produce stem cells of all cell lines (pancytopenia).
- It is classified into *congenital*, *idiopathic*, and *secondary*.
- The most common causes are autoimmunity, medication, chemotherapy, radiotherapy, etc.
- The signs and symptoms have a great spectrum and depend on the functions affected by the red and white cells and the platelets.
- Oral manifestations are common and include mainly ulceration and hemorrhage.

Introduction

Aplastic anemia is a hematologic disease that is characterized by bone marrow failure of all stem cell lines (pancytopenia). The disease may be *idiopathic* (possible of autoimmune nature), *secondary* (due to medication, radiotherapy, chemicals, viruses, systemic lupus erythematosus, etc.), and rarely *congenital* (dyskeratosis congenita and Fanconi's anemia).

Clinical features

As all the hematologic cell lines are involved, the signs and symptoms are present within a great spectrum. The patients may present with weakness, fatigue, headache, tachycardia, and dyspnea due to reduction of red blood cells. Neutropenia is responsible for bacterial infections and mycoses and thrombocytopenia results in hemorrhage of various organs.

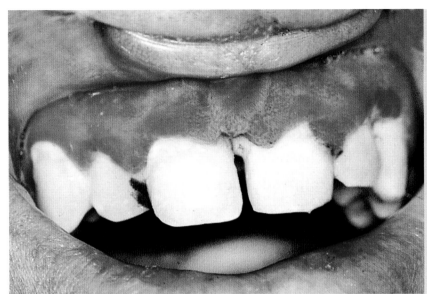

Fig. 27.15 Agranulocytosis, early manifestations with gingival ulceration and inflammation.

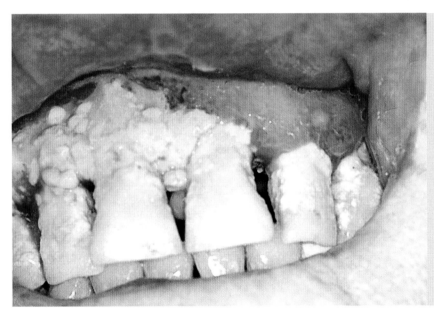

Fig. 27.16 Agranulocytosis, extensive periodontal lesions.

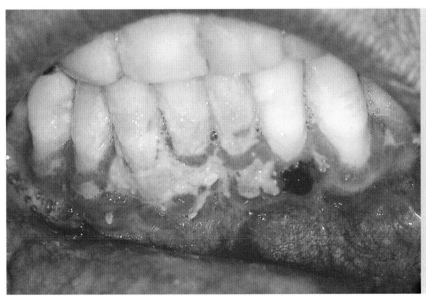

Fig. 27.17 Agranulocytosis, necrosis of the mandibular gingiva of the patient in **Fig. 27.16**.

Clinically, the oral mucosa appears pale with petechiae, ecchymoses, and hematomas. Spontaneous bleeding is also observed, particularly from the gingiva (**Fig. 27.18**). The neutropenia can cause ulceration in various oral sites with characteristic absence of surrounding inflammation (**Figs. 27.19, 27.20**). Additionally, there is hemorrhage, petechiae, and ecchymoses on the skin and other mucosae. Patients with severe aplastic anemia have a poor prognosis if left untreated.

The diagnosis is based on the history, the clinical features, and mainly the hematologic investigations of the peripheral blood and the bone marrow.

Differential diagnosis

- Agranulocytosis
- Neutropenias
- Acute leukemia
- Myelodysplastic syndromes
- Thrombocytopenia
- Infections: tuberculosis, HIV, leishmaniasis
- Systemic lupus erythematosus
- Megaloblastic anemia

Laboratory tests

The hallmark of aplastic anemia is pancytopenia. There is a great reduction or even absence of red and white blood cells as well as platelets in the peripheral blood. The bone marrow aspirate and biopsy appear hypocellular with only scant amounts of normal hematopoietic progenitors.

Treatment

The hematologist is responsible for the treatment of aplastic anemia that requires hospital admission. The treatment may include red blood and platelet transfusions and antibiotics to treat infections. In severe cases, bone marrow transplantation, immunosuppressive medication, corticosteroids, may be used.

Thrombocytopenia

Key points

- A great reduction of platelets in the peripheral blood, usually less than 20,000 to 30,000 µL.
- A characteristic clinical sign is hemorrhage from the skin, the mucosae, and other organs and systems.
- Gingival bleeding is a very common finding.

Introduction

Thrombocytopenia is a hematologic disorder characterized by a reduction of the platelet counts to less than 20,000 to 30,000/µL. The causes of thrombocytopenia are classified into four major categories:

a. *Decreased platelets production* that may reflect a congenital or acquired bone marrow failure (i.e., Fanconi's anemia, aplastic anemia, myelodysplasia, chemotherapeutic agents, radiation, bone marrow neoplasia, infections, nutritional deficiency such as vitamin B_{12}, folic acid, iron, alcohol).
b. *Increased platelets destruction* (medication, immune thrombocytopenic purpura, heparin, thrombotic microangiopathy, systemic lupus erythematosus, HIV infection, von Willebrand's disease [vWD], etc.)
c. *Increased retention* and inactivation of platelets in the spleen (hypersplenism).
d. *Other conditions causing thrombocytopenia* (gestational thrombocytopenia, Bernard-Soulier syndrome, pseudo-thrombocytopenia).

Clinical features

Mucocutaneous bleeding manifestations depend on the platelet count. Hemorrhage usually does not occur until the platelet count is less than 20,000 to 30,000/µL.

Thrombocytopenia is clinically characterized by spontaneous hemorrhage, petechiae, ecchymoses, and hematomas on the skin, the mucosae, and other tissues and organs. Epistaxis

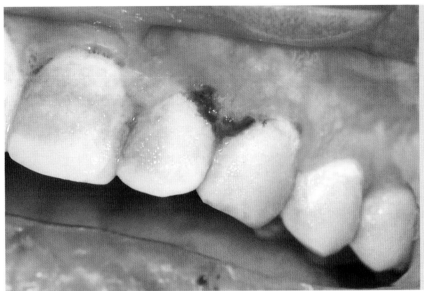

Fig. 27.18 Aplastic anemia, early hemorrhagic ulceration of the maxillary gingiva.

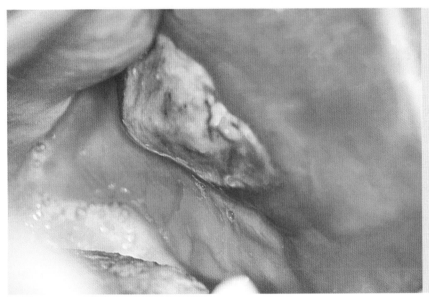

Fig. 27.19 Aplastic anemia, ulceration on the buccal mucosa.

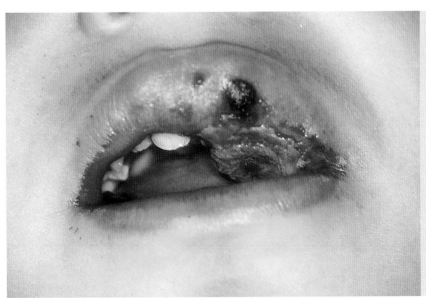

Fig. 27.20 Aplastic anemia, large hemorrhagic ulceration on the upper lip.

and bleeding from the gastrointestinal and uropoietic systems are also common. Intraorally, gingival bleeding is a common and early sign. Additionally, there may be petechiae and ecchymoses and even hematomas and hemorrhagic bullae mainly on the palate, buccal mucosa, and gingiva (**Figs. 27.21–27.23**). Any dental extraction or dental procedure with bleeding risk should be postponed until the platelet level is improved.

Differential diagnosis

- Aplastic anemia
- Leukemia
- Agranulocytosis
- Polycythemia vera

Laboratory tests

The level of platelets in the peripheral blood is usually less than 20,000 to 30,000/µL. Bone marrow should be examined.

Treatment

Only patients with platelet counts less than 20,000 to 30,000/µL or those with significant bleeding should be treated. The remainder may be monitored serially for progression.

The hematologist is responsible for the treatment of the disease. The cause of the thrombocytopenia should be determined and dealt with. The mainstay of treatment includes blood transfusion, corticosteroids, intravenous immunoglobulin (IVIg), and splenectomy.

Polycythemia Vera

Key points

- An acquired myeloproliferative disorder characterized by increased red blood cell count.
- A mutation in *JAK2* gene has been demonstrated in 95% of cases.
- The hematocrit is elevated over 54% in males and 51% in females.
- Oral lesions mainly include gingival bleeding and a deep erythematous color of the oral mucosa.
- Thrombosis is the most common and severe complication of the disease.

Introduction

Polycythemia vera is a myeloproliferative bone marrow disorder characterized by autonomous overproduction of red blood cells. However, overproduction of the two other hematopoietic cell lines may also be observed. This leads to an increase in the volume of red blood cells in the peripheral blood. The exact etiology remains unknown. It is believed that *JAK2* gene mutation is certainly involved in the pathogenesis, as it has been observed in 95% of cases. Polycythemia vera is more common in males older than 60 years.

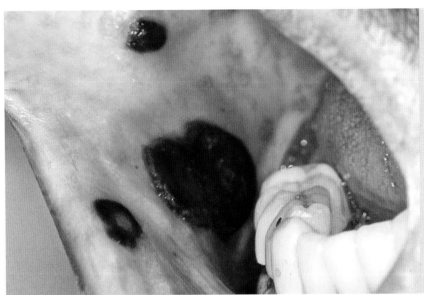

Fig. 27.21 Thrombocytopenia, hemorrhagic bullae on the buccal mucosa.

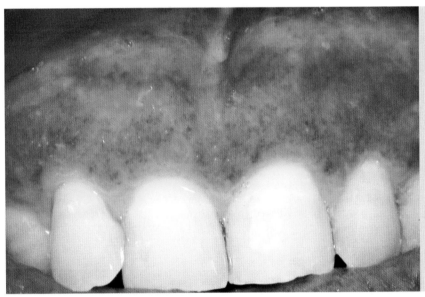

Fig. 27.22 Thrombocytopenia, petechiae on the maxillary gingiva, and alveolar mucosa.

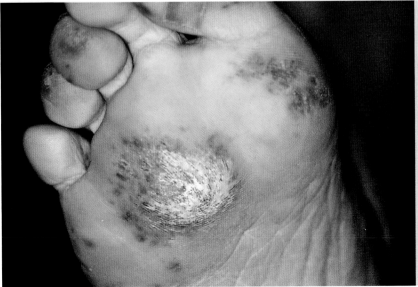

Fig. 27.23 Thrombocytopenia, petechiae and ecchymoses on the sole.

Clinical features

The main signs and symptoms include headache, tinnitus, vertigo, fatigue, visual disturbances, hyperhidrosis, generalized pruritus, dyspnea, hemorrhage, thrombosis, abdominal pain, and splenomegaly. The skin and oral mucosa take a deep red color. Clinically, oral manifestations include petechiae, ecchymoses, and hematomas (**Fig. 27.24**). Gingival bleeding and enlargement is a common finding (**Fig. 27.25**). Thrombosis is the most common complication and the major cause of morbidity and death. Over time, polycythemia vera may convert to chronic or acute myeloid leukemia. The spleen is palpable in 75 to 80% of cases.

Differential diagnosis

- Secondary polycythemia from other causes
- Thrombocytopenia
- Other myeloproliferative disorders

Laboratory tests

The hallmark of polycythemia vera is the increase of hematocrit greater than 54% in men and 51% in women. Red blood cell morphology is normal. There is also an increase of white cells from 10,000 to 20,000/μL and the platelet exceeding 1,000,000/μL while the morphology of both are normal. The diagnosis should be confirmed with the finding of the *JAK2* mutation. The bone marrow is hypercellular.

Treatment

The treatment of polycythemia vera is the responsibility of the hematologist. The treatment of choice is phlebotomy. Myelosuppressive therapy (hydroxyurea), low-dose aspirin (upto 80–100 mg/d), pegylated α-interferon, and allopurinol may also be used as an alternative therapy.

Plasminogen Deficiency

Key points

- A disease transmitted through the autosomal recessive pattern of inheritance.
- It is caused by mutation of the *PLG*, plasminogen encoding gene.
- Common affected sites are the conjunctivae, oral mucosa, and mucosa of the larynx and the cervix.

Introduction

Plasminogen deficiency is a rare disorder that affects clot formation and hemostasis. It is caused by mutation of the *PLG*, plasminogen encoding gene and is transmitted through the autosomal recessive trait. Plasminogen is a serum protein that converts into the active plasmin by a variety of enzymes. Plasmin is a protease that acts to dissolve fibrin blood clots, to avoid its expansion. Plasminogen deficiency leads to accumulation and deposition of fibrin in the form of nodules and plaques mainly on the mucosae of the eye, mouth, larynx, and cervix. The lesions become apparent toward the end of first decade of life.

Clinical features

The conjunctivae are most commonly affected by recurrent, fibrin-rich chronic membranous lesions of wood-like consistency (*ligneous conjunctivitis*). Second in frequency are the gingival lesions, since childhood, that are characterized by irregular, ulcerated swelling, giving the gingiva a verrucous-like appearance and may extend to more than one quadrants (**Figs. 27.26, 27.27**). Occasionally, lesions in the larynx and vocal cords appear causing hoarseness. The nose and cervix may be affected. In severely affected patients, prognosis is poor. In other cases, if there is good control and prevention of clots formation, prognosis can be better.

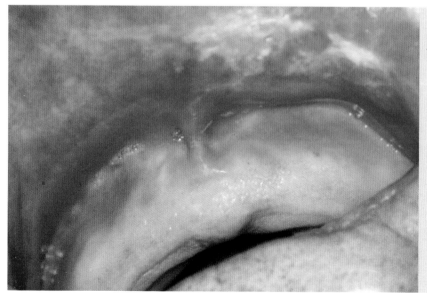

Fig. 27.24 Polycythemia vera, deep erythematous color on the upper vestibule.

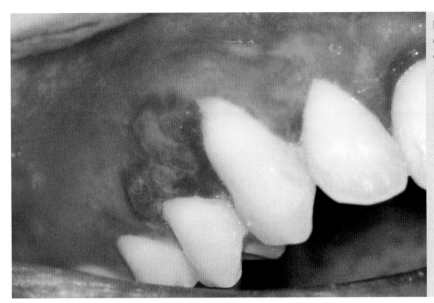

Fig. 27.25 Polycythemia vera, hemorrhagic gingival enlargement, and deep erythematous color on the upper vestibule.

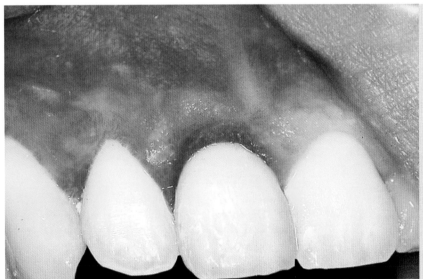

Fig. 27.26 Plasminogen deficiency, localized, early erythematous enlargement of the upper gingiva.

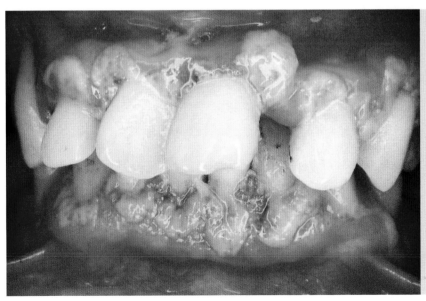

Fig. 27.27 Plasminogen deficiency, generalized, enlargement and ulceration of the upper and lower gingiva.

Differential diagnosis

- Hereditary gingival fibromatosis
- Lipoid proteinosis
- Amyloidosis
- Mucopolysaccharidoses
- Crohn's disease
- Leukemias

Pathology

Histopathologic examination of the gingival lesions reveals accumulation of fibrin in an amorphous, eosinophilic, acecullar, amyloidaceous material that fails to stain for amyloid, glycogen, and lipoid material. In interproximal areas, granular tissue is detected. In addition, the determination of plasminogen quantity in the peripheral blood and functionality is required.

Treatment

The systemic treatment of the disease is the responsibility of hematologist. For the gingival lesions, topical application of heparin is used together with systemic prednisolone at 20 to 30 mg/d.

von Willebrand's Disease

Key points

- The most common inherited bleeding disorder.
- The gene responsible for von Willebrand's factor (vWF) and vWD is located in the short arm of chromosome 12.
- It is classified into three types: *type I*, *type II*, and *type III* depending on the vWF serum levels.
- The main clinical sign of the disease is hemorrhage.

Introduction

vWD is the most common, inherited bleeding disorder with 30 to 100 cases per 1,000,000 of population. It is predominantly transmitted via the autosomal dominant pattern of inheritance (types I and II) and with the autosomal recessive pattern of inheritance (type III). The gene responsible for both, vWF and ultimately for the disease, is located on chromosome 12. vWF is responsible for platelet adhesion and binds to factor VIII which protects it from proteolysis. Depending on the degree of vWF reduction, the disease is classified into three types: *type I*, *type II*, and *type III*. Type I is the most common, seen in 75 to 80% of patients; they usually have mild or moderate platelet type, and are asymptomatic. Type II is seen in 15 to 20% of patients and they usually have moderate-to-severe bleeding that presents in childhood or adolescence. Type III is rare and has severe bleeding during infancy or childhood.

Clinical features

The hallmark of clinical feature is bleeding disposition in different degree, depending on the type. This occurs either spontaneously from the skin and mucosae, or after surgery. Intraorally, erythema and gingival bleeding is common (**Figs. 27.28, 27.29**). Persistent bleeding may be observed after a tooth extraction and gingival or other oral surgical procedure. The diagnosis is based on the clinical features and should be confirmed by laboratory findings.

Differential diagnosis

- Hemophilia
- Other clotting disorders
- Antithrombotic therapy

Laboratory tests

Clotting time tests are useful. Partial thromboplastin time (PTT) is prolonged. Additionally, vWF activity—ristocetin cofactor is performed. Finally, factor VIII levels and activity test are performed, as it binds to vWF.

Treatment

The treatment is absolutely the responsibility of the hematologist.

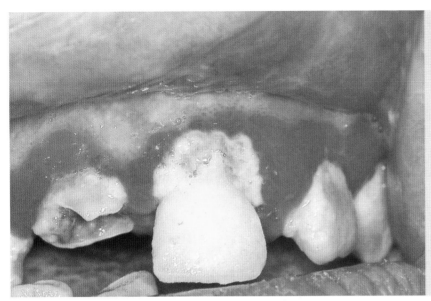

Fig. 27.28 von Willebrand's disease, erythema and hemorrhagic diathesis on the upper gingiva.

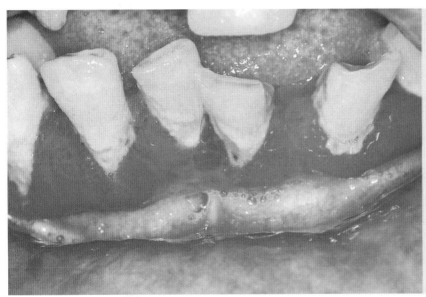

Fig. 27.29 von Willebrand's disease, erythema and hemorrhagic diathesis on the lower gingiva.

Myelodysplastic Syndromes

Key points

- A heterogeneous group of acquired disorders of the hematopoietic stem cells.
- They are characterized by quantitative and qualitative changes in two or more hematopoietic cell lines.
- The clinical manifestations include anemia, infections, and hemorrhage.
- Oral mucosal ulcerations and hemorrhage are common.

Introduction

Myelodysplastic syndromes is a heterogeneous group of acquired clonal disorders of the hematopoietic stem cells. They are characterized by a constellation of cytopenias, a usually hypercellular bone marrow, and several morphologic and cytogenetic disorders. Ineffective hematopoiesis leads to refractory anemia, thrombocytopenia, neutropenia, and monocytosis. In most cases, the disorders are idiopathic, although it may develop secondary to radiotherapy and chemotherapy and is more frequent in patients older than 60 years. Myelodysplastic syndromes are classified into seven groups by the World Health Organization (WHO) (2008) depending on cell lines criteria in the peripheral blood and the bone marrow and clinical features. These are as follows: (1) Refractory cytopenia with unilineage dysplasia (RCUD), (2) Refractory anemia with ring sideroblasts (RARS), (3) Refractory cytopenia with multilineage dysplasia (RCMD), (4) Refractory anemia with excess blasts 1 (RAEB-1), (5) Refractory anemia with excess blasts 2 (RAEB-2), (6) Myelodysplastic syndrome—unclassified (MDS-U), (7) MDS associated with isolated del(5q). Chronic myelomonocytic leukemia (CMML) was considered a type of MDS in the FAB classification, but the WHO classification includes it in another group of diseases. Finally, an International Prognostic Scoring System (IPSS) has been developed that classified patients by risk status based on the percentage of bone marrow blasts, cytogenetics, and the severity of cytopenias.

Clinical features

Clinically, MDSs are characterized by systemic symptoms (fatigue, fever, muscular weakness, etc.), anemia, multiple recurrent bacterial infections, and hemorrhage caused by the neutropenia and thrombocytopenia. The oral manifestations include persistent and recurrent ulceration, hemorrhage, usually gingival bleeding, candidiasis, and periodontitis (**Figs. 27.30–27.35**). Most patients are pale, while splenomegaly (30–50%) and lymphadenopathy may be present. The course may be indolent and the disease may present as a wasting illness. However, myelodysplastic syndromes are ultimately fatal disease. The diagnosis is based on clinical and laboratory criteria.

Differential diagnosis

- Acute myeloblastic leukemia
- Aplastic anemia
- Agranulocytosis
- Other causes of cytopenias
- Megaloblastic anemia
- Sweet's syndrome

Laboratory tests

Bone marrow and peripheral blood examination reveals both quantitative and morphologic disorders of all the blood cell lines.

Treatment

The treatment is the responsibility of the hematologist. It may include growth factors (G-CSF, GM-CSF), erythropoietin, immunosuppressive and chemotherapeutic agents, and allogenic stem cell transplantation.

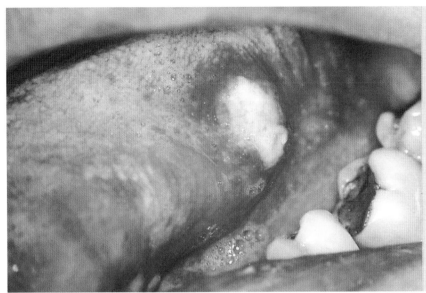

Fig. 27.30 Myelodysplastic syndrome, ulceration on the lateral border of the tongue.

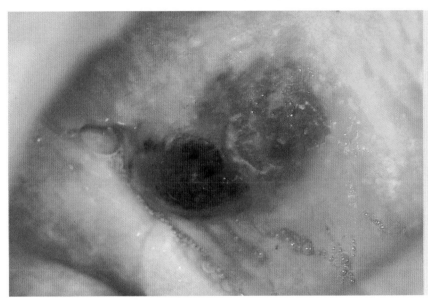

Fig. 27.31 Myelodysplastic syndrome, ulceration and hematoma on the buccal mucosa.

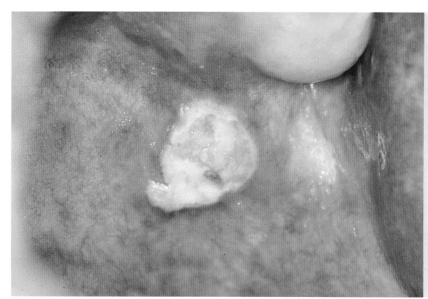

Fig. 27.32 Myelodysplastic syndrome, ulceration on the buccal mucosa.

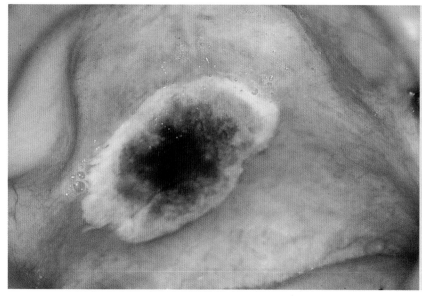

Fig. 27.33 Myelodysplastic syndrome, ulceration on the palatal mucosa.

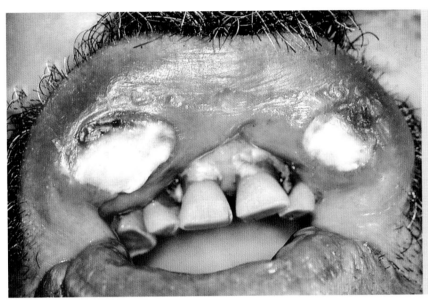

Fig. 27.34 Myelodysplastic syndrome, two ulcers on the mucosa of the upper lip.

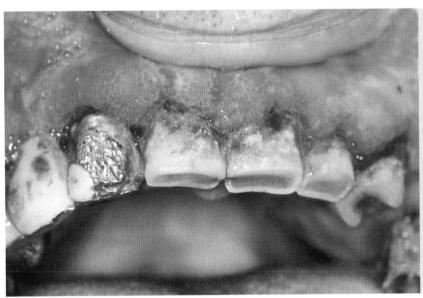

Fig. 27.35 Myelodysplastic syndrome, ulceration and bleeding of upper gingiva.

28 Gastrointestinal Diseases

Celiac Disease

Key points

- Celiac disease is an immune-mediated reaction to gluten.
- Gluten is a protein found in wheat and related grains such as rye and barley.
- The disorder has a genetic base as it develops in patients with genotype HLA-DQ2 (95%) and HLA-DQ8 (5%).
- The clinical spectrum includes *symptomatic* as well as silent cases.
- Aphthous or aphthous-like ulcers and dental enamel defects are the most common oral manifestations.

Introduction

Celiac disease is a common dietary disorder caused by an immunologic response to gluten, a storage protein found in wheat and related grains such as rye and barley, that results in damage to the proximal small intestinal mucosa with malabsorption of nutrients. Gluten intolerance only develops in people with the HLA-DQ2 (95%) and/or HLA-DQ8 (5%) class II molecules, which are present in 40% of the population. The worldwide prevalence is estimated to be 0.6 to 1% of the population. Gluten is broken in the intestine into *gliadin* (a gluten protein). Upon exposure to gliadin, the enzyme *tissue transglutaminase* modifies the protein. This results into anti-immunoglobulin A (anti-IgA) autoantibodies production against the above and a subsequent inflammatory reaction. Lesions are within the small intestine (villous atrophy) which leads to ineffective absorption of nutrients such as fat, proteins, vitamins, and minerals.

Clinical features

The severity of clinical manifestations depends on the extent of the small intestine that is affected. The clinical spectrum of celiac disease includes symptomatic cases with either intestinal or extraintestinal features as well as silent cases revealed only by serologic screening. Intestinal manifestations include indigestion, diarrhea, steatorrhea, abdominal distention, weight loss, and constipation. Extraintestinal manifestations include chronic fatigue, anemia, reduced bone mineral density, amenorrhea, joint and muscle pain, growth retardation, peripheral neuropathy, cutaneous and oral lesions. However, many patients may only experience mild symptoms or even be asymptomatic. The oral lesions include aphthous-like ulceration (20–30%) and less frequently atrophic glossitis, reduction of salivary flow, and enamel defects (**Fig. 28.1**).

In more than 10% of the patients, celiac disease coexists with dermatitis herpetiformis that is regarded as a cutaneous variant of the disease (**Fig. 28.2**). Additionally, most patients with dermatitis herpetiformis have intestinal histologic lesions that are compatible with celiac disease even if they are free of symptom and sign. Celiac disease may coexist with other autoimmune conditions such as Sjögren's syndrome, scleroderma, Addison's disease, diabetes mellitus type 1, and atrophic gastritis. A small percentage of patients who do not respond well to a gluten-free diet might develop T-cell non-Hodgkin's lymphoma. The final diagnosis of celiac disease should be based on a comprehensive evaluation of clinical, serologic, histologic, and genetic elements.

Differential diagnosis

- Other types of malabsorption
- Dermatitis herpetiformis
- Crohn's disease
- Ulcerative colitis

Laboratory tests

Measurement of serum IgA tissue transglutaminase (tTG) antibodies has the best diagnostic sensitivity. Also, the detection of IgA anti-endomysial antibodies (EMA) is nearly 100% specific for celiac disease. Antibodies to deamidated gliadin peptides (DGP) of the IgG class may also be useful in diagnosis. Additionally, biopsy and subsequent histopathologic examination of the small intestine reveal loss or blunting of intestinal villi, hypertrophy of the intestinal crypts, and extensive infiltration of the lamina propria with lymphocytes and plasma cells. Screening tests in children have also been tried during the last few years by detecting salivary anti-tTG IgA by serum radioimmunoassay (RIA). The presence of HLA-DQ2 or HLA-DQ8 alleles is an additional diagnostic criterion.

Treatment

The treatment is the responsibility of the gastroenterologist. The treatment of choice, usually with excellent results, is lifelong gluten-free diet. Additionally, supplements might be required such as iron, folic acid, calcium, and vitamins A, B, C, D.

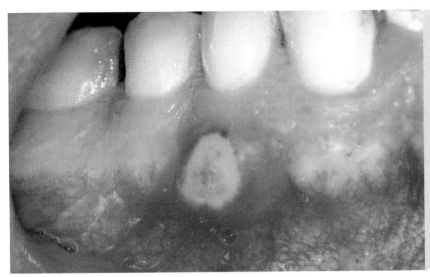

Fig. 28.1 Celiac disease, aphthous-like ulcer on the alveolar mucosa.

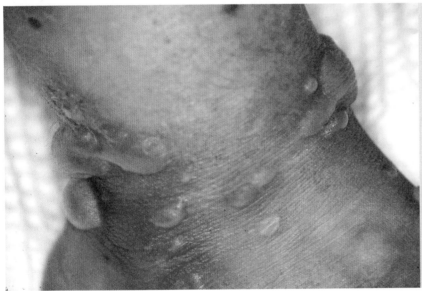

Fig. 28.2 Celiac disease, typical skin bullae in a child with dermatitis herpetiformis.

Crohn's Disease

Key points

- A chronic inflammatory bowel disorder.
- Can affect the ileum, colon, upper intestinal tract, and perianal area.
- Ulcerations, strictures, narrowing of the intestine, abscesses, and fistulas are common.
- The oral mucosa is affected in approximately 10 to 20% or more of the cases.

Introduction

Crohn's disease is a chronic, inflammatory bowel disease characterized by granulomatous inflammation. The disease may affect any part of the gastrointestinal system from the mouth to the anus and can cause strictures and narrowing of the ileum. In 30 to 40% of the cases, it is confined in the ileum; in 20% of the cases, in the colon; in 5%, in the upper intestinal tract; while in 30%, there is also perianal pathology (fissures, abscesses, fistulas). The etiology remains unknown. However, research findings suggest that immunologic reaction against microbial antigens may involve in the pathogenesis, combined with genetic, psychogenic, and dietary factors. The incidence of Crohn's disease is estimated in approximately 4 to 10 cases per 100,000 of the population.

Clinical features

The disease usually appears between 15 and 30 years. The main signs and symptoms are abdominal pain, diarrhea, rectal hemorrhage, weakness, weight loss, vomiting, and low-grade fever. More than 50% of the patients have extraintestinal manifestations such as arthralgias, arthritis, spondylitis, iritis or uveitis, liver and spleen involvement, and oral and cutaneous manifestations. The signs and symptoms depend on the organs affected by the disease and also the activity. The oral lesions may either precede or follow the intestinal involvement and occur in 10 to 20% or more of the patients. A wide spectrum of oral manifestations may be observed with more characteristic, the edema and granulomatous enlargements, that can be ulcerated. Multiple raised nodules of the buccal mucosa result in "*cobblestone*" appearance. Other common lesions include granulomatous lip swelling, angular cheilitis, gingival enlargement, nodules and ulceration in different parts of the mouth, aphthous-like ulcers, mucosal tags, taste disturbances, erythema, and exfoliation (**Figs. 28.3–28.6**). Cutaneous manifestations include erythema nodosum, pyoderma gangrenosum, and Sweet's syndrome. The oral lesions usually regress when the intestinal symptoms are in remission. The clinical diagnosis should be confirmed by the laboratory tests.

Differential diagnosis

- Ulcerative colitis
- Celiac disease
- Orofacial granulomatosis
- Cheilitis granulomatosa
- Melkersson-Rosenthal syndrome
- Cheilitis glandularis
- Sarcoidosis
- Tuberculosis
- AIDS

Laboratory tests

There is a pure correlation between the clinical features and laboratory findings. Blood tests are usually nonspecific as they reveal anemia, iron deficiency, leukocytosis, low albumin, and increased erythrocyte sedimentation rate (ESR) and C-reactive protein (CRP). Colonoscopy, bowel radiology, and histopathologic examination are more reliable investigations. Histologically, there is initially inflammatory infiltrate around the intestinal crypts, followed by epithelial ulceration. Gradually, the inflammation extends to the deeper layers forming noncaseating granulomas. Crypt microabscesses eventually form that lead to crypt atrophy and destruction. The granulomas

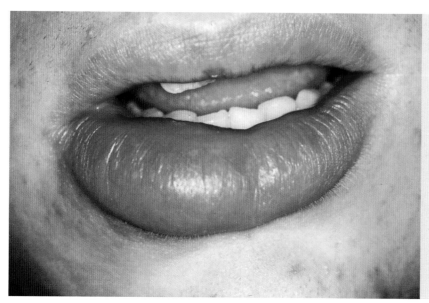

Fig. 28.3 Crohn's disease, cheilitis granulomatosa.

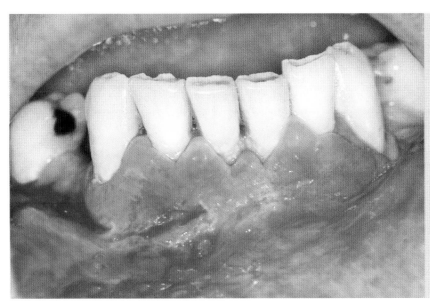

Fig. 28.4 Crohn's disease, gingival enlargement and vegetative ulceration of the mandibular vestibular mucosa.

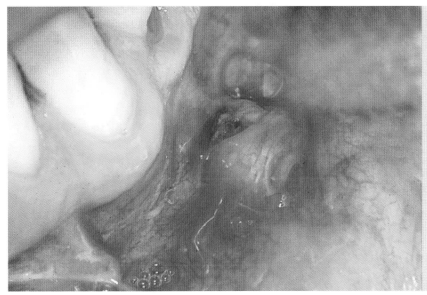

Fig. 28.5 Crohn's disease, ulcerated nodule on the lower vestibule.

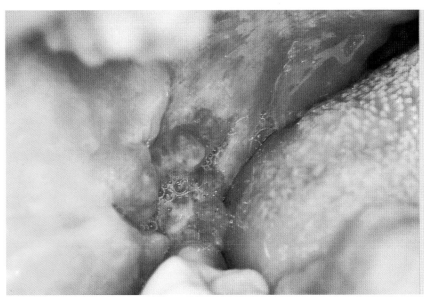

Fig. 28.6 Crohn's disease, vegetative ulceration on the retromolar area and the buccal mucosa.

are considered pathognomonic for the disease; however, their absence does not exclude it. Finally, immunologic test for perinuclear antineutrophil cytoplasmic antibodies (P-ANCA) and against intestinal microbiota helps toward the diagnosis.

Treatment

The treatment is the responsibility of the gastroenterologist. It may include exclusion diet, symptomatic treatment, and disease-specific treatment. The latter includes corticosteroids, immunosuppressive drugs, antibiotics (metronidazole, ciprofloxacin, etc.), 5-aminosalicylic acid agents (mesalamine), and lately, anti–tumor necrosis factor α [anti–TNF-α] treatment (infliximab, adalimumab, certolizumab). Surgical intervention is required for some complications.

Ulcerative Colitis

Key points
- A chronic inflammatory disorder of the colon mucosa.
- It is more common in nonsmokers and former smokers.
- The main symptoms and signs include bloody diarrhea, abdominal pain, and tenesmus.
- Oral manifestations are relatively rare.

Introduction

Ulcerative colitis is an idiopathic, chronic, inflammatory disease that involves the mucosa of the colon resulting in diffuse viability and erosions with bleeding. The etiology remains unclear. It is believed that the patient's immune system reacts abnormally to the bacteria present in the gastrointestinal system. Using clinical and laboratory criteria, it is classified into *mild*, *moderate*, and *severe*. It is more common in nonsmokers, while the signs and symptoms deteriorate when smokers cease the habit. Together with aphthous, ulcers are the only disorders where cigarette smoking appears to have a protective effect.

Clinical features

The clinical profile in ulcerative colitis is variable. The disease can affect individuals of any age and sex and seems to have familial predisposition. Usually, the symptoms appear between 15 and 30 years. The main clinical sign is hemorrhagic diarrhea. Other signs and symptoms include tenesmus, abdominal pain, bowel sensitivity, low-grade fever, nausea, weight loss, arthralgia, anemia, etc. The severity of signs and symptoms depends on the disease activity and the extent of the intestinal involvement. Intraorally, aphthous or aphthous-like ulcers that tend to recur are common as angular cheilitis (**Figs. 28.7, 28.8**). Rarely, pyostomatitis vegetans may be observed. Cutaneous lesions may include pyodermatitis vegetans, pyoderma gangrenosum, erythema nodosum, and

vasculitis (**Fig. 28.9**). Finally, in 5 to 10% of the patients, temporomandibular joint arthritis may occur.

Differential diagnosis
- Other types of colitis
- Crohn's disease
- Celiac disease

Laboratory tests

The degree of abnormality of the hematocrit, sedimentation rate, and serum albumin reflects disease activity. Colonoscopy or sigmoidoscopy, biopsy and histopathologic examination as well as imaging can be useful toward the diagnosis.

Treatment

The treatment is the responsibility of the gastroenterologist. It aims to the acute phase control and of the recurrences thereafter. Medication of treatment includes mesalamine, sulfasalazine, corticosteroids, immunosuppressives, and anti–TNF-α agents (infliximab). If the conservative approach fails, surgical intervention is recommended.

Pyostomatitis Vegetans

Key points
- It is associated with inflammatory bowel diseases, usually ulcerative colitis and rarely Crohn's disease.
- The disease affects the oral mucosa and is considered as the equivalent of the cutaneous pyodermatitis vegetans.
- Clinically, multiple small vesicles on an erythematous, inflamed surface in a snail-track arrangement is the prominent feature.

Introduction

Pyostomatitis vegetans is a rare, noninfectious, benign, oral mucosal vesicular bullous disease of unknown etiology. The disease often coexists with ulcerative colitis and rarely with Crohn's disease. It is believed that immunologic and microbial factors play a role in the pathogenesis.

Clinical features

The disease affects most commonly males than females (ratio 3:1) with a preference for young and middle-aged individuals. Clinically, pyostomatitis vegetans is characterized by multiple, small, gray-to-yellow pustules, in a linear pattern, that coalesce

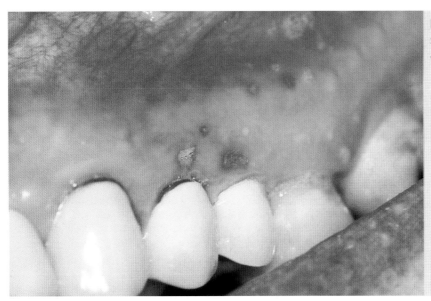

Fig. 28.7 Ulcerative colitis, multiple small ulcers on the upper gingiva and alveolar mucosa.

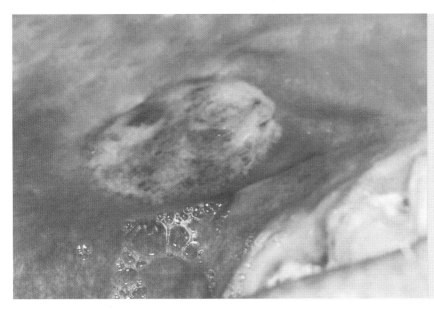

Fig. 28.8 Ulcerative colitis, large, aphthous-like ulcer on the upper labial mucosa.

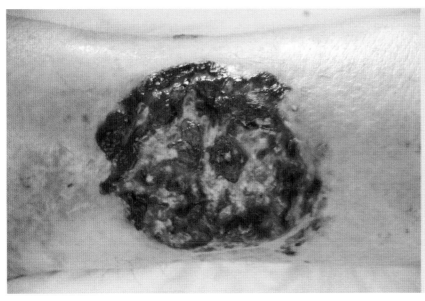

Fig. 28.9 Ulcerative colitis, pyoderma gangrenosum on the skin.

and develop on an erythematous surface (**Figs. 28.10, 28.11**). The pustules then rupture, leaving painful shallow "*snail-track*" ulceration. The most commonly affected sites are the buccal mucosa, gingiva, soft palate, uvula, and labial and vestibular mucosa. The oral lesions usually appear at the same time or after the intestinal symptoms and very rarely may precede them. Rarely, in patients with ulcerative colitis and Crohn's disease cutaneous lesions appear that are defined as *pyodermatitis vegetans* and *pyoderma gangrenosum*. The clinical diagnosis of the oral lesions has to be confirmed by histology and diagnosis of the intestinal disease.

Differential diagnosis
- Herpetiform aphthous ulceration
- Adamantiades-Behçet's disease
- Herpetic gingivostomatitis
- Dermatitis herpetiformis
- Pemphigus vulgaris
- Bullous pemphigoid
- Drug reactions

Pathology

Histologically, pyostomatitis vegetans is characterized by the presence of intraepithelial or subepithelial microabscesses that contain multiple eosinophils and neutrophils. The underlying lamina propria presents with eosinophilic, neutrophilic, and lymphocytic inflammatory infiltrate. Direct immunofluorescence is negative for deposits of IgA, IgG, and C3 and this result is helpful in distinguishing from pemphigus and pemphigoid.

Treatment

The control of the underlying intestinal disease is of great importance toward the treatment of pyostomatitis vegetans. The oral lesions respond well to systemic corticosteroids. A suggested course would be 30 to 40 mg/d of prednisolone, for 7 to 10 days, gradually decreasing, completed within 3 to 4 weeks. Azathioprine or dapsone can be used in parallel with corticosteroids as sparing agents. The oral lesions are likely to recur with intestinal disease exacerbation.

Acrodermatitis Enteropathica

Key points
- It is caused by zinc deficiency (< 50 µg/dL).
- The zinc deficiency may be *genetic* (acrodermatitis enteropathica) or *acquired*.
- Common clinical characteristics are dermatitis, alopecia, and diarrhea.
- Cheilitis and stomatitis are common.

Introduction

Zinc plays a critical function in more than 200 enzymes that regulate protein, lipid, and nucleic acids, synthesis, and degradation. Zinc deficiency may be *genetic* or *acquired*. The genetic form referred to as *acrodermatitis enteropathica*. It is a rare autosomal recessive disease, caused by a defect in the intestinal absorption of zinc, due to mutation in the gene that encodes the zinc transporter, *SLC39A4*.

The acquired form is the result of reduced zinc intake or absorption and may occur in alcoholic disease, HIV infection, malignancies, cystic fibrosis, pregnancy, and drugs. The clinical features and the disease progression may be similar in both forms.

Clinical features

Acrodermatitis enteropathica usually starts within days or weeks from birth and is characterized by lesions on the skin and nails, alopecia, and diarrhea. The cutaneous lesions start as erythematous areas, followed by clusters of vesicles and bullae. As these are eventually covered by crust-forming scabs, the skin takes an eczematous, psoriasiform appearance. *Candida albicans* and bacteria superinfection is common. The dermatitis is characteristically located around the natural orifices, the eyelids, the elbows and knees, the extremities, and around the nails (**Fig. 28.12**). Classically, the perioral area and commissures are affected, while the oral mucosa is rarely involved with erosive lesions (**Fig. 28.13**). Photophobia, apathy, anorexia, hypogeusia, anemia, and developmental disorders are common. The clinical diagnosis should be confirmed by laboratory tests.

Differential diagnosis
- Epidermolysis bullosa
- Bullous diseases of infancy
- Staphylococcal scalded skin syndrome

Laboratory tests

A low plasma zinc, usually less than 50 µg/dL (normal range 70–150 µg/dL), is observed. A low serum alkaline phosphatase is also present.

Treatment

The first line of treatment in acrodermatitis enteropathica is the administration of zinc sulfate or zinc gluconate (2–3 mg/kg/d). For the acquired form, 1 to 2 mg/kg/d is suggested. Lifelong zinc supplements and repeated serum zinc determination are required in acrodermatitis enteropathica.

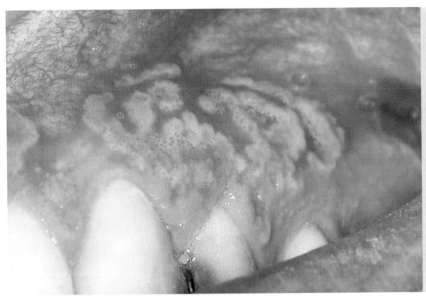

Fig. 28.10 Pyostomatitis vegetans, multiple coalescing pustules on the gingiva and alveolar mucosa.

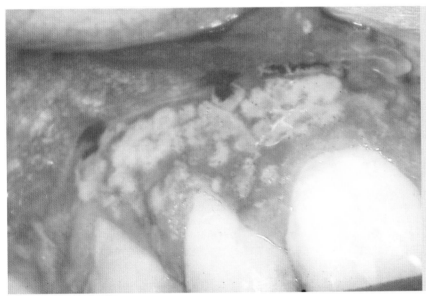

Fig. 28.11 Pyostomatitis vegetans, multiple coalescing pustules on the gingiva and alveolar mucosa.

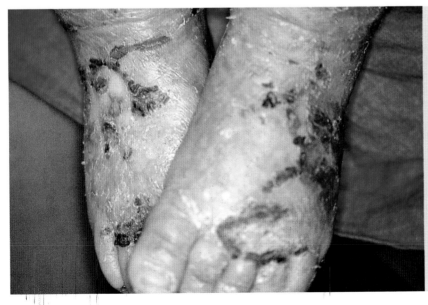

Fig. 28.12 Acrodermatitis entero-pathica, eczematous lesions, bullae, and ulceration on the feet.

Peutz-Jeghers Syndrome

Key points
- An autosomal dominant condition in 70%, while 30% of the cases are caused by new mutations.
- Clinically, it is characterized by multiple melanotic macules on the oral mucosa, lips, and the skin.
- A characteristic finding is the hamartomatous polyps in the gastrointestinal tract.
- Development of neoplasia is relatively common after the 50th year of life.

Introduction

Peutz-Jeghers syndrome, also known as hereditary intestinal polyposis syndrome, is a rare genetic disorder transmitted by an autosomal dominant inheritance in 70% of the cases. In 30% of the cases, the disease is caused by new mutations. Where the autosomal dominant type is involved, the mutation is on the *STK11* gene (66–94%), on chromosome 19p13.3, which is responsible for the serine/threonine kinase 11. Several other genes are involved in the syndrome that lead to various clinical phenotypes (number of polyps, melanotic macules, neoplasias).

Clinical features

Clinically, multiple hamartomatous intestinal polyps are the most important finding. They are benign hamartomas of approximately 0.5 to 7 cm in diameter (**Fig. 28.14**). They may cause intestinal bleeding, abdominal pain, and rarely ischemic necrosis, usually during the second or third decade of life. However, the polyps occasionally may remain asymptomatic. Despite the benign nature of polyps, in patients with Peutz-Jeghers syndrome, an increased risk of malignant neoplasms in the gastrointestinal tract, pancreas, lungs, breast, and ovaries, usually after the 50th year of life, may occur. The cutaneous lesions present with multiple, small, round, ovoid, or irregular shape of brown, or black-brown macules of 1 to 10 mm in diameter. These favor the perioral region, the nose and the eyes, as well as the cheeks (**Fig. 28.15**). Similar pigmented macules can be found on the lips and the oral mucosa, especially on the tongue and buccal mucosa, and rarely on the palate and gingiva (**Fig. 28.16**). The conjunctivae may also be affected. The perioral and oral lesions are the most early and characteristic signs of the disease, occurring in more than 90% of the cases, and usually appear after the first year of life. The clinical diagnosis should be confirmed by laboratory tests.

Differential diagnosis
- Addison's disease
- Ephelides
- Laugier-Hunziker syndrome
- Albright's syndrome
- Gardner's syndrome
- Cowden's disease
- Normal oral pigmentation

Pathology

Histopathologic examination of the mucocutaneous lesions reveals increased melanin production, while the number of melanocytes remains normal. The intestinal polyps are a benign adenomatous hyperplasia without cellular atypia. Stomach and intestinal endoscopy is important for the diagnosis.

Treatment

Treatment is not required for the mucocutaneous lesions. The intestinal polyps are surgically removed if they cause symptoms. Regular monitoring of the known cases is recommended due to the increased risk of malignancies.

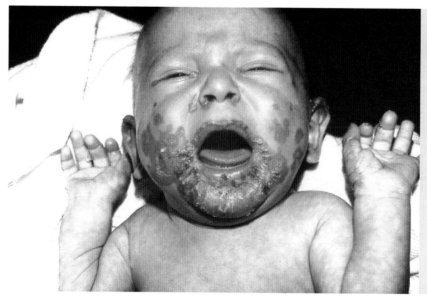

Fig. 28.13 Acrodermatitis enteropathica, characteristic eczematous lesions affecting the perioral skin, lips, and commissures.

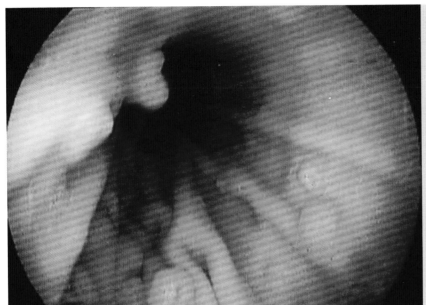

Fig. 28.14 Peutz-Jeghers syndrome, intestinal polyps.

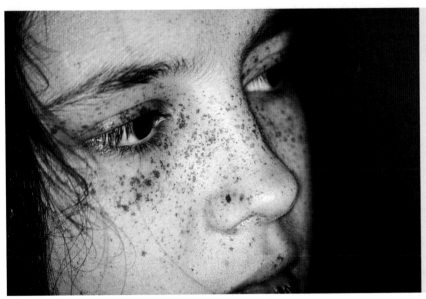

Fig. 28.15 Peutz-Jeghers syndrome, multiple brown-black macules on the face.

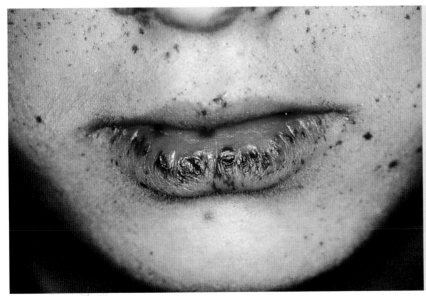

Fig. 28.16 Peutz-Jeghers syndrome, multiple brown-black macules on the lower lip and the skin.

29 Renal Diseases

Uremic Stomatitis

Key points

- Uremic stomatitis occurs in severe acute or chronic renal failure.
- It is caused by salivary urea breakdown and the production of ammonia.
- On the oral mucosa, thick, white plaques are formed, and ulceration is rare.

Introduction

Uremic stomatitis is a relatively rare complication of renal failure. Patients with acute or chronic renal failure have increased levels of urea and other nitrogen-containing products in the peripheral blood. Uremic stomatitis usually occurs when the urea levels in the blood exceed 300 mg/100 mL. It is believed that the urea produced by the microbial flora is deposited and breaks down the salivary urea. This leads to ammonia production that damages the oral mucosa.

Clinical features

Two forms of uremic stomatitis are recognized, the *ulcerative* and *nonulcerative*. The ulcerative form is characterized by painful, superficial, and irregular ulcers of different sizes. These are covered by a white-brown or black pseudomembrane (**Fig. 29.1**). The nonulcerative form presents with creased, thick, white plaques that are painful and develop on an inflammatory surface. The floor of the mouth, buccal mucosa, tongue, and rarely the gingiva are more frequently affected (**Figs. 29.2, 29.3**). Hemorrhage and hematomas may also be observed. Candidiasis and other opportunistic bacterial and viral infections are common. Unpleasant taste, xerostomia, and halitosis with characteristic of ammonia or urea smell in the breath are common symptoms. The clinical diagnosis should be confirmed by laboratory tests.

Differential diagnosis

- Pseudomembranous candidiasis
- Cinnamon contact stomatitis
- Hairy leukoplakia
- Leukoplakia
- White sponge nevus
- Stomatitis due to drugs
- Necrotizing ulcerative stomatitis

Laboratory tests

The blood and urine levels of urea should be determined.

Treatment

The oral lesions improve after 2 to 4 weeks of hemodialysis and improvement of the renal function occurs. Topically, good oral hygiene and the use of oxygen-releasing mouthwashes are recommended. Antifungal or antibiotics are administered only where superinfection is present.

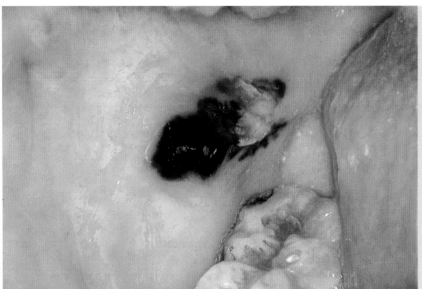

Fig. 29.1 Uremic stomatitis, ulceration covered by a necrotic black pseudomembrane on the buccal mucosa.

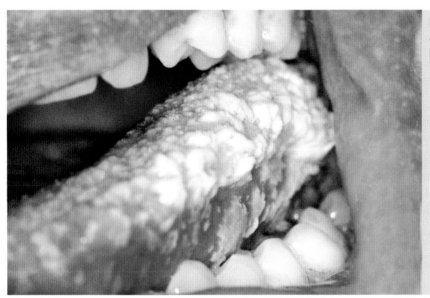

Fig. 29.2 Uremic stomatitis, white, elevated, creased plaques on the lateral border of the tongue.

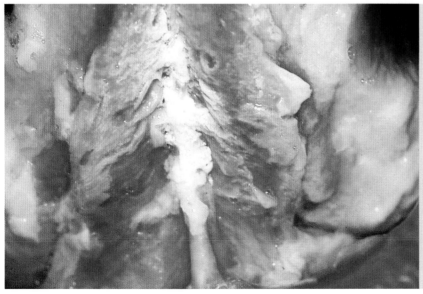

Fig. 29.3 Uremic stomatitis, white, creased surfaces on the ventral aspect of the tongue and the frenum.

30 Metabolic Disorders

Amyloidosis

Key points

- A heterogeneous group of metabolic disorders due to abnormal deposition of amyloid within tissues.
- Clinically, amyloidosis is classified into two major forms: the *systemic* and the *localized*.
- The most common and severe form is primary systemic amyloid light chain (AL) amyloidosis which may be associated with multiple myeloma.
- The oral mucosa is involved often and at the early stages of primary systemic (AL) amyloidosis.
- Positive staining of amyloid material with Congo red with a characteristic green, birefringence under polarized light is the prominent histologic pattern.

Introduction

Amyloidosis is a relatively rare, heterogeneous group of metabolic disorders that is characterized by abnormal extracellular deposition of amyloid, an amorphous fibrillar proteinaceous material, within various tissues and organs. The origin of amyloid is not exactly known, as well as the precise epidemiology. Amyloidosis is clinically classified into (1) *systemic (generalized)* forms (primary systemic [AL], secondary systemic [AA], hemodialysis-related, and genetic-inherited] with involvement of several tissues and organs and (2) *localized forms* (cutaneous, endocrine, cerebral) in which amyloid deposits are limited to a single organ. Amyloidosis may be classified on the basis of the specific precursor protein—chemical classification (named using an abbreviation of the precursor protein with the letter A).

Clinical features

Primary systemic (AL) amyloidosis is the most severe and most common form of the disease and in 10 to 20% of the cases is associated with multiple myeloma. It affects individuals older than 50 years and has male predilection with a ratio of 3:1. The prognosis is poor as death follows approximately 2 years after the disease commences usually due to renal or heart failure. Clinically, it can affect the gastrointestinal tract, heart, kidneys, joints, skeletal muscles, central nervous system, vessels, skin, oral mucosa, and rarely other organs. The most common presenting symptoms are fatigue, weakness, weight loss, edema, dyspnea, hoarseness, bleeding, pain, carpal tunnel syndrome, etc. Cutaneous and oral mucosa manifestations may occur in approximately 30 to 50% of patients. The most common cutaneous lesions are purpura, petechiae, papules, nodules, rarely bullous eruptions, ulcers, alopecia, and waxy discoloration of the skin (**Fig. 30.1**). The oral mucosa is involved early in the course of the disease, and the most frequent manifestations are petechiae, ecchymoses, papules, nodules (**Fig. 30.2**), macroglossia (**Fig. 30.3**), ulcers, minor and major salivary gland infiltration, xerostomia, regional lymph node enlargement, and rarely hemorrhagic bullae formation (**Fig. 30.4**). The tongue is characteristically enlarged, firm, and indurated with red-yellowish nodules along the lateral border. The gingiva is usually clinically normal. The deep red hue of oral lesions is a typical feature of oral amyloidosis, due to amyloid deposition on the vascular wall that causes their rupture. The main oral symptoms include dysphagia, dysphonia, and xerostomia.

In secondary systemic (AA) amyloidosis nodules are noticed in the oral cavity. The diseases that are associated with secondary systemic amyloidosis are tuberculosis, sarcoidosis, osteomyelitis, rheumatoid arthritis, ulcerative colitis, hemodialysis, Hodgkin's disease, and other malignancies. In this form, amyloid is mainly deposited in the liver, kidneys, spleen, and the adrenals. The localized (organ limited) amyloidosis is very rare in the oral tissues, and common in the skin, thyroid gland, diabetes mellitus type 2, cerebral disease, Alzheimer's disease. It does not have systemic manifestations and is of good prognosis. The clinical diagnosis of all forms of amyloidosis has to be confirmed by histologic and immunohistochemical criteria.

Differential diagnosis

- Crohn's disease
- Multiple neurofibromatosis
- Lipoid proteinosis
- Mucopolysaccharidosis
- Kaposi's sarcoma
- Pemphigus
- Bullous pemphigoid
- Macroglossia due to other causes

Pathology

Histopathologic examination is required for the clinical diagnosis of amyloidosis. In hematoxylin-eosin stained sections, amyloid appears as amorphous, eosinophilic material. With Congo red staining amyloid had an orange-red color and it has a characteristic green birefringence under polarized light (*dichroism*). Additionally, other special stains of amyloid are methyl violet that stains amyloid red (metachromasia) and the fluorescent thioflavin T that gives a characteristic green stain. Immunohistochemical techniques can be used to determine other specific proteins.

Treatment

There is no specific therapy and the treatment is usually aimed at alleviating the symptoms and does not lead to amyloid dissolution.

The types of treatment that have been used include corticosteroids, colchicine, melphalan, anthracycline, chlorambucil, dimethyl sulfoxide (DMSO), bortezomib, autologous hematopoietic stem cell transplantation, but with poor results.

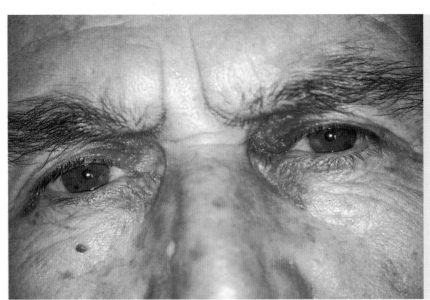

Fig. 30.1 Amyloidosis, multiple papules and nodules on the eyelid.

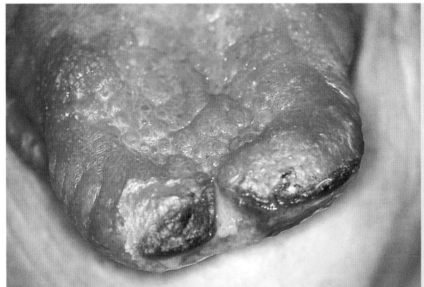

Fig. 30.2 Amyloidosis, two red-brown nodules on the tip of the tongue.

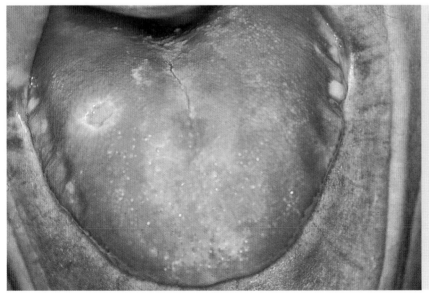

Fig. 30.3 Amyloidosis, macroglossia.

Lipoid Proteinosis

Key points

- A rare autosomal recessive disorder due to mutations in the extracellular matrix protein 1 (*ECM1*) gene.
- It is caused by the deposition of an amorphous hyaline-like material around blood vessels and in the connective tissues.
- The disease primarily affects the skin, oral mucosa, larynx, and the brain.
- An early clinical sign is hoarseness and the inability of the baby to cry.

Introduction

Lipoid proteinosis, or hyalinosis cutis et mucosae, or Urbach-Wiethe disease, is a rare, autosomal, recessive, metabolic disorder due to mutations in the *ECM1* gene. It is characterized by the deposition of an amorphous hyaline-like material around blood vessels and in the connective tissues of the mucous membranes and skin. The disease primarily affects the skin, oral mucosa, larynx, and rarely other organs.

Clinical features

The first and early clinical sign of lipoid proteinosis is hoarseness and the inability of the baby to cry, due to the deposition of a glycoprotein and lipids containing amorphous material on the vocal cords and the larynx. Cutaneous lesions usually appear during the second year of life. Initially, blisters and hemorrhagic crusts appear mainly on the skin of the face and extremities. Subsequently, papules, nodules, and plaques are observed of a few millimeters to 0.5 cm in diameter. These are of yellow discoloration and predominantly affect the face (**Fig. 30.5**), eyelids, neck, axillae, hands and elbows, scrotum, knees, and scalp (**Fig. 30.6**). Later, scars are formed that are the typical cutaneous changes. Verrucous hyperkeratotic lesions may develop on the extensor surfaces of the elbows, knees, and hands. The oral manifestations are early, common, and may become more severe with aging. In early stage, oral vesicles and hemorrhagic crusts may often develop in association with trauma. Induration of the lip mucosa and diffuse infiltration of the tongue are common. By the second decade, nodular lesions appear on the lip and papular lesions on the palate and tongue. Progressively, the affected mucosa becomes paler and pitted in structure. The lingual frenulum becomes indurated, thick, and short, resulting in reduced mobility of the tongue (**Fig. 30.7**). Finally, the oral mucosa becomes firm and glossy with increased induration, fissures, and scarring. Stenosis of the major salivary gland ducts and openings, hypodontia, and enamel hypoplasia or aplasia have also been reported. Dysphagia and difficulty in swallowing may also be encountered due to oral, pharyngeal, or esophageal involvement. The mucosa of the vagina and the anus is less often involved. Finally, neurologic disorders such as seizures and abnormal behavior are common. Usually, the disease has a slowly progressive course that is compatible with a normal life. The diagnosis is predominantly based on the history and the clinical features and less on the laboratory findings.

Differential diagnosis

- Systemic sclerosis
- Amyloidosis
- Mucopolysaccharidosis
- Erythropoietic protoporphyria
- Pseudoxanthoma elasticum
- Papular mucinosis

Pathology

Histologic examination reveals great deposition of amorphous, eosinophilic hyaline-like material around the vascular wall and within the connective tissues. This becomes more obvious with the periodic acid–Schiff (PAS) stain. In mature lesions, hyperkeratosis and papillomatosis is observed.

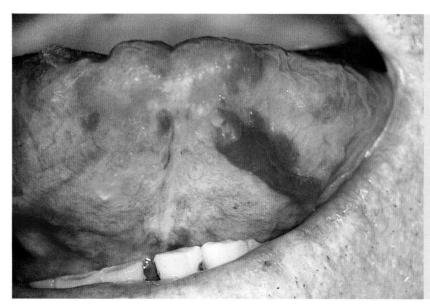

Fig. 30.4 Amyloidosis, hemorrhagic bullae, and ecchymoses on the tongue.

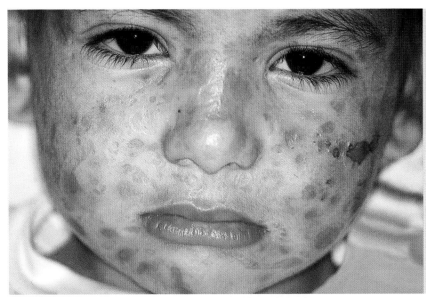

Fig. 30.5 Lipoid proteinosis, nodules and scars on the face.

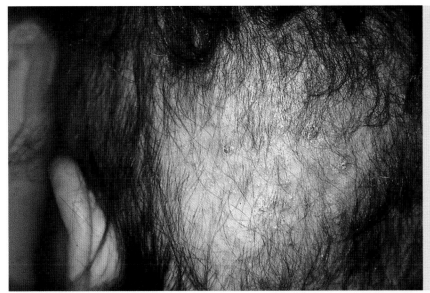

Fig. 30.6 Lipoid proteinosis, atrophy and alopecia of the skull.

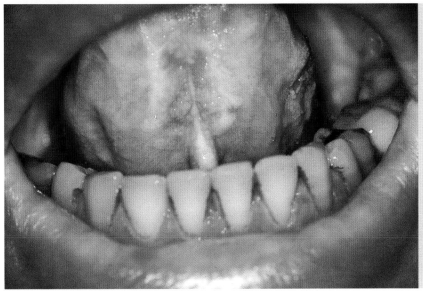

Fig. 30.7 Lipoid proteinosis, short and thick frenum and enlargement of the tongue.

449

Type IV collagen, laminin, and neutral mucopolysaccharides and hyaluronic acid may be demonstrated by Alcian blue and hyaluronidase staining. Radiographic imaging of the skull can offer diagnostic help as there can be symmetrical, bilateral calcification within the temporal lobes.

Treatment

There is no effective therapy. Treatment is symptomatic. Poor results have been recorded from the systemic use of retinoids, D-penicillamine, and oral dimethyl sulfoxide. Plastic surgery can offer help in selected patients.

Mucopolysaccharidoses—Hurler's Syndrome

Key points
- A group of genetic disorders characterized by a deficiency of lysosomal enzymes that participate in the catabolism of glycosaminoglycans.
- Hurler's syndrome is the most severe form and is caused by a deficiency in α-L-iduronidase that results in the accumulation of heparan sulfate and dermatan sulfate within the tissues.
- Oral lesions are common.

Introduction

Mucopolysaccharidoses are due to mutation in several genes that encode the enzymes that participate in the catabolism of glycosaminoglycans. Hurler's syndrome is the most common and severe form of the group, inherited as an autosomal recessive trait. The basic defect is the lack of the enzyme α-L-iduronidase, resulting in the accumulation and deposition of heparan sulfate and dermatan sulfate within the tissues. That manifests through various disorders in several tissues and organs.

Clinical features

The most common clinical signs and symptoms are coarse facies, developmental delay and mental retardation, skeletal abnormalities, joint stiffness, chondrodystrophy, corneal clouding, cardiovascular anomalies, hepatosplenomegaly, and hematologic disorders (**Fig. 30.8**). The oral manifestations are multiple and include macroglossia, macrocheilia, and gingival overgrowth that may cover the crowns of the teeth particularly in the anterior part of the jaws (**Fig. 30.9**). Numerous impacted teeth, large interdental spaces, teeth dislocation and abrasion, and diminished temporomandibular joint mobility may occur. Cutaneous manifestations may include thickening of the skin, hypertrichosis, and dermal melanocytosis. The clinical diagnosis should be confirmed by laboratory tests.

Differential diagnosis
- Other forms of mucopolysaccharidoses
- Amyloidosis

Laboratory tests

Screening tests include urine examination for increased amounts of mucopolysaccharides. The histochemical profile indicates the presence of lymphocytes or skin fibroblasts with characteristic vacuoles or granules in the peripheral blood. Finally, genetic mutation analysis can offer diagnostic help before birth.

Treatment

There is no effective systemic treatment. Symptomatic and supportive interventions play a role in the treatment. However, nowadays bone marrow transplants have been reported to improve some features of the disease. Enzyme replacement therapies are additional therapeutic options and currently a lot of interest is in gene therapy.

Glycogen Storage Disease, Type 1b

Key features
- The glycogen storage diseases are a group of genetic disorders involving the metabolic pathways of glycogen.
- Eleven types have been recognized depending on the specific enzyme deficiency.
- Type 1b is caused by a transporter deficiency of the glucose-6-phosphate.
- Glycogen is deposited mainly in the liver and the muscles and to a lesser degree in the kidneys, the bowel, and the red and white blood cells.
- Oral manifestations occur in type 1b.

Introduction

The glycogen storage diseases are a group of genetic disorders involving the metabolic pathways of glycogen. They are classified into 11 types (I-XI) depending on the type of enzyme deficiency. Type I represents 25% of all types and is implicated in 1 in 100,000 births. There are two subtypes, Ia and Ib. Type Ia is caused by deficiency of the enzyme glucose-6-phosphatase in the liver, kidneys, and other organs while type Ib is caused by a deficiency of glucose-6-phosphatase transporter. Both enzymes functions revolve around the breakdown of glycogen and its subsequent conversion into free glucose molecules to be used for the body's energy needs. This deficiency results in glycogen accumulation, leading to a plethora of disorders of various systems and organs. Glycogen storage disease type Ib is transmitted through the autosomal recessive pattern of inheritance.

Clinical features

The disease is first noticed during infancy and its main manifestations include hypoglycemia, hyperlipidemia, hepatomegaly, enlarged kidneys, bleeding diathesis, delayed physical development, and a characteristic facial appearance known as "*doll's face*" (**Fig. 30.10**). The patients present with quantitative

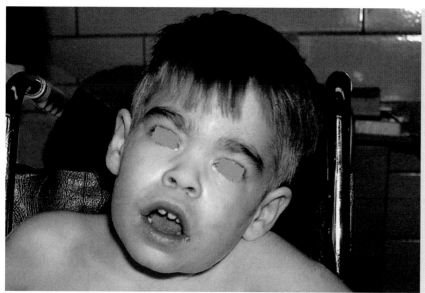

Fig. 30.8 Hurler's syndrome, characteristic facial appearance with depressed nasal bridge, open mouth, hypertelorism, and large ears.

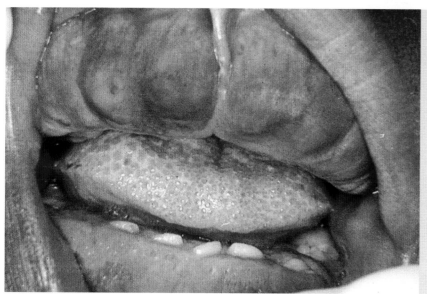

Fig. 30.9 Hurler's syndrome, prominent enlargement of the upper and lower gingiva that result in burying the clinical crown of teeth.

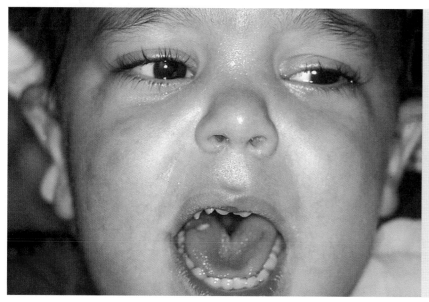

Fig. 30.10 Glycogen storage disease type Ib, characteristic "doll's face."

and functional disorders of the peripheral neutrophils that make the patient prone to recurrent bacterial and fungal infections. Chronic pancreatitis, ulcerative colitis, and Crohn's disease may also occur.

Oral manifestations include gingivitis and aggressive periodontal disease and recurrent ulceration. The oral ulcers appear as deep punched-out lesions, a few millimeters to several centimeters in size, covered by a white pseudomembrane (**Fig. 30.11**). Other features may include macroglossia, deep arched palate, viral, bacterial, and fungal infections (**Fig. 30.12**).

Differential diagnosis

- Acatalasia
- Hypophosphatasia
- Cyclic neutropenia
- Congenital neutropenia
- Chédiak-Higashi syndrome
- Mediterranean fever
- Diabetes mellitus (type 1)

Pathology

Liver biopsy and subsequent histologic examination confirms the clinical diagnosis. Blood tests reveal hypoglycemia and increased triglycerides, cholesterol, transaminases, uric acid, and creatine kinase.

Treatment

The treatment is symptomatic and is best to be left to pediatricians and other specialists. High level of oral hygiene and the use of antiseptic mouthwashes are recommended. Antibiotics and antifungals are administered in the case of oral infections.

Cystic Fibrosis

Key points

- Transmitted via the autosomal recessive type of inheritance.
- The mutation of the gene responsible for the coding of CFTR protein which is responsible for the chloride ion transport across the cell membrane.
- It affects almost all exocrine glands with emphasis on the lungs and the digestive system.
- Rarely affects the salivary glands.

Introduction

Cystic fibrosis is a genetic disease of poor prognosis that is transmitted by an autosomal recessive type of inheritance. The disease is caused by mutation in the cystic fibrosis transmembrane conductance regulator (*GFTR*) gene located on chromosome 7 that results in altered chloride ion transport and water flow across the apical surfaces of epithelial cells. More than 1,000 mutations in the gene that encodes CFTR have been described and at least 250 can cause clinical abnormalities. The disease is characterized by a dysfunction of almost all exocrine glands, but mainly the pulmonary and gastrointestinal systems and more rarely the salivary glands. It is the most common cause of pulmonary disease during childhood and puberty. The median survival age is more than 35 years.

Clinical manifestations

The main features include manifestations from the pulmonary and gastrointestinal tracts and include a dry cough, sputum production, great reduction of pulmonary secretions, hemoptysis, and recurrent pulmonary infections, mainly due to *Pseudomonas aeruginosa*. Hepatic and pancreatic disorders, fat-soluble vitamin deficiencies, sinusitis, purulent nasal discharge, constipation, abdominal pain, bulky, foul-smelling and greasy stools, excess sweating, with a characteristic salty taste, and finger clubbing are also common (**Fig. 30.13**). Developmental delay,

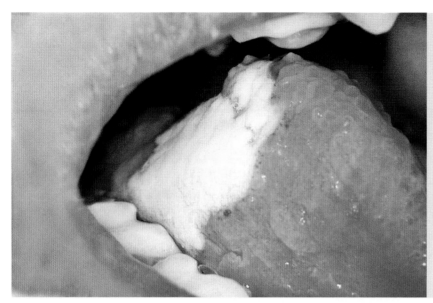

Fig. 30.11 Glycogen storage disease type Ib, large ulceration on the lateral border of the tongue.

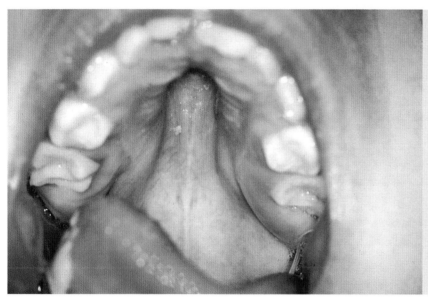

Fig. 30.12 Glycogen storage disease type Ib, high-arched palate.

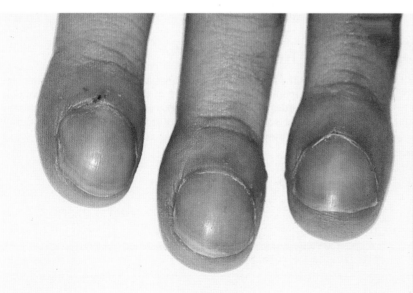

Fig. 30.13 Cystic fibrosis, finger clubbing.

loss of appetite and weight loss, and nausea may also be seen. Enlargement of the lower lip can be a common finding due to involvement of the minor salivary glands. Xerostomia and gingivitis can also be noticed (**Fig. 30.14**). Patients with cystic fibrosis have an increased risk of malignancies of the gastrointestinal tract, osteopenia, and arthropathies. The diagnosis is usually done within the first 2 to 3 years of life. However, in more than one-third, the diagnosis is made during the adult life.

Differential diagnosis

- Mucopolysaccharidosis
- Lipoid proteinosis
- Cheilitis granulomatosa
- Cheilitis glandularis

Laboratory tests

Special biochemical analysis is required. The measurement of immunoreactive trypsinogen (IRT) is used for screening in newborn babies, where increased amounts will require further investigation. The quantitative pilocarpine iontophoresis sweat test reveals elevated chloride and sodium level (> 60 mEq/L) in the sweat of patients. Genotyping diagnostic investigation should be pursued if the sweat test is repeatedly negative, but there is a high clinical suspicion of cystic fibrosis. Chest radiograph and other biochemical investigations of the lungs, stools, and pancreas can also help toward the definite diagnosis.

Treatment

The treatment is symptomatic and supportive and consists of many different elements. It is performed by a group of specialists and needs to be supervised by a specialist pediatrician. Lung transplantation is currently the only definitive treatment for advanced cystic fibrosis. Gene therapy had been pursued and could be the therapy of the future.

Xanthomas

Key points

- Common lesions due to a lipid metabolism disruption that are subsequently stored in macrophages.
- They are caused by either topical dysfunction on a cellular level or are the result of a systemic disruption in lipid metabolism.
- The lesions appear mainly on the skin and rarely on the oral mucosa.
- Cutaneous and oral xanthomas can signal the presence of an underlying hyperlipidemia or monoclonal gammopathy.

Introduction

Xanthomas present as macules and papules to nodules and plaques of yellowish color and develop as a result of intracellular and dermal deposition of lipid. The major lipid stored is usually cholesterol ester, although primarily triglycerides may be present. Their presence indicates a systemic disruption in lipid metabolism or a topical dysfunction on a cellular level. Xanthomas affect both sexes at any age.

Clinical features

Cutaneous xanthomas that are linked with hyperlipidemia are classified into six types. The most common is *xanthelasma palpebrarum*, usually affecting the eyelids. They are bilateral and asymptomatic, appearing as soft yellow papules or nodules around the eyelids (**Fig. 30.15**). Xanthomas occur often in cutaneous areas that are subject to mild pressure or friction and repeated minor trauma. They are rare in the oral mucosa and when present may affect the labial mucosa, buccal mucosa, and the gingiva. Clinically, oral xanthomas present as asymptomatic and well-circumscribed yellowish plaques or nodules that may be localized or scattered in multiple sites (**Fig. 30.16**). The presence in the oral cavity might be a clinical indication of hyperlipidemia that requires further investigation. The clinical diagnosis should be confirmed by histologic examination.

Differential diagnosis

- Verruciform xanthoma
- Fordyce's granules
- Lipomas
- Fibromas
- Focal epithelial hyperplasia
- Mucosal and skin grafts

Pathology

Histopathologic examination of oral lesions reveals numerous macrophages containing lipids within their cytoplasm—*foam cell*.

Treatment

The treatment of xanthomas associated with hyperlipidemia requires the identification of the underlying lipoprotein disorder and other possible exacerbating factors, but it is beyond the scope of this book. Localized oral lesions can be surgically removed.

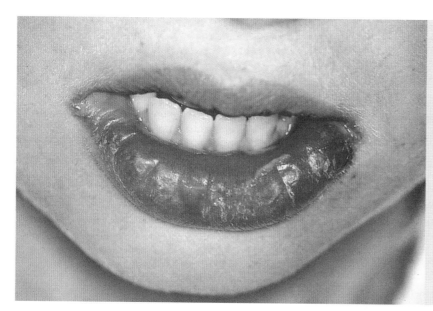

Fig. 30.14 Cystic fibrosis, lower lip enlargement.

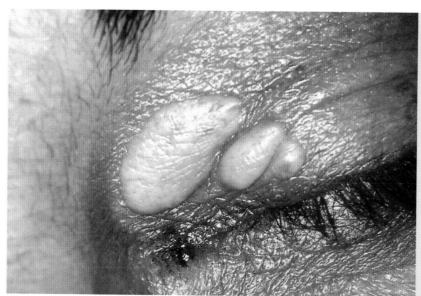

Fig. 30.15 Xanthelasmas on the skin of the eyelids.

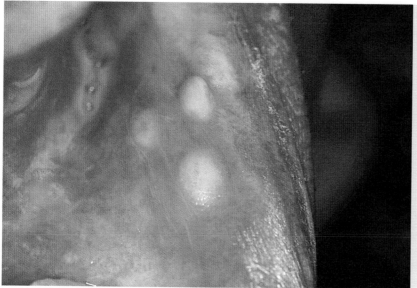

Fig. 30.16 Multiple xanthomas of the labial mucosa.

Porphyrias

Key points

- A group of metabolic disorders that mainly affects the skin, the nervous system, or both.
- The porphyrias result from enzyme dysfunctions involved in heme biosynthesis.
- They are classified into either *acute* and *nonacute* or *cutaneous* and *noncutaneous*.
- Life-threatening neurologic disorders can occur in the acute porphyrias.
- Oral lesions are relatively rare and do not occur in all types.

Introduction

Porphyrias are a group of mostly genetic metabolic disorders characterized by a deficiency of one of the eight enzymes of the porphyrin-heme biosynthetic pathway. Classically, porphyrias are subdivided into *erythropoietic* and *hepatic* forms, according to the site of expression of the enzyme defect. Recently, it has been proposed a new classification either into *acute* and *nonacute* or *cutaneous* and *noncutaneous* forms.

Every type of the disorder is characterized by an enzyme deficiency from the heme biosynthesis that translates to the relevant metabolic expression (**Table 30.1**).

Clinical features

The clinical signs and symptoms of porphyrias depend on the form. In cutaneous forms (porphyria cutanea tarda, erythropoietic protoporphyria, variegate porphyria, hereditary coproporphyria, congenital erythropoietic porphyria, hepatoerythropoietic porphyria, X-lined dominant protoporphyria), light-exposed areas of the skin are primarily affected presenting with photo-sensitivity in almost all types of porphyria. Characteristically, the skin is fragile and there can be erythema, vesicles, bullae, erosions, hyperpigmentation, hypertrichosis, scars, scarring alopecia and milia (**Figs. 30.17, 30.18**). Oral manifestations may occur in congenital erythropoietic porphyria or Günther's disease and may include the presence of red-brown teeth, due to incorporation of porphyrins into the developing deciduous and permanent teeth. Under ultraviolet light, the teeth exhibit a characteristic reddish-pink fluorescence. The oral mucosa is rarely affected in porphyrias. However, erythema, vesicles, bullae, ulcers, atrophy but no scarring may appear occasionally in congenital erythropoietic porphyria and porphyria cutanea tarda. The oral lesions usually develop on the vermilion

Table 30.1 Classification of the porphyrias into acute and nonacute forms

Form	Mode of inheritance	Gene locus	Protein product (enzyme deficiency)
	Acute		
Acute intermittent porphyria	AD	11q23.3	Porphobilinogen (PBGD)
Variegate porphyria	AD	1q22–23	Protoporphyrinogen oxidase (PPOX)
Hereditary coproporphyria	AD	3q12	Coproporphyrinogen oxidase (CPO)
ALA-D deficiency porphyria	AR	9q34	δ-Aminolevulinic acid dehydratase (ALAD)
	Nonacute		
Porphyria cutaneous tarda	AD > 25% or acquired	1p34	Uroporphyrinogen decarboxylase (UROD)
Erythropoietic protoporphyria	AD	18q21.3	Ferrochelatase (FECH)
Congenital erythropoietic porphyria	AR	10q25.2–q26.3	Uroporphyrinogen III synthase (UROS)
Hepatoerythropoietic porphyria	AR	1p34	Uroporphyrinogen decarboxylase (UROD)
X-linked dominant protoporphyria	XLD	Xp11.21	δ-Aminolevulinic acid synthase 2 (ALAS2)

Abbreviations: AD, autosomal dominant; AR, autosomal recessive; XLD, X-linked dominant. Adapted from Bolognia JL, Jorizzo JL, Schaffer JV: Dermatology 3rd ed 2012, Elsevier; partly modified.

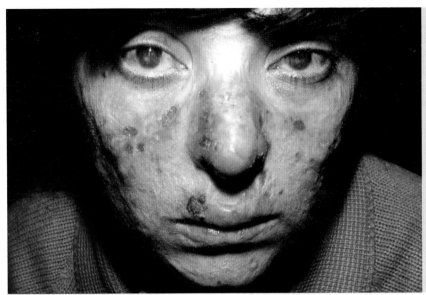

Fig. 30.17 Congenital erythropoietic porphyria, extensive lesions (erosions and scars) on the face.

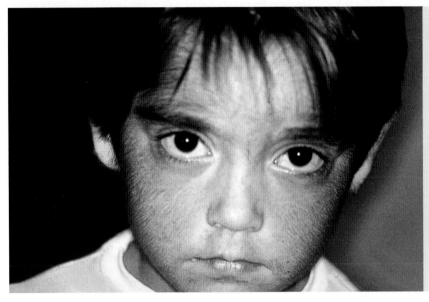

Fig. 30.18 Latent porphyria cutanea tarda, hypertrichosis, and pigmentation on the face.

border of the lips, commissures, labial mucosa, anterior vestibular alveolar mucosa, and gingiva (**Figs. 30.19, 30.20**). Signs and symptoms from the central nervous system are common in acute porphyrias. The clinical diagnosis should be confirmed by the laboratory tests.

Differential diagnosis
- The different types of porphyrias
- Lipoid proteinosis
- Epidermolysis bullosa
- Scleroderma
- Pellagra
- Drug-induced photosensitivity

Laboratory tests

Biochemical examination of blood, urine, and stools is required, followed by more specific immunohistochemical and immunologic examinations depending on the form suspected. Molecular and genetic investigation is suggested for affected families.

Treatment

The treatment can be challenging and must be left to the dermatologist and internal medicine specialist. Each type of porphyria requires a different course of action and the specifics are outside the scope of this book. The oral lesions are treated symptomatically.

Hemochromatosis

Key points
- A genetic iron metabolic disorder that subsequently leads to iron deposits in tissues and organs.
- Hepatic abnormalities and cirrhosis, congestive heart failure, hypogonadism, and arthritis.
- Generalized pigmentation of skin and oral mucosa.

Introduction

Hemochromatosis is an autosomal, recessive, genetic iron-storage disorder resulting in deposition of large amounts of iron in the internal organs. In many cases, it is caused by mutation in *HFE* gene, most commonly *C282Y* on chromosome 6.

Clinical features

The symptoms and signs usually begin after the age of 50 years. Clinically, early symptoms are nonspecific (fatigue, arthralgias). Later, the disorder is usually characterized by the coexistence of diabetes mellitus, liver cirrhosis, hyperpigmentation, and less frequently, gonadal deficiency, heart failure, supraventricular arrhythmias, and joint disorders. Hyperpigmentation may appear both on the skin and mucous membranes (oral and conjunctiva) due to the deposition of hemosiderin or melanin or both. The skin acquires a generalized gray-brown hyperpigmentation in almost all cases. The oral mucosa shows diffuse homogeneous pigmentation of gray-brown or deep brown hue in approximately 20% of the cases. The buccal mucosa and the attached gingiva are the most frequently involved sites (**Fig. 30.21**). In addition, major and minor salivary gland involvement has been reported.

Differential diagnosis
- Addison's disease
- Drug-induced hyperpigmentation
- Normal pigmentation in dark-skinned people

Laboratory test

There is an elevated serum iron, transferrin, and ferritin. Blood glucose levels are also elevated. Liver function tests should also be performed if hepatic problems are suspected. Genetic testing is available for *HFE* gene mutations.

Treatment

Phlebotomy to reduce iron stores is first-line therapy. In addition, an oral chelator (e.g., deferasirox or deferoxamine) may be used. Symptomatic treatment of any other complications is required.

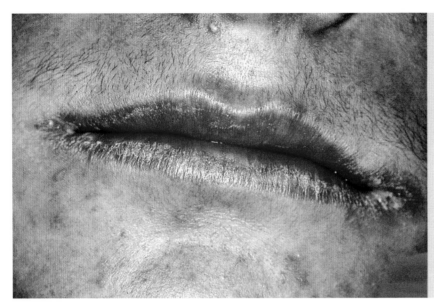

Fig. 30.19 Latent porphyria cutanea tarda, erythema, and ragades on the lips.

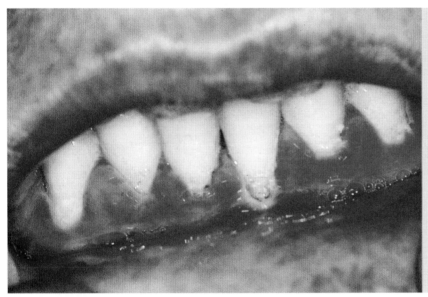

Fig. 30.20 Latent porphyria cutanea tarda, erythema, and mild enlargement of the mandibular gingiva.

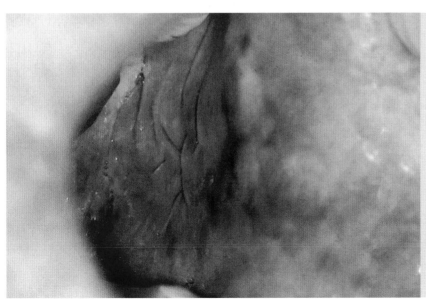

Fig. 30.21 Hemochromatosis, prominent pigmentation of the buccal mucosa.

31 Vitamin Deficiency

General considerations

- Vitamins are required constituents of the human diet as they are essential organic nutrients required for development and maintenance of bodily functions.
- They are classified into *water-soluble* (B_1, B_2, B_3, B_5, B_6, B_7, B_9, B_{12}) and *fat-soluble* (A, D, E, and K).
- Most of water-soluble vitamins appear to serve as cofactors for enzyme while none of the fat-soluble vitamins do.
- Vitamin deficiency in the developing world occurs through reduced intake as a result of a poor diet.
- The oral symptoms and signs of most vitamin deficiencies are similar.

Vitamin B₁ Deficiency

Key points

- Caused by the lack of thiamine (vitamin B_1).
- Other risk factors may be present such as B_1-deficient diet, chronic alcoholism, malabsorption diseases, hemodialysis, leukemia.
- Neurologic disorders and mucocutaneous lesions.
- The oral lesions usually occur on the tongue.
- B_1 deficiency is also known as *Beriberi*, which is divided into "*wet*" and "*dry*" forms.

Introduction

Vitamin B_1 or thiamine is a coenzyme that plays a significant role in carbohydrate metabolism. It can be found in vegetables, meat, liver, eggs, cereal grains etc. It usually manifests in chronic alcoholism, diabetes mellitus, pregnancy, and other causes of chronic protein–caloric undernutrition. B_1 deficiency is also known as *Beriberi* which is divided into "*wet*" form which primarily affects the cardiovascular system and "*dry*" form which involves the nervous system.

Clinical features

Early clinical signs and symptoms include loss of appetite, weakness, irritability, constipation, and abdominal pain. Late manifestations include memory loss, peripheral neuropathy, cardiac failure, growth retardation. Ophthalmic and cutaneous disorders are also present. Intraorally, there is erythema and mild edema and atrophy of the lingual papillae (**Fig. 31.1**). The patient may complain of taste disturbances and glossodynia. The diagnosis is based on the history, the clinical features, and a variety of biochemical tests.

Differential diagnosis

- B_2, B_6, and B_{12} deficiency
- Iron deficiency anemia
- Plummer-Vinson syndrome
- Megaloblastic anemia

Laboratory tests

The most frequently used biochemical diagnostic tests are measurement of erythrocyte transketolase activity and urinary thiamine excretion. A transketolase activity coefficient greater than 15 to 20% suggests thiamine deficiency. In addition, decreased circulating plasma–thiamine levels are diagnostic.

Treatment

Treatment of the existing causative factor/disease and administration of 50 to 100 mg/d intravenous of thiamine for the first few days, followed by daily oral administration of 5 to 10 mg/d. Foods rich in thiamine are also recommended.

Vitamin B₂ Deficiency

Key points

- Decrease of vitamin B_2 through either reduced intake or absorption.
- Ophthalmic, neurologic, and mucocutaneous abnormalities.
- Oral lesions are common and include angular cheilitis and glossitis.

Introduction

Riboflavin or vitamin B_2 is an essential vitamin for the transfer of electrons in the cellular oxidation-reduction reactions that lead to energy production. It is also required in the early stages of protein synthesis. B_2 can be found in dairy products, milk, liver, meat, cereal grains, and leafy green vegetables. Riboflavin deficiency can be caused through reduced intake due to dietary habits or a variety of medications or malabsorption due to achlorhydria or hypochlorhydria malabsorption syndrome, chronic alcoholism, etc. The disorder, almost always occurs in combination with deficiencies of other vitamins.

Clinical features

Clinically, vitamin B_2 deficiency may result in seborrheic dermatitis, conjunctivitis, and corneal vascularization, and, in advanced stages, keratitis, anemia, cognitive decline, and oral lesions. The most frequent oral manifestation is angular cheilitis, which may be unilateral or bilateral. The lips are dry and cracked. In most cases atrophy of the filiform papillae results in a smooth red tongue (**Fig. 31.2**). The diagnosis is mainly based on the medical history and the clinical features, but it should be confirmed by laboratory tests.

Differential diagnosis

- Vitamins B_1, B_6, B_7, and B_{12} deficiency
- Iron deficiency anemia
- Plummer-Vinson syndrome
- Megaloblastic anemia

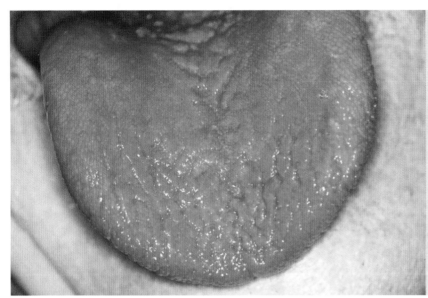

Fig. 31.1 B$_1$ deficiency, erythema, and edema of the tongue.

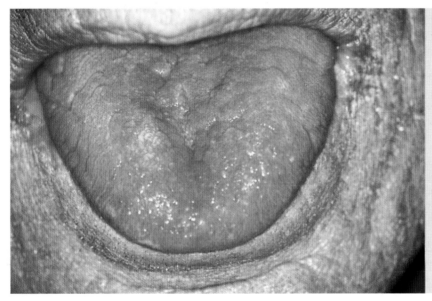

Fig. 31.2 B$_2$ deficiency, erythema of the tongue, and angular cheilitis.

Laboratory tests

Measuring the riboflavin-dependent enzyme erythrocyte glutathione reductase can confirm the diagnosis. Activity coefficients greater than 1.2 to 1.3 are suggestive of riboflavin deficiency. Urinary riboflavin excretion and serum levels of red cell and plasma flavins are also useful.

Treatment

Any underlying disease has to be treated. Administration of riboflavin 5 to 15 mg/d orally until clinical findings are resolved. Food rich in vitamin B_2 is also recommended.

Vitamin B₃ Deficiency—Pellagra

Key points
- Severe vitamin B_3 deficiency results in *pellagra*.
- The classic triad of pellagra is dermatitis, diarrhea, and dementia.
- Oral manifestations are common.

Introduction

Pellagra is a deficiency of vitamin B_3 or niacin or nicotinic acid. Niacin is an essential component of the coenzymes nicotinamide adenine dinucleotide and nicotinamide adenine dinucleotide phosphate which are involved in oxidation-reduction reactions. Among others, it also helps with the biosynthesis of epidermal lipids and it facilitates DNA repair. The vitamin is mainly found in foods such as red meat, liver, salmon, and dairy products. Lack of B_3 is caused by reduced intake due to malnutrition, intestinal malabsorption, chronic alcoholism, medication (isoniazid), and carcinoid syndrome.

Clinical features

Early clinical symptoms and signs can be loss of appetite and weight loss, abdominal pain, diarrhea, indigestion, and a burning sensation in various parts of the body. The main clinical manifestations include gastrointestinal disorders (esophagitis, gastritis, proctitis, abdominal pain, diarrhea), nervous system manifestations (such as apathy, restlessness, anxiety, irritability, paresthesias, hallucinations, amnesia, depression, disorientation), and symmetric dermatitis, particularly on areas exposed to sunlight and friction. The dermatitis is characterized by sharply outlined erythema with scaling and vesiculobullous lesions. With time, the skin becomes hard and pigmented with a marginated darker edge (**Fig. 31.3**). The oral mucosa is involved with edema, generalized erythema, and intense burning sensation. The tongue is smooth due to desquamation of the papillae, while painful ulcers may appear (**Figs. 31.4, 31.5**). Gingivitis, dry and fissured lips, angular cheilitis, and dysphagia are also prominent features. Advanced pellagra without treatment can result in death. The diagnosis is based mainly on the history and the clinical features.

Differential diagnosis
- Vitamins B_1, B_6, B_7, and B_{12} deficiency
- Porphyrias
- Drug reactions
- Nutritional deficiency

Laboratory tests

There are no specific or sensitive serum assays. A relatively reliable test is urinary excretion of niacin metabolites: N-methylnicotinamide and N-methyl-2-pyridone-5-carboxamide.

Treatment

The underlying cause responsible for the niacin deficiency has to be treated. Therapeutically, oral nicotinamide 50–150 mg/d for approximately 2 to 3 weeks is the treatment of choice.

Vitamin B₆ Deficiency

Key points
- Most commonly occurs as a result of interactions with medications or alcoholism.
- It may coexist with other vitamin deficiencies.
- Cutaneous, mucosal, and rarer neurologic disorders are the prominent features.

Introduction

Vitamin B_6 or pyridoxine acts as cofactor for multiple enzymes involved in lipids and protein metabolism, gluconeogenesis, heme biosynthesis, and normal nerve function. Deficiency of B_6 is rare and usually coexists with other vitamin and protein deficiencies and interactions with medications such as isoniazid, D-penicillamine, hydralazine, and contraceptives. Finally, liver cirrhosis, renal failure, and inflammatory bowel disease can lead to its depletion. The vitamin B_6 is mainly found in plant foods and meat.

Clinical features

Vitamin B_6 deficiency results in clinical features similar to that seen in other vitamin B deficiencies. Early signs and symptoms can be loss of appetite, nausea, weakness, irritability, and symptoms of iron deficiency anemia. Cutaneous manifestations include seborrheic dermatitis that predominantly occurs around the natural body openings. The oral mucosa can be erythematous and edematous with mild papillary atrophy, ulcerations, and angular cheilitis

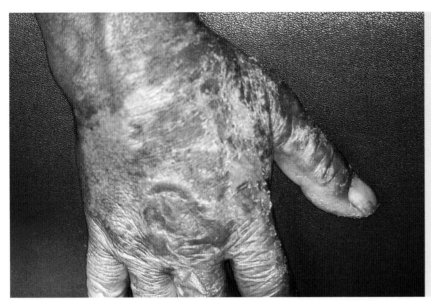

Fig. 31.3 Pellagra, erythema, exfoliation, and atrophy of the skin.

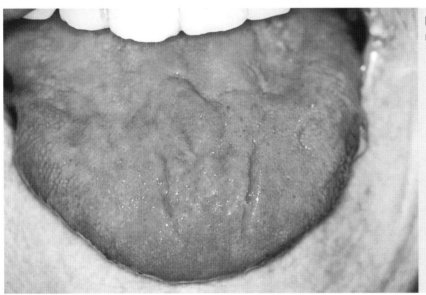

Fig. 31.4 Pellagra, erythema, and mild edema of the tongue.

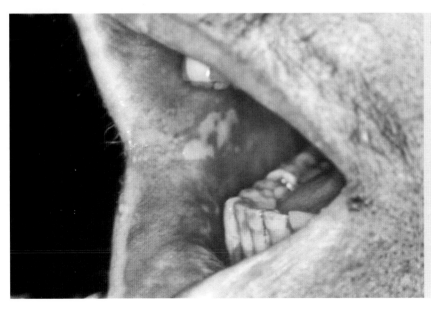

Fig. 31.5 Pellagra, erythema, and erosion of the buccal mucosa.

(**Fig. 31.6**). The patients complain of glossodynia or stomatodynia. Other clinical signs can be conjunctivitis and rarely neurologic disorders such as peripheral neuropathy and confusion. The diagnosis is based on the history, the clinical features, and laboratory tests.

Differential diagnosis

- Vitamin B$_1$, B$_2$, B$_{12}$ deficiency
- Protein deficiency
- Iron deficiency anemia
- Plummer-Vinson syndrome
- Megaloblastic anemia

Laboratory tests

The diagnosis of vitamin B$_6$ deficiency can be confirmed by measurement of pyridoxal phosphate in blood (normal levels > 50 ng/mL).

Treatment

Treatment of the underlying cause that has caused the deficiency is required. For elevation of vitamin B$_6$ levels, administration of pyridoxine per os (50–100 mg/d for 3–4 weeks) is advised.

Vitamin B$_{12}$ Deficiency

Key points

- Caused by lack of vitamin B$_{12}$ due to reduced dietary intake, but mainly due to malabsorption from the small bowel.
- B$_{12}$ deficiency leads to megaloblastic anemia due to disruption of folic acid metabolism.
- Oral lesions are early and common.

Introduction

Vitamin B$_{12}$ or cyanocobalamin plays an important role in DNA synthesis. It can be found in fish, meat, and dairy products. Deficiency can occur in vegetarians. Other causes include reduced absorption from the gastrointestinal tract. That can be due to gastrectomy or operations elsewhere in the intestine, pancreatic dysfunction, parasitic diseases, diseases of the ileum, and medication (metformin). It can also be due to a decrease in gastric intrinsic factor production. A megaloblastic anemia occurs.

Clinical features

The hallmark of symptomatic vitamin B$_{12}$ deficiency is megaloblastic anemia. Early signs and symptoms include weakness, loss of appetite, graying of the hair, and other symptoms of megaloblastic anemia. Diffuse or patchy skin hyperpigmentation and alopecia are common. The oral mucosa, particularly the tongue appears erythematous, edematous, and smooth

due to atrophy of the lingual papillae (**Fig. 31.7**). Glossodynia and burning mouth syndrome can be prominent and there might be pain due to superficial erosions. Angular cheilitis is also common. The diagnosis is based on the history, clinical features, and vitamin B$_{12}$ plasma levels.

Differential diagnosis

- Megaloblastic anemia
- Folic acid deficiency
- Vitamins B$_1$, B$_2$, and B$_6$ deficiency
- Iron deficiency anemia

Laboratory tests

The diagnosis of vitamin B$_{12}$ deficiency is based on an abnormally low vitamin B$_{12}$ (cobalamin) serum level (normal level: > 240 pg/mL). The diagnosis is best to be confirmed by elevated level of serum methylmalonic acid greater than 1000 nmol/L.

Treatment

Intramuscular injections of 100 µg of vitamin B$_{12}$ are adequate for each dose. The complete treatment regimen must be left to specialists of hematology or gastroenterology.

Vitamin C Deficiency—Scurvy

Key points

- Scurvy is caused by vitamin C deficiency.
- Most cases are due to dietary inadequacy in patients with chronic alcoholism or chronic illnesses.
- Oral lesions are characteristic and common.

Introduction

Scurvy is caused by the deficiency of vitamin C or ascorbic acid. Vitamin C can be found in high quantities in citrus fruits but also in other fresh fruits and vegetables. Vitamin C plays an important role in collagen composition, folic acid metabolism, iron absorption, and immune stimulation. The deficiency is mainly caused by inadequate dietary intake and chronic alcoholism or chronic illnesses. Scurvy traditionally occurred in sailors that had to rely on preserved food. Nowadays, it is very rare in adults.

Clinical features

Early clinical manifestations of scurvy include malaise and weakness. In more advanced stages, perifollicular hyperkeratotic papules, petechiae, hematomas, and hemorrhages (on the skin, conjunctiva, muscles, joints, and gastrointestinal tract), susceptibility to infections, skin ecchymoses, delayed wound healing, and oral lesions are the prominent features. The oral manifestations include swelling and redness of the interdental and marginal gingiva that may be accompanied by spontaneous hemorrhage and sometimes ulceration (**Figs. 31.8, 31.9**).

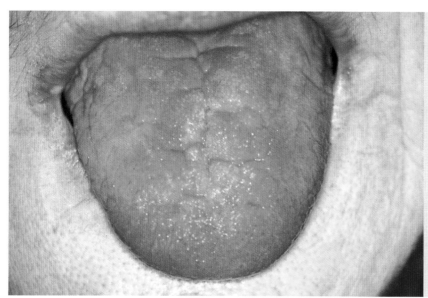

Fig. 31.6 Vitamin B$_6$ deficiency, angular cheilitis, edema, and mild atrophy of the lingual papillae.

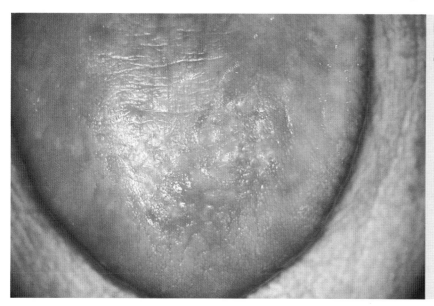

Fig. 31.7 Vitamin B$_{12}$ deficiency, mildly edematous and smooth tongue due to papillary atrophy.

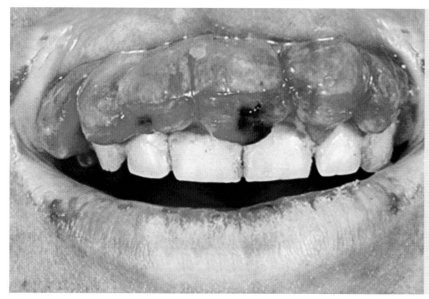

Fig. 31.8 Scurvy, prominent gingival enlargement, and erythema.

Petechiae, ecchymoses, and hemorrhages are commonly seen in other oral mucosal sites. In late stages, generalized edema, oliguria, neuropathy, intracerebral hemorrhage, and death may occur. The diagnosis is based on the history, clinical features, and the vitamin C plasma levels.

Differential diagnosis

- Leukemia
- Agranulocytosis
- Neutropenia
- Protein deficiency
- Necrotizing ulcerative gingivitis

Laboratory tests

The diagnosis can be confirmed by low plasma levels of vitamin C (L-ascorbic acid), typically below 0.1 mg/dL.

Treatment

For immediate results ascorbic acid can be administered orally 1 to 2 g/d. A diet rich in fresh fruits and vegetables is recommended. Improvement occurs within few days.

Protein Deficiency

Key points

- Protein deficiency usually coexists with vitamin deficiency.
- It can be the result of starvation, metabolic disorders, malignancies, and gastrointestinal conditions that cause malabsorption.
- The oral mucosa is commonly affected.
- Protein–energy malnutrition classified as two syndromes: *Kwashiorkor* and *Marasmus*.

Introduction

Protein deficiency often coexists with vitamin deficiency and is usually associated with several severe systemic conditions, such as malignant diseases, nutritional disorders, metabolic diseases, malabsorption, and inadequate diet. When only protein deficiency occurs, it is characterized as *Kwashiorkor* syndrome while when protein and energy deficiency occurs, it is named as *Marasmus*.

Clinical features

Clinically, protein deficiency is characterized by weight loss, edema, muscle wasting, weakness, hypoglycemia, anemia, and hypotension. The oral manifestations are atrophic glossitis with loss of papillae, redness and atrophy of the oral mucosa, angular cheilitis, and burning mouth (**Fig. 31.10**). The skin appears dry, anelastic and atrophic with areas of hyperpigmentation. There is also alopecia, impaired nail growth and fissured nails, hemorrhage, hyperkeratosis, etc. The diagnosis is based on the history, clinical features, and laboratory tests.

Differential diagnosis

- Vitamin deficiencies (especially of the B complex)
- Megaloblastic anemia
- Iron deficiency anemia
- Plummer-Vinson syndrome

Laboratory tests

Biochemical studies that reveal plasma protein and vitamin levels can be helpful. The serum protein level typically declines and the serum albumin is often less than 2.5 g/dL.

Treatment

Treatment requires a complete and balanced diet that includes proteins, vitamins, and minerals, as well as treatment of any underlying condition.

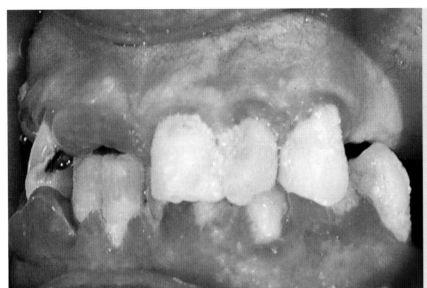

Fig. 31.9 Scurvy, gingival enlargement, and prominent erythema.

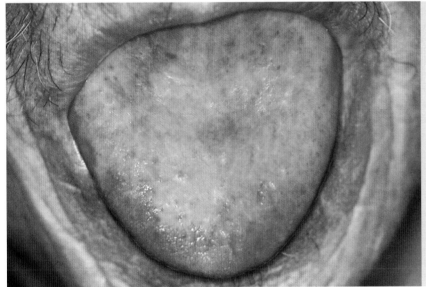

Fig. 31.10 Protein deficiency, smooth tongue with absence of papillae.

32 Endocrine Diseases

Diabetes Mellitus

Key points

- A group of metabolic disorders caused either by a reduced production of insulin from the pancreas or by reduced activity of insulin, or both.
- Classified into two main types: *type 1 diabetes mellitus* (*DM*) and *type 2 DM*.
- Gestational diabetes occurs in pregnancy in women without a history of diabetes.
- Oral lesions are often observed, mainly in type 1.

Introduction

Diabetes mellitus is the most common of the endocrine diseases. It is characterized by abnormalities in the metabolism, not only of carbohydrates, but also of proteins and fat. It has a multifactorial etiology. However, the main abnormalities are reduced production of insulin from the pancreas, insufficient response of the cells to it, or both. This ultimately results in the increase of blood glucose levels. Diabetes mellitus is classified into two main types: *types 1 and 2*. There are other "*specific types*" of diabetes and also *gestational* diabetes that occurs during pregnancy without any previous history.

Clinical features

The main clinical features include polydipsia, polyuria, polyphagia with weight loss and generalized weakness. These can be followed by increased susceptibility to infections, neuropathy and microvasculopathy and other complications. Early oral manifestations may include dryness of the mouth, angular cheilitis, taste change, and burning mouth syndrome. In poorly controlled diabetes mellitus (mainly type 1), there can be gingival enlargement, bleeding, gingivitis, and rapidly progressive periodontitis that may lead to teeth loss (**Fig. 32.1**). Other oral complications can be delayed healing, candidiasis, and rarely mucormycosis and even noma (**Fig. 32.2**).

Differential diagnosis

- Chronic gingivitis
- Aggressive periodontal disease
- Chronic periodontitis
- Mucopolysaccharidoses

Laboratory tests

A plasma glucose level of 126 mg/dL or higher on more than one occasion after at least 8 hours of fasting is diagnostic of diabetes mellitus. Fasting plasma glucose levels of 100 to 125 mg/dL are associated with an increased risk of diabetes.

There are also additional laboratory tests that are out of the scope of this book. Oral glucose tolerance test should be performed.

Treatment

Control of diabetes mellitus, by a specialist, with insulin, per os medication and diet, as required is essential. The management of the oral lesions includes oral hygiene, periodontal treatment, and systemic antibiotics or antifungal agents for any fungal and bacterial infections.

Addison's Disease

Key points

- Chronic adrenocortical insufficiency classified as primary and secondary.
- Addison's disease is usually caused by distraction or dysfunction of the adrenal cortices.
- Weakness, anorexia, weight loss, fatigability, nausea, diarrhea, muscle and joint pains, and amenorrhea are common symptoms.
- An early sign is cutaneous and oral mucosal pigmentation.

Introduction

Addison's disease is a form of chronic adrenal insufficiency caused by destruction or dysfunction of the adrenals. Autoimmune destruction of the adrenals is the most common cause. Other causes may include HIV infection, tuberculosis, systemic fungal infections, amyloidosis, hemochromatosis, adrenal cancer, and adrenal hemorrhage. It is more common in women between 20 and 40 years, resulting in insufficient secretion of glucocorticoids and mineralocorticoids. To counterbalance the low levels of hormones secreted, there is an increase of adrenocorticotropic hormone (ACTH) and melanocyte-stimulating hormone (MSH) secreted by the pituitary gland.

Clinical features

Clinically, Addison's disease can manifest acutely or in a more chronic form. It is characterized by weakness, fatigue, weight loss and loss of appetite, nausea, hypotension, tachycardia and gastrointestinal disorders, muscle and joint pains, amenorrhea, and mental irritability. A typical sign is increased mucosal and cutaneous pigmentation especially in areas that are subject to friction and pressure. This occurs because of melanocyte stimulation from the overly secreted MSH. Dark brown pigmentation of the oral mucosa is an early and common feature of the disease (**Figs. 32.3, 32.4**). It may be spotty or diffuse and involves the buccal mucosa, palate, lips, and gingiva. The clinical diagnosis has to be confirmed by the appropriate investigations.

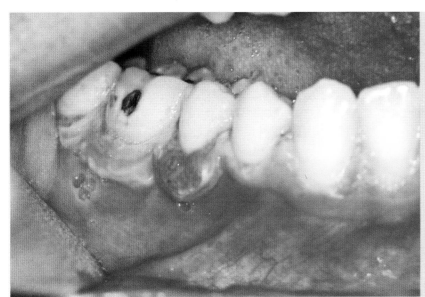

Fig. 32.1 Diabetes mellitus, localized periodontal disease in the molar area.

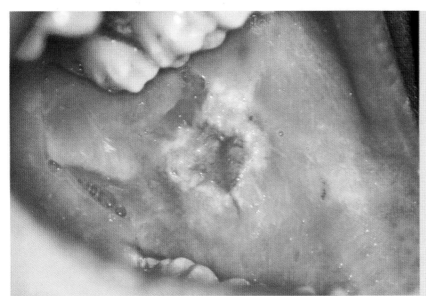

Fig. 32.2 Diabetes mellitus, delayed healing on the buccal mucosa.

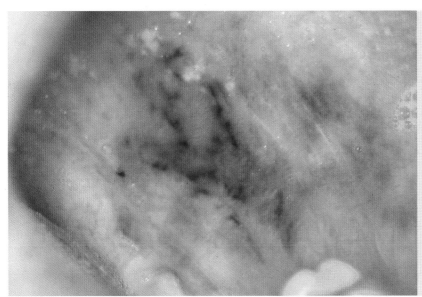

Fig. 32.3 Addison's disease, pigmentation of the buccal mucosa.

Differential diagnosis

- Normal pigmentation
- Smoker's pigmentation
- Pigmentation due to drugs
- Peutz-Jeghers syndrome
- Pigmented nevi
- Lentigo maligna
- Malignant melanoma

Laboratory tests

To establish diagnosis, a series of tests is required. ACTH stimulation test is performed whereby adrenal hormone levels remain low after synthetic pituitary ACTH hormone is administered. The rapid ACTH test is also performed. Additionally, increased ACTH levels (usually > 200 pg/mL) combined with low cortisol levels (< 3 µg/dL) in an early morning blood test is diagnostic. Antiadrenal antibodies are found in the serum in approximately 50% of cases in autoimmune Addison's disease. In nonautoimmune disease, a chest radiograph is necessary to search for tuberculosis or other causes.

Treatment

The treatment is performed by the specialist endocrinologist. It consists of hormone replacement therapy to correct the levels of corticosteroid and mineralocorticoids. Supportive treatment of the signs and symptoms is also performed.

Cushing's Syndrome

Key points

- Caused by the prolonged action of elevated plasma glucocorticoids.
- The etiology can be *iatrogenic* (corticosteroid treatment) or *noniatrogenic* (adrenal neoplasia, high production of ACTH).
- Elevated serum cortisol and urinary free cortisol.

Introduction

Cushing's syndrome or hypercorticolism is caused by an increase of the plasma glucocorticoid levels. Rarely, it is caused by an endogenous increase of corticosteroids due to adrenal and pituitary or nonpituitary tumors (*noniatrogenic Cushing*). Most commonly, it is the result of chronic use of corticosteroids for therapeutic reasons (*iatrogenic Cushing*).

Clinical features

The most common clinical manifestations include obesity, fat redistribution, including collection around the face and neck that causes the characteristic "*moon face*" (**Fig. 32.5**). Other features can be hirsutism, thinning skin with red or purple striated atrophic areas, hypertension, osteoporosis, increase

of blood sugar, weakness, amenorrhea, polyuria, and psychiatric disorders. In iatrogenic Cushing, the diagnosis is based on the history, the clinical features, and the laboratory tests.

Differential diagnosis

- Antiretroviral therapy for HIV infection
- Chronic alcoholism
- Obesity of other etiology

Laboratory tests

The most common tests include the 24-hour urinary free cortisol test, the dexamethasone suppression test, and measurement of midnight plasma cortisol.

Treatment

The treatment plan is performed by the specialists, endocrinologist, and internal medicine physician. In iatrogenic Cushing, there has to be an adjustment in the treatment regime and supportive treatment.

Hypothyroidism

Key points

- The result of thyroid hormones deficiency.
- Classified into *primary* and *secondary*.
- Hypothyroidism in children causes delay in development which in severe cases can be characterized as *cretinism*.
- Severe hypothyroidism in adults results in *myxoedema*.
- Common oral findings are enlarged tongue and lips.

Introduction

Hypothyroidism may be *primary*, due to the inability of thyroid gland to secrete sufficient hormones, or *secondary*, caused by reduced thyroid-stimulating hormone (TSH) secretion by the pituitary gland. Low thyroid function results in reduced thyroid hormone secretion.

Clinical features

Congenital hypothyroidism, also known as *cretinism*, manifests with facial edema, poor feeding, sluggishness, hoarse crying, and jaundice in the newborn. If left untreated, it manifests with severe mental retardation with or without seizures, poor growth and development, weakness, fatigue, cold intolerance, and constipation. Macroglossia, delayed dental development, thick lips, and enamel hypoplasia are the cardinal oral clinical findings (**Fig. 32.6**). In adults (myxoedema), myxedematous pale, carotenemic skin accompanied by weight increase, mental sluggishness, constipation, cold intolerance, muscle cramps, myalgias and arthralgias, dry skin, hypercholesterolemia, and gonadal dysfunction are the most characteristic findings. Macroglossia and thickening of the lips are common oral manifestations.

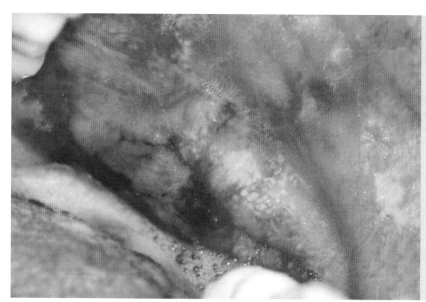

Fig. 32.4 Addison's disease, pigmentation of the sulcus and the buccal mucosa.

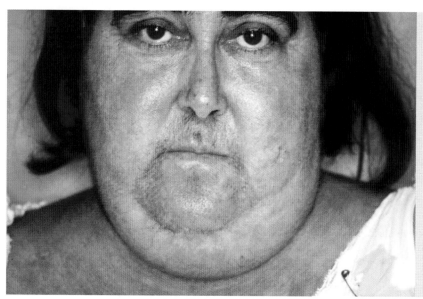

Fig. 32.5 Cushing's syndrome, characteristic "*moon face*" resulting from chronic use of high doses of corticosteroids.

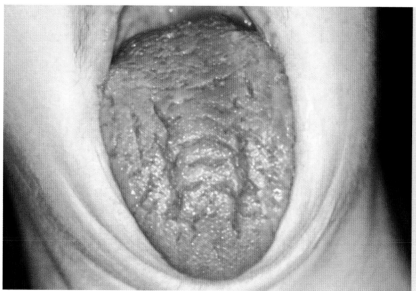

Fig. 32.6 Congenital hypothyroidism, large and fissured tongue.

Differential diagnosis
- Mucopolysaccharidoses
- Hurler's syndrome
- Lipoid proteinosis
- Down's syndrome

Laboratory tests

Initial screening tests includes the serum TSH and thyroid hormone measurements. In patients with autoimmune thyroiditis, titers of antibodies against thyroperoxidase and thyroglobulin are high. Serum antinuclear antibodies (ANAs) are usually present.

Treatment

The treatment is performed by the endocrinologist. It typically consists of replacement therapy with thyroxine.

Hyperparathyroidism

Key points
- Overproduction and secretion of parathormone.
- Classified into *primary* and *secondary* forms.
- Renal calculi, polyuria, hypertension, constipation, bone pain, fatigue, mental disorders.
- Oral lesions are observed in the primary type.

Introduction

Primary hyperparathyroidism is an endocrine disorder characterized by chronic poorly regulated excessive secretion of parathyroid hormone (PTH—parathormone) that results in hypercalcemia. Parathyroid adenoma (80%) and less commonly hyperplasia or carcinoma are the causes. In *secondary* hyperparathyroidism, the excessive secretion of PTH results as a response to hypocalcemia (mostly due to renal failure). The primary form affects more often women over 60 years.

Clinical features

Primary hyperparathyroidism may occur alone or as part of multiple endocrine neoplasia type 1 or type 2 syndrome. The clinical manifestations depend on the severity and chronicity. The disease presents with polydipsia and polyuria, hypertension, lassitude, mental dysfunction, muscular weakness, osteoporosis, osteitis fibrosa cystica, duodenal ulceration, renal calculi, subperiosteal bone resorption, and "brown" giant cell tumors in different bones. "Brown" giant cell tumors may appear in the jaws and may be an early sign of the disease, along with loss of lamina dura. Rarely, the tumor may protrude

as a soft mass in the oral cavity due to bone destruction (**Fig. 32.7**). A characteristic oral radiographic finding is the absence of lamina dura. The diagnosis is based on the clinical features and the laboratory tests.

Differential diagnosis
- Central giant cell granuloma
- Peripheral giant cell granuloma
- Pyogenic granuloma
- Kaposi's sarcoma
- Hemangioendothelioma
- Hemangiopericytoma
- Hypercalcemia of other etiology

Laboratory tests

The hallmark is the serum calcium greater than 10.5 mg/dL, the serum phosphate (< 2.5 mg/dL), the urine calcium may be high or normal. The alkaline phosphatase is elevated only if bone disease is present. Elevated serum levels of intact PTH confirm the diagnosis. Skeletal and dental radiographs may be helpful. Histologically, the "*brown*" tumor is characterized by a proliferation of vascular granulation tissue with numerous multinucleated giant cells.

Treatment

Excision of the "*brown*" tumor is curative only if the underlying disease is treated simultaneously.

Estrogen Disorder

Key points
- Mucocutaneous lesions are common.
- Oral lesions include gingivitis, pyogenic granuloma, and glossodynia.

Introduction

Estrogen disorder during puberty, menstruation, pregnancy, and menopause can give rise to several oral manifestations.

Clinical features

The female sex hormones (estrogens and progesterone) play an important role in the maintenance of oral health. Several disorders can affect the gingiva during the menstrual cycle, puberty, pregnancy, menopause, and the use of oral contraceptives. The most classic example is gingivitis during pregnancy or exaggeration of gingival inflammation before or during menstruation (**Figs. 32.8, 32.9**). In addition, the so-called (*pregnancy tumor* or *granuloma*) is not an unusual

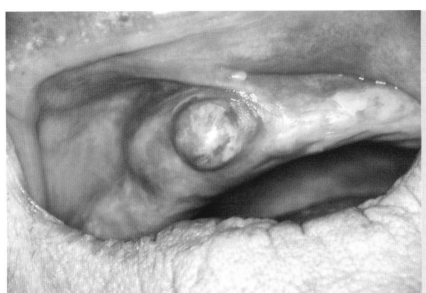

Fig. 32.7 Hyperparathyroidism, "*brown*" giant cell tumor of the maxilla that protrudes intraorally.

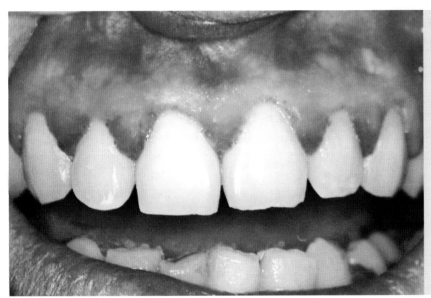

Fig. 32.8 Chronic gingivitis during pregnancy.

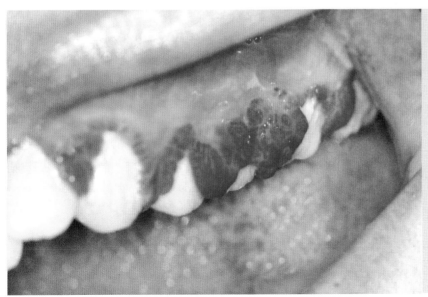

Fig. 32.9 Hyperplastic gingivitis and granulomas during pregnancy.

finding during pregnancy (**Figs. 32.10, 32.11**). Atrophy and sensitivity of the oral mucosa, glossodynia, and dysgeusia are common during the menopausal and postmenopausal periods of life. During pregnancy, cutaneous alterations may include pigmentation, chloasma or melasma, nail and hair lesions.

Differential diagnosis
- Plaque-related gingivitis
- Pyogenic granuloma of other etiology
- Peripheral giant cell granuloma
- Scurvy
- Diabetes mellitus

Laboratory tests

Measurement of the levels of plasma estrogens is required.

Treatment

The treatment of the oral lesions includes high level of oral hygiene. Surgical excision of granulomas after childbirth is possible, but rarely required.

Acromegaly

Key points
- Excessive production of growth hormone by the anterior pituitary.
- In most cases, the etiology is a benign pituitary adenoma.
- Internal organs are affected in their morphology and function.
- Macroglossia and enlarged lips are common features.

Introduction

Acromegaly is a rare endocrine disorder caused by an increased production of growth hormone after closure of the epiphyseal plates. This usually results from a benign pituitary adenoma. It affects both sexes, usually between 40 and 60 years.

Clinical features

Clinically, acromegaly is characterized by enlarged hands and feet, nasal bone hypertrophy, frontal bossing, coarsening facial features, and laryngeal and vocal cord hypertrophy leading to a hollow-sounding voice. Neurologic disturbances, decreased vision, musculoskeletal symptoms, cardiorespiratory and genitourinary disorders, myopathy, skin tags and acanthosis nigricans, and general symptoms (fatigue, increased sweating, heat intolerance) are also common. The oral manifestations include macroglossia, enlarged lips, mandibular overgrowth (prognathism), and widened interdental spaces (**Fig. 32.12**).

Differential diagnosis
- Hypothyroidism
- Amyloidosis
- Lipoid proteinosis
- Hurler's syndrome
- Down's syndrome

Laboratory tests

Measurement of serum growth hormone levels, usually after oral administration of glucose, is suggested. Magnetic resonance imaging may identify the pituitary adenoma.

Treatment

If caused by an adenoma, surgical excision or radiotherapy is recommended.

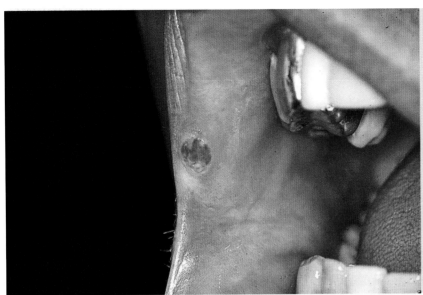

Fig. 32.10 Small pyogenic granuloma on the buccal mucosa in a 6-month pregnant patient.

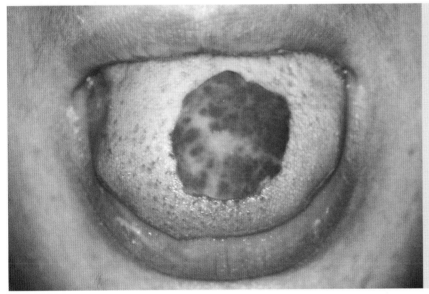

Fig. 32.11 Large pyogenic granuloma on the dorsum of the tongue in a 7-month pregnant patient.

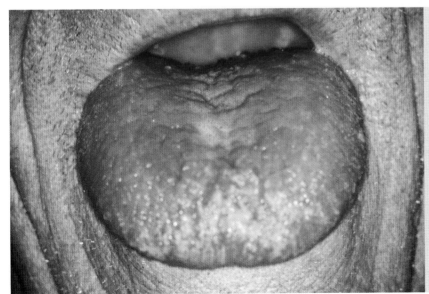

Fig. 32.12 Acromegaly, enlarged tongue.

33 Peripheral Nervous System Disorders

Facial Nerve Palsy

Key points

- The most common type of palsy in the head and neck area.
- The causes can be infection, trauma in the area, tumors, HIV infection, cold stroke, and systemic diseases.
- The disorder usually has an acute onset.

Introduction

Peripheral facial nerve palsy is the most common cause of weakness of the muscles of facial expression. Different etiology has been implicated, such as reactivation of herpes simplex virus infection in the geniculate ganglion, trauma, systemic diseases, tumors, and exposure to cold. Malignant tumors of the parotid gland invariably induce facial nerve paralysis by invasion of the nerve. Occasionally, the facial disorder may occur after tooth extraction or local anesthesia of the oral tissues or section of the facial nerve during surgical procedures in the parotid gland. Facial nerve palsy may also occur in Melkersson-Rosenthal syndrome, Lyme disease, AIDS, and multiple sclerosis. In case of unknown etiology, the palsy is considered idiopathic and the term *Bell's palsy* is used.

Clinical features

The facial nerve palsy is usually unilateral and has an acute onset manifesting within hours or being noticed first thing in the morning. It is more common in middle-aged women and often occurs during the spring and autumn. Clinically, it is characterized by dropping of the angle of the mouth of the involved side, the inability to close the eyelid, grin or whistle, or sudden dribbling (**Fig. 33.1**). When the patient attempts to smile, the affected side remains motionless, whereas the healthy side shows wrinkling of the skin. On attempts to close the eyes, the eyeball on the affected side is seen to deviate upward (*Bell's phenomenon*). The facial expressions can be absent while there can be problems with speech, mastication, salivary outflow, and taste. In the milder forms of the palsy, the patients recover spontaneously within 1 to 2 months. If the symptoms and signs persist for more than 1 year, it is likely that the palsy will be permanent. The diagnosis is based on the clinical features.

Differential diagnosis

- Melkersson-Rosenthal syndrome
- Heerfordt's syndrome
- Multiple sclerosis
- Angioneurotic edema
- Guillain-Barré syndrome
- Cerebral vasculitis

Laboratory tests

No laboratory tests are required to support the diagnosis, unless there is a need to establish an underlying disease. Radiologic imaging may be helpful.

Treatment

The first line of treatment is corticosteroids. Treatment with prednisolone, 50 to 60 mg daily for 5 to 6 days, followed by tapering of the dose over the next 8 to 10 days, is a suggested regimen within the first 5 days of onset. Antiherpes antivirals do not confer any additional benefit. If trauma of the nerve has occurred, surgery may be performed to repair or replace the damaged nerve.

Hypoglossal Nerve Paralysis

Key points

- Unilateral paralysis of the hypoglossal nerve affects the ipsilateral side of the tongue.
- The cause may be central or peripheral.

Introduction

The hypoglossal nerve supplies motor fibers to most of the muscles of the tongue. Unilateral lesions of this nerve cause paralysis and atrophy of the ipsilateral (same side) of the tongue. The etiology may be *central* or *peripheral* and caused by infectious polyneuritis, syringomyelia, poliomyelitis, nerve trauma and trauma to the head, neurofibromatosis, multiple sclerosis, tumors, etc.

Clinical features

In peripheral lesions, there is deviation of the tongue toward the affected side, during protrusion (**Figs. 33.2, 33.3**). That causes the tongue to appear sickle-shaped. Movements toward the unaffected side are either limited or completely absent. When the tongue rests on the floor of the mouth, a mild deviation toward the unaffected side may be observed (**Fig. 33.4**). In central lesions, involvement is often bilateral. The patient cannot protrude the tongue, and attempted movement of the tongue posteriorly is defective and uncoordinated. When atrophy is present, the affected side is smaller and firm. The diagnosis is based on the clinical features.

Differential diagnosis

- Postsurgical tongue dysmorphia
- Hemifacial atrophy

Laboratory tests

Special tests are not really required, except when radiologic imaging may be helpful when an underlying etiology needs investigation.

Treatment

This is aimed toward the underlying cause of the lesion of the hypoglossal nerve, or the lesion in the brain.

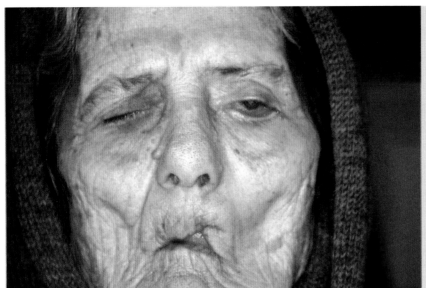

Fig. 33.1 Facial nerve palsy of the left side.

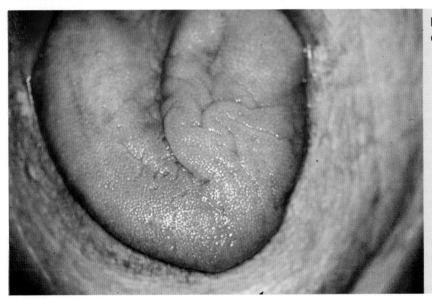

Fig. 33.2 Hypoglossal nerve paralysis of the left side.

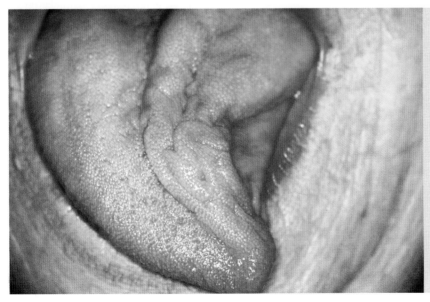

Fig. 33.3 Hypoglossal nerve paralysis of the left side with the tongue taking the characteristic sickle shape.

Trigeminal Neuralgia

Key points
- The most common and painful neuralgia in the face.
- Pain is in the territory of the second and third division of the trigeminal nerve.
- The pain is acute and very severe, lasts for 1 to 2 minutes, and is precipitated when pressure is applied to certain trigger zones.
- The disease is classified into *idiopathic* and *secondary*.

Introduction

Trigeminal neuralgia is the most common and painful neuralgia in the face. The exact etiology remains unclear. It is classified into *idiopathic* (*tic douloureux*) when a cause cannot be determined and *secondary* when the cause is known (i.e., tumor of the posterior cranial fossa). The incidence is four to six new cases per 100,000/annum. It is believed to be caused by vascular compression at the trigeminal nerve root. Arterial hypertension, atherosclerosis, and multiple sclerosis can contribute to the above.

Clinical features

Trigeminal neuralgia is more common in females, usually above 50 years, with a ratio of 2:1. It predominantly affects unilaterally the second and third branches of the facial nerve and rarely the first. The pain is acute and severe, described by the patient as stabbing and lancinating, almost like an electric shock. It may last from a few seconds to two minutes. The pain is distributed across the trigeminal nerve's affected branch. During the acute phase, there might be muscular spasm of the affected side and the patient may be seen to bring his hand over the area (**Fig. 33.5**). The pain recurs and can have triggers such as contact with cold air, mastication, swallowing, speech, palpation, tooth brushing, face washing, shaving, etc. The pain is so severe that can lead the patients to despair and even suicide. Following the paroxysmal phase, there can be a period of calm. Spontaneous recession periods may occur that can last between 6 and 8 months before a new episode of pain occurs. The diagnosis is mainly based on clinical criteria.

Differential diagnosis
- Postherpetic neuralgia
- Chronic paroxysmal hemicrania
- Atypical facial pain
- Multiple sclerosis
- Brainstem neoplasm
- Raeder's syndrome

Laboratory tests
Magnetic resonance imaging (MRI) and magnetic resonance tomographic angiography can help determine an underlying cause.

Treatment

The treatment can be medication or surgery. The drug of choice is carbamazepine 400 to 800 mg/d. In addition, diazepam 2 to 5 mg/d in association with prednisolone 20 to 30 mg/d may control the pain. Other treatment options include gabapentin, phenytoin, baclofen, lamotrigine, and clonazepam. If the noninvasive approach is not effective, the surgical procedures include Gamma knife surgery, percutaneous procedures, and microvascular decompression. Alcohol or phenol injection in the ganglion or in various locations along the nerve can also be performed, but the success rate is low and there will be permanent anesthesia of the affected area.

Tonic–Clonic Spasm of Masseter

Key points
- A disorder of neuromuscular nature.
- It can follow chronic muscular pain and may affect different muscles.
- Spasm of the masseter is rare.

Introduction

The muscular pain, if chronic, may cause episodes of muscular spasm and contraction that can spread to several muscles. The most common is blepharospasm. It is caused by muscle spasm of the orbicularis oculi and its adjacent muscles. The exact etiology remains unclear. Several conditions have been implicated for the muscular spasm, such as central nervous system (CNS) disorders, brain tumors, temporal bone dysplasia, focal seizures, facial nerve palsy, stress, and pregnancy. However, occasionally, no cause can be identified and the muscular spasm is then defined as idiopathic. Finally, occlusal disorders can lead to muscular fatigue and eventually spasm.

Clinical features

Clinically, masseter's spasm and contraction presents as a sudden enlargement of the cheek that is usually unilateral and becomes obvious with the jaw movements and particularly when the teeth come into occlusion (**Fig. 33.6**). Five to twenty spasm episodes may occur within an hour and can last for a few minutes. Spasms are not observed throughout sleep. Automatic dysfunction, such as transient salivation, unilateral lacrimation, and sweating, may accompany muscle spasms. Additionally, the referral pain occurs from stimulation of trigger areas in hypersensitive muscles of mastication.

Differential diagnosis
- Masseteric hypertrophy
- Facial hemihypertrophy
- Parotid gland and other tumors
- Sjögren's syndrome
- Mikulicz's syndrome
- Heerfordt's syndrome

Laboratory tests

Electromyography, brain MRI and any other specialized tests are required to identify an underlying cause.

Treatment

Systemic treatment is best left to the neurologist. Topical use of Botox and correction of the occlusion may be helpful.

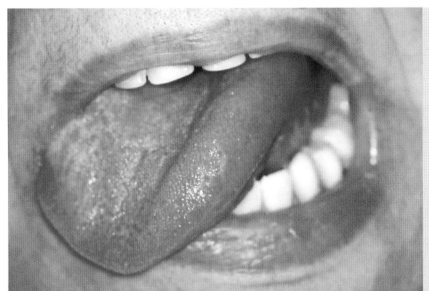

Fig. 33.4 Hypoglossal nerve paralysis, deviation toward the nonaffected side.

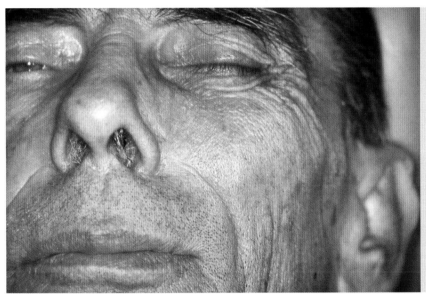

Fig. 33.5 Idiopathic trigeminal neuralgia of the second branch, muscular spasm of the affected side.

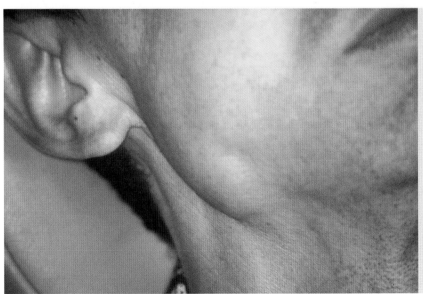

Fig. 33.6 Ipsilateral masseter spasm due to hypersensitive mastication muscle disorder.

34 Benign Tumors

1. Epithelium

1a. Surface Epithelium

Papilloma

Key points

- A benign tumor of the surface epithelium.
- In 50 to 60% of papillomas, human papillomavirus (HPV), types 6 and 11, are detected within the tumor.
- It has a characteristic clinical presentation, comprising of multiple, small projections with a "*cauliflower-like*" appearance.
- The final diagnosis is based on the histologic pattern.

Introduction

Papillomas are relatively common benign neoplasms of the stratified squamous epithelium that are frequently associated with the HPV types 6 and 11. These viral subtypes have been found in 50 to 60% of the cases, while in healthy mucosal cells these are found in less than 5%. The exact mode of transmission is not well known.

Clinical features

Papilloma affects both sexes equally, most commonly between the ages of 30 and 50 years. Clinically, it presents as an exophytic, well-circumscribed, pedunculated or sessile tumor, consisting of multiple, small projections that give the tumor a *cauliflower-like* appearance (**Figs. 34.1, 34.2**). The color varies between white, pale pink, or even normal mucosal, depending on the degree of keratinization. The size usually ranges between 3 and 6 mm and rarely grows above 1 cm. Papillomas are usually solitary, occurring more commonly on the tongue and the soft palate and less frequently in other sites.

Differential diagnosis

- Verruca vulgaris
- Condyloma accuminatum
- Verruciform xanthoma
- Verrucous carcinoma
- Sialadenoma papilliferum
- Focal dermal hypoplasia syndrome
- Focal epithelial hyperplasia

Pathology

On histologic examination, the papilloma is characterized by hyperplasia of the epithelial layers that give rise to characteristic multiple, finger-like projections with a slender fibrovascular core. Koilocyte-like cells can be observed in the prickle cell layer and are indicative of viral infection.

Treatment

The treatment of choice is conservative surgical excision.

Verruca Vulgaris

Key points

- Verruca vulgaris is associated with HPV, mainly types 1, 2, and 4.
- Lesions are very common on the skin, but are rarely observed in the mouth.
- It is transmitted intraorally through self-inoculation from the existing lesions of the fingers.
- The final diagnosis is based on the histologic pattern.

Introduction

Verruca vulgaris is a common, benign, skin hyperplasia caused by the HPV, mainly types 1, 2, and 4. Most often it presents on children's fingers, from where it can potentially be autoinoculated on the oral mucosa.

Clinical features

Oral verruca vulgaris is rare. When it occurs intraorally, the sites most commonly affected are the lips, tongue, and gingiva. Clinically, they present as small, painless, exophytic lesions with a "*cauliflower-like*" surface and white or pink-white color (**Figs. 34.3, 34.4**). They may be sessile or pedunculated, multiple or solitary. The clinical diagnosis has to be confirmed histopathologically.

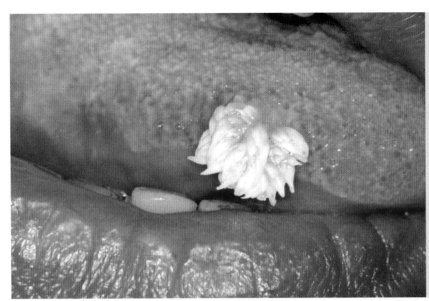

Fig. 34.1 Papilloma on the lateral aspect of the tongue.

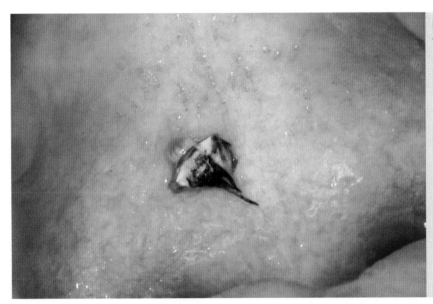

Fig. 34.2 Papilloma of black color on the palate due to increased melanin production.

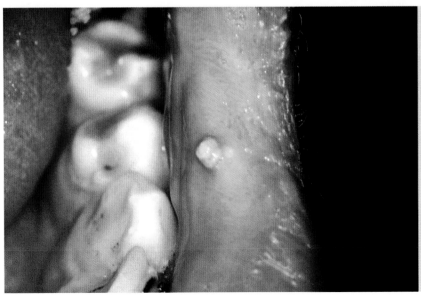

Fig. 34.3 Solitary verruca vulgaris on the lower lip.

Pathology

Histologically, the lesion is characterized by papillomatous projections of hyperplastic and hyperkeratotic squamous epithelium supported by a thin fibrous core. The rete ridges are elongated and tend to converge toward the center of the lesion (cupping effect). In the prominent granular cell layer, coarse, clumped keratohyalin granules are typically found, along with abundant koilocytes.

Treatment

Conservative surgical or electrosurgical excision of the oral lesions is the treatment of choice.

Condyloma Accuminatum

Introduction

Condyloma accuminatum is a common, sexually transmitted disease, observed mainly on the perianal skin and mucosa. It is caused by HPV, mainly types 6 and 11 and more rarely from other benign types. In most cases, it occurs at a young age through sexual transmission. Condyloma accuminatum is rare in the oral mucosa, where it can be caused from either direct orogenital contact or from self-inoculation with the hands being the vehicle of the viral transmission from the genitals to the mouth. Quite often, they can be observed on both the genitals and the oral mucosa.

Clinical features

Clinically, condyloma accuminatum appears as a sessile, painless, well-circumscribed exophytic tumor with a "*cauliflower-like*" surface and normal mucosal or pale pink color (**Figs. 34.5, 34.6**). The lesions are usually multiple, with size that ranges between 1 and 3 cm and have a tendency to coalesce and recur. Most commonly affected sites are the lips, buccal mucosa, tongue, lingual frenum, and soft palate. The clinical diagnosis has to be confirmed by the histologic examination.

Pathology

Histologically, condyloma accuminatum is characterized by parakeratosis, acanthosis, and elongation of the rete ridges. Koilocytes are frequently observed (small pyknotic nuclei surrounded by a clear cytoplasmic halo), indicating a microscopic feature of HPV infection. Verification of the virus infection can be proved by in situ hybridization and polymerase chain reaction (PCR) techniques.

Treatment

Conservative surgical excision or electrosurgery would be the preferred treatment for the oral lesions.

Focal Epithelial Hyperplasia

Introduction

Focal epithelial hyperplasia or Heck's disease is a benign hyperplastic condition of the oral mucosa, first described by Archard et al. in 1965. It is predominantly observed in Eskimos, American Indians, and South Africans. Sporadic cases have been reported in Europe and other ethnic groups. It is caused by HPV types 13 and 32. The familial presentation and predilection to certain ages suggests that a genetic factor might be implicated. Additionally, cases have been reported in patients with AIDS. It is more commonly observed in children, but it can also appear in adults.

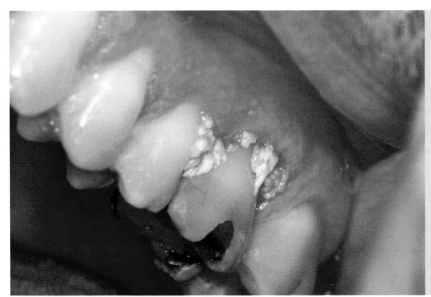

Fig. 34.4 Multiple verruca vulgaris on the gingiva.

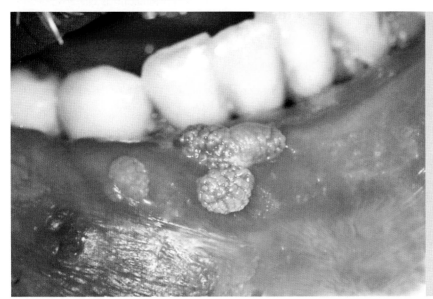

Fig. 34.5 Multiple condylomata acuminata on the lower lip mucosa.

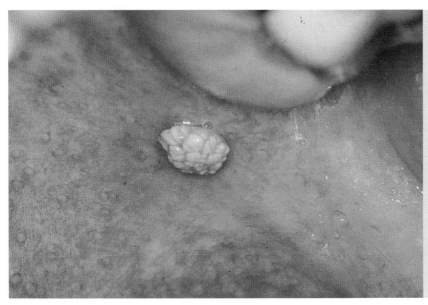

Fig. 34.6 Condyloma accuminatum on the palate.

Clinical features

Clinically, focal epithelial hyperplasia presents as multiple, sessile, painless, and slightly elevated nodules of 1 to 10 mm in diameter and normal mucosa, pale pink, or white color (**Figs. 34.7, 34.8**). The surface is smooth or mildly granular. Characteristically, when the mucosa is stretched, the lesions tend to disappear. The most commonly affected sites are the lower lip, tongue, and buccal mucosa, followed by the upper lip, gingiva, and palate. Rarely, conjunctival involvement may occur. The diagnosis is based on the clinical features, but has to be confirmed by a biopsy and the histopathologic pattern.

Differential diagnosis

- Condyloma accuminatum
- Multiple verruca vulgaris
- Multiple papillomas
- Multiple fibromas
- Cowden's disease
- Focal dermal hypoplasia syndrome

Pathology

On histologic examination, the lesions show prominent acanthosis and elongated broad rete ridges. Koilocytes and sporadic mitoses may be observed particularly on the upper epithelial layers. HPV virus has been found with DNA in situ hybridization and PCR techniques.

Treatment

The lesions may spontaneously reverse after a few months and up to 2 years. For lesions that cause esthetic problem, conservative surgical excision or CO_2 laser, or electrosurgery can be suggested. Recurrences after therapy rarely occur.

Keratoacanthoma

Key points

- It is often observed on the face and areas exposed to sunlight.
- About 10% of the cases appear on the lips.
- The tumor is rarely observed on the oral mucosa.
- It has characteristic clinical picture and behavior.
- Clinically and histologically, it can imitate squamous cell carcinoma.

Introduction

Keratoacanthoma is a fairly common benign skin tumor that occurs on exposed skin and arises from the hair follicles. The exact etiology is still unknown. However, the sunlight and HPV seem to play an important role in the pathogenesis.

Clinical features

Keratoacanthoma is more common in males than females (ratio 1.8:1) usually affecting older than 50 years. Clinically, it appears as a painless, well-circumscribed, dome- or bud-shaped tumor of 1 to 2 cm in diameter, with a characteristic keratin crater at the center (**Fig. 34.9**). Based on histogenesis and biological behavior, two types of keratoacanthoma are recognized. *Type I* (*bud-shaped*) occurs in the upper layers of the epidermis. It arises as a result of thickening and elongation of the walls of the superficial parts of hair follicles. *Type II* (*dome-shaped*) is seen deep in the epidermis and arises from the hair germ or the deeper part of the hair follicles. Characteristically, the tumor grows rapidly and within 4 to 8 weeks reaches the final size. For a period of 1 to 2 months, it persists without change and may then undergo spontaneous regression over the next 6 to 8 weeks. About 10% of keratoacanthomas are located on the lips

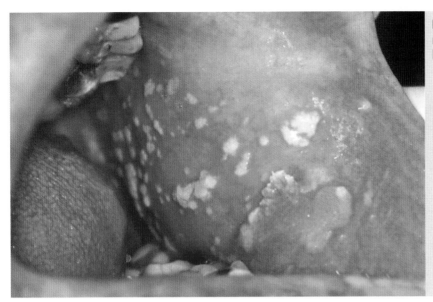

Fig. 34.7 Focal epithelial hyperplasia, multiple white-pink nodules on the buccal mucosa.

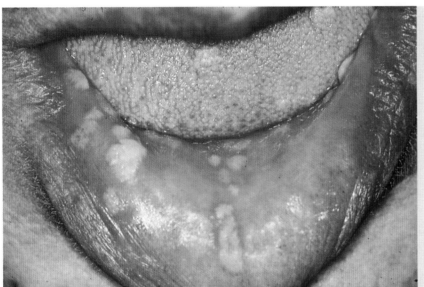

Fig. 34.8 Focal epithelial hyperplasia, multiple white-pink nodules on the mucosa of the lower lip and the tongue.

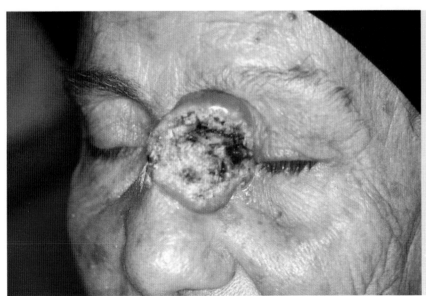

Fig. 34.9 Keratoacanthoma on the skin of the nose.

whereas very few cases have been reported intraorally (**Fig. 34.10**). The presence of oral hair and follicles may offer an explanation for the rare development of keratoacanthoma intraorally.

Differential diagnosis

- Squamous cell carcinoma
- Warty dyskeratoma
- Basal cell carcinoma
- Cutaneous and mucosal horn
- Molluscum contagiosum

Pathology

There is prominent epithelial hyperplasia with a characteristic keratin crater in the center of the lesion while the epithelium at the base of the crater exhibits a downward "pushing" pattern. There are different histologic changes depending on the stage of the tumor. At the early stages, cellular atypia and mitoses are observed. Pseudoepithelial hyperplasia is also present, mimicking the histologic pattern of squamous cell carcinoma. At later stages, the cellular atypia and mitoses are reduced and the keratinization is more prominent.

Treatment

Although some keratoacanthomas may regress spontaneously, the treatment of choice is surgical excision. Alternative therapies include electrosurgery, cryotherapy, topical imiquimod, and low dose of radiation. Recurrences are rare.

Mucosal Horn

Key points

- The oral equivalent of the cutaneous horn.
- It is very rare intraorally.
- An increased keratin production is the cause.

Introduction

Mucosal and cutaneous horns are both descriptive, clinical terms. The lesions are characterized by a prominent conical projection caused by keratin accumulation, usually in older people. On the skin, the lesion usually occurs on actinic keratosis, actinic cheilitis, seborrheic keratosis, verruca vulgaris, keratoacanthoma, basal cell carcinoma, squamous cell carcinoma, and lupus erythematosus. The oral lesions develop as an isolated disorder unrelated with other oral diseases.

Clinical features

Clinically, cutaneous horns present as straight or slightly convex keratin projection of just a few millimeters to many centimeters. Its color can be white-brown or yellow-brown (**Fig. 34.11**). It usually occurs on the face and rarely on the lower lip. A similar lesion can be observed on the oral mucosa (*mucosal horn*) and the glans penis, due to keratin overdevelopment, which is whitish in color (**Fig. 34.12**). The diagnosis is based on the clinical criteria and there is rarely a need for histologic examination.

Differential diagnosis

- Papilloma
- Verruca vulgaris
- Condyloma accuminatum
- Leukoplakia
- Squamous cell carcinoma

Pathology

On microscopic examination, prominent hyperkeratosis and parakeratosis are observed, as well as different degrees of acanthosis.

Treatment

The treatment of choice is conservative surgical excision.

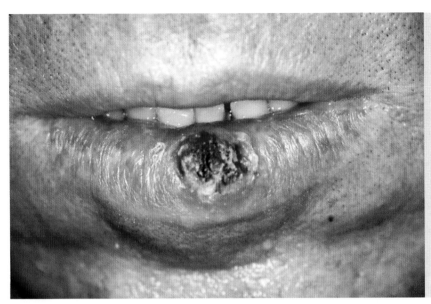

Fig. 34.10 Keratoacanthoma on the vermilion border of the lower lip.

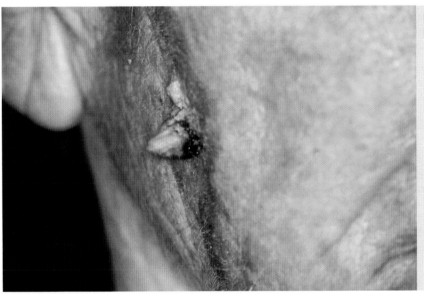

Fig. 34.11 Cutaneous horn on the skin of the cheek.

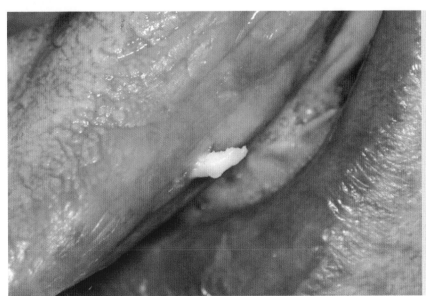

Fig. 34.12 Mucosal horn on the lingual mucosa.

1b. Glandular Epithelium

Pleomorphic Adenoma

Key points
- The most common benign tumor of the major and minor salivary glands.
- The palate is affected in 40 to 50% of all cases.
- It develops slowly to a painless, hard swelling.
- Commonly pose problems in diagnosis.
- Diagnosis should be histologically confirmed.

Introduction

The benign tumors of the salivary glands belong to either pleomorphic or monomorphic adenomas. Pleomorphic adenoma is the most common neoplasm of the major and minor salivary glands and is derived from the myoepithelial and glandular cells of the salivary duct accompanied by variable amounts of characteristic stroma. It represents 53 to 75.6% of all major salivary gland tumors and 33 to 43% of the minor salivary gland tumors.

Clinical features

Pleomorphic adenoma of minor salivary glands most commonly develops in the posterior aspect of the palate (60–65%), followed by the upper lip, retromolar area, buccal mucosa, and rarely the tongue. In the major salivary glands, 90% of the cases are observed in the parotids (**Fig. 34.13**). It equally affects both sexes, usually between 40 and 60 years. Clinically, pleomorphic adenoma of minor salivary glands presents as an asymptomatic slow-growing firm swelling with a size of 2 to 3 cm in diameter. The tumor is covered by normal mucosa and is rarely ulcerated (**Figs. 34.14, 34.15**). It might cause problems with mastication, speech, and even denture retention. The clinical picture is similar when the major salivary glands are affected; however, the tumor size can take much bigger dimensions. Bilateral development of tumor on the parotid glands may rarely occur. Diagnosis is based on the clinical feature but must be confirmed by a biopsy and the histologic examination.

Differential diagnosis
- Monomorphic adenomas
- Malignant tumors of the salivary glands
- Schwannoma
- Leiomyoma
- Lipoma
- Fibroma
- Necrotizing sialadenometaplasia
- Non-Hodgkin's lymphoma
- Chronic abscess

Pathology

Microscopically, the tumor consists of epithelial and myoepithelial cells with tubular, solid, trabecular, papillary, or cystic architecture. The epithelial cells are usually cuboidal, while the myoepithelial cells display spindle, epithelioid, plasmacytoid, oncocytic, or clear cell morphology. The stroma may be myxoid, hyaline, chondroid, and occasionally osseous. The tumor is surrounded by an incomplete fibrous capsule of variable thickness. However, microscopic satellite tumor nodules may be seen beyond the capsule. There is no significant mitotic activity.

Treatment

The treatment of choice is surgical excision. Recurrence after complete excision ranges between 3.5 and 6%.

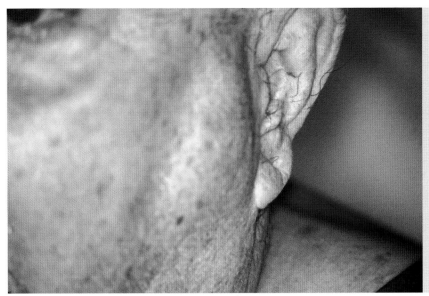

Fig. 34.13 Pleomorphic adenoma, swelling of the parotid.

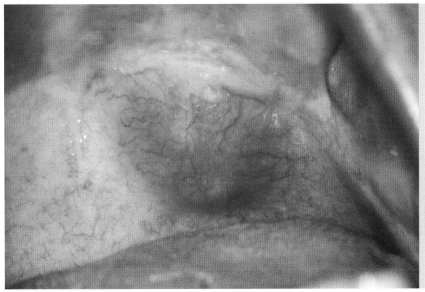

Fig. 34.14 Pleomorphic adenoma, swelling on the palate.

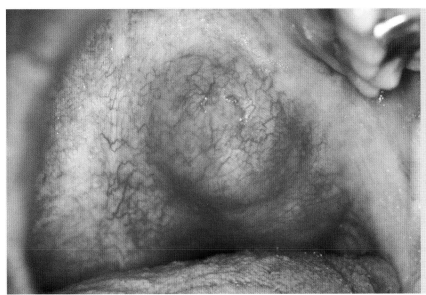

Fig. 34.15 Pleomorphic adenoma, swelling on the palate.

Myoepithelioma

Key points

- A benign tumor composed exclusively of neoplastic cells exhibiting myoepithelial differentiation.
- It has no pathognomonic clinical characteristics.
- Diagnosis is based exclusively on histopathologic examination.

Introduction

Myoepithelioma is a relatively rare benign tumor of the salivary glands, originating from the myoepithelial cells. Myoepithelioma, basal cell adenoma, and pleomorphic adenoma can be envisaged to lie on a continuous spectrum.

Clinical features

Myoepithelioma most frequently affects the parotid gland and the minor salivary glands of the palate, mainly between the ages of 30 and 50 years with no sex predilection. Clinically, myoepitheliomas of minor salivary glands present as a painless, slowly developing, well-circumscribed, firm enlargement that may be covered by normal mucosa. It can be ulcerated when trauma is involved (**Fig. 34.16**). The most commonly affected site is the palate. The clinical features are not pathognomonic; therefore, the diagnosis should be confirmed by histopathologic examination.

Differential diagnosis

- Pleomorphic adenoma
- Monomorphic adenomas
- Malignant salivary gland tumors
- Fibroma
- Neurofibroma
- Schwannoma
- Necrotizing sialadenometaplasia

Pathology

The characteristic histologic feature of myoepitheliomas is the presence of myoepithelial cells (spindled, plasmacytoid hyaline, epithelioid, clear, or oncocytic) in various formations, but without the creation of tubular (ductal) structures. The stroma ranges from being scanty to myxoid, hyaline, or sclerotic.

Treatment

The treatment of choice is surgical excision.

Papillary Cystadenoma Lymphomatosum

Key points

- It mainly affects the parotid gland.
- Rarely occurs in the minor salivary glands.
- The tumor has characteristic histopathologic pattern.

Introduction

Papillary cystadenoma lymphomatosum, also known as adenolymphoma or Warthin's tumor, is a relatively common benign tumor of the salivary glands, almost exclusively occurring in the parotids. A few cases have been reported in the submandibular gland and the minor salivary glands. It is the second most common benign parotid tumor (5–15%) after the pleomorphic adenoma. The histogenesis is not well understood. Its origin is believed to be heterotopic adrenal epithelium that remained inside the lymphatic tissue of the gland or may derive from a proliferation of ductal epithelium that is associated with lymphoid tissue.

Clinical features

Papillary cystadenoma lymphomatosum affects males to a higher ratio (5:1–7:1), predominantly between the ages of 50 and 70 years. Intraorally, the most commonly affected site is the palate, followed by buccal mucosa and the upper lip. Clinically, it appears as a painless swelling covered by normal mucosa (**Fig. 34.17**). On palpation, it may be firm or soft. It develops slowly and can reach 1 to 4 cm in diameter. When the parotid is affected, the presentation is usually unilateral, but bilateral involvement may occur in approximately 5 to 15% (**Fig. 34.18**). The clinical features are not characteristic and the final diagnosis should be confirmed by histologic examination.

Differential diagnosis

- Other benign tumors of the salivary glands
- Malignant tumors of the salivary glands
- Non-Hodgkin's lymphoma
- Cystadenoma
- Mucocele
- Lymphoepithelial cyst
- Sialadenosis (sialosis)

Pathology

Microscopically, the epithelial cells are arranged in two rows, surrounding cystic spaces. The cells have abundant granular eosinophilic cytoplasm with centrally placed hyperchromatic

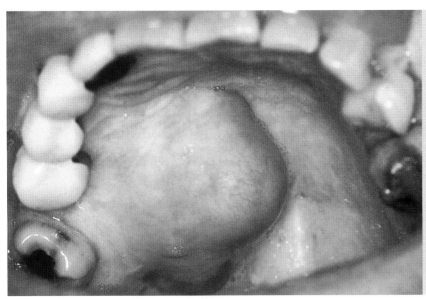

Fig. 34.16 Myoepithelioma on the palate.

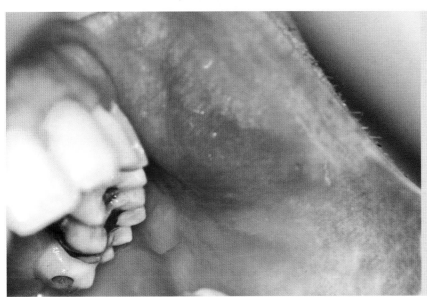

Fig. 34.17 Papillary cystadenoma lymphomatosum, swelling with unclear borders in the buccal mucosa.

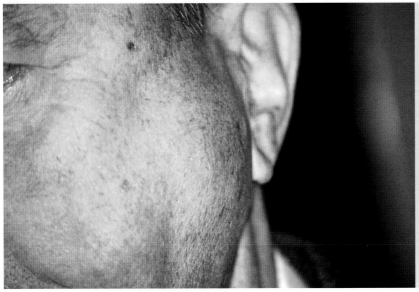

Fig. 34.18 Papillary cystadenoma lymphomatosum, swelling of the parotid.

nuclei. Multiple papillary projections into the cystic spaces are usually observed. The epithelium is characteristically supported by a lymphoid stroma containing scattered germinal centers.

Treatment

The treatment of choice is surgical excision.

Basal Cell Adenoma

Key points

- A rare benign tumor of the salivary glands.
- It represents 1 to 2% of all salivary gland tumors.
- Mainly affects the parotid glands (60–80%) and rarely the minor salivary glands.
- The diagnosis is based on the histologic pattern.

Introduction

Basal cell adenoma is a rare benign tumor of the salivary glands. It belongs to the groups of monomorphic adenomas. Histologically, it is characterized by the basaloid pattern of the tumor cells. It develops more frequently in the parotid glands (60–80%), followed by the minor salivary glands, the submandibular and sublingual glands.

Clinical features

Basal cell adenoma is more commonly observed in females with a predilection of 2:1. The age group that is predominantly affected is the 50 to 70 years old. About 70% occur in the parotid glands. Intraorally, it affects the upper lip more frequently (10–20%) and rarely the palate and buccal mucosa. Clinically, basal cell adenoma presents as a painless, slowly developing, well-circumscribed, firm small tumor 1 to 3 cm in size that may be ulcerated (**Figs. 34.19, 34.20**). The clinical features are not sufficiently diagnostic. Therefore, histologic examination is always required for the definite diagnosis.

Differential diagnosis

- Pleomorphic adenoma
- Canalicular adenoma
- Other monomorphic adenomas
- Malignant tumors of the salivary glands
- Non-Hodgkin's lymphoma
- Fibroma
- Neurofibroma
- Schwannoma

Pathology

Histologically, the tumor is often surrounded by a fibrous capsule. There are three main types of the basal cell adenoma, the *solid*, *trabecular*, and *membranous*. The solid type is characterized by multiple islands and strands of epithelial cells that are supported by a small amount of connective tissue. Basal cell adenoma comprises of two cell types: basaloid and larger polygonal cells. The cells are characteristically arranged in a palisading, tubular or lobular, or trabecular pattern, resembling the skin basal cell carcinoma.

Treatment

The treatment of choice is complete surgical excision. Recurrences are rare.

Canalicular Adenoma

Key points

- A rare tumor of the salivary glands.
- It mainly affects the minor salivary glands.
- The clinical features are not characteristic and the diagnosis must be confirmed histologically.

Introduction

Canalicular adenoma is a rare benign tumor mainly affecting the minor salivary glands. It is rare in the parotid, the submandibular, or sublingual glands.

Clinical features

Canalicular adenoma more commonly affects females between 60 and 70 years. Intraorally, the most commonly affected site is the upper lip (approximately 80%), followed by the buccal mucosa (10%) and palate. Clinically, it presents as a painless, slowly developing, circumscribed painless tumor that is covered by normal epithelium (**Fig. 34.21**). On palpation, it may be firm or fluctuant mimicking a cyst. The size ranges between 0.5 and 2 cm. Occasionally, multifocal lesion may be seen, particularly on the upper lip. The clinical features are not diagnostic and histopathologic examination is required for the definite diagnosis.

Differential diagnosis

- Basal cell adenoma
- Other types of monomorphic adenomas
- Pleomorphic adenoma
- Cystadenoma
- Basal cell carcinoma
- Mucoepidermoid carcinoma
- Adenoid cystic carcinoma
- Mucocele
- Neurofibroma

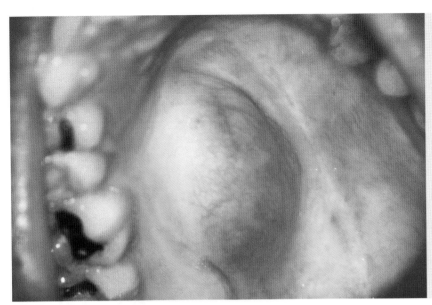

Fig. 34.19 Basal cell adenoma on the palate.

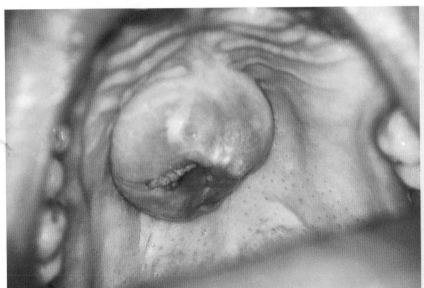

Fig. 34.20 Basal cell adenoma on the palate.

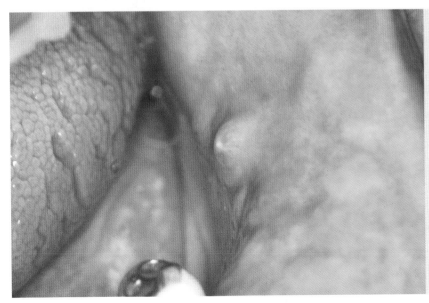

Fig. 34.21 Canalicular adenoma on the buccal mucosa.

Pathology

Histologic examination is necessary for a definitive diagnosis. Microscopically, a monomorphic cellular population, consisting of cylindrical or cuboidal cells with basophilic nuclei, arranged in tubular pattern or forming cystic spaces is the prominent histologic pattern. The tumor cells are supported by a vascular connective tissue substrate. The tumor is encapsulated by a thin fibrous capsule of connective tissue.

Treatment

The treatment of choice is complete surgical excision. Recurrences are rare.

Sebaceous Adenoma

Key points

- A benign neoplasm that originates from the sebaceous glands' epithelium.
- More commonly is seen on the skin of the scalp and the neck.
- It is very rarely seen intraorally.
- The diagnosis is based on the histologic pattern.
- Approximately 50% of the tumor develops in the parotid gland.

Introduction

Sebaceous adenoma is a rare, benign skin tumor, originating from the dermal sebaceous glands. It appears on the scalp and the face of elderly patients without sex preponderance. On the lips and intraorally, the lesion is extremely rare and when present, it is believed to originate from the ectopic sebaceous glands (Fordyce's granules) of the oral mucosa.

Clinical features

Clinically, oral sebaceous adenoma presents as a solitary, well-circumscribed, round and firm painless mass (**Fig. 34.22**). It has a yellow-pink color, smooth or slightly granulated surface, and size between 0.5 and 1 cm. The diagnosis is based on the histologic pattern.

Differential diagnosis

- Xanthoma
- Verruciform xanthoma
- Lipoma
- Myxoma
- Fibroma
- Cystadenoma

Pathology

On histologic examination, oral sebaceous adenoma is characterized by multiple, scattered, immature sebaceous elements arranged in nests, together with normal sebaceous cells with vacuolated cytoplasm. Sporadic mitoses may be seen.

Treatment

The treatment of choice is surgical excision.

Papillary Syringadenoma

Key points

- A benign neoplasm that originates from the epithelium of the skin's apocrine glands.
- It develops on the skin, mainly of the scalp and the neck.
- In the oral area, it can only occur around the mouth.
- Diagnosis is based on the histologic pattern.

Introduction

Papillary syringadenoma or syringocystadenoma papilliferum is a rare benign tumor of apocrine sweat glands of the skin. It usually appears at birth or during childhood and puberty. It is more frequently observed on the skin of the scalp, the neck, and rarely on the face. Extremely rare, it develops on the lips while it is not observed intraorally.

Clinical features

Clinically, papillary syringadenoma appears as a solitary, well-circumscribed, and asymptomatic nodule or plaque with a slightly depressed center (**Fig. 34.23**). The size varies between 0.5 and 1.5 cm. The clinical findings are not pathognomonic; hence, the diagnosis is based on the histologic pattern.

Differential diagnosis

- Keratoacanthoma
- Basal cell carcinoma
- Squamous cell carcinoma
- Cutaneous horn

Pathology

Histologically, papillary projections are observed that are lined by two cell layers, an outer or luminal cylindrical cells with apocrine differentiation and an inner of basal-like cells. The connective tissue stem of the projections has a lymphocytic and plasma cell infiltrate.

Treatment

The treatment of choice is complete surgical excision.

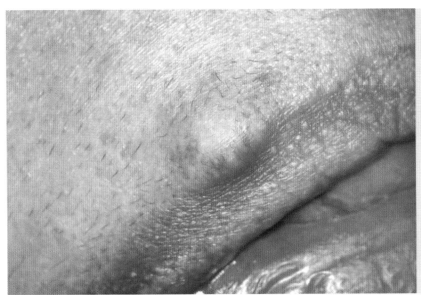

Fig. 34.22 Sebaceous adenoma on the border of the skin and the vermilion border of the upper lip.

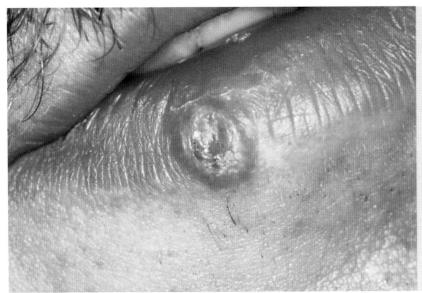

Fig. 34.23 Papillary syringadenoma on the border of the skin and the vermilion border of the lower lip.

Chondroid Syringoma

Key points

- A hamartoma that is classified as an adenoma of the skin components.
- It has a benign behavior and usually does not regress after its excision.
- Histologically, it is similar with pleomorphic adenoma of the salivary glands.
- The oral mucosa is not affected.

Introduction

Chondroid syringoma or mixed tumor of the skin is a hamartoma from a follicular–sebaceous apocrine unit of the skin component, adenomas type. Histologically, it has similarities with the pleomorphic adenoma (mixed tumor) of the salivary glands. It has a good biological response and rarely recurs after the surgical excision.

Clinical features

Clinically, chondroid syringoma appears as a firm, painless, slowly developing skin nodule of 0.5 to 1 cm in diameter. It usually occurs in the head and neck area (nose, cheeks, upper lip) and more rarely on the trunk, axilla, and perigenital area (**Fig. 34.24**). The clinical characteristics are not pathognomonic; hence, the diagnosis has to be based on the histologic pattern.

Differential diagnosis

- Trichoepithelioma
- Sebaceous adenoma
- Syringoma
- Other skin tumors

Pathology

The histologic examination of the lesion is a prerequisite for the definitive diagnosis. The tumor consists of epidermal cells forming a network of tubular structures, or small ducts or both. The epidermal component of the tumor contains follicular and sebaceous elements. The epidermal structures are surrounded by connective tissue which contains collagen in abundance with myxomatous degeneration and cartilage formation.

Treatment

The treatment of choice is the conservative excision of the tumor. The risk for recurrence is rare.

2. Connective Tissue

Fibroma

Key points

- The most common intraoral benign tumor.
- The cause is usually chronic trauma or irritation.
- Diagnosis is frequently based on the clinical features.

Introduction

Fibroma is the most common benign intraoral tumor. It originates from the connective tissue. In most cases, it is not a true neoplasm but a reactive hyperplasia of the connective tissue to chronic local irritation or trauma.

Clinical features

Fibromas affect equally, both sexes, usually between 30 and 50 years. Clinically, it presents as a well-circumscribed, usually sessile or with a broad base, asymptomatic nodule. The tumor is covered by normal mucosa and has a firm consistency (**Figs. 34.25–34.27**). Not uncommonly, the surface has a white appearance and is rarely ulcerated due to continuous mechanical irritation. Fibroma is usually solitary with a diameter of approximately 0.5 to 1 cm, although in rare cases it may reach several centimeters. Most commonly, it occurs on the buccal mucosa, gingiva, tongue, lips, and palate. The diagnosis is based on the clinical features, but it has to be supported by the histologic findings.

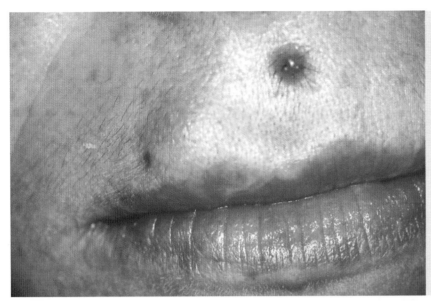

Fig. 34.24 Chondroid syringoma, enlargement on the border of the skin, and the vermilion border of the upper lip.

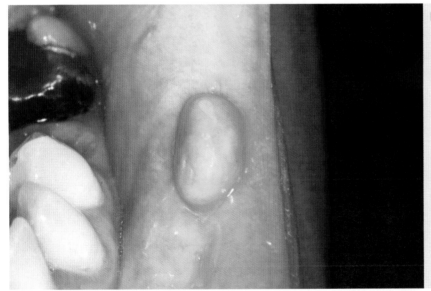

Fig. 34.25 Fibroma on the lower lip.

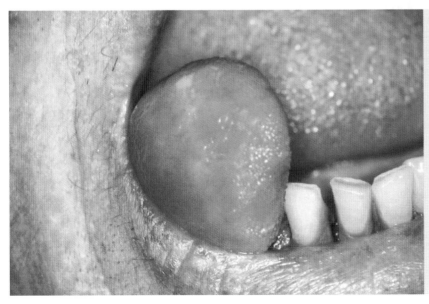

Fig. 34.26 Large fibroma on the buccal mucosa.

Differential diagnosis

- Peripheral gingival fibroma
- Giant cell fibroma
- Neurofibroma
- Schwannoma
- Lipoma
- Myxoma
- Oral focal mucinosis
- Fibrous histiocytoma
- Fibrous developmental hyperplasia

Pathology

Histologically, fibroma is predominantly characterized by abundant connective tissue varying in cellularity with mild inflammation. The tumor is covered by a thin and atrophic epithelium with absence of rete ridges. Occasionally, hyperkeratosis may be present as a result of friction.

Treatment

The treatment of choice is conservative surgical excision. Electrosurgery, cryotherapy, and laser surgery can also be used as alternative methods. Recurrences are uncommon.

Giant Cell Fibroma

Key points

- A variation of fibroma.
- It is not associated with mechanical irritation.
- Diagnosis is based mainly on the histologic pattern.

Introduction

Giant cell fibroma is a connective tissue tumor with specific clinical and histologic features that do not associate with chronic irritation or trauma. The tumor is histologically characterized by the presence of numerous stellate and multinucleated fibrous cells. It accounts for approximately 3 to 5% of the intraoral, benign, connective tissue tumors.

Clinical features

Clinically, giant cell fibroma appears as a painless, well-circumscribed, usually pedunculated tumor, of normal color and slightly nodulated surface (**Fig. 34.28**). The size of the tumor varies from a few millimeters up to 1 cm. It affects both sexes and usually occurs in the first three decades of life. The gingivae are predominantly affected, followed by the tongue,

palate, buccal mucosa, and lips. The clinical diagnosis has to be confirmed histologically.

Differential diagnosis

- Fibroma
- Neurofibroma
- Peripheral gingival fibroma
- Granular cell tumor

Pathology

Histologically, giant cell fibroma is characterized by abundant and vascular fibrous connective tissue. The most characteristic findings are the presence of numerous, large stellate fibroblasts with multiple nuclei. The covering epithelium is usually atrophic and thin with narrow and elongated rete ridges.

Treatment

The treatment of choice is conservative surgical excision. Recurrences are uncommon.

Peripheral Ossifying Fibroma

Key points

- It originates from the periodontal ligament or the periosteum.
- Appears exclusively on the gingiva.
- The tumor has characteristic clinical and histomorphologic features.
- The diagnosis is predominantly based on the histologic pattern.

Introduction

Peripheral ossifying fibroma or peripheral fibroma of the gingiva is a relatively common benign tumor. It occurs exclusively on the gingiva and has specific clinical and histologic features. The exact histogenesis is unclear, but it is believed to derive from either the periodontal membrane or the periosteum.

Clinical features

The peripheral ossifying fibroma is usually seen in teenagers and young adults. It affects females more commonly to a ratio of 2:1. The tumor equally affects the maxilla and mandible, usually in the incisor–cuspid region. The size varies between 0.5 and 2 cm. Clinically, it presents as a circumscribed gingival growth, sessile or pedunculated that is covered by normal mucosa (**Fig. 34.29**). However, frequently the surface

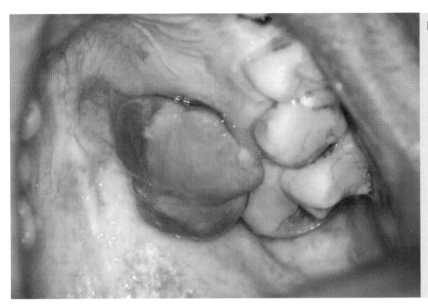

Fig. 34.27 Fibroma on the palate.

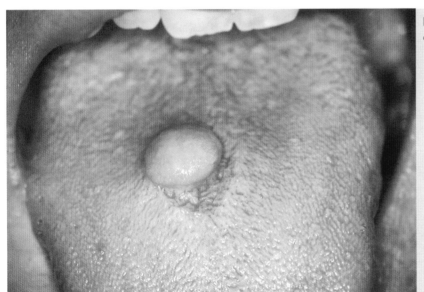

Fig. 34.28 Giant cell fibroma on the dorsum of the tongue.

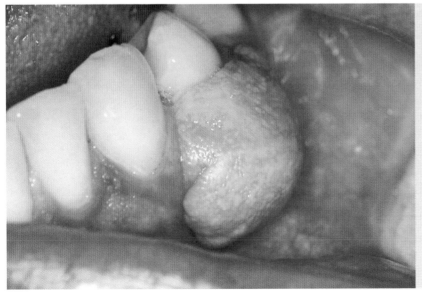

Fig. 34.29 Peripheral ossifying fibroma on the lower gingiva.

can be erythematous, or even ulcerated due to mechanical trauma (**Fig. 34.30**). The clinical diagnosis has to be confirmed histologically.

Differential diagnosis

- Fibroma
- Giant cell fibroma
- Pyogenic granuloma
- Pregnancy granuloma
- Peripheral odontogenic tumor
- Peripheral giant cell granuloma

Pathology

Histologically, peripheral ossifying fibroma is characterized by the presence of abundant cellular and vascular connective tissue. Usually, it is associated with mineralization of osteoid and bone formation. The epithelium is usually thin, atrophic, and usually ulcerated.

Treatment

The treatment of choice is surgical excision. The tumor should be excised beneath the periosteum to avoid recurrences.

Denture Fibrous Hyperplasia

Key points

- It is due to chronic mechanical irritation from the ill-fitting denture flanges.
- The lesions usually occur in the vestibules.
- The term epulis fissuratum should be avoided as the teeth and gingiva do not exist in these patients.

Introduction

Denture fibrous hyperplasia or epulis fissuratum is a common mucosal reaction caused by poorly fitting dentures in individuals who have been wearing dentures usually for a long period of time. The chronic irritation may be due to a sharp margin of the denture or overextended flags.

Clinical features

Clinically, denture fibrous hyperplasia presents as multiple or solitary inflamed elongated mucosal papillary folds usually on the facial aspect of the mucolabial or mucobuccal grooves (**Figs. 34.31, 34.32**). The size may vary between 0 and 5 cm and up to several centimeters. The lesions are mobile and firm to palpation and their continued growth may cause problems in maintaining denture retention. Painful ulcerations are common at the base of the folds. The fibrous hyperplasia may affect either the maxilla or mandible. The diagnosis is based on the clinical features and rarely a biopsy and histologic explanation are necessary to rule out other oral lesions.

Differential diagnosis

- Multiple fibromas
- Neurofibromatosis
- Squamous cell carcinoma
- Verrucous hyperplasia
- Fibromatosis
- Gardner's syndrome
- Non-Hodgkin's lymphoma

Pathology

Histologically, the denture fibrous hyperplasia shows severe hyperplasia of the fibrous connective tissue. The overlying epithelium demonstrates parakeratosis, acanthosis, and elongation of the rete ridges. Sometimes pseudoepitheliomatous hyperplasia can be observed. Areas of ulceration may also be seen. A chronic inflammatory reaction may also occur on the connective tissue stroma.

Treatment

The treatment of choice is surgical excision followed by the construction of new dentures.

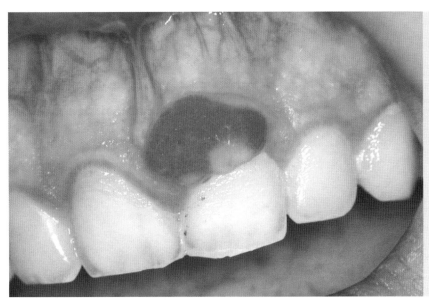

Fig. 34.30 Peripheral ossifying fibroma with an erythematous surface, on the upper gingiva.

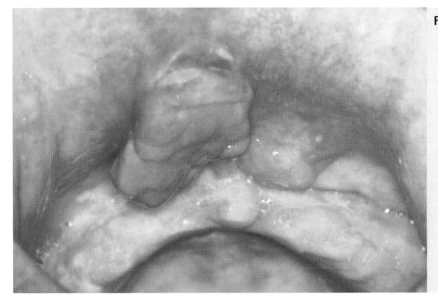

Fig. 34.31 Denture fibrous hyperplasia.

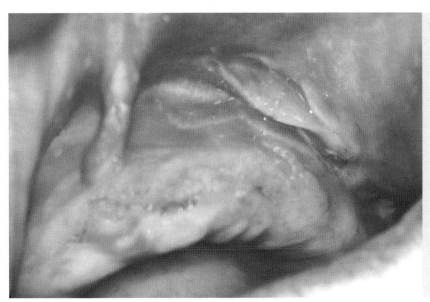

Fig. 34.32 Denture fibrous hyperplasia.

Oral Focal Mucinosis

Key points

- Mucinoses are a group of diseases caused by an increased mucous production and deposition, mainly on the skin.
- They are classified into two groups: *primary* and *secondary*.
- They are rarely seen in the mouth and when present, the lesions belong to the focal primary, degenerative–inflammatory type.
- The gingiva is the most commonly affected oral site.
- The diagnosis is based on the histologic pattern.

Introduction

Mucinoses are heterogeneous groups of diseases that affect the production and deposition of mucous on the skin. They are classified into *primary* and *secondary*. The primary group is divided into two categories: the *degenerative–inflammatory* and the *hamartomatous–neoplastic*. Focal dermal mucinosis belongs to the primary degenerative–inflammatory type. Oral focal mucinosis is rare and of unknown etiology. It is believed to be caused by a functional disorder that leads to increased production of hyaluronic acid from the connective tissue fibroblasts.

Clinical features

Oral focal mucinosis affects females to males in a ratio of 2:1, usually between the ages of 30 and 50 years. Clinically, it presents as a circumscribed and painless tumor that might be sessile or pedunculated and is covered by smooth normal mucosa (**Fig. 34.33**). The size varies between 0.5 and 2 cm. In over 70% of the cases, it occurs on the gingiva, followed by the palate, buccal mucosa, and tongue. The clinical features are not pathognomonic and the diagnosis is based on the histologic pattern.

Differential diagnosis

- Fibroma
- Peripheral ossifying fibroma
- Lipoma
- Myxoma
- Mucocele
- Cystadenoma

Pathology

Histologically, oral focal mucinosis is characterized by an abundance of loose connective tissue dominated by mucous deposition that is surrounded by dense connective tissue. Vimentin positive, stellate and fusiform fibroblasts are observed. There is absence of elastic and reticular fibers. The epithelium is thin and presents with flattened rete ridges. Histochemical stains (i.e., Alcian blue) demonstrate the hyaluronic acid nature of the myxomatous tissue.

Treatment

The treatment of choice is conservative surgical excision.

Lipoma

Key points

- A benign tumor of the adipose tissue.
- Clinically, it presents as an exophytic tumor with yellowish or pink-yellow color and soft consistency.
- The clinical diagnosis has to be confirmed by the histologic examination.

Introduction

Lipoma is a benign tumor of the adipose tissue. It is one of the most common mesenchymal benign tumor. It is relatively rare intraorally. The exact pathogenesis of lipomas is not well known.

Clinical features

Oral lipoma equally affects both sexes, usually between 40 and 60 years. Clinically, it presents as a well-defined, painless tumor, usually sessile, of yellow or pink-yellow color (**Figs. 34.34, 34.35**). It is covered by a thin mucosal layer with visible blood capillaries. On palpation, it is usually soft and occasionally fluctuant and may be misdiagnosed as a cyst, especially if seated deep within the submucosal tissues. The buccal mucosa and vestibule and less often the tongue and palate, lips, and gingiva are the sites most commonly affected. The size of tumor varies between 1 and 3 cm or more.

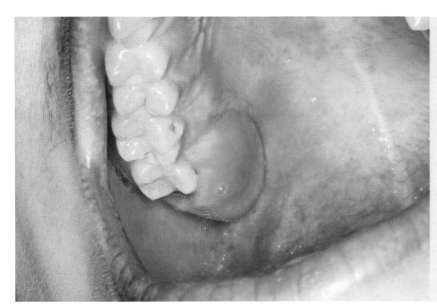

Fig. 34.33 Oral focal mucinosis, circumscribed tumor on the palatal gingiva.

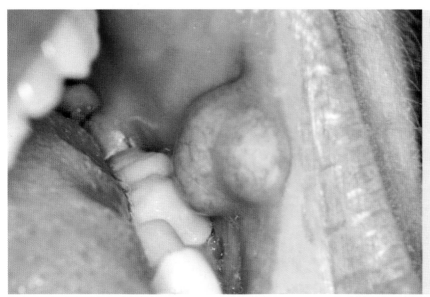

Fig. 34.34 Bilobular lipoma on the buccal mucosa.

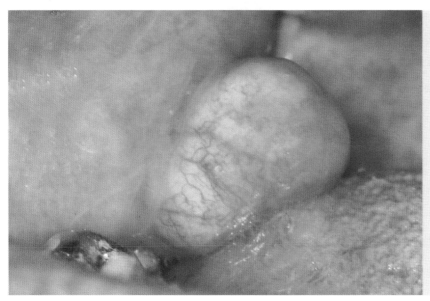

Fig. 34.35 Lipoma on the buccal mucosa.

Differential diagnosis

- Fibroma
- Myxoma
- Oral focal mucinosis
- Mucocele
- Dermoid cyst
- Cystadenoma

Pathology

Histologically, abundant mature adipose tissue is present. The tumor is usually encapsulated by a thin layer of connective tissue. When large proportion of connective tissue is present, the term fibrolipoma is used while the term angiolipoma is applied when a rich vascular component is seen. The covering epithelium appears normal.

Treatment

The treatment of choice is conservative surgical excision.

Myxoma

Key points

- A benign tumor that rarely occurs in the mouth.
- The clinical features are not pathognomonic.
- The diagnosis is based on the histologic pattern.

Introduction

Myxoma is a benign tumor of the mesenchyme and is rare in the soft tissues. It is extremely rare in the oral mucosa and most of the lesions represent a myxoid degeneration of the connective tissue rather than a true neoplasm. Odontogenic myxoma of the jaws is derived from odontogenic mesenchyme and should not be confused with soft tissue myxoma.

Clinical features

Clinically, myxoma presents as a well-circumscribed tumor covered by normal mucosa and soft on palpation (**Figs. 34.36, 34.37**). It can occur at any age and equally affects both sexes. It appears mainly on the buccal mucosa and less often on the floor of the mouth, palate, and gingiva. The diagnosis is based exclusively on the histologic pattern.

Differential diagnosis

- Lipoma
- Oral focal mucinosis
- Fibroma
- Mucocele
- Cystadenoma

Pathology

Histologically, myxomas are composed of stellate and spindle-shaped cells in a loose myxoid stroma. Histochemically, myxoid matrix is positive with Alcian blue, mucicarmine, and colloidal iron. Immunohistochemically, spindle cells are vimentin positive and in 50% of the cases CD34 is also positive.

Treatment

The treatment of choice is conservative surgical excision. Recurrences are uncommon.

Fibrous Histiocytoma

Key points

- A benign tumor derived from histiocytes.
- Common on the skin and rare on the oral mucosa.
- The diagnosis is based exclusively on the histologic pattern.

Introduction

Fibrous histiocytoma is a benign cellular tumor primarily composed of histiocytes and fibroblasts producing reticulum fibers. The tumor develops more often on the skin of the neck and the extremities and very rarely on the oral mucosa.

Clinical features

Fibrous histiocytoma equally affects both sexes, usually between 50 and 70 years. Clinically, it presents as a painless, mildly mobile, and firm tumor covered by normal or ulcerated mucosa (**Fig. 34.38**). The size varies between 0.5 and 2 cm in diameter. It most commonly occurs on the buccal mucosa followed by the tongue, lips, and gingiva. Intraosseous fibrous histiocytoma on the jaws may also rarely occur. The diagnosis is predominantly based on the histologic pattern.

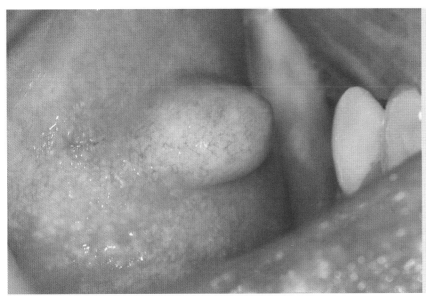

Fig. 34.36 Myxoma on the buccal mucosa.

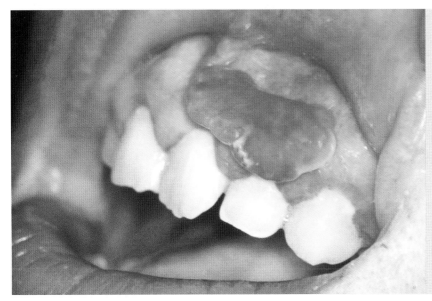

Fig. 34.37 Fibromyxoma on the maxillary alveolar mucosa.

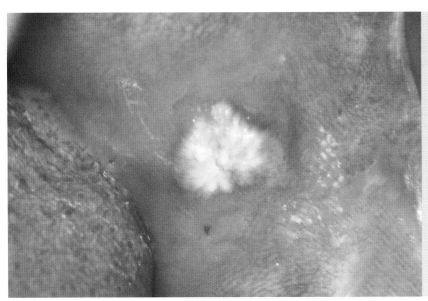

Fig. 34.38 Fibrous histiocytoma on the buccal mucosa.

Differential diagnosis

- Fibroma
- Neurofibroma
- Schwannoma
- Granular cell tumor
- Myxoma
- Lipoma
- Lymphoepithelial cyst

Pathology

Histologically, fibrous histiocytoma is characterized by multiple spindle-shaped fibroblasts with vesicular nuclei. There are also round histiocytes, xanthomatous cells containing lipids, and some sporadic multinucleated giant cells. The stroma may demonstrate areas with myxoid degeneration. Storiform pattern is commonly seen with hyperplasia of the overlying epithelium.

Treatment

The treatment of choice is surgical excision. Recurrences are uncommon.

Verruciform Xanthoma

Key points

- A rare lesion of unclear cause.
- Intraorally, it occurs mainly on the gingiva and alveolar mucosa.
- Clinically, it has a characteristic mild papillary surface.
- Histologically, it is characterized by lipids-containing histiocytes.

Introduction

Verruciform xanthoma is a rare oral hyperplasia of unknown cause and histogenesis that was first described by Shafer in 1971. Histologically, the lesion demonstrates a characteristic pattern with similarities to other xanthomas. However, it is not associated with systemic metabolic diseases.

Clinical features

Clinically, verruciform xanthoma presents as a painless, sessile, well-demarcated, and slightly elevated lesion with a papillary surface and normal or red-yellowish color (**Figs. 34.39, 34.40**). It equally affects both sexes, usually between the fifth and seventh decade of life. The size ranges between 0.2 and 2 cm in diameter. It most commonly develops on the alveolar mucosa and the gingiva and less often on the vestibule, palate, floor of the mouth, tongue, lips, and buccal mucosa. The clinical diagnosis has to be confirmed histologically.

Differential diagnosis

- Papilloma
- Condyloma accuminatum
- Verruca vulgaris
- Verrucous hyperplasia
- Verrucous leukoplakia
- Verrucous carcinoma
- Sialadenoma papilliferum

Pathology

Histologically, verruciform xanthoma is characterized by numerous large, foamy, lipid-containing histiocytes (*xanthomatous cells*) in the connective tissue. These cells do not characteristically extend beyond the elongated rete ridges. The epithelium appears thickened with significant acanthosis, parakeratosis, and enlargement of the rete ridges to a uniform pattern. After immunohistochemical stains, the xanthomatous cells are positive for specific markers such as cathepsin B and CD68 (KP1).

Treatment

The treatment of choice is conservative surgical excision. Recurrences are uncommon.

Soft Tissue Chondroma

Key points

- A very rare tumor on the oral mucosa.
- The tongue is the most commonly affected.
- The diagnosis is based on the histologic pattern.

Introduction

Chondroma is a benign tumor of chondroid tissue that may exceedingly rarely develop in the oral soft tissues. In those cases, it is characterized as a soft tissue chondroma or a cartilaginous choristoma (normal tissue in the wrong place). The tumor is believed to derive from remnants of ectopic chondroid tissue or from polyvalent mesenchyme cells.

Clinical features

Clinically, soft tissue chondroma appears as a painless, sessile, or pedunculated spherical and firm enlargement that is covered by normal mucosa (**Fig. 34.41**). It varies in size between 0.5 and 1 cm in diameter. The lateral borders and the dorsum of the tongue are the most commonly affected sites (80–90%), followed by the buccal mucosa, palate, and gingiva. The clinical features are not pathognomonic and diagnosis should be confirmed by the histologic examination.

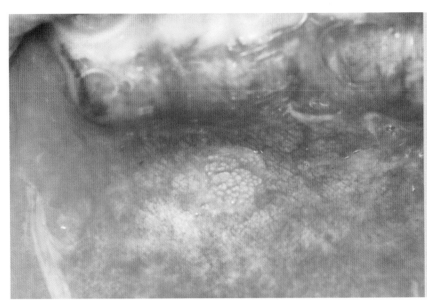

Fig. 34.39 Verruciform xanthoma on the mucosa of the lower lip.

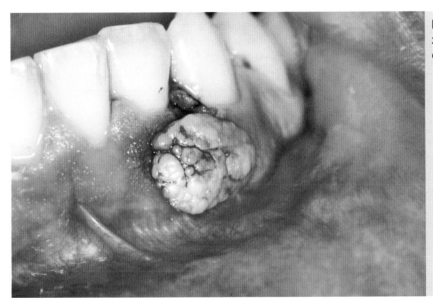

Fig. 34.40 Exophytic verruciform xanthoma with unusual presentation, on the lower gingiva.

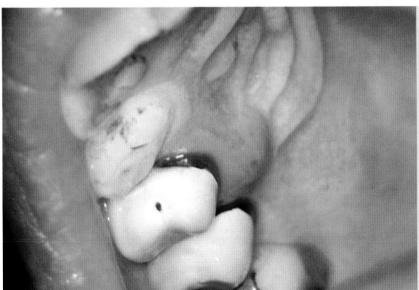

Fig. 34.41 Chondroma, the palatal gingiva respectively with the premolars.

Differential diagnosis

- Fibroma
- Neurofibroma
- Schwannoma
- Peripheral ossifying fibroma
- Granular cell tumor
- Lipoma

Pathology

Histologically, soft tissue chondroma shows lobules of mature cartilage, containing numerous small chondrocytes, surrounded by dense fibrous connective tissue layers.

Treatment

The treatment of choice is conservative surgical excision.

Soft Tissue Osteoma

Key points

- A very rare tumor on the oral mucosa.
- The tongue is more frequently affected.
- The diagnosis is based on the histologic examination.

Introduction

Osteoma is a benign tumor caused by proliferation of osseous cells in the oral soft tissues (*choristoma*). It can develop in different parts of the skeleton and rarely on the maxilla or the mandible. Multiple osteomas of the jaws are a common manifestation of Gardner's syndrome. It is more common in males aged between 30 and 50 years. Oral soft tissue osteoma is exceedingly rare and belongs to choristomas.

Clinical features

Clinically, oral soft tissue osteoma appears as a painless, well-circumscribed, and hard enlargement, covered by thin, smooth, and normal mucosa. The size ranges from 0.5 to 2 cm in diameter. The lesion has been described on the tongue, palate, buccal mucosa, and alveolar mucosa (**Fig. 34.42**). Osteoma of the jaws is more common on the maxilla. The clinical diagnosis has to be confirmed histologically.

Differential diagnosis

- Torus palatinus
- Torus mandibularis
- Other exostoses
- Chondroma
- Fibroma
- Gardner's syndrome

Pathology

Histologically, soft tissue osteoma exhibits a well-circumscribed, dense, normal osseous tissue that is surrounded by dense fibrous connective tissue. The epithelium is thin with absence of rete ridges.

Treatment

The treatment of choice is conservative surgical excision.

3. Nervous Tissue

Neurofibroma

Key points

- A benign tumor of the peripheral nerves that rarely occurs in the mouth.
- Might be solitary or may be component of von Recklinghausen's disease.
- The clinical diagnosis should be confirmed histologically.

Introduction

Neurofibroma is a common benign tumor of the peripheral nerves. It derives from Schwann cells, the perineural fibroblasts, or the endoneurium. Intraorally, the tumor is rare and can be either *solitary* or *multiple* as part of von Recklinghausen's disease (**Fig. 34.43**).

Clinical features

Clinically, neurofibroma appears as a slowly developing, well-circumscribed, usually pedunculated, and painless tumor of relatively firm consistency that is covered by normal mucosa (**Fig. 34.44**). Neurofibromas vary in size from several millimeters to several centimeters. It is most commonly seen on the buccal mucosa and followed by the tongue, palate, and alveolar mucosa. Very rarely, the tumor may appear on the jaw bone. The clinical diagnosis has to be confirmed histologically.

Differential diagnosis

- Neurofibromatosis, type 1
- Schwannoma
- Fibroma
- Leiomyoma
- Fibrous histiocytoma
- Granular cell tumor

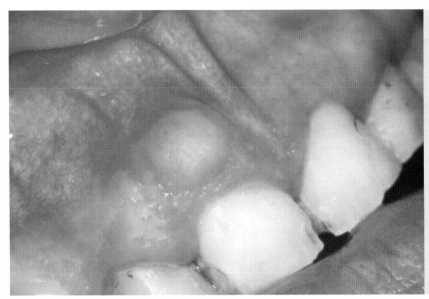

Fig. 34.42 Soft tissue osteoma on the alveolar mucosa.

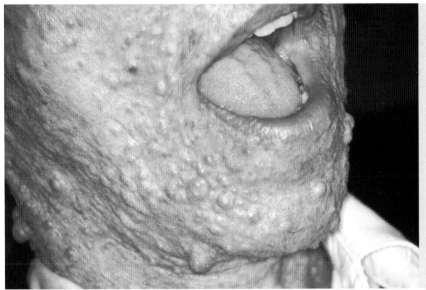

Fig. 34.43 Neurofibromatosis, multiple neurofibromas of the skin, as part of von Recklinghausen's disease.

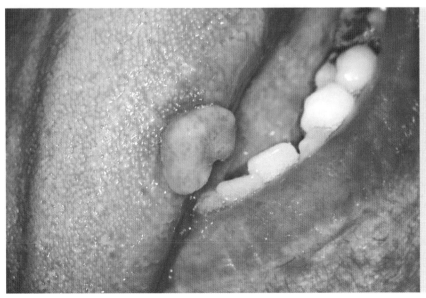

Fig. 34.44 Solitary neurofibromas in the side of the tongue.

Pathology

Histologically, the neurofibroma is composed of multiple collagen fibers that undergo myxomatous degeneration peripherally. Abundant spindle-shaped cells with wavy nuclei are present. Characteristically, numerous mast cells are almost always present. Immunohistochemically, the tumor cells are positive for S100 protein. The covering epithelium is thin and atrophic.

Treatment

The treatment of choice is conservative surgical excision.

Schwannoma

Key points

- A benign tumor of nervous tissue.
- It might be solitary or be part of neurofibromatosis, type 2.
- The tongue is the site of predilection.
- The diagnosis is mainly based on the histologic pattern.

Introduction

Schwannoma or neurilemmoma is a relatively rare, benign neoplasm of the nervous tissue that derives from the Schwann cells. The tumor is usually solitary, but it may be part of neurofibromatosis, type 2.

Clinical features

Schwannoma can equally affect either sex, usually between 20 and 40 years. Clinically, it appears as a slowly growing, solitary, well-circumscribed, sessile tumor that is covered by normal mucosa and lacks specific characteristics (**Fig. 34.45**). It is usually painless and firm and the size can range from 0.5 to 2 cm in diameter. The most commonly affected site is the tongue, followed by the palate, floor of the mouth, buccal mucosa, gingiva, and lips. Rarely, the tumor may develop centrally in the jaws, frequently in the posterior mandible. The clinical diagnosis has to be confirmed by the histopathologic examination.

Differential diagnosis

- Neurofibroma
- Traumatic neuroma
- Leiomyoma
- Fibrous histiocytoma
- Fibroma
- Granular cell tumor
- Pleomorphic adenoma
- Other salivary gland tumors

Pathology

Microscopically, schwannoma consists of two histologic types: *Antoni A* (cellular) and *Antoni B* (containing fewer cells). *Antoni A* type is characterized by an abundance of spindle-shaped cells whose nuclei are arranged in a double palisaded pattern around central acellular, eosinophilic areas (*Verocay bodies*). *Antoni B* type has fewer cells that are scattered in the connective tissue stroma which undergoes myxomatous degeneration. The lesion is usually well encapsulated.

Treatment

The treatment of choice is conservative surgical excision. Recurrences are very rare.

Traumatic Neuroma

Key points

- It is not a true neoplasm but a hyperplasia of neural nervous tissue following trauma.
- Often it is located close to the mental foramen of the mandible.
- The clinical diagnosis has to be confirmed by histologic examination.

Introduction

Traumatic neuroma or amputation neuroma is not a true neoplasm, but a reactive hyperplasia of the nervous tissue and the surrounding tissues to trauma or incision of the nerve.

Clinical features

Clinically, traumatic neuroma appears as a small nodule, usually movable, covered by smooth normal oral mucosa. It grows slowly and rarely exceeds 1 cm in diameter. The lesion is accompanied by pain in approximately 40 to 50% of the cases, particularly on palpation or hypoesthesia. It occurs most commonly around the mental foramen, alveolar mucosa of edentulous patients, lips, and tongue (**Fig. 34.46**). It affects females, usually over 50 years. Traumatic neuroma is also a common complication following trauma or incision of the auricular nerve that occurs during parotid surgery. The clinical diagnosis should be confirmed by histopathologic examination.

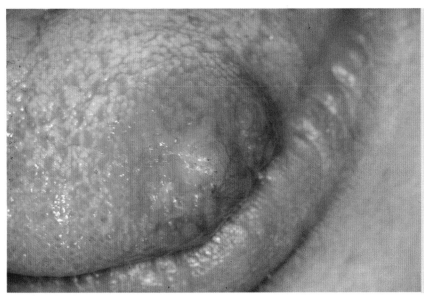

Fig. 34.45 Schwannoma of the tongue.

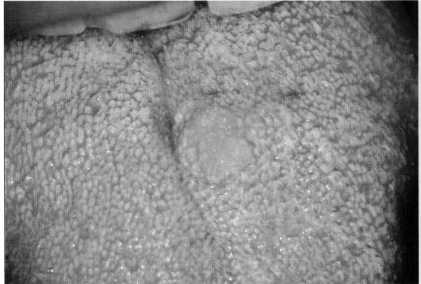

Fig. 34.46 Traumatic neuroma on the dorsum of the tongue.

Differential diagnosis

- Schwannoma
- Neurofibroma
- Granular cell tumor
- Fibroma
- Lipoma
- Multiple endocrine neoplasia syndrome, type 2B
- Salivary gland tumors
- Foreign body reaction

Pathology

Histologically, traumatic neuroma demonstrates multiple bundles of neurofibers within a fibrous connective tissue stroma collagenous to myxomatous in nature. Mild chronic inflammatory cells may be present.

Treatment

The treatment of choice is conservative surgical excision, including a small proximal part of the associated nerve.

Granular Cell Tumor

Key points

- A benign tumor probably originated from Schwann cells.
- It usually appears in the oral mucosa and on the skin.
- The tongue is the most common intraoral site of development.
- The diagnosis has to be confirmed by the histologic examination.

Introduction

Granular cell tumor is a benign tumor with unclear histogenesis. It is believed to derive from Schwann cells or undifferentiated mesenchymal cells rather that from striated muscle.

Clinical features

The granular cell tumor usually affects females (ratio 2:1) between 40 and 60 years. Clinically, it appears as a small, well-circumscribed, sessile, and painless nodule of pale, erythematous, or whitish or normal color. The tumor might be slightly elevated and is usually firm and solitary, although multiple lesions may occur. It mostly develops on the dorsum and lateral borders of the tongue (**Figs. 34.47, 34.48**) and less commonly on the buccal mucosa and palate (**Fig. 34.49**). It may also be found on the skin, breast, and very rarely in viscera. The clinical diagnosis has to be confirmed by histology.

Differential diagnosis

- Schwannoma
- Neurofibroma
- Fibrous histiocytoma
- Fibroma
- Lipoma
- Traumatic neuroma
- Rhabdomyoma
- Granular cell tumor of the newborn

Pathology

Histologically, granular cell tumor is composed of large, polygonal cells with abundant eosinophilic and granular cytoplasm and small nuclei. The overlying epithelium usually displays significant pseudoepitheliomatous hyperplasia, which occasionally mimics squamous cell carcinoma. Histochemically, the cells are positive for the S100 protein.

Treatment

The treatment of choice is conservative surgical excision. Recurrences are very rare.

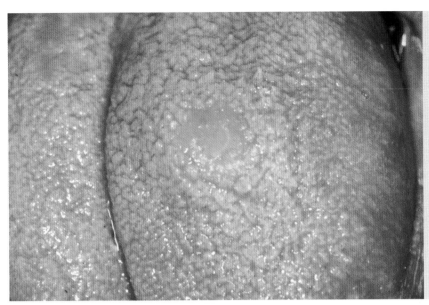

Fig. 34.47 Granular cell tumor on the dorsum of the tongue.

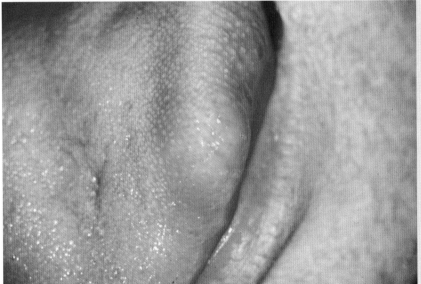

Fig. 34.48 Granular cell tumor on the lateral border of the tongue.

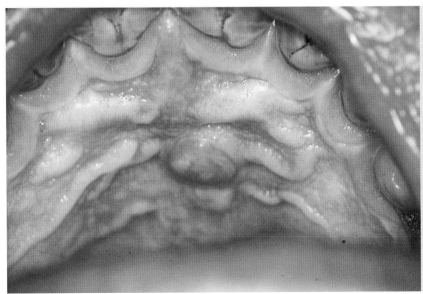

Fig. 34.49 Granular cell tumor in the middle of the hard palate.

Granular Cell Tumor of the Newborn

Key points

- A rare benign tumor, exclusively seen in newborns.
- It occurs exclusively on the alveolar ridges.
- The clinical diagnosis should be confirmed by the histologic examination.

Introduction

Granular cell tumor of the newborn, or congenital epulis of the newborn, is a reactive tumor of unclear histogenesis. It is believed to originate from primitive mesenchymal cells. Despite the fact that it histologically appears similar to the granular cell tumor, there are immunohistochemical and structural differences between the two lesions.

Clinical features

The granular cell tumor of the newborn occurs exclusively on the alveolar mucosa of newborns, more commonly on the maxilla than the mandible. It has a female predilection (80–90%). Clinically, it appears at birth as an asymptomatic, solitary, pedunculated, erythematous, or of normal color tumor with smooth or slightly papillomatous surface (**Figs. 34.50, 34.51**). The size varies from 0.5 to 2 cm. The diagnosis is based on the history and the clinical features, but it has to be supported by histopathologic examination.

Differential diagnosis

- Melanotic neuroectodermal tumor of infancy
- Hamartomas
- Gingival cyst of the newborn
- Hemangioma
- Pyogenic granuloma
- Fibroma

Pathology

Histologically, granular cell tumor of the newborn is characterized by large, round, or polygonal cells with abundant eosinophilic and granular cytoplasm and small basophilic nuclei. Characteristically, the covering epithelium, unlike in granular cell tumor, is thin, atrophic with flat rete ridges. Immunohistochemical analysis demonstrates that the cells are negative for S100 protein.

Treatment

The treatment of choice is conservative surgical excision. The tumor may rarely regress spontaneously.

Melanotic Neuroectodermal Tumor of Infancy

Key points

- A rare benign tumor that occurs in infants.
- It derives from the neural crest cells.
- Most commonly affects the anterior part of the maxilla.
- The clinical diagnosis should be confirmed by the histologic examination.

Introduction

Melanotic neuroectodermal tumor of infancy is a rare benign tumor of neuroectodermal origin with a propensity to appear in tooth-bearing areas. It occurs exclusively in newborns and babies usually below 12 months. It has no sex predilection.

Clinical features

The melanotic neuroectodermal tumor of infancy mostly appears on the maxilla (75–80%). The mandible is more rarely affected. Cases have also been reported on the skull, the skin, the mediastinum, the brain, the epididymis, the testicles, and the uterus. Clinically, oral tumor presents as a rapidly growing and painless mass of erythematous-brown or normal color and elastic consistency that is covered by normal mucosa (**Figs. 34.52, 34.53**). The tumor may lead to osseous destruction which together with the rapid development can give the impression of malignancy. The clinical diagnosis has to be confirmed histologically and histochemically.

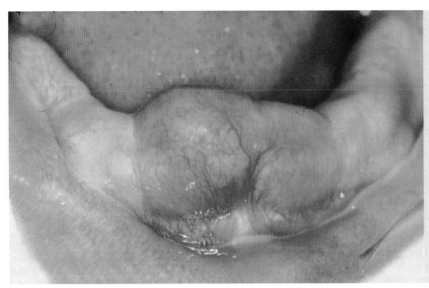

Fig. 34.50 Granular cell tumor of the newborn.

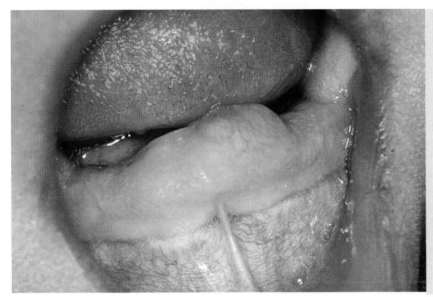

Fig. 34.51 Granular cell tumor of the newborn.

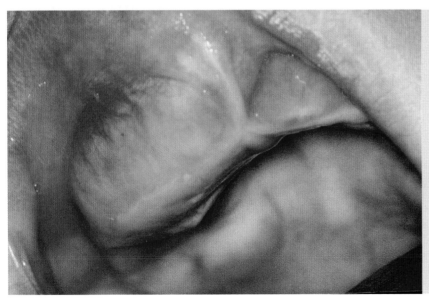

Fig. 34.52 Melanotic neuroectodermal tumor of infancy on the maxilla.

Differential diagnosis

- Granular cell tumor of the newborn
- Hamartomas
- Osteosarcoma
- Schwannoma
- Chondrosarcoma
- Neuroblastoma
- Odontogenic tumors
- Eruption cyst
- Malignant melanoma

Pathology

Histologically, melanotic neuroectodermal tumor of infancy is characterized by two cellular populations that form nests and tubular structures within the connective tissue stroma. There are nests consisting of small round cells with hyperchromatic nuclei and a little cytoplasm (neuroblasts), while around the nests large cuboidal, epithelial cells with vesicular nuclei and melanin-containing cells are seen. Immunohistochemically, both types of cells are positive for vimentin, while large epithelial and melanin-containing cells are positive for cytokeratin AE1/AE2, EMA, and HMB45. Synaptophysin is present in small neuroblast-like cells. Mitoses are rarely observed. Additional diagnostic aids are the dental panoramic tomography and the increase of vanillylmandelic acid in urine.

Treatment

The treatment of choice is surgical excision.

4. Muscle Tissue

Leiomyoma

Key points

- A benign tumor that originates from smooth muscle tissue.
- It is rare in the oral cavity.
- Classified into *solid*, *vascular*, and *epithelioid* type.
- The clinical diagnosis should be confirmed by the histologic examination.

Introduction

Leiomyoma is a benign tumor of smooth muscle that usually develops in the uterus, the gastrointestinal tract, and the skin. Oral leiomyoma is rare and originates from the smooth muscles of blood vessel walls or the circumvallate papillae of the tongue. Histologically, leiomyomas are classified into three types (*solid*, *vascular*, and *epithelioid*). The majority of oral lesions are the solid and vascular in type and rarely the epithelioid type.

Clinical features

Oral leiomyoma affects both sexes equally and usually over the age of 30 years. Clinically, it appears as a slowly developing, usually painless, well-circumscribed nodule, of red-brown or normal color, depending on its vascularity. It may rarely ulcerate (**Figs. 34.54, 34.55**). The tumor is usually movable and fairly soft on palpation. The most commonly affected site is the tongue, followed by alveolar mucosa, buccal mucosa, palate, and lips. The clinical diagnosis has to be confirmed by the histologic examination.

Differential diagnosis

- Myofibroma
- Hemangioma
- Hemangiopericytoma
- Hemangioendothelioma
- Rhabdomyoma
- Granular cell tumor
- Schwannoma
- Squamous cell carcinoma

Pathology

Histologically, leiomyoma is classified into three types: *solid*, *vascular* or *angioleiomyoma*, and *epithelioid*. The first two are the commonest types. The solid type consists of bundles of spindle-shaped smooth muscle cells with elongated pale-staining nuclei and rounded ends. Mitotic figures are rare. The vascular type is characterized by well-circumscribed fascicles of smooth muscle cells surrounding vascular lumina. The epithelioid type is composed primarily of epithelioid cells rather than spindle-shaped ones. Special stains are required, such as Masson trichrome stain, or even immunohistochemical techniques (positive for smooth muscle actin, vimentin, and desmin) are usually helpful to confirm the final diagnosis.

Treatment

The treatment of choice is surgical excision.

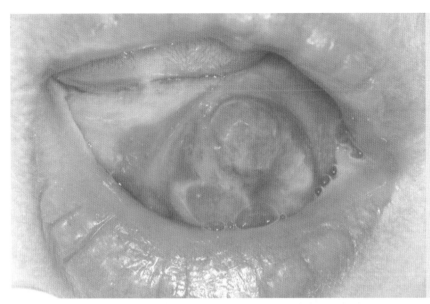

Fig. 34.53 Melanotic neuroectodermal tumor of infancy on the mandible.

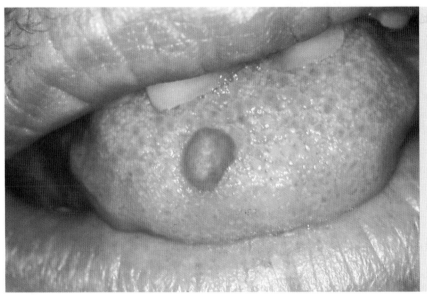

Fig. 34.54 Leiomyoma on the dorsum of the tongue.

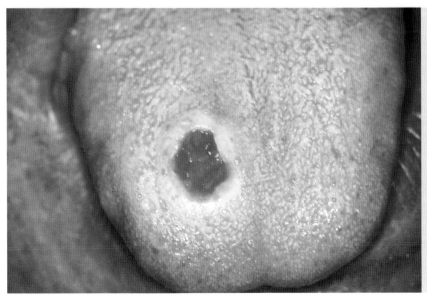

Fig. 34.55 Ulcerated leiomyoma on the dorsum of the tongue.

517

Rhabdomyoma

Key points
- A benign tumor originating from striated muscle.
- Rhabdomyomas of the head and neck are subclassified as *fetal* and *adult* types.
- It is very rare in the oral cavity.
- The clinical diagnosis has to be confirmed by the histologic examination.

Introduction

Rhabdomyoma is a rare benign neoplasm of striated muscle origin. The tumor may in particular occur in the heart, although in this case is a hamartoma. The extracardiac rhabdomyomas are histologically subclassified into two types: *fetal* and *adult*. The adult type usually occurs on the head and neck, while fetal type commonly develops on the face and periauricular area.

Clinical features

Adult rhabdomyoma exhibits a predilection for the head and neck areas and is more common in males between 50 and 70 years. Clinically, oral rhabdomyoma, appears as a slowly growing, well-circumscribed asymptomatic mass with size that may vary between a few and many centimeters (**Fig. 34.56**). The most commonly affected oral sites are the buccal mucosa, tongue, floor of the mouth, and soft palate. It may also occur in the larynx and pharynx occasionally creating airway problems. The clinical features are not pathognomonic, hence histopathologic examination is required for the definitive diagnosis.

Differential diagnosis
- Leiomyoma
- Actinomycosis
- Rhabdomyosarcoma
- Other malignant tumor
- Amyloidosis

Pathology

Histologically, rhabdomyoma is characterized by well-circumscribed lobules of large polygonal or round cells with abundant eosinophilic and granular cytoplasm and small hyperchromatic nucleus. They are either scattered or arranged in lobular formations. Immunohistochemical examination demonstrates cell positivity to desmin, muscle-specific actin, and myoglobin.

Treatment

The treatment of choice is surgical excision. Recurrences are rare.

5. Vascular Tissue

Hemangioma and Vascular Malformations

Key points
- Vascular tissue anomalies are classified into vascular tumors, vascular malformations, and unclassified vascular anomalies.
- Hemangioma is the most common benign vascular neoplasm of infancy and childhood due to endothelial cells proliferation.
- Vascular malformations are not neoplasms but dysplastic anomalies of the blood vessels that are not associated with endothelial cell proliferation.

Introduction

Neoplasms and vascular tissue malformations present within a broad spectrum and have been reclassified and reviewed during the last few years. In 2014, a new classification was approved in Melbourne, by the General Assembly of the International Society for the Study of Vascular Anomalies. Vascular anomalies are now divided into (1) *vascular tumors* (benign: include hemangiomas, locally aggressive or borderline and malignant), (2) *vascular malformations* (simple, combined, anomalies of major named vessels and vascular malformations associated with other anomalies), and (3) provisionally *unclassified vascular anomalies*.

Vascular malformations are not neoplasms, but dysplastic anomalies of the blood vessels that are not accompanied by proliferation of endothelial cells. Hemangioma is a benign neoplasm of childhood, characterized by a great proliferation of endothelial cells. It is the most frequent tumor of infancy and childhood, most commonly seen on the skin of the head and neck. In approximately 50 to 90% of the cases, it regresses spontaneously within 5 to 10 years.

Clinical features

Infantile hemangioma is less common in the mouth than on the skin. Clinically, it is characterized by an early phase of great proliferation of endothelial cells that is followed by a progressively regressive phase. However, the oral lesions regress less than the skin ones. Most commonly, vascular malformations in the mouth occur during childhood or puberty and remain for life.

Clinically and histologically, hemangiomas are divided into *superficial*, also called capillary and *deep*, also called cavernous and *mixed* lesions. Capillary hemangioma consists of multiple, small capillaries and clinically appears as a flat or slightly elevated erythematous macule (**Fig. 34.57**). Cavernous hemangioma consists of large vascular, blood-filled spaces. Clinically, an elevated tumor is observed of deep red or brown-red color (**Fig. 34.58**). The size varies between a few to many centimeters and may grow to cause organ deformity (**Fig. 34.59**).

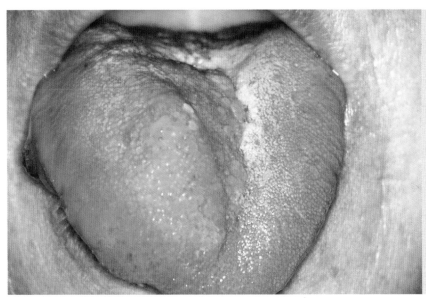

Fig. 34.56 Rhabdomyoma on the right lateral aspect of the tongue.

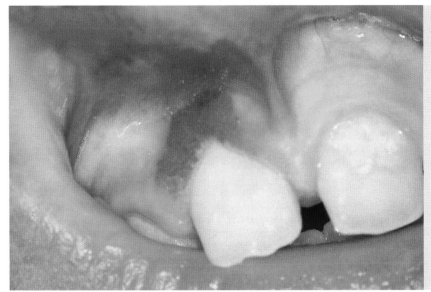

Fig. 34.57 Capillary hemangioma on the gingiva.

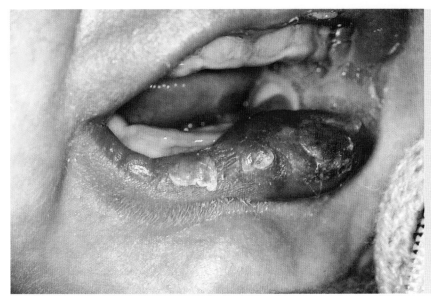

Fig. 34.58 Cavernous hemangioma on the lower lip.

A characteristic clinical sign is blanching with pressure. Hemangiomas are much more common in females than males.

The most commonly affected site is the lips, followed by tongue and palate, while it may also rarely occur in the jaws. It is usually asymptomatic and nonprogressive, the only risk possibly being bleeding. The diagnosis is mainly based on the history and the clinical features.

Differential diagnosis

- Pyogenic granuloma
- Leiomyoma
- Hemangioendothelioma
- Hemangiopericytoma
- Kaposi's sarcoma
- Angiosarcoma
- Syndromes associated with vascular anomalies
- Pigmented lesions

Pathology

Histologically, hemangioma is characterized by numerous vascular spaces that are lined with plump endothelial cells. If a biopsy is performed, great care is needed because of bleeding.

Treatment

Possible treatments include surgical excision, laser, cryotherapy, embolization, and sclerotherapy. Some infantile hemangiomas regress spontaneously, particularly on the skin, but very unusual on the oral cavity.

Angiolymphoid Hyperplasia with Eosinophilia

Key points

- A reactive vascular hyperplasia.
- It commonly occurs on the skin of the head and neck, in particular periauricularly.
- It is rare intraorally.
- The diagnosis is based on the histologic examination.

Introduction

Angiolymphoid hyperplasia with eosinophilia or epithelioid hemangioma is a benign, reactive, vascular anomaly first described in 1969. Trauma is believed to be the cause of the disorder.

Clinical features

Angiolymphoid hyperplasia with eosinophilia occurs usually between 30 and 50 years and is more common in females. The lesion is common on the skin of the head and neck, in particular, in the periauricular area, while it is rare intraorally. Clinically, it appears as a red-brown, usually painless, small nodule or papule. Intraoral lesions have been described on the lips, buccal mucosa, tongue, palate, and gingiva (**Figs. 34.60, 34.61**). Other nonskin locations include the muscles, salivary glands, and the bones. The diagnosis is exclusively based on the histologic pattern.

Differential diagnosis

- Kimura's disease
- Pyogenic granuloma
- Benign lymphoid hyperplasia
- Kaposi's sarcoma
- Angiosarcoma
- Hemangioendothelioma
- Non-Hodgkin's lymphoma
- Squamous cell carcinoma

Pathology

Histologically, angiolymphoid hyperplasia with eosinophilia is characterized by proliferation of the capillaries usually around major blood vessels. Lymphocytic and eosinophilic perivascular infiltrates are common findings. There are also lymphoid infiltrates with or without germinal centers. Many of the major vessels are lined with plump, "epithelioid" endothelial cells.

Treatment

The treatment of choice is conservative surgical excision.

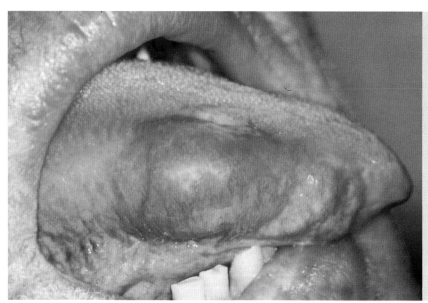

Fig. 34.59 Large cavernous hemangioma that has caused deformity of the tongue.

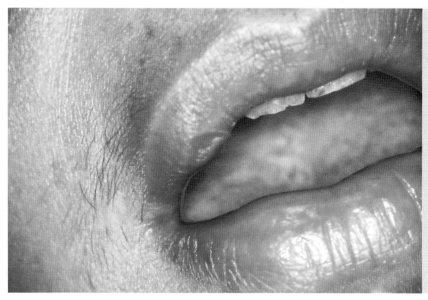

Fig. 34.60 Angiolymphoid hyperplasia with eosinophilia presenting as a mild enlargement on the upper lip.

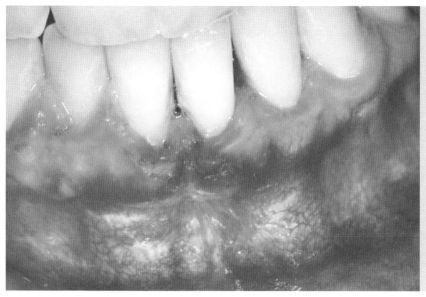

Fig. 34.61 Angiolymphoid hyperplasia with eosinophilia presenting as a red plaque on the lower gingiva.

Lymphangioma

Key points

- A benign dysplastic anomaly of the lymphatic system.
- It becomes obvious during birth or infancy.
- The lesion commonly occurs intraorally and in the head and neck area.
- It is classified into *microcystic*, *macrocystic*, and *mixed*.

Introduction

Lymphangioma is a relatively common oral lesion caused by hyperplasia of the lymphatic system. It is believed to be a developmental malformation rather than a true neoplasm. Depending on the size of the lymphatic spaces, lymphangiomas are classified into three types: *capillary* or *microcystic*, *cavernous* or *macrocystic*, and *mixed* or *micro-macrocystic*. A special type of macrocystic lymphangioma is the *cystic hygroma*.

Clinical features

About half of all lymphangiomas are present at birth while 95% of the lesions develop before the second year of life. The head and neck region is the most commonly affected. All types of lymphangiomas may develop in the oral cavity while cystic hygroma can be seen in the neck area, extending sometimes into the mouth. Clinically, oral lymphangioma appears as small, soft, irregular nodules that resemble small cysts or vesicles and are of yellow-brown color, or even red if the lymphatic spaces contain red blood cells (**Fig. 34.62**). When the lesions are situated deep within the tissues, a diffuse soft ill-defined mass is present with normal color. The size ranges from a few millimeters up to many centimeters, or even very extensive lesions that cause generalized enlargements and organ deformities (**Fig. 34.63**). The dorsum of the tongue is the most common site for oral lymphangiomas, causing macroglossia when the lesion is extensive (**Fig. 34.64**). Less often lymphangiomas may be found on the lips, buccal mucosa, soft palate, and very rarely on gingiva. It is usually asymptomatic; however, very extensive lesions may cause pain and discomfort during speech, chewing, and swallowing. Infection of the lesions is commonly associated with pain and other symptoms constitute a serious problem. The diagnosis is based on clinical and histopathologic features.

Differential diagnosis

- Vascular malformations
- Hemangioma
- Median rhomboid glossitis
- Papillary hyperplasia of the palate
- Lymphoepithelial cyst
- Lingual thyroid
- Acquired lymphangiectasia
- Lymphoedema
- Deep lymphangiomas may be confused with mesenchymal neoplasms

Pathology

Histologically, lymphangiomas are characterized by enlarged lymphatic spaces of different size, depending on the type of the lesion. The lymphatic spaces contain proteinaceous fluid, lymphocytes, and occasional red blood cells. The lymphatic vessels are situated directly beneath the epithelium. The cover epithelium is thin and atrophic.

Treatment

Surgical excision is recommended for small lesions. Larger lymphangiomas pose treatment difficulties where different techniques might prove ineffective.

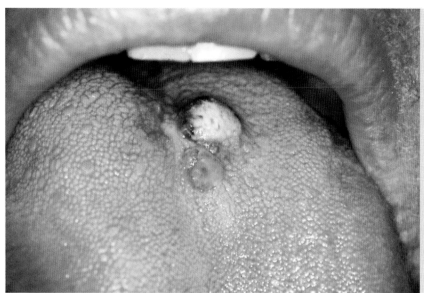

Fig. 34.62 Small lymphangioma on the dorsum of the tongue.

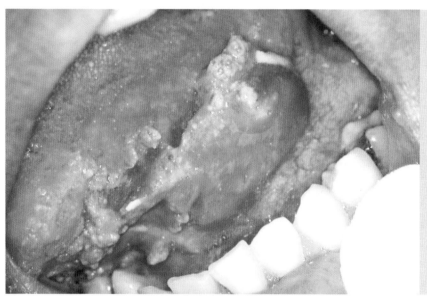

Fig. 34.63 Large lymphangioma on the lateral border and the ventral aspect of the tongue.

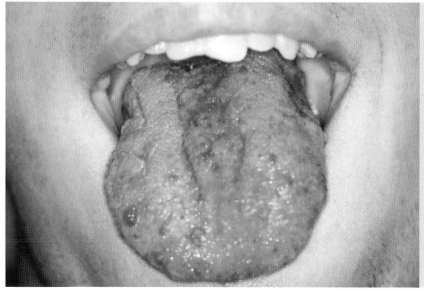

Fig. 34.64 Generalized lymphangioma causing macroglossia.

Cystic Hygroma

Key points
- A type of macrocystic lymphangioma.
- Characteristically, it develops on the side of the neck.
- It may be unilateral or bilateral.

Introduction

Cystic hygroma is a type of macrocystic lymphangioma formed by large lymphatic spaces, which primarily develops on the side of the neck. It occurs during infancy and childhood.

Clinical features

Clinically, cystic hygroma presents as an extensive soft enlargement in the head and neck area, extending into the submandibular and sublingual spaces and occasionally to the buccal mucosa and the parotid space causing aesthetic or even respiratory problems (**Fig. 34.65**). The lesion may be unilateral or bilateral. The diagnosis is based on the clinical and histopathologic features.

Differential diagnosis
- Branchial cyst
- Dermoid cyst
- Diffuse lymphadenopathy
- Sialadenoma
- Infectious parotitis
- Thyroid cyst
- Hodgkin's disease
- Sjögren's syndrome
- Heerfordt's syndrome

Treatment

The treatment of choice is surgical excision.

6. Pigmented Tissue

Ephelides

Key points
- Ephelides are caused by increased melanocyte activity and deposition of melanosomes in the cells of the basal layer.
- They most often appear on sun-exposed skin.
- In the mouth, they are seen mainly on the lower lip.

Introduction

Ephelides are caused by increased melanocyte activity and deposition of melanosomes in the epithelial cells, predominantly of the basal layer. The number of melanocytes is normal. Ephelides almost exclusively occur on sun-exposed skin and usually appear during the first 3 years of life. Rarely, ephelides may appear on the vermilion border of the lips and intraorally as well.

Clinical features

Clinically, ephelides appear as multiple, usually brown, or red-brown discrete round or oval macules less than 5 mm in diameter. Rarely, solitary lesion may be seen. It is relatively uncommon to appear on the lips or intraorally (**Figs. 34.66, 34.67**). The clinical diagnosis should be confirmed histologically.

Differential diagnosis
- Lentigo
- Melanocytic nevi
- Oral melanoacanthoma
- Peutz-Jeghers syndrome
- Albright's syndrome
- Malignant melanoma
- Amalgam tattoo

Pathology

Histologically, ephelides are composed of increased melanin amount, especially within the cells of the basal layer. There are also melanin granules in the upper parts of the connective tissue. The melanocyte number is normal. However, they might be larger in size and have more dendrites due to increased cellular activity.

Treatment

Treatment is not required. However, for esthetic reasons, local surgical excision or laser treatment can be recommended.

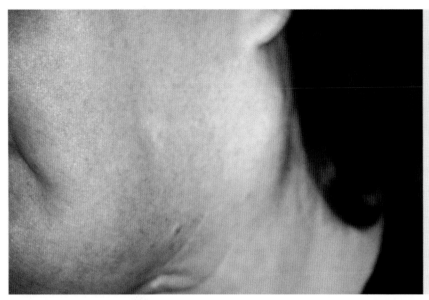

Fig. 34.65 Cystic hygroma, enlargement in the submandibular area and the neck.

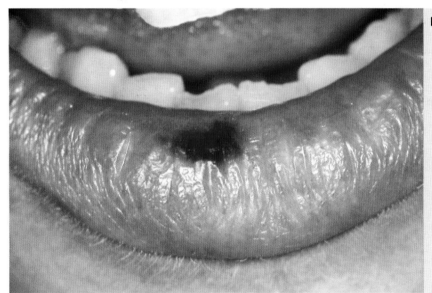

Fig. 34.66 Ephelis on the lower lip.

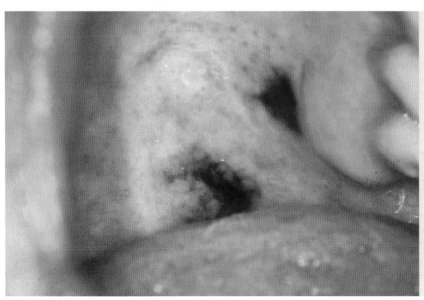

Fig. 34.67 Ephelides on the palatal mucosa.

Lentigo Simplex

Key points

- Lentigo simplex is caused by an increase in the number of melanocytes in the basal layer and increased melanin production.
- It is not related to sunlight exposure.
- Oral lesions are rare.

Introduction

Lentigo simplex is caused by an increased number of melanocytes in the basal layer. There is also increase in melanin. It is more common on the skin than the oral mucosa. It is not associated with sunlight and occurs usually after the third year of life.

Clinical features

Clinically, oral lentigo simplex appears as sharply demarcated, flat, round macule of brown or black-brown color, usually less than 0.5 cm in diameter (**Fig. 34.68**). The most commonly affected oral sites are the lower lip, buccal mucosa, and gingiva. They can also occur in the genital area. Solitary lesions of lentigo simplex are clinically indistinguishable from melanocytic nevus. The clinical diagnosis should be confirmed by a biopsy and histologic examination.

Differential diagnosis

- Ephelides
- Melanocytic nevi
- Oral melanoacanthoma
- Peutz-Jeghers syndrome
- Albright's syndrome
- LEOPARD syndrome
- Malignant melanoma
- Amalgam tattoo

Pathology

Histologically, lentigo simplex is characterized by an increased number of melanocytes within the basal layer of the epithelium. Increased melanin is distributed among the melanocytes and basal cells as well as within the upper part of connective tissue.

Treatment

Usually, no treatment is required, except for esthetic reasons. However, if lentigo simplex is in an area of the mouth that comes under constant mechanical friction, surgical excision is recommended.

Oral Melanoacanthoma

Key points

- A benign, rare, acquired pigmentation disorder caused by an increased number of dendritic melanocytes dispersed throughout the epithelium.
- Common on the skin where it is believed to be a melanocytic variant of seborrheic keratosis.
- It is rare intraorally.

Introduction

Melanoacanthoma is usually seen on the skin and is believed to be a variant of seborrheic keratosis with considerable melanosis. It is caused by an increase in both melanocytes and melanin. The mechanism is an obstruction of the transport of melanin from the melanocytes to the epithelial cells that results in its retention in the melanocytes. Oral melanoacanthoma is usually associated with chronic mechanical irritation.

Clinical features

Melanoacanthoma is usually observed in blacks and rarely in Caucasians and is more commonly found in those aged between 30 and 50 years. Clinically, it manifests as a flat, slightly raised macule or plaque of black or brown-black color (**Fig. 34.69**). The size varies from a few to many centimeters. The most commonly affected oral sites are the buccal mucosa followed by gingiva, lips, and palate. The diagnosis is based on the histologic pattern.

Differential diagnosis

- Lentigo simplex
- Ephelides
- Melanocytic nevi
- Malignant melanoma
- Amalgam tattoo
- Smoker's melanosis
- Drug-induced melanosis

Pathology

Histologically, oral melanoacanthoma is characterized by an increased number of dendritic melanocytes throughout the epithelial layers and melanin overproduction. In addition, mild acanthosis, spongiosis, and mild inflammatory reaction in the connective tissue are observed.

Treatment

Conservative surgical excision is recommended, if troubling the patient.

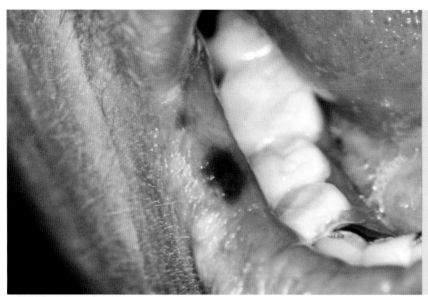

Fig. 34.68 Lentigo simplex on the lower lip.

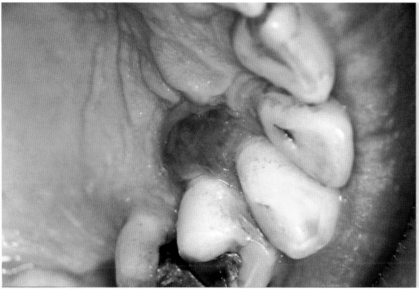

Fig. 34.69 Melanoacanthoma on the palatal gingiva in the canine–premolar area.

Melanocytic Nevi

Key points

- These are developmental malformations.
- Derived from melanoblasts that migrate from the neural crest into the epidermis and the epithelium.
- They are caused by proliferation of modified melanocytes or nevus cells in the epidermis, dermis, or both.
- Genetic factors seem to play a role in the development of nevi. Additionally, other factors such as environmental, hormonal, and immunological seem to take part into their neogenesis.
- There are two main varieties of nevi: *congenital* and *acquired*.
- Acquired melanocytic nevi begin to develop on the skin during childhood.
- Intraoral acquired nevi are histologically classified into four types: *intradermal (intramucosal), junctional, compound*, and *blue* depending on location of nevus cells and the presence or absence of junctional activity.
- Some nevi have an increased risk of malignant transformation into a malignant melanoma.
- The clinical features are not pathognomonic and the diagnosis has to be based on the histologic pattern.

Intradermal Nevus

Introduction

Intradermal (intramucosal) nevus is the most common type intraorally, representing 55% of all oral nevi. It is characterized by several nevus cells within the lamina propria that are separated from the epithelium by a band of collagen. It is more common in females and can be found at any age group.

Clinical features

Clinically, oral intradermal nevus appears as an asymptomatic, flat, or slightly raised macule and is observed of black or black-brown color (**Fig. 34.70**). Very rarely, an intradermal nevus might present with normal color (*achromatic nevus*) making the clinical diagnosis almost impossible (**Fig. 34.71**). It occurs most commonly on the palate and buccal mucosa and less often on the gingiva and lips. Intradermal oral nevi have little capacity for malignant transformation into malignant melanoma. The diagnosis is exclusively based on the histologic pattern.

Differential diagnosis

- Compound nevus
- Junctional nevus
- Blue nevus
- Lentigo simplex
- Ephelides
- Melanoacanthoma
- Lentigo maligna
- Malignant melanoma
- Amalgam tattoo
- Hematoma

Pathology

Histologically, intradermal nevus is characterized by several nevus cells within the connective tissue. Characteristically, nevus cells lack the dendritic processes that melanocytes possess and tend to be organized into nests or chords. The cells are round and small with small uniform nuclei and eosinophilic cytoplasm. These cells have a variable capacity to produce melanin.

Treatment

Conservative surgical excision is recommended when the oral intradermal nevus lies in an area sustaining mechanical friction or pressure.

Junctional Nevus

Introduction

Junctional nevus is the least frequent oral nevi, accounting for 3 to 5.5% of all oral nevi. Histologically, it is characterized by nests of nevus cells along the basal layer of the epithelium. Junctional nevus has an increased risk for malignant transformation to melanoma.

Clinical features

Clinically, junctional nevus does not present with any special characteristics. It appears as an asymptomatic black or brown macule that may be flat or slightly elevated. The size varies between 0.1 and 0.5 cm in diameter (**Fig. 34.72**). It mainly occurs on the palate, buccal mucosa, and alveolar mucosa. It has an increased risk for malignant transformation to malignant melanoma. Generally, any change in color, size, and texture of oral nevi should be regarded with suspicion and the possibility of transformation to malignant melanoma should not be excluded. The diagnosis of junctional nevus is exclusively based on the histologic pattern.

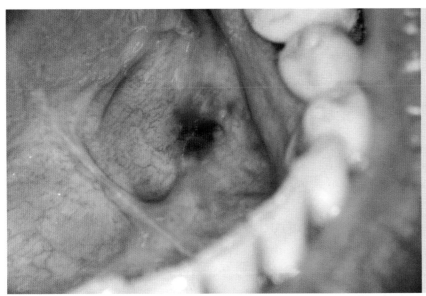

Fig. 34.70 Intradermal nevus on the floor of the mouth.

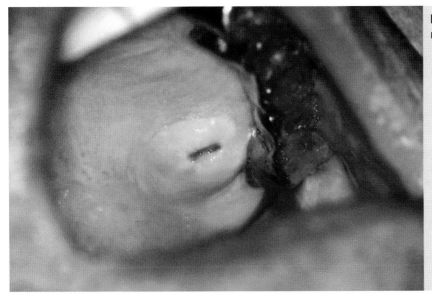

Fig. 34.71 Achromatic intradermal nevus on the palate.

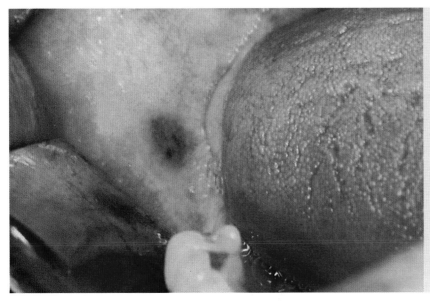

Fig. 34.72 Junctional nevus on the retromolar area.

Differential diagnosis

- Intradermal nevus
- Compound nevus
- Blue nevus
- Lentigo simplex
- Ephelides
- Melanoacanthoma
- Lentigo maligna
- Malignant melanoma
- Amalgam tattoo

Pathology

Histologically, junctional nevus is characterized by a cluster of nevus cells that form nests along the epithelial–connective tissue junction. Characteristically, as the nevus cells proliferate, group of cells appear to "*drop off*" into the underlying connective tissue. Some of nevus cells demonstrate mitotic activity.

Treatment

The treatment of choice is surgical excision.

Compound Nevus

Introduction

Compound nevus is characterized by clusters of nevus cells located both along the epithelial–connective tissue junction and deeper into the underlying connective tissue.

Clinical features

Compound nevus is rare in the oral cavity, representing approximately 6 to 8.5% of all oral nevi. It can affect either sex at any age. Clinically, it appears as an asymptomatic slightly raised macule of red-brown or black-brown color and is 0.5 to 1 cm in diameter (**Figs. 34.73, 34.74**). It occurs more often on the buccal mucosa, palate, and gingiva. Compound nevus may rarely be transformed into malignant melanoma.

Differential diagnosis

- Intradermal nevus
- Junctional nevus
- Blue nevus
- Lentigo simplex
- Ephelides
- Melanoacanthoma
- Lentigo maligna
- Malignant melanoma
- Amalgam tattoo

Pathology

Histologically, compound nevus is characterized by clusters of nevus cells located both along the epithelial–connective tissue junction and within the underlying connective tissue. Histologic features of both intradermal and junctional nevi patterns are seen.

Treatment

The treatment of choice is surgical excision.

Blue Nevus

Introduction

Blue nevus is the second most frequent nevus in the oral mucosa, representing approximately 30.5 to 36% of all oral nevi. It comprises of melanocytes that are filled with melanin. These form clusters in a parallel form deep within the connective tissue. There are two types of blue nevi, the *common*, that can occur in the oral cavity and the *cellular*, which only occurs on the skin.

Clinical features

Blue nevus affects equally males and females at any age and becomes obvious during adulthood. Clinically, it appears as an asymptomatic, flat or slightly raised or flat macule. The color may be blue or brown and the shape may be oval or irregular (**Fig. 34.75**). It frequently occurs on the hard palate (60%) and more rarely elsewhere on the oral mucosa. Malignant transformation of orally common blue nevus has not been reported. The clinical diagnosis has to be supported by histology.

Differential diagnosis

- Intradermal nevus
- Junctional nevus
- Compound nevus
- Nevus of Ota
- Lentigo simplex
- Ephelides
- Lentigo maligna
- Malignant melanoma
- Amalgam tattoo

Pathology

Histologically, blue nevus is characterized by the presence of numerous elongated slender and melanin-containing melanocytes arranged in a pattern parallel to the epithelium, in the middle and lower parts of the lamina propria. Characteristically, the cells have branching dendritic extensions and melanin granules, while junctional activity is absent.

Treatment

Treatment is usually not required. However, if it is located in a place sustaining trauma or if it poses a diagnostic problem, surgical excision is recommended.

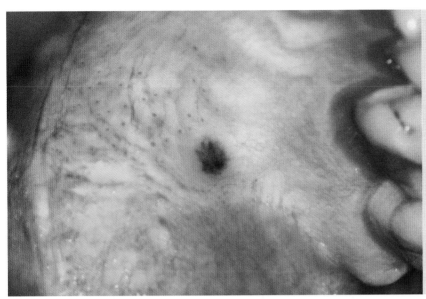

Fig. 34.73 Compound nevus on the palate.

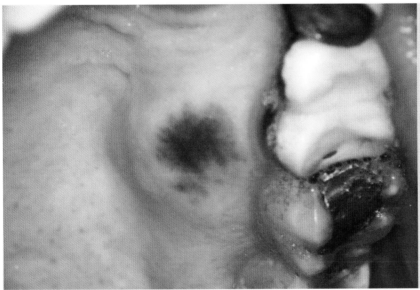

Fig. 34.74 Compound nevus on the palate.

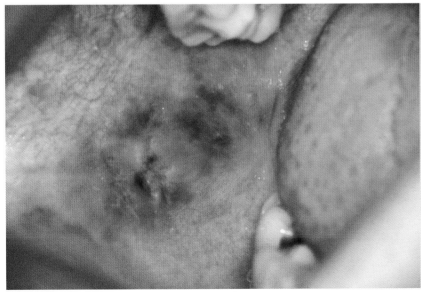

Fig. 34.75 Blue nevus on the buccal mucosa.

Nevus of Ota

Key points

- Nevus of Ota is characterized by increased melanin production from melanocytes in the connective tissue as the blue nevus.
- It is distributed along areas of the face that are innervated by the first and second branches of the trigeminal nerve.
- Very rarely undergoes malignant transformation.
- The diagnosis is based on the clinical and histologic features.

Introduction

Nevus of Ota is a pigmentation disorder that is histologically characterized by scattered melanocytes on the upper layers of the connective tissue, similar to blue nevus. It is most common in Japanese and Africans and African-Caribbeans and rare in other ethnologic groups.

Clinical features

Nevus of Ota appears predominantly in childhood and is more common in females (ratio 5:1). The lesions are usually unilateral, although bilateral involvement may also occur. Characteristically, the affecting areas are innervated by the first and second branches of the trigeminal nerve. Typically, the pigmentation occurs on the eyeball (**Fig. 34.76**), the skin of the face (**Fig. 34.77**), and more rarely the nasal mucosa, the pharyngeal mucosa, and the oral mucosa. Oral lesions most commonly appear on the palate and buccal mucosa (**Fig. 34.78**). Clinically, the pigmentation appears as flat or slightly raised mottled macules, of blue, blue-black, brown, or brownish-gray color. Very rarely, it may undergo malignant transformation to malignant melanoma. The diagnosis is based on the clinical features but has to be confirmed histologically.

Differential diagnosis

- Blue nevus
- Other melanocytic nevi
- Sturge-Weber syndrome
- Lentigo maligna
- Malignant melanoma

Pathology

Histologically, in the connective tissue, there are large dendritic melanocytes intertwined with collagen fibers. There is also an increase in melanocyte presence in the basal cell layer as well as an increased melanin production.

Treatment

The treatment can be problematic due to the extent of the lesions. In the last few years, Q-switched lasers have been used successfully. (Ruby: 694 nm wavelength, Alexandrite: 755 nm wavelength, Nd:YAG: 1064 nm wavelength.)

Spitz Nevus

Key points

- Mainly, it is observed on the skin of the face and the extremities.
- It does not occur in the oral cavity.
- Clinically, it appears as a red or red-brown solitary nodule during childhood.
- Histologically, it consists of spindled and epithelioid melanocytes.

Introduction

Spitz nevus or nevus with spindled and epithelioid melanocytes is a rare melanocytic skin nevus, usually observed in children and younger adults, under 30 years.

Clinical features

Clinically, Spitz nevus appears as a well-defined solitary, dome-shaped, reddish-brown nodule of 0.5 to 2 cm in diameter (**Figs. 34.79, 34.80**). The most commonly affected site is the skin of the face, followed by neck, trunk, and the extremities. The oral mucosa is not affected. It does not undergo malignant transformation into malignant melanoma. The diagnosis is exclusively based on the histologic pattern.

Differential diagnosis

- Malignant melanoma
- Melanocytic nevi
- Hemangioma
- Pyogenic granuloma
- Skin fibroma
- Mastocytoma

Pathology

Histologically, the tumor is characterized by the presence of spindle-shaped elements intermixed with epithelioid cells. These cells extend from the basal cell layer deep into the connective tissue. Mitoses may be seen but are not atypical. Vascular dilatation is usually present forming the reddish color of the lesion.

Treatment

Conservative surgical excision is recommended.

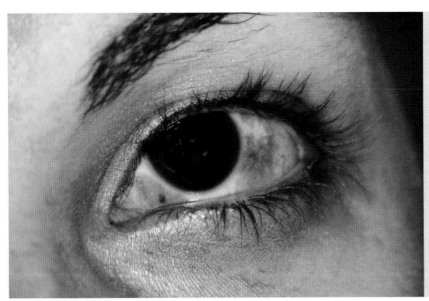

Fig. 34.76 Nevus of Ota, pigmentation in the eye.

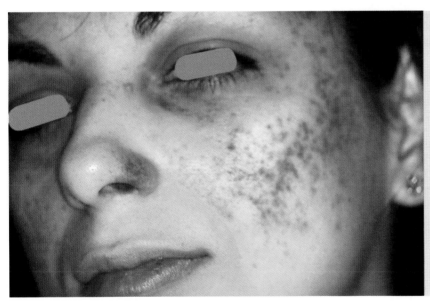

Fig. 34.77 Nevus of Ota, black-brown macules on the skin of the face.

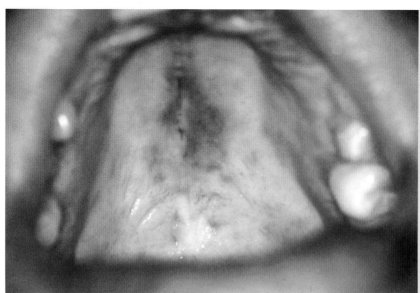

Fig. 34.78 Nevus of Ota, blue nevus in the palatal midline.

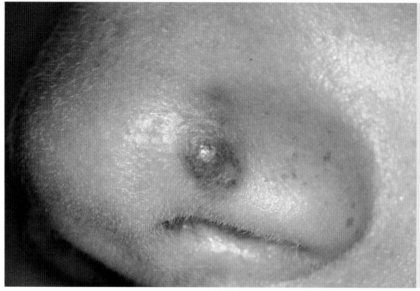

Fig. 34.79 Spitz nevus on the skin of the nose.

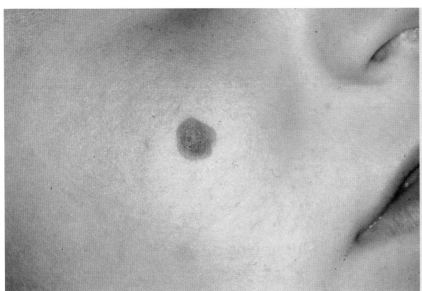

Fig. 34.80 Spitz nevus on the skin of the face.

35 Reactive Tumors

Pyogenic Granuloma

Key points
- Pyogenic granuloma is a reactive lesion.
- It commonly occurs on the gingiva.
- Clinically, it appears as a nodule that easily bleeds.
- Histologically, it is characterized by great neoangiogenesis and cellularity.

Introduction

Pyogenic granuloma is a common tumor of the oral mucosa. It is not a true neoplasm but a reactive overgrowth of vascular tissue (capillary neoangiogenesis) to topical irritation or mild trauma. Despite the name, it is not associated with any infection.

Clinical features

Clinically, pyogenic granuloma appears as a painless, sessile, or pedunculated exophytic nodule with smooth or slightly lobulated surface and deep red color. The surface is often ulcerated and covered by a white-yellow membrane. It has elastic consistency and bleeds easily, either spontaneously or under light pressure. The tumor usually grows rapidly and the size varies between a few millimeters up to 1 to 2 cm. In more than 70% of the cases, it occurs on the gingiva (**Figs. 35.1, 35.2**) and more rarely on the tongue (**Figs. 35.3, 35.4**), lips (**Figs. 35.5, 35.6**), buccal mucosa, palate (**Fig. 35.7**), or elsewhere. The tumor is more common in females (ratio 2:1) and can affect any age group. However, over 60% of the patients are between 11 and 40 years.

Differential diagnosis
- Peripheral giant cell granuloma
- Peripheral ossifying fibroma
- Peripheral "*brown*" tumor
- Hemangioma
- Leiomyoma
- Bacillary angiomatosis
- Kaposi's sarcoma
- Hemangioendothelioma
- Hemangiopericytoma
- Metastatic neoplasms

Pathology

Histologically, pyogenic granuloma is characterized by prominent vascular proliferation and increased cellularity. Multiple vascular formations are observed of varied size that are lined by endothelial cells and contain many red blood cells. The surface is usually ulcerated and covered by a thick membrane consisting of fibrin mixed with inflammatory cells (neutrophils, lymphocytes, plasma cells) and microorganisms. Mature lesions demonstrate more fibrin and less vascular formations and inflammation.

Treatment

The treatment of choice is conservative surgical excision.

Pregnancy Granuloma

Pregnancy granuloma or pregnancy tumor is a variant of pyogenic granuloma which frequently develops during pregnancy. It has the same clinical and histologic characteristics with the classic pyogenic granuloma. It is believed to be caused by an increase in estrogens and progesterones during pregnancy in combination with local mechanical and microbial factors. Clinically, it appears as a single pedunculated mass with a smooth surface and red color. Rarely, more than one lesion develops on the gingiva, and not infrequently, it is associated with gingivitis (*pregnancy gingivitis*). It most commonly occurs during the second trimester (**Figs. 35.8, 35.9**).

Treatment

The recommended treatment is conservative excision usually after childbirth. However, in cases where it is causing irritation, excision can be performed during pregnancy. After delivery, the tumor may sometimes regress or disappear.

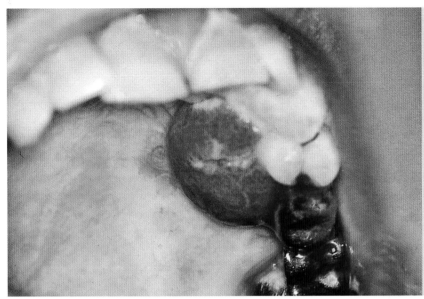

Fig. 35.1 Pyogenic granuloma on the palatal gingiva.

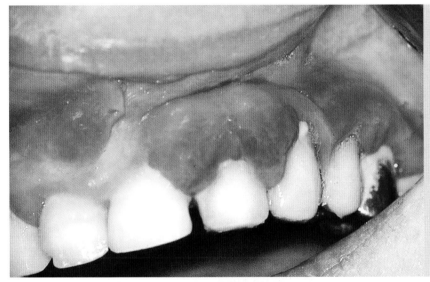

Fig. 35.2 Pyogenic granulomas on the upper anterior gingiva.

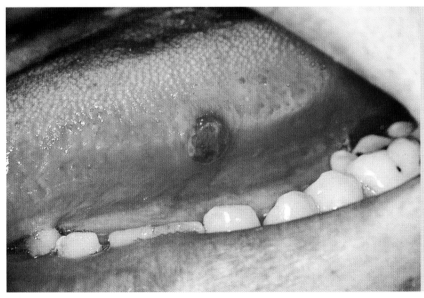

Fig. 35.3 Pyogenic granuloma on the lateral border of the tongue.

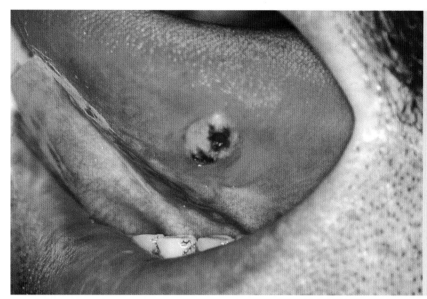

Fig. 35.4 Pyogenic granuloma on the ventral aspect of the tongue.

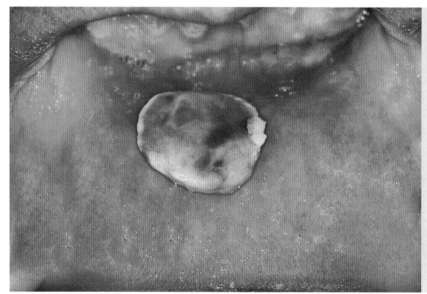

Fig. 35.5 Large pyogenic granuloma on the mucosa of the lower lip.

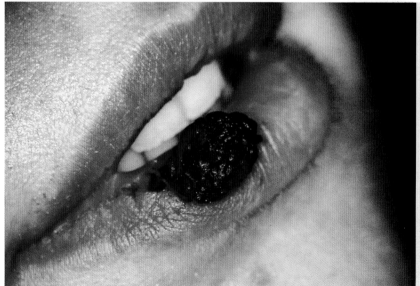

Fig. 35.6 Pyogenic granuloma, hemorrhagic, on the lower lip.

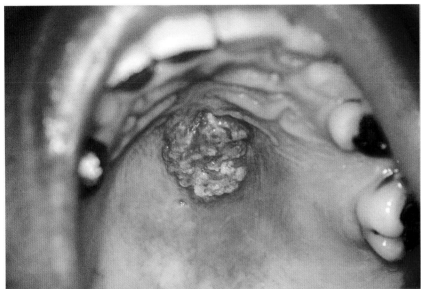

Fig. 35.7 Pyogenic granuloma on the palate.

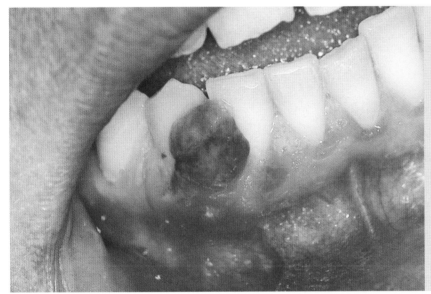

Fig. 35.8 Pregnancy granuloma on the gingiva.

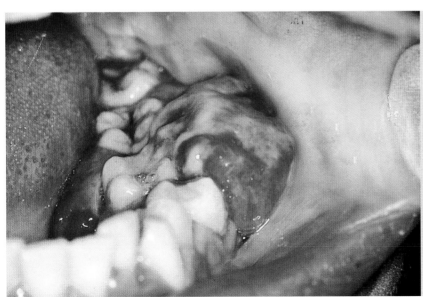

Fig. 35.9 Large pregnancy granuloma on the gingiva.

Postextraction Granuloma

Postextraction granuloma or epulis granulomatosa is a variant of pyogenic granuloma that characteristically develops in the tooth socket following tooth extraction. It is caused by tooth, osseous remnants, or remnants of restoration materials left in the socket following the extraction of the tooth (**Fig. 35.10**). The clinical and histologic characteristics are the same as pyogenic granuloma.

Treatment

Extraction socket debridement and curettage.

Fistula Granuloma

It is a variant of pyogenic granuloma. It characteristically develops at the opening of the duct of a dental or periodontal fistula (**Fig. 35.11**).

Treatment

Endodontic treatment of the responsible tooth or periodontal treatment/scaling.

Peripheral Giant Cell Granuloma

Key points
- A reactive tumor of uncertain histogenesis.
- It occurs exclusively on the gingiva and the edentulous alveolar ridge.
- Clinically, it appears as an exophytic tumor of deep red color and smooth surface that easily bleeds.
- It has a characteristic histologic pattern.

Introduction

Peripheral giant cell granuloma is a relatively common, re-active, tumor-like lesion with characteristic clinical and histologic picture. It occurs exclusively on the gingiva or edentulous alveolar ridge. It is the result of tissue reaction to chronic mechanical irritation, dental plaque, or mild trauma. The histogenesis remains unclear. The dominant belief is that it originates from mononuclear phagocytes or osteoclasts.

Clinical features

Clinically, peripheral giant cell granuloma presents as a well-circumscribed pedunculated or sessile tumor with deep red color and elastic consistency and size between 0.5 and 2 cm or more. It can easily bleed and is often ulcerated (**Fig. 35.12**). It usually occurs close to a tooth, especially of the anterior areas, but it can also be seen on an edentulous area of the alveolar mucosa. It can affect any age group with a peak between 30 and 40 years of life. It is also common during mixed dentition. During childhood, the tumor mostly affects boys, while after the 16th year, it is twice more common in females. The lesion may cause mild osseous destruction of the underlying alveolar bone. The clinical diagnosis should be confirmed by histopathologic examination.

Differential diagnosis
- Pyogenic granuloma
- Peripheral ossifying fibroma
- Peripheral "*brown*" tumor
- Central giant cell granuloma
- Bacillary angiomatosis
- Kaposi's sarcoma
- Hemangioendothelioma
- Hemangiopericytoma
- Hemangioma
- Leiomyoma

Pathology

Histologically, peripheral giant cell granuloma is characterized by numerous multinucleated giant cells, mixed with large oval and spindled mesenchymal cells and inflammatory cells. The giant cells may contain a few or several nuclei. Abundant hemorrhage is found throughout the lesion along with hemosiderin granules deposition. The overlying epithelium is frequently ulcerated.

Treatment

The treatment of choice is surgical excision, down to the underlying bone.

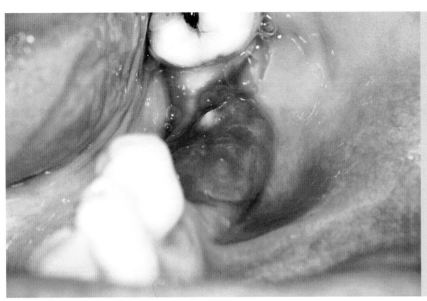

Fig. 35.10 Post extraction granuloma of the mandible.

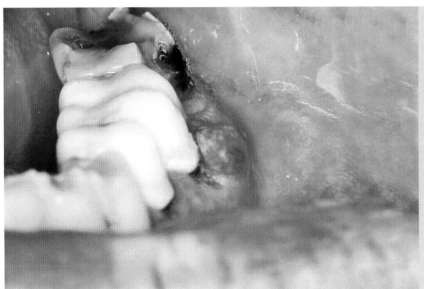

Fig. 35.11 Granuloma at the opening of a periodontal fistula.

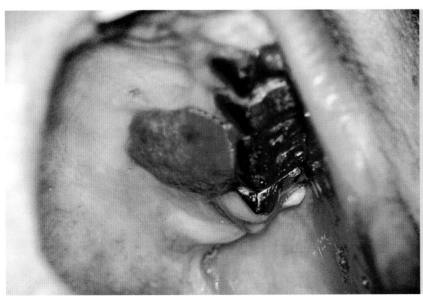

Fig. 35.12 Peripheral giant granuloma on the palatal gingiva.

36 Nonneoplastic Lesions of the Salivary Glands

Necrotizing Sialadenometaplasia

Key points

- A painless enlargement that then evolves into a deep painful ulceration with a crater.
- It mainly occurs on the posterior part of the palate.
- Clinically and histologically mimics a malignant neoplasm.

Introduction

Necrotizing sialadenometaplasia is a relatively rare, benign self-healing inflammatory lesion of the salivary glands, first described in 1973. The cause is unknown, but the dominant theory suggests a vascular damage of the involved salivary gland.

Clinical features

Necrotizing sialadenometaplasia is more common in males (ratio 2:1), usually between 30 and 50 years. About 75–80% of the cases occur on the posterior part of the hard palate and less frequently on lower lip, buccal mucosa, and retromolar region. Sporadic cases have also been described in the parotid gland and very rarely in the submandibular and sublingual salivary glands. Clinically, the lesion appears acutely, as a painless enlargement that then evolves within 1 to 2 weeks to a painful crater-like ulceration with raised, infiltrated border and diameter of 0.5 to 5 cm (**Figs. 36.1, 36.2**). It is usually unilateral as isolated lesion, but more than one lesions may present even in bilateral pattern (**Fig. 36.3**). Destruction of the underlying palatal bone may rarely occur. Clinically and histologically, the condition mimics squamous cell carcinoma and adenocarcinoma.

Differential diagnosis

- Squamous cell carcinoma
- Mucoepidermoid carcinoma
- Other adenocarcinomas
- Nasal natural killer (NK)-T non-Hodgkin's lymphoma
- Syphilitic chancre
- Aspergillosis
- Mucormycosis
- Necrosis in the palate following local anesthetic injection
- Traumatic ulcer

Pathology

Histologically, there is necrosis of the acini in early lesion followed by metaplasia of the excretory duct epithelium to squamous epithelium. Additionally, trapped mucous is observed as well as neutrophilic, plasmacytic, and lymphocytic inflammatory infiltrate. The overlying epithelium may exhibit pseudoepitheliomatous hyperplasia. The histologic pattern occasionally resembles that of squamous cell carcinoma or mucoepidermoid carcinoma.

Treatment

The lesion is self-limiting and usually heals within 4 to 6 weeks. However, systemic prednisolone in 20 to 30 mg/d for 1 week with another week of tapering schedule and completion of treatment reduces the healing time to 2 to 3 weeks and most importantly prevents a possible osseous destruction. Additionally, oxygen-releasing topical agents three times per day help in cleaning the ulcerated area from debris, necrotic tissue, and microbes.

Sialolithiasis

Key points

- Submandibular gland sialoliths are most common.
- It allows infection of the salivary gland.
- Clinically, it presents as painful swelling, especially during a meal.
- Radiographic examination usually reveals a radiopacity.

Introduction

Sialoliths are relatively common in the secretory ducts or in the parenchyma mainly of the major salivary glands. They are caused by the deposition of calcium salts around a nidus of debris, e.g., epithelial cells, thick mucus, bacteria, etc. inside the duct. Additionally, the formation of sialoliths is helped by inflammatory conditions and partial obstruction of the glands. In approximately 70 to 80%, they occur in the submandibular gland and less often in the parotid, the sublingual, and the minor salivary glands. Sialoliths may occur at any age, but it is more often in middle age without any sex predilection.

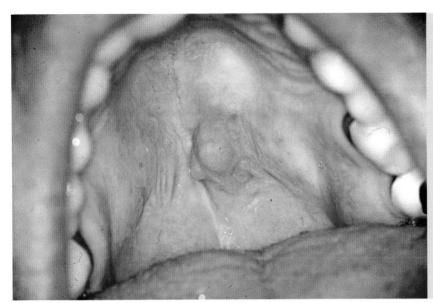

Fig. 36.1 Necrotizing sialadenometaplasia, early lesion presenting as a small enlargement.

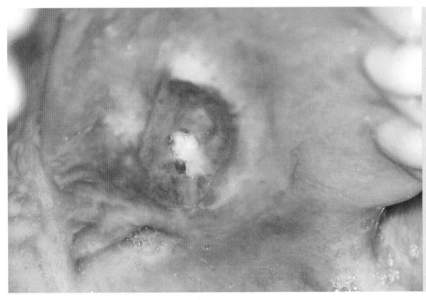

Fig. 36.2 Necrotizing sialadenometaplasia, large, crater-like ulceration on the posterior part of the hard palate.

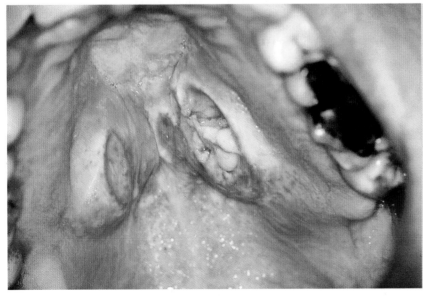

Fig. 36.3 Necrotizing sialadenometaplasia, two ulcerations on either side of the palatal midline.

Clinical features

Clinically, major salivary glands sialoliths present as a painful enlargement of the salivary gland especially during the mealtimes. When the sialolith is located at a more peripheral part of the duct, it can cause significant edema and inflammation. In those cases, it can be palpated and occasionally can be visible through the secretory duct opening (**Figs. 36.4, 36.5**). The blockage of salivary flow promotes salivary gland infections.

Differential diagnosis
- Infectious sialadenitis
- Tumors of the salivary glands
- Ranula

Pathology

Radiographic examination is important for the diagnosis. Sialoliths usually appear as radiopaque area, although not all sialoliths are visible on routine radiographs. The more useful radiation techniques to be used are occlusal radiography, panoramic radiography, dental scan, and recently sialendoscopy. Sialendoscopy is currently regarded as the first-choice test for most cases of obstructive sialadenitis. It may be used in combination with ultrasonography. Ultrasonography is a well-established method in patients with a clinical suspicion of sialolithiasis and should be used as a primary imaging modality. On histologic examination, sialolith exhibits central laminations which usually surround a nidus of amorphous material.

Treatment

During the acute phase, antibiotics and sialogogues are recommended followed by surgical excision of the lith. Recently, lithotripsy and/or sialoendoscopic-guided basket retrieval can also be used.

Mikulicz's Syndrome

Key points
- It is not an independent entity but a clinical manifestation of other diseases.
- The disorder is characterized by bilateral enlargement of the major salivary glands and the lymph nodes of the head and neck area.
- The treatment of underlying disease is the first decision.
- The fine-needle aspiration cytology (FNAC) investigation is important tool for diagnosis.

Introduction

Mikulicz's syndrome is characterized by an inflammatory enlargement of mainly the major salivary glands, frequently associated with swelling of the lymph nodes. It is not an independent disease, but the result of systemic conditions such as tuberculosis, sarcoidosis, leukemias, lymphomas, amyloidosis, and bulimia nervosa. Therefore, the meaning of the syndrome is theoretical, and the diagnosis of the underlying disease has to be established.

Clinical features

Clinically, Mikulicz's syndrome presents as a bilateral, symmetrical, usually painless enlargement of the major salivary glands. It can rarely be unilateral. The full syndrome is accompanied by enlargement of the submandibular and cervical lymph nodes forming a characteristic moon-like face (**Fig. 36.6**).

Differential diagnosis
- Sjögren's syndrome
- Heerfordt's syndrome
- Tuberculosis
- Leukemias
- Non-Hodgkin's lymphoma
- Primary systemic amyloidosis
- Sialadenosis
- Benign lymphoepithelial lesion
- Bulimia nervosa
- HIV infection and AIDS
- Graft-versus-host disease
- Orofacial granulomatosis

Pathology

Investigations appropriate to each different disease that might be implicated are recommended. FNAC is a well-established diagnostic technique and it is used in patients with the swelling of major salivary glands. The cytologic findings should be used in conjunction with the patient's medical history, the clinical features, and other imaging methods (e.g., ultrasound-guided core-needle biopsy). In difficult cases, surgical biopsy and histologic examination are necessary.

Treatment

The treatment of Mikulicz's syndrome consists of cure of the underlying disease.

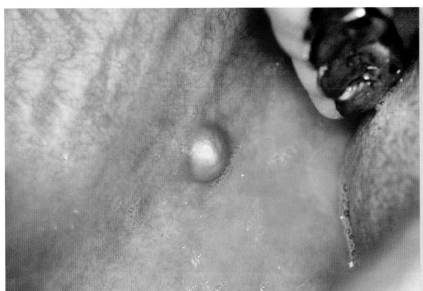

Fig. 36.4 Sialolith at the parotid duct opening.

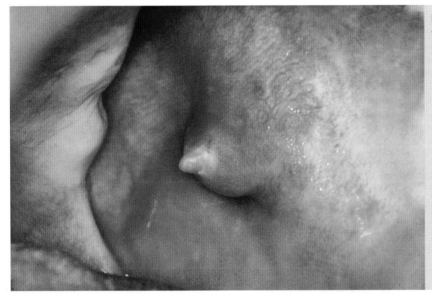

Fig. 36.5 Large sialolith appearing at the parotid duct opening.

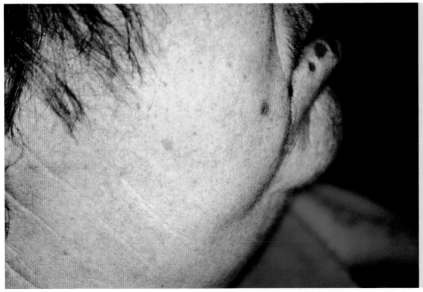

Fig. 36.6 Mikulicz's syndrome, enlargement of the submandibular salivary glands and lymph nodes in a patient with chronic lymphoblastic leukemia.

Sialadenosis

Key points

- A rare, noninflammatory disorder mainly of the parotid glands.
- It causes parotid enlargement and rarely enlargement of other major salivary glands.
- The disorder is frequently associated with several systemic disorders.

Introduction

Sialadenosis is an unusual noninflammatory disorder, characterized by enlargement of the major salivary glands, mainly involving the parotid glands, that is caused by hypertrophy of the acinar cells. The exact etiology is not understood. The disorder coexists with systemic conditions such as hepatic cirrhosis, diabetes mellitus, alcoholism, thyroid gland disorders, ovarian insufficiency, obesity, bulimia nervosa, and occasionally medication.

Clinical features

Sialadenosis, clinically presents as a painless, slowly developing enlargement of the parotid glands. Submandibular, sublingual, and minor salivary glands' involvement may rarely occur. The enlargement is usually bilateral and rarely unilateral (**Figs. 36.7, 36.8**). It is relatively soft on palpation and is accompanied by a small reduction in salivary flow. It is more common in patients over 50 years.

Differential diagnosis

- Sjögren's syndrome
- Mikulicz's syndrome
- Heerfordt's syndrome
- Benign and malignant tumors of the salivary glands
- Bacterial parotitis
- Bulimia nervosa
- Amyloidosis

Pathology

Histologically, sialadenosis is characterized by hypertrophy of the gland parenchyma and acinar cells enlargement with cytoplasm containing zymogen granules and small displaced nuclei. This phenomenon is due to retention of the granules and is explained by neuropathy compromising their release. Sialography can be diagnostic. In ultrasonic examination, the gland is hyperechoic with a poorly visible deep lobe without focal lesions and increased blood flow. Ultrasound-guided core-needle biopsy should be used as an important diagnostic tool in cases of sialadenosis.

Treatment

The treatment is symptomatic. The treatment of the underlying disease will also improve the salivary gland enlargement. Low-dose corticosteroids can offer little help.

Xerostomia

Key points

- Xerostomia (dry mouth) is the most common salivary complaint.
- It can be both a subjective symptom or a sign (hyposalivation) confirmed by the physician objectively.
- Hyposalivation is the low salivary flow rate confirmed by measurement.
- About 20 to 30% of the general population older than 60 years, mainly females, complain about a feeling of dryness in the mouth.
- Stimulation of salivary secretion influences both the quantity and composition of saliva.
- It can be a local problem or represent systemic disease.
- The most common cause of xerostomia is medications.

Introduction

Xerostomia is the feeling of dryness in the mouth that may be caused by (1) a reduction of the saliva produced, (2) a qualitative alteration in the saliva composition, and (3) dehydration. Xerostomia is usually a subjective symptom, but it can equally represent a sign confirmed by the physician (hyposalivation). Over the last decades there has been an increase of the problem. This has been attributed to both an increase in life span and also the extensive use of medication that can produce xerostomia as a side effect. Etiologically, xerostomia is often linked to medication such as anticholinergic, sympathomimetic. It is believed that over 500 different medications can cause xerostomia. Drug-related xerostomia is usually due to adverse side effects of anticholinergic medication taken to treat several diseases. Second in frequency regarding etiology are systemic diseases such as Sjögren's syndrome, graft-versus-host-disease, HIV disease, Heerfordt's syndrome, diabetes mellitus, stress, and various genetic conditions. Radiotherapy in the head and neck area for the treatment of solid tumors follows in frequency, as well as topical causes (candidiasis, mouth breathing, smoking) and finally salivary gland developmental disorders (aplasia, hypoplasia).

Clinical features

Clinically, the oral mucosa, and particularly the tongue, appears dry, thin, shiny, and erythematous (**Figs. 36.9–36.11**). Additionally, there is a decrease of the saliva that is thick,

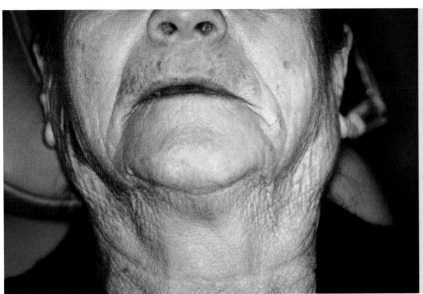

Fig. 36.7 Sialadenosis, bilateral parotid enlargement.

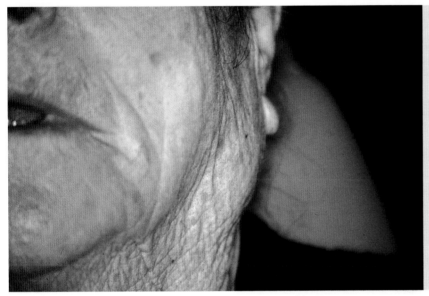

Fig. 36.8 Sialadenosis, unilateral parotid enlargement.

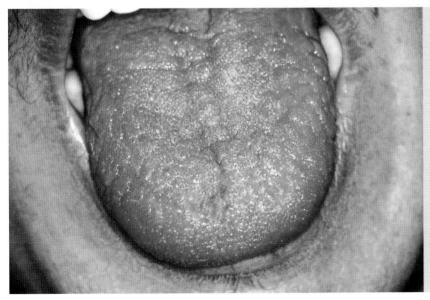

Fig. 36.9 Xerostomia, dry and shiny tongue.

sticky, and many times "frothy." The patients often complain of a burning sensation, taste alteration, difficulty in eating, speech and swallowing, speech impairment, and controlling dentures. Chronic oral complications of a dry mouth are *Candida* infection, gingivitis, and dental caries (**Fig. 36.12**). In **Table 36.1**, xerostomia complications are listed. Females, usually above the age of 50 years, seem to present mostly with symptoms.

Differential diagnosis

- Sjögren's syndrome
- Xerogenic drugs
- Head and neck radiotherapy
- Connective tissue diseases
- Endocrine disorders
- Neurologic disorders
- Metabolic disturbances
- Genetic disorders
- Graft-versus-host disease
- Heerfordt's syndrome
- HIV infection
- Systemic condition and cause that might involve salivary glands
- Bulimia nervosa
- Anorexia nervosa
- Cancer-associated disturbances
- Metabolic disturbances

Table 36.1 Xerostomia: oral complications

- Dry and atrophic mucosa
- Glossodynia
- Increase in dental caries
- Gingivitis
- Periodontitis
- Reduced denture retention
- Salivary gland infections
- Candidiasis
- Taste alterations
- Difficulty in eating and swallowing
- Speech problems

Pathology

Quantitative measuring of saliva (i.e., whole salivary flow) stimulated or unstimulated salivary flow rates can be determined. Other special investigations may be required if there is suspicion of an underlying disease (serology, histology, ultrasound scan, sialography, sialendoscopy, etc.).

Treatment

Before any treatment, it is important the exact cause of the dry mouth is determined. Topical saliva substitutes can be prescribed. However, these help moisturize the mucosa for a limited

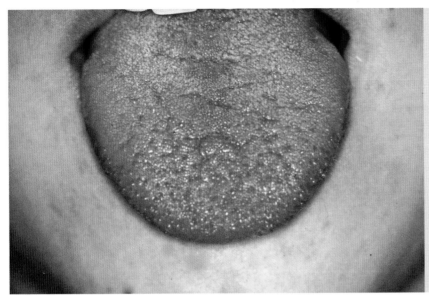

Fig. 36.10 Xerostomia, dry tongue.

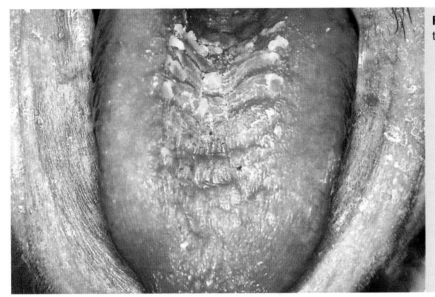

Fig. 36.11 Xerostomia, extremely dry tongue with scale formation.

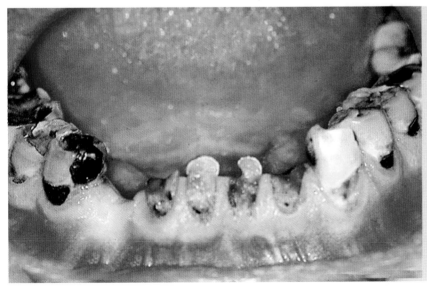

Fig. 36.12 Xerostomia, multiple dental caries.

time and have to be repeated. Sialagogue medication that stimulates the salivary glands (parasympathomimetic agents) can be useful, such as pilocarpine (Salagen tablet 5 mg) 10 to 15 mg/d or cevimeline (Evoxac capsule 30 mg) three times per day. For the sialagogue medication to have an effect, there needs to be some functioning gland parenchyma. Importantly, one has to consider their side effects, especially after prolonged use. Bethanechol (Urecholine) and anethol trithione (Sialor) have also been used as stimulation of salivation. Further in the book, there are references to the treatments of the different systemic diseases that cause xerostomia. Prevention and treatment of oral complications of xerostomia is important.

Sialorrhea

Key points

- It is an increase in saliva quantity that may be actual or subjective.
- In most cases, it does not reflect a true increase in saliva, but a secondary condition due to either reduced swallowing, or neuromuscular failure to retain the saliva in the mouth.
- It has serious psychological and social implications and may cause topical and systemic problems.

Introduction

Sialorrhea is defined as the increased saliva quantity in the mouth that can often cause drooling. It might be *real*, caused by true excess production or *ostensible*, caused by failure to retain the saliva in the mouth due to neuromuscular weakness. The main causes of sialorrhea are classified into five groups: *topical*, *systemic*, *medications*, *psychopathic*, and *idiopathic paroxysmal* (**Table 36.2**).

Clinical features

Depending on the severity of each case, clinically excess saliva production produces choking and drooling, usually through the commissures, wetting the skin periorally (**Fig. 36.13**). As a result, angular cheilitis may be caused, as well as cheilitis and perioral dermatitis. These can then often be infected from *Candida albicans* or bacteria.

The most common problems that sialorrhea can cause are psychological embarrassments, wetting of clothes, difficulty in speech, angular cheilitis, cheilitis, candidiasis, and in very serious cases even dehydration and electrolyte imbalance. Idiopathic paroxysmal sialorrhea is characterized by short episodes of excessive saliva overproduction lasting 3 to 6 minutes. The diagnosis in mainly based on the clinical history and the clinical examination.

Differential diagnosis

- Causative links to sialorrhea
- Neuromuscular weakness, in ostensible sialorrhea
- Heavy metal poisoning

Pathology

Usually, the diagnosis is clinical. The salivary flow and quantitative analysis helps in determining the true or apparent nature.

Treatment

The main concern is the treatment of any possible topical or systemic disease. In cases of excessive sialorrhea, anticholinergic medication can be prescribed, but may produce several side effects, anxiolytics, or scopolamine has been given with partial success. Recently, intraglandular injection of botulinum toxin has been tried. Surgical operations have also been used to control severe drooling, particularly in patients with weak neuromuscular control. Speech and language therapy can help in the cases of neuromuscular dysfunction of the lips and tongue.

Table 36.2 Sialorrhea: causative classification

I.	Local diseases: oral lesions causing pain or irritation (i.e., aphthous ulcers, herpetic stomatitis, erythema multiforme, pemphigus, new dentures causing mucosal irritation)
II.	Systemic diseases: such as Parkinson's disease, Alzheimer's disease, amyotrophic lateral sclerosis, Down's syndrome, epilepsy, gastroesophageal reflux disease, stomach and esophageal cancer, etc.
III.	Medication: clozapine, clonazepam, pilocarpine, lithium, iodine medication, heavy metals (bismuth, mercury)
IV.	Psychogenic
V.	Idiopathic paroxysmal

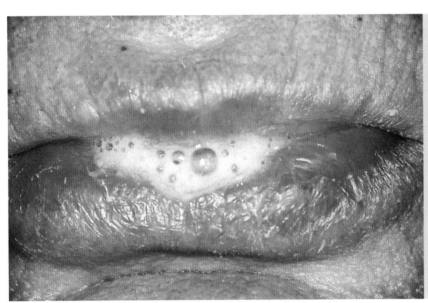

Fig. 36.13 Sialorrhea, great salivary flow from the mouth.

Major Salivary Gland Aplasia

Key points

- A developmental anomaly that may involve one or more of the major salivary glands.
- It may coexist with lacrimal gland aplasia or other ectodermal anomalies.
- Intraorally, the orifices of the affected glands are absent.

Introduction

Major salivary gland aplasia is a very rare dysplasia that may involve only the parotid, the submandibular gland, or sublingual gland, or all three. It can be unilateral or bilateral. It is important that the minor salivary glands are not affected. Occasional ectopia or duplication abnormality of the ducts may occur. In human patients, mutations in *FGF10* gene are responsible for agenesis of the salivary and lacrimal glands and lacrimoauriculodentodigital (LADD) syndrome.

Clinical features

Major salivary gland aplasia is more common in boys than girls with a ratio of 2:1. A clinical characteristic is the absence of the parotid duct opening or the submandibular opening. There is also severe oral dryness with all the usual complications. The tongue and the lips appear rough (**Fig. 36.14**). Common oral complications may include candidiasis, gingivitis, and dental caries. There is some saliva in small quantities due to the minor salivary glands function. The degree of xerostomia depends on the number of the major salivary glands involved. Additionally, if there is lacrimal gland aplasia,

great ocular dryness can be caused conjunctivitis and other ocular complications (**Fig. 36.15**). Finally, other ectodermal dysplasias or oral birth defects might coexist. The diagnosis is based on the clinical features and the results of various investigations.

Differential diagnosis

- Sjögren's syndrome
- Graft-versus-host-disease
- Sarcoidosis
- LADD syndrome
- Treacher Collins syndrome
- Hypohidrotic ectodermal dysplasia
- Facial hemiatrophy

Pathology

Salivary quantitative measuring, sialography, sialendoscopy, ultrasound scan, scintigraphy, computed tomography (CT), and magnetic resonance imaging (MRI) are recommended for the confirmation of diagnosis.

Treatment

The first-line treatments are salivary substitutes, good oral hygiene, salivary flow stimulation, and sialagogue drugs such as pilocarpine and cevimeline may be used to increase salivary production in cases that residual salivary gland mesenchyme is still active. The ophthalmologist has to manage the ocular problems.

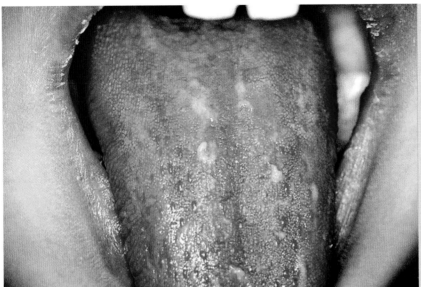

Fig. 36.14 Major salivary gland aplasia, severe dryness of the tongue.

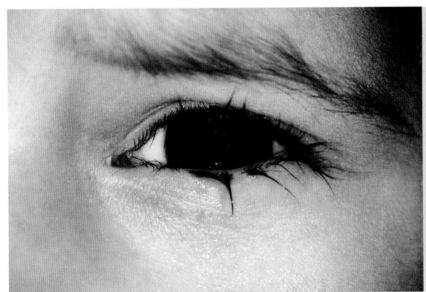

Fig. 36.15 Major salivary gland aplasia, severe ocular dryness due to lacrimal gland aplasia.

37 Potentially Malignant Disorders

1. Precancerous Lesions

Leukoplakia

Key points

- The most common precancerous lesion[a] in the mouth (90–95%).
- It is characterized by biological heterogeneity, since only some lesions have malignant potential while others do not.
- Smoking and alcohol consumption are the main environmental causative factors.
- Leukoplakia is classified into two main groups applying clinical criteria: *homogeneous* and *nonhomogeneous*, which is subdivided into *speckled* or *nodular* and *verrucous* forms.
- Biopsy of the lesion and histopathologic examination are required to determine the risk of malignant transformation.
- The first-line treatment is surgical excision and cessation of the smoking habit.

Introduction

Leukoplakia is the commonest and most studied precancerous lesion of the oral mucosa, since it represents approximately 90 to 95% of all precancerous lesions. Leukoplakia is purely a *clinical* term without any histologic significance. The clinical criteria of leukoplakia have to therefore be determined.

Leukoplakia is defined as a white patch or plaque that cannot be rubbed off and cannot be characterized clinically or histologically as any other condition or disease. It is therefore a definition by exclusion that does not include other known oral diseases or disorders that do not meet the above criteria and that carry no increased risk for malignancy.

It is also important to recognize that leukoplakia is characterized by biological heterogeneity since several leukoplakias present with a risk of malignant transformation to squamous cell carcinoma, but others do not. This is possibly associated with gene variations in combination with environmental factors. The latter can be divided into *primary* (smoking, alcohol, human papillomavirus [HPV] types 16, 18) and *secondary* (chronic mechanical irritation, atrophic epithelium, *Candida* species, herpes viruses, diet, etc.). Smoking is one of the most important causative factors, since more than 90% of the patients that present with leukoplakia are smokers. The prevalence rate of leukoplakia ranges from 0.1 to 5% of the general population. However, a more realistic prevalence figure is between 0.1 and 1%.

Clinical features

Leukoplakia occurs almost equally between males and females during the past 20 years. The age groups affected are usually between 40 and 60 years in countries where women are smoking in a similar pattern to men. Based on clinical criteria, leukoplakia is classified in two main types: *homogeneous*, that is the most common (93–97%) and is characterized by a white, thin, flat uniform white plaque (**Fig. 37.1**) and *nonhomogeneous*. The nonhomogeneous group is subdivided into *speckled* or *nodular type* that is rare (2–3%) and is characterized by a red surface with multiple, small, white nodules or macules and is often infected by *Candida albicans* (**Fig. 37.2**) and *verrucous* that is very rare (0.2–1%) and is characterized by an exophytic, irregular, wrinkled, or corrugated white plaque (**Fig. 37.3**). *Proliferative verrucous leukoplakia* is a subtype of verrucous leukoplakia which is presented by multifocal location, tendency to recur after surgical excision, and a high rate of malignant transformation. It is more common in elderly women (ratio 4:1). The classification of leukoplakia is of practical, clinical importance in recognizing the lesions with the highest percentage in malignant transformation (i.e., speckled leukoplakia is four to five times more likely to transform into a malignancy than the homogenous type). Also verrucous leukoplakia has an increased risk of malignant transformation. The annual malignant transformation rate is approximately 1% for all types of leukoplakia together. The total risk of malignant transformation of leukoplakia in 5 years is 3 to 6% independent of the type. The size may vary from being a few millimeters to several centimeters, and it does not correlate with the risk of malignant transformation. The most commonly affected sites are the buccal mucosa and commissures (**Figs. 37.4–37.6**), followed by gingiva (**Figs. 37.7, 37.8**) and alveolar mucosa (**Fig. 37.9**),

---

[a] **Precancerous lesion** *is the morphologically altered (clinical and histopathologic) epithelium that presents an increased risk of malignant transformation to squamous cell carcinoma, when compared with normal epithelium. Recently, (WHO, 2005) the term* **potentially malignant disorders** *has been suggested to be used in order to describe all precancerous oral lesions and conditions.*

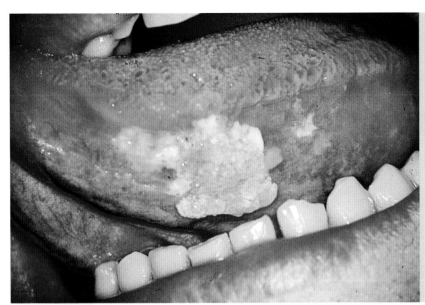

Fig. 37.1 Homogeneous leukoplakia on the tongue.

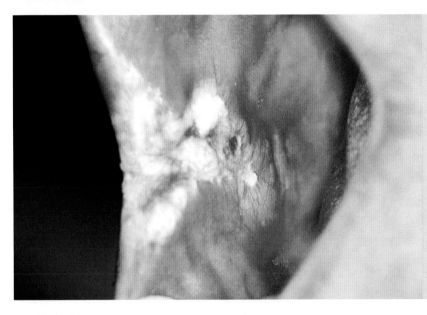

Fig. 37.2 Speckled leukoplakia on the buccal mucosa.

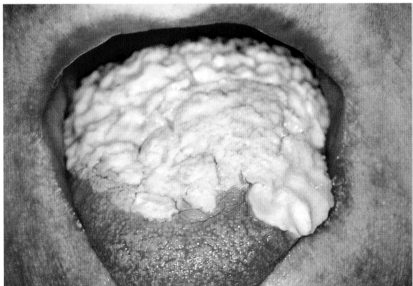

Fig. 37.3 Verrucous leukoplakia on the dorsum of the tongue.

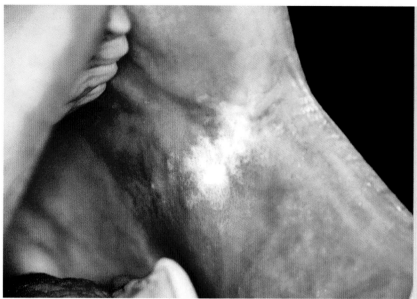

Fig. 37.4 Homogeneous leukoplakia on the buccal mucosa.

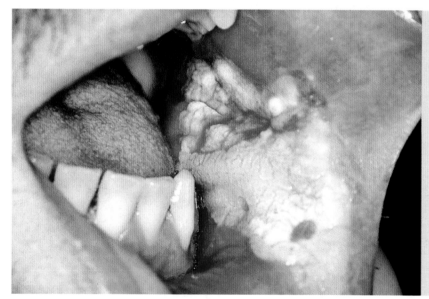

Fig. 37.5 Speckled leukoplakia on the buccal mucosa.

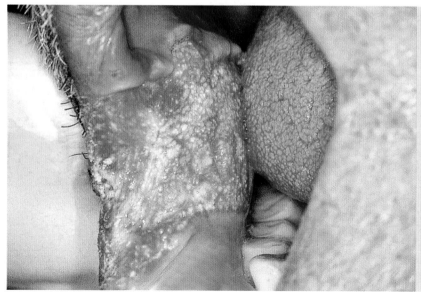

Fig. 37.6 Speckled leukoplakia on the buccal mucosa.

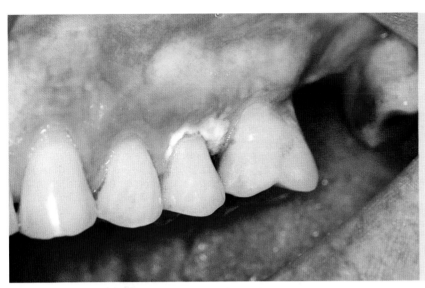

Fig. 37.7 Homogeneous leukoplakia on the upper gingiva.

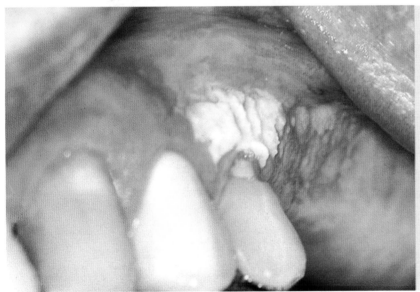

Fig. 37.8 Homogeneous leukoplakia on the upper gingiva.

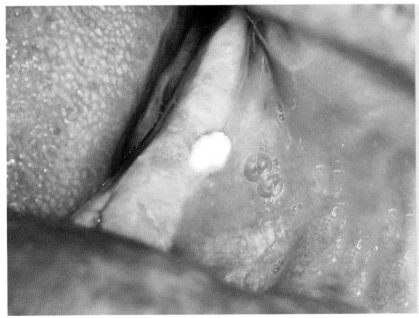

Fig. 37.9 Homogeneous leukoplakia on the alveolar mucosa.

tongue (**Fig. 37.10**), floor of the mouth (**Fig. 37.11**), lips (**Fig. 37.12**), and palate. Some of the locations represent areas of higher risk of malignant transformation such as the floor of the mouth, lateral borders and ventral surface of the tongue, and lower lip. Clinically, suspicion of malignant transformation can be raised by the speckled and verrucous types, erosion or ulceration within the lesion, the development of nodules, peripheral hardening, and the location of the leukoplakia. For these reasons, biopsy is recommended for any leukoplakia. The clinician has to carefully (1) select the right site for the biopsy (the most suspicious), (2) take a sufficient sample, and if required, take more than one samples from multiple areas, and (3) accompany the sample with relevant clinical information. Upon receipt of the histopathologic results, the combination of the histologic and clinical features has to be taken into account. The clinicians should remember that the histologic results represent only the site of biopsy taken in a specific time frame (the time of the biopsy) and do not have a long-time value.

Differential diagnosis

- Lichen planus
- Pseudomembranous and nodular candidiasis
- Hairy leukoplakia
- Cinnamon contact stomatitis
- Uremic stomatitis
- Chronic mechanical friction
- Chronic mucosal biting
- Chemical injury
- Nicotinic stomatitis
- Leucoedema
- Skin graft
- Discoid lupus erythematosus
- White sponge nevus
- Dyskeratosis congenita
- Pachyonychia congenita
- Focal palmoplantar and oral mucosa hyperkeratosis syndrome

Pathology

Histopathologic examination is the most reliable laboratory test to determine the risk of malignant transformation. Histologically, approximately 16 changes in the epithelium (architecture and cytology) are included in the term *epithelial dysplasia*. Depending on the histologic findings, we classified the lesions as *without epithelial dysplasia* (low risk) and *with epithelial dysplasia* (high risk). The degree of epithelial dysplasia is then characterized as *mild, moderate,* or *severe* and if it spreads throughout the epithelium as carcinoma in situ. The associated risk correlates with the degree of epithelial dysplasia. However, there are lesions without epithelial dysplasia or with only mild epithelial dysplasia that have the potential of malignant transformation, and equally, there are leukoplakias with moderate and severe epithelial dysplasia that do not undergo malignant transformation.

Recently, other techniques have been adopted to determine the risk of malignant transformation even in lesions that do not have any epithelial dysplasia or with mild epithelial dysplasia. These are molecular techniques that include detection of suprabasal expression of the tumor suppressor gene *p53*, loss of heterozygosity, DNA ploidy analysis, expression of podoplanin and cytokeratin, and the presence of high-risk HPV types (e.g., 16 and 18). However, all of these molecular markers cannot reliably predict malignant transformation of leukoplakia in an individual patient.

Treatment

The treatment of choice of leukoplakia is surgical excision, followed by electrosurgery, cryosurgery, and lasers. The width of the margin that should be taken into account is 3 to 5 mm. Topical or systemic use of medication, i.e., retinoids, has not produced good results. Photodynamic therapy has also been used. Independent to the treatment followed, smoking cessation and reduction in alcohol consumption are strongly recommended. The patients have to be followed up every 6 months for 3 to 5 years. It should be kept in mind that oral leukoplakia may occasionally regress after discontinuation of tobacco use. This event is more common in leukoplakia of the floor of the mouth.

Erythroplakia

Key points

- It is second in frequency but first in malignant transformation risk of the precancerous lesions.
- It was first described by Queyrat on the glans penis.
- In over 90% of the cases, at detection time, it presents with severe epithelial dysplasia, carcinoma in situ, or early squamous cell carcinoma.

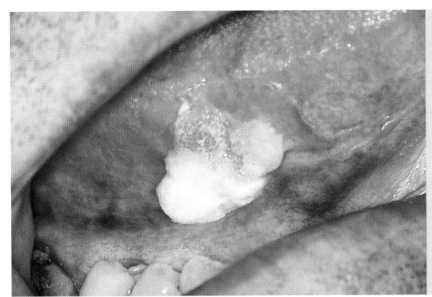

Fig. 37.10 Homogenous leukoplakia on the tongue.

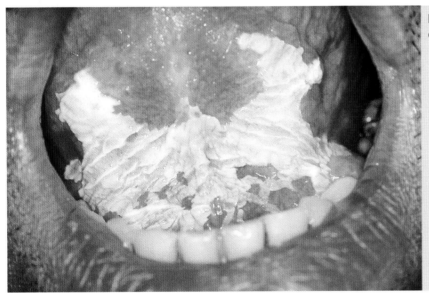

Fig. 37.11 Homogenous leukoplakia on the floor of the mouth.

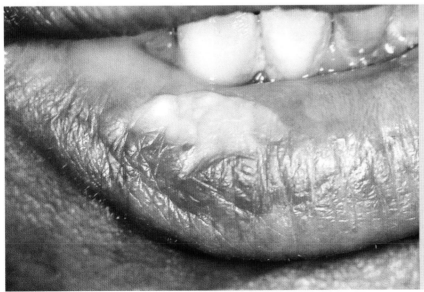

Fig. 37.12 Homogenous leukoplakia on the lower lip.

Introduction

Erythroplakia or erythroplasia of Queyrat is a lesion mainly presenting on the glans penis (**Fig. 37.13**) and rarely in the mouth. When the term erythroplakia is used in oral lesion, it refers to its clinical features, describing nonspecific fiery erythematous patch that is adherent and cannot be attributed to a specific condition or disease, by clinical or histopathologic criteria. The exact etiology is not well known. However, the factors that relate to leukoplakia and squamous cell carcinoma (tobacco and alcohol) are also involved in the occurrence of erythroplakia.

Clinical features

Clinically, erythroplakia presents as an asymptomatic, red patch, of varied size, and smooth or granular surface that may be flat or slightly elevated (**Figs. 37.14, 37.15**). Small white spots or macules can be observed inside the lesion (**Fig. 37.16**). The most commonly affected sites are the buccal mucosa, floor of the mouth, palate, retromolar area, and rarely, tongue. Erythroplakia is the most dangerous precancerous lesion of the mouth because over 90% of the cases at the time of diagnosis have histologically severe epithelial dysplasia, carcinoma in situ, or even early squamous cell carcinoma. Without treatment, the majority of erythroplakias will undergo malignant transformation. The lesion equally affects both sexes between 50 and 70 years. The clinical diagnosis should be confirmed histopathologically.

Differential diagnosis

- Erythematous candidiasis
- Erosive lichen planus
- Discoid lupus erythematosus
- Squamous cell carcinoma
- Verrucous leukoplakia
- Desquamative gingivitis
- Plasma cell stomatitis
- Plasmacytoma
- Reiter's disease
- Cinnamon contact stomatitis

Pathology

Histologically, the epithelium appears thin and atrophic with absence of keratin. Usually, there is moderate-to-severe epithelial dysplasia while carcinoma in situ or early invasive squamous cell carcinoma can also be seen.

Treatment

The treatment of choice is surgical excision. The surgical criteria depend on histopathologic findings. Smoking and alcohol cessation is strongly recommended. The patients have to be followed up every 3 months for 2 to 3 years. There are no data about the recurrence rate after treatment of erythroplakia.

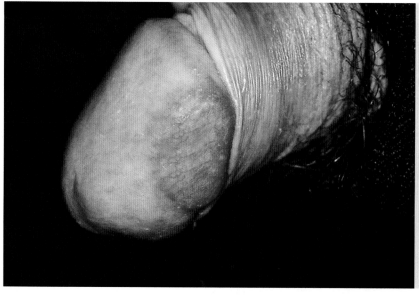

Fig. 37.13 Erythroplakia on the glans penis.

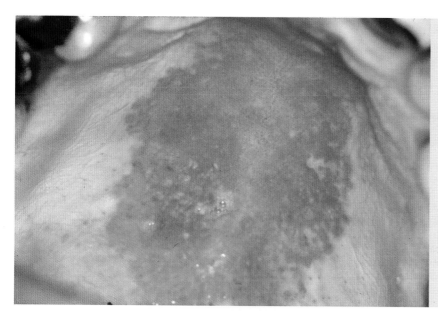

Fig. 37.14 Erythroplakia on the palate.

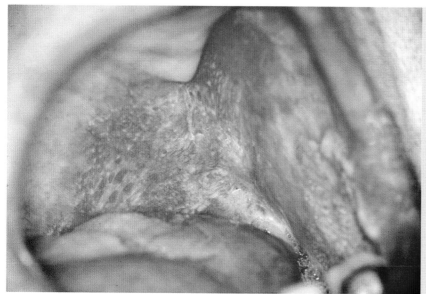

Fig. 37.15 Erythroplakia on the soft palate and buccal mucosa.

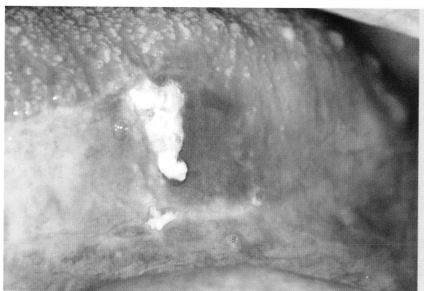

Fig. 37.16 Erythroplakia in conjunction with leukoplakia on the lateral border of the tongue.

38 Potentially Malignant Disorders

2. Precancerous Conditions

Plummer-Vinson Syndrome

Plummer-Vinson syndrome is considered a precancerous condition[a] of the oral mucosa. Its correlation with squamous cell carcinoma was first described in Sweden by Ahlbon in 1936. It was noticed in females who presented with squamous cell carcinoma and iron deficiency in a percentage of approximately 25%. However, the malignant transformation does not appear to be as great in Europe as in Sweden in particular.

Clinically, Plummer-Vinson syndrome is characterized by epithelial atrophy of the oral mucosa and in particular of the tongue (**Fig. 38.1**). It is believed that atrophic epithelium is more vulnerable to the action of carcinogens that results in an increased risk of carcinoma development.

Syphilitic Glossitis

In the past, syphilis was considered to be an important risk factor for the development of leukoplakia and squamous cell carcinoma in the mouth. This role had actually been exaggerated. The only connection that exists is between syphilitic atrophic glossitis and squamous cell carcinoma of the tongue. Syphilitic atrophic glossitis is a manifestation of the third stage of the disease and is characterized by epithelial atrophy and loss of the lingual papillae due to endoarteritis. It is believed that atrophic epithelium is more vulnerable to the action of carcinogens that results in the development of leukoplakia and squamous cell carcinoma (**Fig. 38.2**). Nowadays, due to early detection and most importantly, successful treatment of syphilis, we very rarely see syphilitic glossitis.

Submucous Fibrosis

Key points
- A precancerous condition that is almost exclusively seen in people of Asian origin.
- Sporadic cases have been described in other parts of the world.
- It is linked to keeping in the mouth and chewing of betel quid, areca nut, paan, and gutka.
- They cause atrophy and inflexibility of the oral tissues.

Introduction

Submucous fibrosis is a chronic disorder of unknown etiology. It affects the epithelium and connective tissue of the mouth and sometimes the pharynx and esophagus. It was first described by Schwartz in 1952 and affects almost exclusively the people of Asian origin. Sporadic cases have been described in other parts of the world (United Kingdom, South Africa, Greece). The exact etiology remains unknown. However, the habits of keeping in the mouth and chewing the products of betel quid, areca nut, paan masala, mawa, and gutka have been implicated as etiologic factors. Some of these products may combine with tobacco or contain tobacco. In the past, the increased consumption of chilli had also been incorrectly considered a possible factor.

Clinical features

Clinically, submucous fibrosis in early stage is characterized by an intense burning sensation and development of vesicles and superficial ulceration, mainly on the palate. This can be accompanied by sialorrhea or xerostomia (**Fig. 38.3**). In late stage, the oral mucosa becomes smooth, atrophic, and inelastic, similar to scleroderma. The tongue becomes smooth,

---

[a] ***Precancerous conditions*** *are diseases that may or may not cause alterations (mainly atrophy) of the oral mucosa and predispose to the appearance of squamous cell carcinoma with an increased frequency than those individuals who do not present with these diseases.*

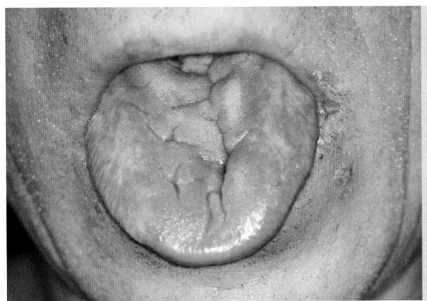

Fig. 38.1 Plummer-Vinson syndrome, atrophy of the papillae and the epithelium of the dorsum of the tongue and angular cheilitis.

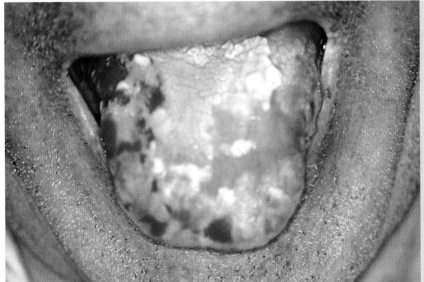

Fig. 38.2 Syphilitic glossitis, atrophic areas and leukoplakia.

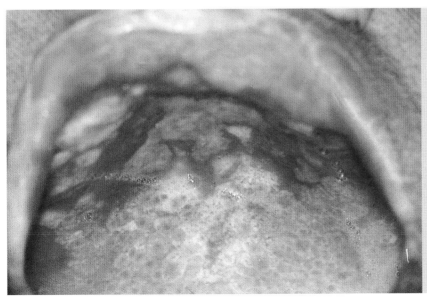

Fig. 38.3 Submucous fibrosis, erosions on the palate.

without papillae, and hard. The uvula is destroyed and many fibrinous creases develop intraorally (**Fig. 38.4**). There is also difficulty in opening (trismus) the mouth, chewing, and swallowing. Beyond the oral cavity, oropharynx and upper third of esophagus may also be involved. The atrophic epithelium predisposes to the development of a squamous cell carcinoma in the presence of different carcinogens. The precancerous nature of the condition is well established because approximately 10 to 14% of the cases exhibit histologically epithelial dysplasia that might transform to squamous cell carcinoma (**Fig. 38.5**). In India, in oral squamous cell carcinoma studies, it was found that submucous fibrosis was co-existing in approximately 40 to 50% of the cases, compared with only 1.2% in the general population.

Oral submucous fibrosis is most frequent in people of 20 to 40 years of age . In a long-term follow-up study, the annual malignant transformation rate was around 0.5%. Biopsy and histopathologic examination is required for diagnosis and the determination of the risk for malignant transformation.

Differential diagnosis

- Systemic scleroderma
- Plummer-Vinson syndrome
- Megaloblastic anemia
- Acquired epidermolysis bullosa
- Mucous membrane pemphigoid
- Lichen planus, atrophic form
- Porphyria

Pathology

Histologically, submucous fibrosis is characterized by an abundance of dense collagen with few cells. The covering epithelium is initially hyperkeratotic and gradually progresses to atrophy in older stage. Various degree of epithelial dysplasia or carcinoma in situ, or even invasive squamous cell carcinoma may be found.

Treatment

There is no specific treatment. Partial result can be achieved by the topical and systemic use of corticosteroids, particularly in patients with early lesions. The habit cessation should be suggested to the patients, although the lesions do not regress.

A program of consequent follow-up is necessary for early diagnosis of possible malignant transformation.

Xeroderma Pigmentosum

Key points

- A genetic disease inherited in an autosomal recessive way.
- It is caused by a defect for DNA repair in the cells of the epidermis after exposure to ultraviolet radiation.
- The disorder is characterized by multiple serious lesions on the skin and the development of multiple malignancies from a young age.
- Squamous cell carcinoma may develop on the lips and rarely intraorally.

Introduction

Xeroderma pigmentosum is a typical precancerous condition of the skin. It is a genetic disease that is inherited through the autosomal recessive trait. It is caused by defective DNA repair in the cells of the epidermis, following damage from ultraviolet sunlight exposure and chemical substances. There are seven different types of xeroderma pigmentosum, depending on the position of the gene mutation and the DNA damage. It is reflected in the different phenotypes of the disease. The prevalence is 1 in 1,000,000 newborns in the West World and 1 in 40,000 to 100,000 births in Japan.

Clinical features

Xeroderma pigmentosum is a systemic disease that usually begins with photosensitivity between the first and third years of life with prominent lesions on the skin, the eyes (photophobia, keratitis, corneal vascularization, and opacification in ~40%), and the central nervous system (20–23%). Clinically, the skin appears edematous, dry, and atrophic, with spider veins, pigmentation, lentigines, scales, and scars. Over 60% of the patients develop multiple malignancies predominantly on sun-exposed skin (squamous cell carcinoma, basal cell carcinoma, melanoma) that result in death, usually before the age of 20 years. Squamous cell carcinoma occasionally develops on the lower lip (**Fig. 38.6**) and rarely intraorally. The diagnosis is based on the medical history and the clinical features.

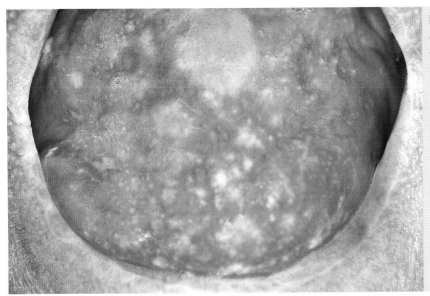

Fig. 38.4 Submucous fibrosis, smooth, atrophic tongue with erythematous and white hearths.

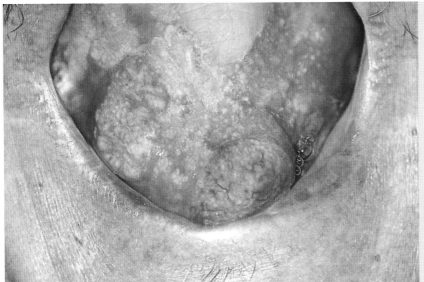

Fig. 38.5 Submucous fibrosis, development of squamous cell carcinoma on the patient of **Fig. 38.4**.

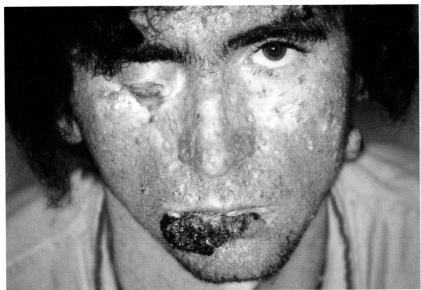

Fig. 38.6 Xeroderma pigmentosum, scars on the face, loss of the right eye, and squamous cell carcinoma of the lower lip.

Differential diagnosis

- Various types of porphyrias
- Genetic types of epidermolysis bullosa
- Gorlin's syndrome
- Cockayne's syndrome
- Bloom's syndrome
- Rothmund-Thomson syndrome

Pathology

Histologically, findings of actinic hyperkeratosis, squamous cell carcinoma, basal cell carcinoma, or melanoma can be seen.

Treatment

Strict photoprotection is recommended. Early diagnosis and surgical excision, or cryotherapy, or electrosurgery of the malignancies are recommended. The systemic use of retinoids has been tried as a chemopreventive agents but with poor results. Topical imiquimod has also been used.

Epidermolysis Bullosa Dystrophica

Epidermolysis bullosa dystrophica is a rare hereditary disease. Both autosomal dominant and recessive variants of the disease lead to severe atrophy and scarring of the skin and mucous membranes. These patients tend to develop neoplasms, usually squamous cell carcinoma of the skin and less frequently of the oral cavity (**Figs. 38.7, 38.8**). It has been suggested that skin scar formation in the recessive variant is associated with a persistent growth-activated immunophenotype of epidermal keratinocytes. This chronic activation state or failure of cells to differentiate in a normal fashion may be linked to the high incidence of squamous cell carcinomas. Oral clinicians should keep in mind the possibility of development of squamous cell carcinoma in the atrophic oral lesions of epidermolysis bullosa dystrophica. More details about the disease (e.g., clinical features, differential diagnosis, pathology, and treatment) could be found in Chapter 25.

Lichen Planus

There is considerable controversy in the literature whether patients with oral lichen planus carry an increased risk of developing squamous cell carcinoma. Many investigators dispute the potential malignant nature of lichen planus while others accept this possibility. The reported data of the malignant transformation varies between 0.4 and 2.5% while the annual transformation rate is below 1%.

It is believed that erosive and atrophic forms of the disease probably have a very small risk of malignant transformation to squamous cell carcinoma (**Fig. 38.9**). Based on personal data of examining over of 40,000 patients with lichen planus, we found only 6 cases of squamous cell carcinoma to coexist with lichen planus lesions. In most reported cases, there is not enough documentation of the diagnosis of lichen planus, lichenoid reaction, or even leukoplakia. Additionally, lichen planus and squamous cell carcinoma are both common oral diseases, a coincidental coexistence is possible. Recent data, which rely on molecular biology, have not confirmed the precancerous nature of lichen planus. On the contrary, the current hypothesis connecting oral lichen planus and squamous cell carcinoma is that chronic inflammation results in crucial DNA damage, which over time produces cancer development. The available data for the potential malignant transformation of lichen planus need further clarification.

Actinic Cheilitis

Actinic cheilitis represents a relatively common potentially malignant condition of the lower lip vermilion.

Ultraviolet light exposure along with tobacco smoking, immunosuppression, and genetic factors increase the risk of transformation to squamous cell carcinoma (see Chapter 13).

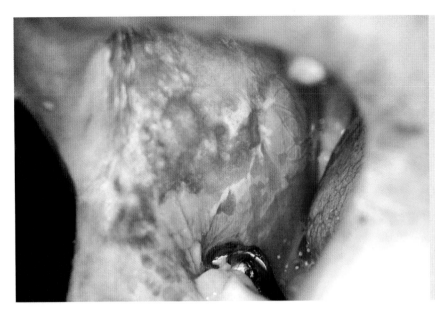

Fig. 38.7 Dystrophic epidermolysis bullosa, development of squamous cell carcinoma on lesions of the buccal mucosa.

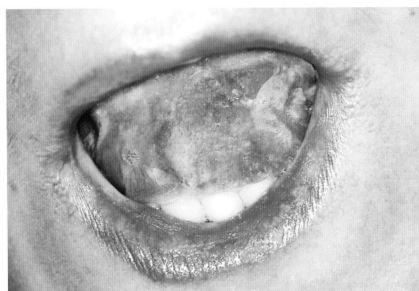

Fig. 38.8 Dystrophic epidermolysis bullosa, development of squamous cell carcinoma on atrophic areas of the tongue.

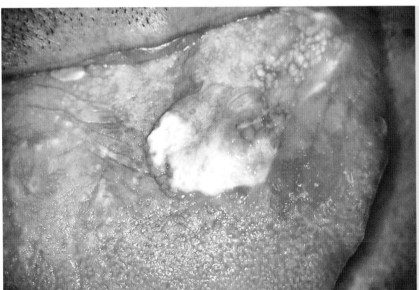

Fig. 38.9 Lichen planus, development of squamous cell carcinoma on lesions on the dorsum of the tongue.

39 Malignant Neoplasms

1. Epithelium

1a. Surface Epithelium

Squamous Cell Carcinoma

Key points

- The most common malignancy of the oral cavity.
- Represents 95% of all malignant neoplasms in the mouth.
- Multifactorial and multifaceted disease.
- Close association with the use of tobacco and alcohol.
- Human papillomavirus (HPV) oral infection, especially types 16 and 18, is now implicated in oral carcinogenesis.
- Over 50% of the cases occur on the lateral borders and the ventral aspect of the tongue.
- Early diagnosis and correct treatment are crucial for survival.

Introduction

Malignant neoplasms of the mouth account for 3 to 5% of all malignancies in humans. Squamous cell carcinoma is the most common malignant neoplasm of the mouth and accounts for 95% of oral malignancies. The annual incidence rate within the European countries and in the United States of America varies between 3–11 new cases per 100,000 individuals. In Greece, the incidence is calculated to 5–7 new cases per 100,000 per year. Despite the fact the exact etiology remains unknown, many intrinsic and extrinsic factors have been implicated. The most important factors are smoking, alcohol consumption, chemicals, sunlight exposure, diet, hepatic cirrhosis, iron deficiency anemia, immunodeficiency, oncogenes and tumor suppressor genes, oncogenic viruses (mainly HPV), chronic trauma, and poor oral hygiene.

Over the last two decades, great importance has been attributed to the role of HPV, mainly of the types 16 and 18 in oral carcinogenesis. Emphasis is given on the viral transmission through the orogenital route as a result of sexual practice. It is believed that the role of HPV, especially types 16 and 18, is crucial in the nonsmokers, under 50 years. In the group over 50 years old, smoking, with or without alcohol consumption are the primary factors for oral carcinogenesis. Genetic predisposition has not been fully studied, but appears not to be strongly linked with oral squamous cell carcinoma. Human cancers share properties referred to as hallmarks, among which sustained proliferation, escape from apoptosis, and genomic instability are the most common. All of them are associated with DNA replication stress and cancer development.

Clinical features

Squamous cell carcinoma is more common in males than females with a ratio of approximately 2:1. However, in Greece, in the past 20 years, there is a tendency of equalization between the two sexes and occurrence in younger groups. Importantly, despite the fact that the mouth is an open cavity and easy to examine, and the patients often visit their dentist for dental problems, diagnosis of oral squamous cell carcinoma is usually late. It has been calculated that at the time of diagnosis there are metastases in over 50% of patients. The responsibility lies with the patients on one hand, who have to be alert regarding possible problems and seek advice and, on the other hand, with the health care professionals, mainly the dentist and the oral medicine physician. The diagnostic methodology is based on good medical and dental history, high index of suspicion, knowledge of clinical characteristics, biopsy, and histopathologic examination. A clinical staging system depending on the tumor size, local lymph nodes' involvement, distant metastasis—TNM, with useful prognostic value, classified oral squamous cell carcinoma into four stages I, II, III, IV. The higher the stage (IV), the worse prognosis, while the lower the stage (I), the better prognosis.

Squamous cell carcinoma presents with great clinical polymorphism. At an *early stage*, it appears as an asymptomatic white or red plaque, or combination of both, erosion, or a small nodule. In the *advanced stage*, it appears as a deep ulcer with irregular, vegetating surface, and elevated hard edges, or as an exophytic ulcerated irregular mass, or an endophytic process with varying degrees of induration. At a *later stage*, it might present with pain if nerves and muscles are involved. The lateral borders and the ventral surface of the tongue (**Figs. 39.1–39.6**) that account for 50% of all intraoral sites and lower lip (**Figs. 39.7, 39.8**) are the most commonly affected sites. They are followed by the buccal mucosa (**Fig. 39.9**), floor of the mouth (**Figs. 39.10, 39.11**), palate (**Figs. 39.12, 39.13**), gingiva (**Figs. 39.14, 39.15**), and alveolar

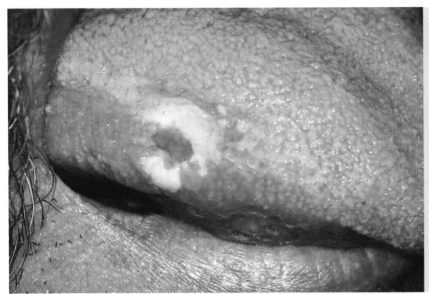

Fig. 39.1 Early squamous cell carcinoma on the lateral border of the tongue.

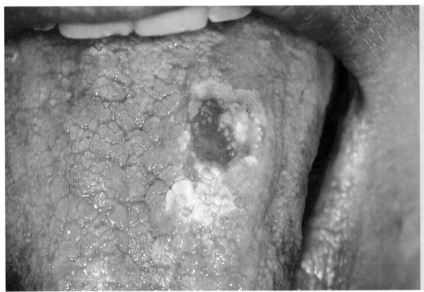

Fig. 39.2 Early squamous cell carcinoma on the dorsum of the tongue with leukoplakia at the periphery.

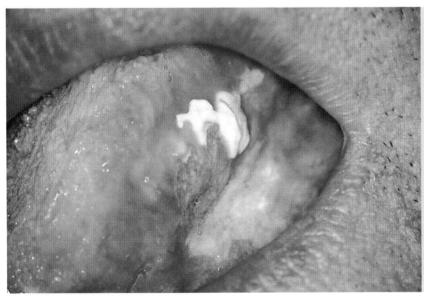

Fig. 39.3 Squamous cell carcinoma on the lateral border of the tongue with areas of leukoplakia at the periphery.

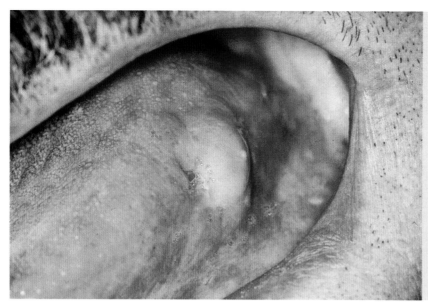

Fig. 39.4 Early squamous cell carcinoma on the lateral border of the tongue.

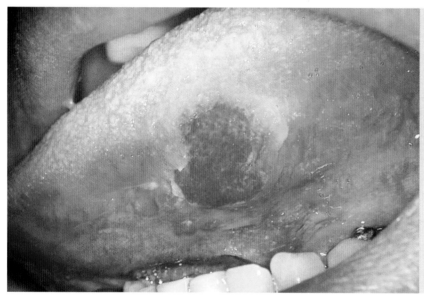

Fig. 39.5 Early squamous cell carcinoma on the lateral border of the tongue.

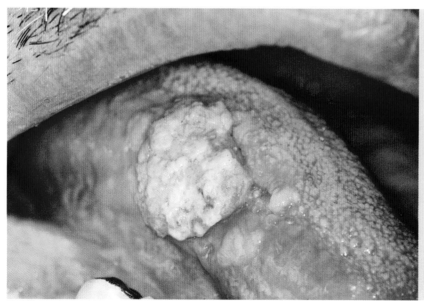

Fig. 39.6 Early squamous cell carcinoma on the lateral border of the tongue.

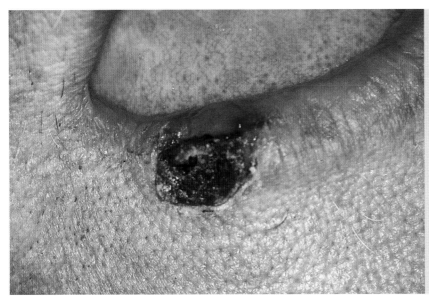

Fig. 39.7 Early squamous cell carcinoma on the lower lip.

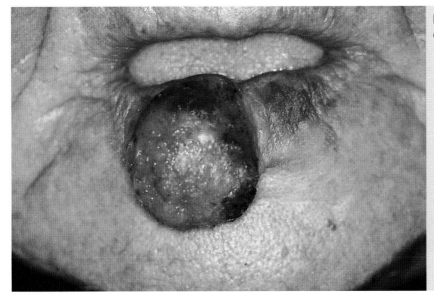

Fig. 39.8 Exophytic squamous cell carcinoma on the lower lip.

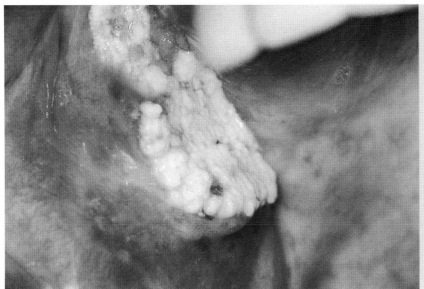

Fig. 39.9 Squamous cell carcinoma on the buccal mucosa with lobulated surface.

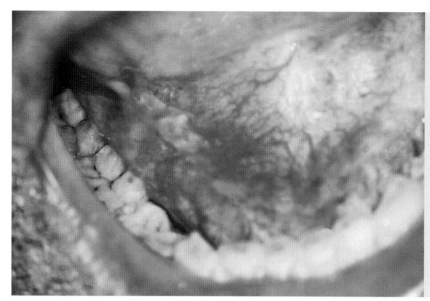

Fig. 39.10 Early squamous cell carcinoma, erythematous plaque on the right aspect of the floor of the mouth.

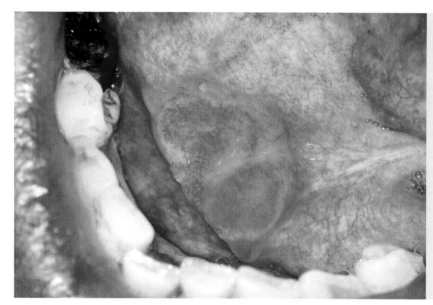

Fig. 39.11 Squamous cell carcinoma on the floor of the mouth.

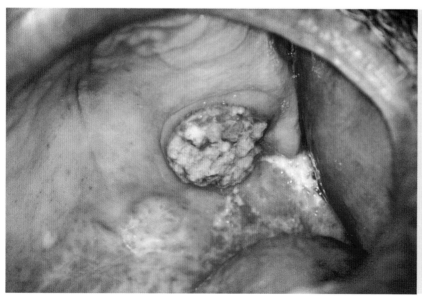

Fig. 39.12 Early squamous cell carcinoma on the palate.

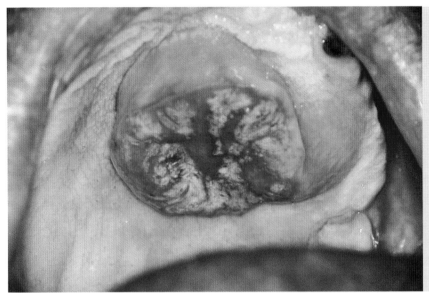

Fig. 39.13 Late, exophytic, squamous cell carcinoma on the palate.

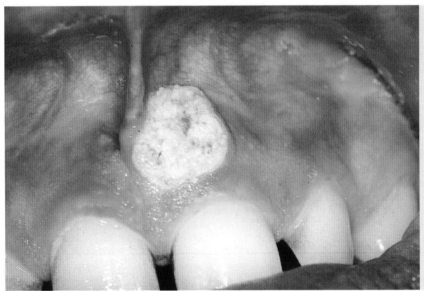

Fig. 39.14 Early squamous cell carcinoma on the gingiva and the alveolar mucosa.

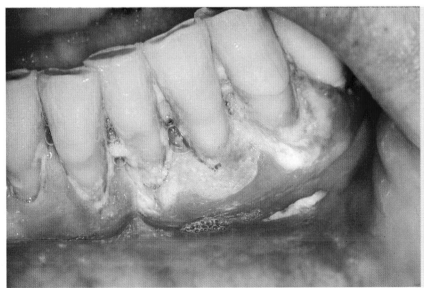

Fig. 39.15 Early squamous cell carcinoma, mimicking leukoplakia, on the lower gingiva.

mucosa (**Fig. 39.16**). As a rule, any oral lesion that persists for more than 10 to 12 days, in the absence of a clear etiologic factor, has to raise suspicion to the clinician for carcinoma. Biopsy and histopathologic examination are strongly recommended in such cases.

Oral squamous cell carcinoma mainly metastasizes through the lymphatics to the ipsilateral submandibular and cervical lymph nodes (**Fig. 39.17**) and less often bilaterally. Distant metastases usually develop only at a later stage and are rare. The prognosis depends greatly on the early diagnosis of the disease and the treatment followed.

Differential diagnosis

- Traumatic ulcer
- Leukoplakia
- Erythroplakia
- Aphthous ulcer
- Tuberculous ulcer
- Eosinophilic ulcer
- Non-Hodgkin's lymphoma
- Wegener's granulomatosis
- Minor salivary gland adenocarcinoma
- Necrotizing sialadenometaplasia
- Any atypical oral lesion that persists for more than 10 days

Pathology

Biopsy and histopathologic examination are required for the definitive diagnosis of squamous cell carcinoma. Upon histologic examination, there is greatly dysplastic epithelium with connective tissue infiltration by groups of malignant cells that form solid keratinized or nonkeratinized islands and/or nests or cords of varied diameter. Depending on the degree of the maturation of the cells as well as the cellular and nuclear polymorphism and the number of mitoses, squamous cell carcinoma is histologically classified into three types: *well-differentiated*, *moderately differentiated*, and *poorly differentiated* or *non-differentiated*. The latter is the most aggressive form of the disease. The majority of squamous cell carcinomas are moderate to well differentiated.

Treatment

The treatment has to be multidisciplinary (i.e., oral medicine physician, oral maxillofacial surgeon, plastic surgeon, pathologist, radiotherapist, oncologist). The first line of treatment is usually radical surgical excision with or without radiotherapy and/or chemotherapy. In advanced disease (stages III and IV), radiochemotherapy may be the first line of treatment, then followed by surgery. The decision for monotherapy or combination of therapies depends on the clinical stage, the age and systemic health of the patient, and the histopathologic cell differentiation.

Lately, targeted treatments have also been applied using monoclonal antibodies. In addition to that, research is now exploring the potential of other treatments that have a molecular basis, such as *cellular apoptosis, neoangiogenesis inhibitors, and viruses* aiming to destroy cancer cells. Techniques that aim at resetting and activating the tumor suppressor gene *p53* and personalized gene-targeted cancer therapy, also known as genetic "*cocktails*," are being developed.

Finally, quite recently, targeted treatments have been tried, using monoclonal antibodies.

Verrucous Carcinoma

Key points

- A low-grade variant of squamous cell carcinoma characterized by slow, persistent growth, and good biological behavior.
- Tobacco usage and HPV 16, 18, and/or 33 seem to play important role in the pathogenesis.
- The oral mucosa, larynx, pharynx, anus, vagina, and skin may be affected.
- The buccal mucosa, palate, tongue, and gingiva are the most common oral sites of involvement.

Introduction

Verrucous carcinoma is an uncommon low-grade variant of squamous cell carcinoma. It was first described by Ackerman in 1948. It differs to squamous cell carcinoma as it clinically presents as an exophytic mass that extends superficially rather than infiltrating deep into the connective tissue. It develops slowly, has a good biological behavior, characteristic pathology, and rarely metastasizes. Outside the mouth, it occurs less frequently in the larynx, pharynx, esophagus, vagina, glans penis, anus, and skin. Most cases are associated with HPV infection, particularly types 16, 18, and/or 33.

Clinical features

Verrucous carcinoma more commonly affects males than females with a ratio of 2:1, older than 60 years, usually smokers. Clinically, the tumor presents as a slow-growing painless exophytic mass with a characteristic cauliflower-like whitish surface (**Figs. 39.18, 39.19**). The size ranges from 1 to several centimeters if left untreated. That is usually due to the fact it has

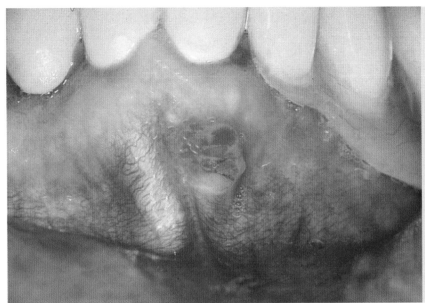

Fig. 39.16 Early squamous cell carcinoma on the alveolar mucosa, mimicking dental/periodontal fistula.

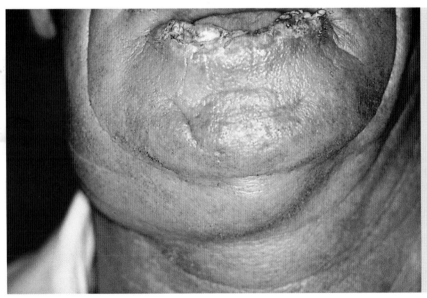

Fig. 39.17 Late squamous cell carcinoma on the lower lip with enlargement of the right submandibular and cervical areas due to metastases.

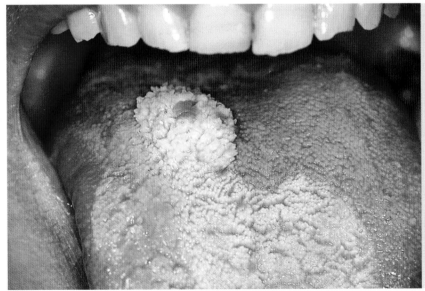

Fig. 39.18 Early verrucous carcinoma on the dorsum of the tongue.

started developing approximately 2 to 4 years prior to the time of definitive diagnosis. The most commonly affected oral sites are the buccal mucosa, gingiva, and alveolar mucosa, followed by tongue, palate, floor of the mouth, and the palate. If the tumor remains untreated for a long time, then it may transform to squamous cell carcinoma (**Fig. 39.20**). The diagnosis is based on the clinical features but has to be confirmed histologically.

Differential diagnosis

- Papilloma
- Verrucous hyperplasia
- Verrucous leukoplakia
- Squamous cell carcinoma
- Verruciform xanthoma
- Cinnamon contact stomatitis
- White sponge nevus

Pathology

Histologically, verrucous carcinoma is characterized by great epithelial hyperplasia with broad, blunt downward-pushing rete ridges, surface protections, and abundant keratin plugging. Normal cellular maturation with mild mitoses are a common pattern. However, there is a need for extra cautiousness during the histopathologic examination of the tissue because it is possible that areas invaded by squamous cell carcinoma may be present.

Treatment

The first line of treatment is surgical excision of the tumor with more conservative surgical margins than those applied to squamous cell carcinoma, with usually excellent results. Chemotherapy combined with radiotherapy is the next preferred treatment when surgery is not indicated in advanced disease.

Spindle Cell Carcinoma

Key points

- A rare variant of squamous cell carcinoma.
- The diagnosis is based on histologic criteria.
- Occurs predominantly in the larynx, esophagus, and mouth.

Introduction

Spindle cell carcinoma is a rare variant of squamous cell carcinoma with a characteristic histologic picture. It usually presents on the upper part of the respiratory and digestive tracts (larynx, esophagus, mouth). The tumor is a little more common in males, 55 to 65 years old.

Clinical features

Oral spindle cell carcinoma most commonly occurs on the lower lip, tongue, and gingiva. Clinically, the tumor presents as a rapidly growing pedunculated or sessile exophytic mass or as a painful or painless ulcer with a size ranging from 0.5 to 5 cm in diameter (**Fig. 39.21**). The clinical features are not pathognomonic and diagnosis is exclusively based on histologic examination. The neoplasm tends to metastasize early and is usually diagnosed in stages III or IV.

Differential diagnosis

- Squamous cell carcinoma
- Adenosquamous carcinoma
- Other variants of squamous cell carcinomas
- Fibrosarcoma

Pathology

Histologically, anaplastic, spindle cells, similar to atypical mesenchymal cells are observed. Numerous mitotic figures are common. These cells have been linked with epithelial origin through immunohistochemical techniques and electron microscope observation. The overlying surface of epithelium usually exhibits severe dysplasia or carcinoma in situ.

Treatment

The treatment of choice is radical surgical excision with lymph node neck dissection. Radiotherapy may also be used as adjuvant therapy.

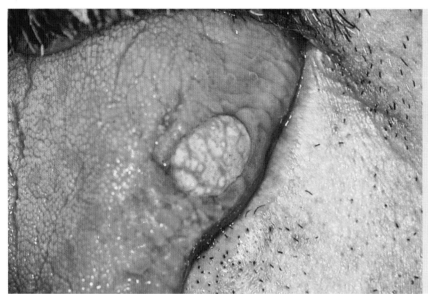

Fig. 39.19 Early verrucous carcinoma on the lateral border of the tongue.

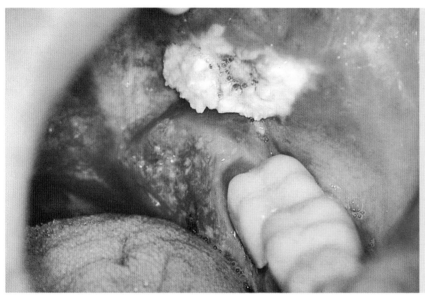

Fig. 39.20 Coexistence of verrucous carcinoma (white exophytic lesion on the buccal mucosa) and squamous cell carcinoma (ulceration in the lingual aspect of the retromolar area).

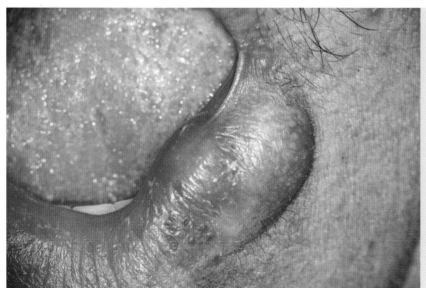

Fig. 39.21 Spindle cell carcinoma on the lower lip.

Adenosquamous Carcinoma

Key points
- A rare variant of squamous cell carcinoma.
- It mainly occurs on the skin of the scalp and neck.
- It is rare in the oral mucosa.
- The diagnosis is exclusively based on the histopathologic pattern.

Introduction

Adenosquamous carcinoma is a rare variant of squamous cell carcinoma that histologically presents with features of both adenocarcinoma and squamous cell carcinoma. It was first described by Lever in 1947.

Clinical features

Adenosquamous carcinoma mainly occurs on the skin of the scalp and the neck. It is very rarely seen in the mouth. The most common affected sites are the lower lip, tongue, and floor of the mouth. It predominantly affects males, usually older than 50 years. Clinically, it presents as a painful ulcer or an exophytic mass with lobulated surface (**Fig. 39.22**). The clinical features mimic the squamous cell carcinoma and metastasizes quickly. The diagnosis is exclusively based on the histologic features.

Differential diagnosis
- Squamous cell carcinoma
- Other variants of squamous cell carcinoma
- Mucoepidermoid carcinoma
- Other adenocarcinomas

Pathology

Histologically, adenosquamous carcinoma is characterized by areas of conventional squamous cell carcinoma arising from the overlying squamous epithelium and areas of glandular adenocarcinoma in the deeper portion of the neoplasm.

Treatment

The treatment of choice is radical surgical excision, with or without radiotherapy.

Lymphoepithelial Carcinoma

Key points
- A rare variant of squamous cell carcinoma or salivary gland carcinoma.
- Intraorally, it occurs in areas rich in lymphatic tissue.
- It is commonly associated with Epstein-Barr virus (EBV).

Introduction

Lymphoepithelial carcinoma was thought to be a rare variant of undifferentiated squamous cell carcinoma with characteristic histologic picture. However, in the revised World Health Organization (WHO) histologic classification in 2005, salivary gland tumors include lymphoepithelial carcinoma in this group of neoplasms, accounting for less than 1% of all salivary gland tumors.

Clinical features

Lymphoepithelial carcinoma presents in younger individuals with a mean age of 26 years. It occurs in intraoral areas with a rich lymphatic component such as the posterior third of the tongue and the nasopharynx. Clinically, it appears as a painless or painful small ulcer or an exophytic mass with lobulated surface (**Figs. 39.23, 39.24**). It metastasizes quickly and is of poor prognosis. The diagnosis is exclusively based on the histologic features.

Differential diagnosis
- Squamous cell carcinoma
- Adenocarcinoma of the salivary glands
- Metastatic undifferentiated carcinoma
- Non-Hodgkin's lymphoma
- Benign lymphoepithelial lesion

Pathology

Lymphoepithelial carcinoma is histologically characterized by syncytial sheets and clusters of neoplastic cells with ill-defined cell borders bearing vesicular nuclei and prominent nucleoli in rich lymphoplasmacytic infiltrate.

Treatment

The treatment of choice is surgical excision and radiotherapy.

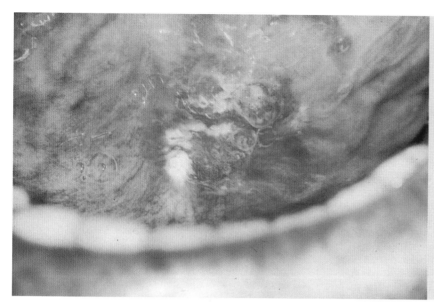

Fig. 39.22 Adenosquamous carcinoma on the floor of the mouth.

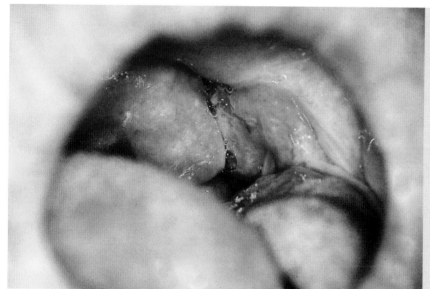

Fig. 39.23 Lymphoepithelial carcinoma on the tonsillar area.

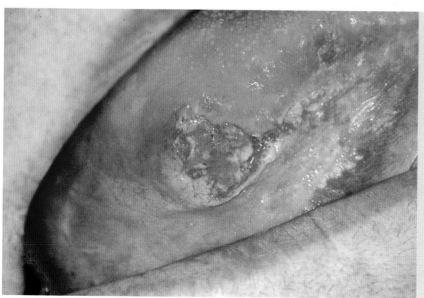

Fig. 39.24 Lymphoepithelial carcinoma on the lateral border of the tongue.

Basal Cell Carcinoma

Key points

- The most common skin neoplasm.
- It does not primarily develop on the oral mucosa, but as a secondary extension of a skin lesion.
- The upper and lower lips are the most common areas of oral involvement.

Introduction

Basal cell carcinoma or basal cell epithelioma is the most common neoplasm of the skin. It stems from the basal layer of the hair follicle and the epidermis. It mostly occurs in areas exposed to sunlight, such as the face and the scalp (85–90%). It is very common in farmers, sailors, and individuals that work outdoors. It usually affects the over-50-year-olds. It has good biological behavior and very rarely metastasizes. The main etiologic factor is sunlight, while predisposing factors considered are the ionizing radiation, carcinogenic chemicals, skin atrophy and scars, HPV viruses, genetic syndromes, immunodeficiency, etc.

Clinical features

Clinically, basal cell carcinoma presents as a slightly raised papule or small nodule that gradually grows and then ulcerates (**Fig. 39.25**). If left untreated, it can cause topical damage. Around the mouth, it can rarely develop on the vermilion border of the lips (**Figs. 39.26, 39.27**). It does not occur in the oral mucosa, unless a skin lesion extends intraorally following topical tissue destruction. The clinical diagnosis has to be confirmed by histology.

Differential diagnosis

- Squamous cell carcinoma
- Keratoacanthoma
- Other malignancies

Pathology

Histologically, basal cell carcinoma is characterized by proliferation of the basal cells of the epidermis in various formations, depending on the type of the tumor. They often lie on a fibromyxomatous background. The neoplastic cells have little cytoplasm and bear uniformly hyperchromatic nuclei. A peripheral palisade is typically present around the rim of the neoplastic lobules or cords.

Treatment

The treatment of choice is surgical excision or radiotherapy.

1b. Glandular Epithelium

Acinic Cell Adenocarcinoma

Key points

- A total of 24 malignant salivary gland neoplasms are described in WHO classification, 2005.
- The majority of patients (60–70%) have one of four types: acinic cell carcinoma, mucoepidermoid carcinoma, polymorphous low-grade adenocarcinoma, and adenoid cystic carcinoma.
- Acinic cell adenocarcinoma is a malignant neoplasm demonstrating at least focal differentiation toward serous acinar cells.
- Eighty percent of the tumors occur in the parotid gland.
- In the minor salivary glands, it represents 8 to 10% of all acinic cell carcinomas.
- The prognosis is better in minor salivary glands than in major salivary glands.

Introduction

Acinic cell adenocarcinoma is a malignant neoplasm of the salivary glands with low malignant potential. It originates from differentiated serous acinar cells or from polyvalent, undifferentiated, acinar cells of the duct. About 80 to 90% of all acinic cell adenocarcinomas develop in the parotid, where they represent approximately 1 to 3% of all tumors. The neoplasm is rare in the submandibular and sublingual glands, while 10 to 15% of all acinic cell adenocarcinomas develop in the minor salivary glands, where they represent approximately 2 to 6% of all tumors.

Clinical features

Acinic cell adenocarcinoma is more common in females than males with a ratio of 1.3:1. The age group predominantly affected is between 40 and 60 years. Acinic cell adenocarcinoma of minor salivary glands more frequently develops in the palate, buccal mucosa, and lips. Clinically, it presents as a slow-growing mass with or without pain and elastic consistency (**Fig. 39.28**). The tumor is slightly mobile and rarely ulcerates. The tumor arising from minor salivary glands is associated with a better prognosis than arising from major salivary glands. As the clinical features are not pathognomonic, biopsy and histopathologic examination are required to confirm the diagnosis.

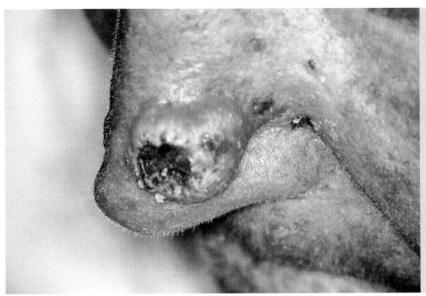

Fig. 39.25 Basal cell carcinoma on the skin of the nose.

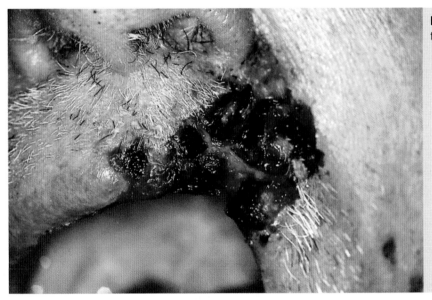

Fig. 39.26 Basal cell carcinoma on the upper lip.

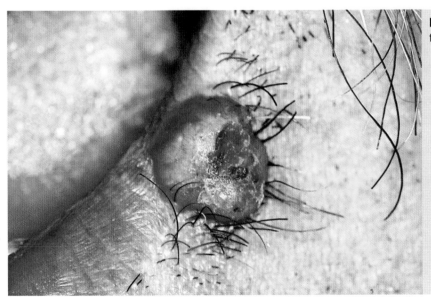

Fig. 39.27 Basal cell carcinoma on the lower lip.

Differential diagnosis

- Pleomorphic adenoma
- Monomorphic adenomas
- Mucoepidermoid carcinoma
- Low-malignancy carcinoma ex pleomorphic adenoma
- Adenoid cystic carcinoma
- Other types of salivary gland adenocarcinomas

Pathology

Histologically, acinic cell adenocarcinoma is characterized by serous acinar cells with abundant granular, basophilic cytoplasm, and round, displaced, hyperchromatic nuclei. The tumor cells appear uniform and commonly arranged in organoid sheets with few mitoses. There are also variable cellular populations, some with characteristics of intercalated duct cells and others of uncommon cell types including vacuolated cells with solitary or multiple clear vacuoles and clear cells. Depending on the dominant morphology, there are different types: *solid, microcystic, papillary cystic, adenomatous, and follicular.*

Treatment

The first-line treatment is complete surgical excision, supplemented by postoperative radiotherapy. The prognosis is usually good, especially when it arises in the minor salivary glands. However, local recurrences and metastases may occur in about 10 to 30% of patients. The overall survival prevalences are 90% at 5 years. A program of lifelong follow-up is necessary because local recurrences and metastases are often delayed.

Mucoepidermoid Carcinoma

Key points

- The most common salivary gland malignancy in children and adults.
- It has characteristic histologic features and broad spectrum of biological behavior.
- Comprises of three cell populations: mucous-secreting cells, squamous cells, and intermediate cells in variable combinations.
- The parotid gland (45%) and the soft palate (85%) are the most common sites of occurrence.
- The minor salivary glands constitute the second most common development site, especially the soft palate and less often the retromolar pad and lips.

Introduction

Mucoepidermoid carcinoma is a common salivary gland malignancy that comprises of three, histologically different, cellular populations. The biological behavior of the tumor can range in a broad spectrum from relatively good to very poor, depending on the dominant cellular type. It represents 2 to 3% of major salivary gland tumors and 6 to 9% of the minor salivary gland tumors. Mucoepidermoid carcinoma is the most common malignant salivary gland tumor in children with increased frequency among children who received radiotherapy for leukemia, lymphoma, and tinea capitis.

Clinical features

Mucoepidermoid carcinoma equally affects both sexes, more commonly between the age of 30 and 50 years. Clinically, intraoral tumors present as a slowly growing, painless enlargement that can have soft or firm consistency and could be ulcerated (**Figs. 39.29, 39.30**). Fluctuation is a characteristic clinical finding due to cystic formation inside the tumor. The tumor produces mucous material and may mimic mucocele. Intraorally, it occurs mainly in the soft palate and retromolar pad and less frequently in the buccal mucosa, lips, tongue, and floor of the mouth. Mucoepidermoid carcinoma in the parotid gland typically presents as a slow-growing painless mass. Progressively, tenderness, pain, trismus, and facial nerve paresis, usually in association with high-grade tumor, may occur. Very rarely, mucoepidermoid carcinomas develop intraosseously in the jaws. The 5-year overall survival of patients with mucoepidermoid carcinoma is about 80%. The diagnosis is based on the histologic findings.

Differential diagnosis

- Warthin's tumor with squamous mucinous metaplasia
- Pleomorphic adenoma
- Mucocele
- Cystadenoma
- Necrotizing sialadenometaplasia
- Acinic cell adenocarcinoma
- Polymorphous low-grade adenocarcinoma
- Low-malignancy carcinoma ex pleomorphic adenoma
- Other types of salivary gland adenocarcinomas

Pathology

Histologically, mucoepidermoid carcinoma comprises of three cellular types: *mucous-secreting, squamous (epidermoid),* and *intermediate* in variable combinations. Biological behavior and prognosis of mucoepidermoid carcinoma is determined by microscopic grading. There are several grading systems based on specific histologic features. According to the Armed Forces Institute of Pathology (AFIP), grading parameters with point values include the following: (1) intracystic component (+2), (2) neural invasion present (+2), (3) necrosis present (+3), (4) mitosis (4 per 10 high-power field [+3]), (5) anaplasia present (+4). Total point scores are 0 to 4 for low grade, 5 to 6 for intermediate grade, and 7 to 14 for high-grade mucoepidermoid carcinoma. Histologic variants of mucoepidermoid carcinomas (clear cell, spindle cell, oncocytic, sclerosing) may also occur. The stroma is sclerotic and abundant with infiltration of chronic inflammatory cells and extravascular mucin. Recent studies in the molecular genetics and specific gene expression have been identified in mucoepidermoid carcinoma cells, such as chromosomal translocation t(11;19) (q14–21, p12–13) and implicated genes *CRTC1–MAML2* and *CRTC3–MAML2*. These are helpful to separate benign salivary gland lesions from malignant.

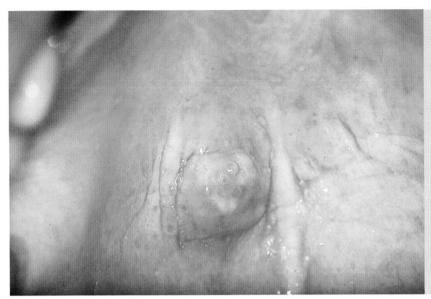

Fig. 39.28 Acinic cell adenocarcinoma of the palate.

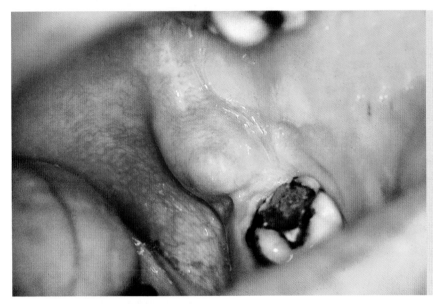

Fig. 39.29 Mucoepidermoid carcinoma in the retromolar area.

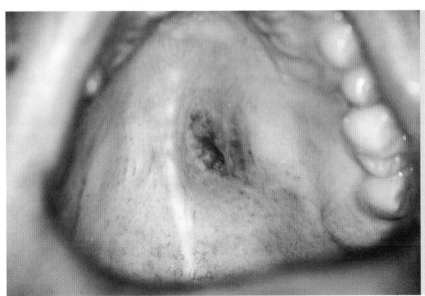

Fig. 39.30 Ulcerated mucoepidermoid carcinoma in the palate.

Treatment

The first line of treatment is surgical excision. The extent of the surgery depends on the location, the tumor's clinical stage, and histopathologic grade. Postoperative radiotherapy may be used for aggressive tumors.

Adenoid Cystic Carcinoma

Key points

- One of the most common malignant neoplasms of the salivary glands.
- More than 50% of the cases develop within the minor salivary glands.
- The palate is the most commonly affected site.
- In the parotid gland, it is relatively rare.
- A high rate of metastasis (30–40%) and is of poor prognosis.
- Pain is a common and early symptom.

Introduction

Adenoid cystic carcinoma or cylindroma is a common invasive malignant neoplasm of the salivary glands with characteristic histologic structure. It represents approximately 2 to 6% of all parotid gland tumors, 15% of submandibular gland tumors, and 20 to 30% of all the minor salivary gland tumors. In over 50% of the cases, the tumor develops in the minor salivary glands. Adenoid cystic carcinoma may occasionally arise in lacrimal glands, respiratory tract, digestive tract, breast, prostate, female genital tract, and skin.

Clinical features

Adenoid cystic carcinoma equally affects both sexes, most commonly between the age of 40 and 60 years. It is uncommon in under 20-year-olds. In minor salivary glands, it mainly occurs in the palate and less commonly in the buccal mucosa, lips, and the tongue. Clinically, adenoid cystic carcinoma of the minor salivary glands presents as slightly painful slow-growing swelling that often ulcerates (**Figs. 39.31, 39.32**) and at the final stages can cause severe pain. Along with the gradual swelling, tenderness, pain, and facial nerve palsy are common findings in patients with parotid tumor. Jaw bone invasion may occur without radiographic changes. The tumor metastasizes in approximately 30 to 40% of the cases and is usually of poor prognosis. The diagnosis is based on the histologic features.

Differential diagnosis

- Pleomorphic adenoma
- Basal cell adenoma
- Carcinoma ex pleomorphic adenoma
- Mucoepidermoid carcinoma
- Polymorphous low-grade adenocarcinoma
- Other tumors of the salivary glands

Pathology

Histologically, adenoid cystic carcinoma is characterized by a mixture of myoepithelial and ductal cells in various formations. There are three characteristic growth patterns: *cribriform*, *solid*, and *tubular* in variable combinations. The cribriform subtype is the most commonly seen and consists of cellular islands in a palisading pattern with many cystic spaces giving rise to a "*Swiss cheese*" appearance. Around the cribriform islands there is abundant eosinophilic material. Nuclear pleomorphism is mild and mitotic figures are usually few. The solid subtype consists of larger islands and sheets of closely packed basaloid cells that do not form any cystic spaces or ducts. The tubular subtype presents with ductal epithelial cells that form multiple small ducts or tubules surrounded by basaloid cells, within an eosinophilic hyalinized stroma. A common finding of adenoid cystic carcinoma is perineural invasion and spread. Immunohistochemically, the basaloid cells exhibit myoepithelial/basal differentiation. These cells express cytokeratin S100 protein, actin, calponin, and p63. The ductal epithelial cells express cytokeratin, CK7, CEA, EMA, and CD117.

Treatment

The treatment of choice is radical surgical excision. Radiotherapy is commonly used as adjunctive therapy. Local recurrence and distant metastases involving the bones and lungs are common.

Polymorphous Low-Grade Adenocarcinoma

Key points

- A malignant tumor of salivary gland with low metastatic potential.
- The second most common malignant neoplasm of the minor salivary glands.
- The palate is the most commonly affected site.
- The diagnosis is based on the histologic features.

Introduction

Polymorphous low-grade adenocarcinoma is a separate clinicopathologic entity that was first described in 1983. It almost exclusively affects the minor salivary glands. It consists 10 to 15% of all minor salivary gland tumors and is the second most common malignant neoplasm after mucoepidermoid carcinoma. Polymorphous low-grade adenocarcinoma may also develop in the nasopharynx, vulva, vagina, lung, and intraosseously.

Clinical features

Polymorphous low-grade adenocarcinoma is more common in females, usually between the age of 60 and 70 years. It commonly occurs in the soft–hard palate junction (60–70%) followed by buccal mucosa, upper lip, and the retromolar pad. Clinically, the tumor appears as a painless, firm slow-growth mass with or without ulceration (**Figs. 39.33, 39.34**). The size

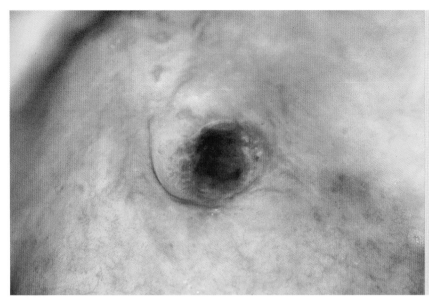

Fig. 39.31 Ulcerated adenoid cystic carcinoma on the palate.

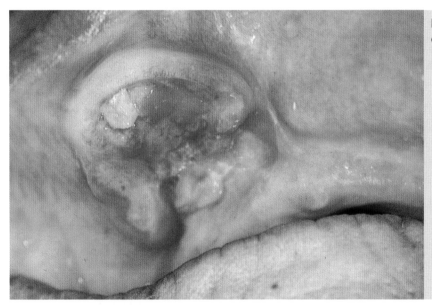

Fig. 39.32 Ulcerated adenoid cystic carcinoma on the upper lip.

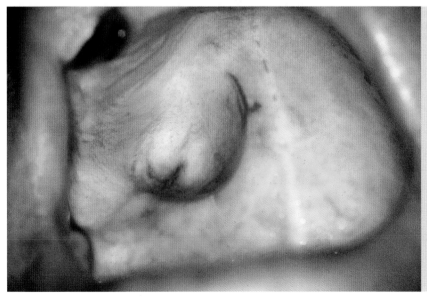

Fig. 39.33 Polymorphous low-grade adenocarcinoma on the palate.

varies from 1 to many centimeters. The overall prognosis is excellent with more than 90 to 95% of patients being alive after a 10-year follow-up. The diagnosis is based on the histologic features.

Differential diagnosis

- Pleomorphic adenoma
- Carcinoma ex pleomorphic adenoma
- Adenoid cystic carcinoma
- Mucoepidermoid carcinoma
- Acinic cell adenocarcinoma
- Other salivary gland tumors

Pathology

Histologically, polymorphous low-grade adenocarcinoma is characterized by variability of the growth pattern. The three most common patterns are *tubular*, *trabecular*, and *solid nests*. The tumor cells may assume cuboidal, spindled, round, columnar, and polygonal morphology with round nuclei and moderate amount of eosinophilic cytoplasm. The neoplastic cells are surrounded by a hyalinized eosinophilic stroma. Immunohistochemically, the cells exhibit reactivity for cytokeratin, S100 protein, vimentin, and epithelial membrane antigen (EMA).

Treatment

The first-line treatment is surgical excision. The prognosis is generally good and metastasis to regional lymph nodes is uncommon.

Carcinoma Ex Pleomorphic Adenoma

Key points

- It represents malignant transformation of a preexisting pleomorphic adenoma.
- About 80% of the cases occur in the major salivary glands, primarily the parotid.
- Nearly 70% of minor salivary gland cases occur on the palate.
- Signs of malignant transformation are rapid growth, fixation to surrounding tissues, ulceration, facial nerve palsy, and regional lymphadenopathy.

Introduction

Carcinoma ex pleomorphic adenoma is a rare tumor of the salivary glands that is histologically characterized by pleo-

morphic adenoma areas and areas of malignancy. It is believed to be the result of malignant transformation of pleomorphic adenoma. It occurs approximately 12 to 15 years later, compared with pleomorphic adenoma. It represents approximately 2 to 4% of all major salivary gland tumors and 3 to 7% of minor salivary glands. Over 95% of the cases occur in the major salivary glands, mainly the parotid, and the remaining 5% in the minor salivary glands.

Clinical features

Carcinoma ex pleomorphic adenoma more commonly affects females, usually between the age of 50 and 70 years. Clinically, the tumor initially appears with the characteristics of pleomorphic adenoma. It appears as a painless swelling that slowly increases in size and may later become painful and ulcerated. Facial nerve palsy and regional lymph node enlargements are common (**Figs. 39.35, 39.36**). Intraorally, the palate is the most commonly affected (70–80%), followed by buccal mucosa, upper lip, and the tongue. The diagnosis is based on the histologic features.

Differential diagnosis

- Pleomorphic adenoma
- Acinic cell adenocarcinoma
- Polymorphous low-grade adenocarcinoma
- Adenoid cystic carcinoma
- Other benign and malignant tumors of the salivary glands

Pathology

Histopathologically, malignant transformation may display three forms of malignancy: *carcinoma in situ*, *intracapsular carcinoma*, and *invasive carcinoma*. Histologically, malignant pleomorphic adenoma is characterized by typical areas of pleomorphic adenoma intermixed with malignant elements showing significant cellular pleomorphism, high mitotic index, atypical mitotic figures, necrosis, and infiltrative pattern. Amplification and overexpression of genes in chromosome 12q13–15, CDK4, HMGIC, and MDM2, represent significant findings for the malignant transformation. HER2 overexpression or gene amplification and S100P overexpression are useful in the differential diagnosis at histologic level. An additional indication of malignant transformation is the infiltration or extention beyond the tumor capsule, so that the tumor can be subclassified into *noninvasive*, *minimally invasive*, and *invasive*. The first two groups usually have better prognosis than the latter one.

Treatment

The first line of treatment is radical surgical excision in conjunction with regional lymph node dissection with or without radiotherapy. Recurrence and metastases are common and the overall 5-year survival is about 30%.

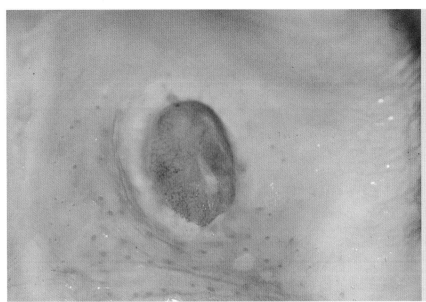

Fig. 39.34 Ulcerated polymorphous low-grade adenocarcinoma on the palate.

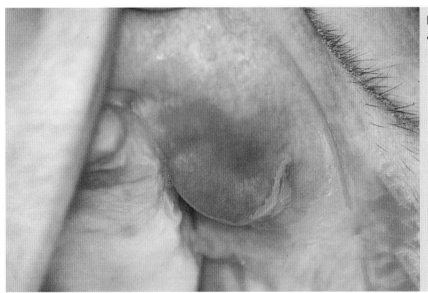

Fig. 39.35 Malignant pleomorphic adenoma on the buccal mucosa.

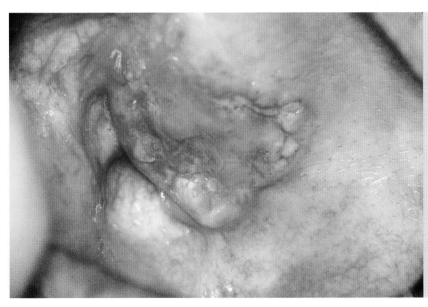

Fig. 39.36 Ulcerated malignant pleomorphic adenoma on the palate.

Clear Cell Adenocarcinoma

Key points
- Rare type of adenocarcinoma.
- The tumor is composed of monomorphic epithelial cells with clear cytoplasm.
- Most of the tumor affects the parotid gland and the minor salivary glands.
- The diagnosis is based on the histologic features.

Introduction

Clear cell adenocarcinoma is a rare malignant salivary gland neoplasm which is histologically characterized by monomorphic epithelial cells with clear cytoplasm without myoepithelial differentiation. The characteristic of other salivary gland neoplasms should be absent.

Clinical features

Clear cell adenocarcinoma affects slightly more commonly females, usually between the age of 50 and 70 years. It mostly occurs in the parotid gland and the minor salivary glands. Clinically, the tumor presents as a painless, hard, slow-growing mass that may ulcerate or cause fixation to adjacent tissues and enlarge (**Fig. 39.37**). Diagnosis cannot be based on the clinical features alone and biopsy with subsequent histopathologic examination is required for final diagnosis.

Differential diagnosis
- Epithelial–myoepithelial carcinoma
- Acinic cell carcinoma
- Mucoepidermoid carcinoma
- Other types of adenocarcinoma
- Clear cell oncocytoma
- Non-Hodgkin's lymphoma
- Wegener's granulomatosis
- Squamous cell carcinoma

Pathology

Histologically, the tumor is composed of sheets, columns, nests, and cords of large, monomorphic clear cells in a variable amount of fibrous stroma. The neoplastic cells exhibit abundant clear cytoplasm and nuclei with granular chromatin. Mild-to-moderate nuclear atypia is common feature, while mitotic figures are rare. The tumor cells are immunoreactive for cytokeratins.

Treatment

The first-line of treatment is radical surgical excision with or without adjunct radiotherapy.

Adenocarcinoma Not Otherwise Specified

Key points
- Malignant neoplasm of the salivary glands that lacks diagnostic criteria of other defined types of salivary carcinomas.
- Most frequently occurs between 60- and 80-year-old individuals.
- The parotid and submandibular glands and the palate are the most common locations.
- The diagnosis is based on the histologic criteria.

Introduction

This is an adenocarcinoma of the major and minor salivary glands that exhibits glandular differentiation and cannot be classified histopathologically under a specific category of other defined types of adenocarcinoma.

Clinical features

Intraorally, these adenocarcinomas affect more frequently males over 50 years. The palate is the most commonly affected site followed by buccal mucosa, upper lip, and tongue. Clinically, the tumors present with all the characteristics of malignant neoplasms such as fast-growing painful mass, ulceration, induration, fixation of the surrounding tissues, and metastases (**Figs. 39.38, 39.39**). The parotid and submandibular salivary glands may also be affected. The clinical features are not diagnostic and biopsy followed by histopathologic examination are required for final diagnosis.

Differential diagnosis
- Pleomorphic adenoma
- All types of adenocarcinoma
- Squamous cell carcinoma

Pathology

Histologically, the tumors are characterized by the presence of neoplastic glandular or ductal cells with great pleomorphism and a spectrum of cellular differentiation (well-moderate-poor) that do not fit to other recognizable patterns diagnostic of any specific salivary gland neoplasm.

Treatment

The first line of treatment is radical surgical excision with or without radiotherapy.

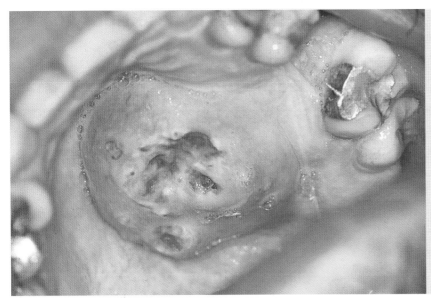

Fig. 39.37 Ulcerated clear cell adeno-carcinoma on the palate.

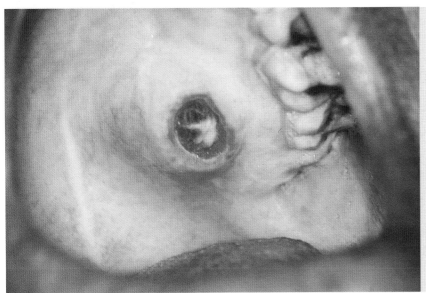

Fig. 39.38 Adenocarcinoma not otherwise specified on the palate.

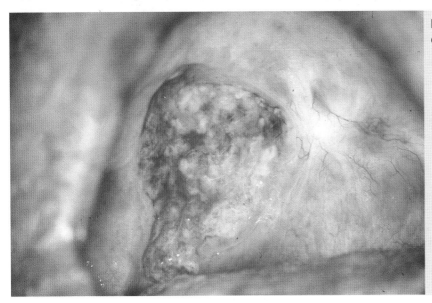

Fig. 39.39 Adenocarcinoma not otherwise specified on the palate.

2. Mesenchyme

Fibrosarcoma

Key points

- Soft tissue sarcomas are very rare in the mouth, representing 0.5 to 1% of all malignant tumors in the area.
- Fibrosarcoma derives from fibroblasts in the connective tissue and the underlying soft tissues.
- Diagnosis is based on the histopathologic features.

Introduction

Soft tissue fibrosarcoma is a rare malignant neoplasm of mesenchymal origin, deriving from fibroblasts. The tumor is most common in the limbs and trunk and only 10% develops in the head and neck region and very rare in the mouth.

Clinical features

Fibrosarcoma usually affects individuals under 50 years and can also affect neonates and older children. Intraorally, it most commonly occurs on the gingiva, buccal mucosa, palate, and the tongue. Clinically, the tumor presents as an exophytic, slow-growing, usually painless mass of soft or firm consistency that adheres to the surrounding tissues with or without ulceration (**Fig. 39.40**). The clinical features are not pathognomonic and the definitive diagnosis is based on histopathologic criteria.

Differential diagnosis

- Malignant fibrous histiocytoma
- Squamous cell carcinoma
- Liposarcoma
- Rhabdomyosarcoma
- Malignant schwannoma
- Kaposi's sarcoma
- Angiosarcoma
- Peripheral giant cell granuloma

Pathology

Histologically, fibrosarcoma is characterized by atypical, spindled fibroblasts with little cytoplasm and large hyperchromatic nuclei. They are arranged in bundles in a crisscross or herringbone pattern. Depending on the degree of differentiation, cellular areas, pleomorphism, atypical nuclei, mitoses of varied number, areas of necrosis, and collagen formation in different degree can be seen.

Treatment

The treatment of choice is radical surgical excision. Radiotherapy and chemotherapy may also be used as adjunctive therapy.

Malignant Fibrous Histiocytoma

Key points

- The most common soft tissue sarcomas in adults.
- Primarily considered to be a neoplasm of late adult life.
- Very rare in the mouth.
- The diagnosis is based on histopathologic criteria.

Introduction

Malignant fibrous histiocytoma is one of the most common soft tissue sarcomas in adults. It is very rare in the head and neck area. It derives from fibroblasts and histiocytes. Lately, the great frequency of the tumor has been questioned and the diagnostic criteria are reconsidered.

Clinical features

Malignant fibrous histiocytoma is extremely rare in the mouth and is usually developing in the jaw bones or the soft tissues. Clinically, the tumor presents as a rapidly developing and painless or painful, exophytic mass, of red-brown color, with or without ulceration (**Figs. 39.41, 39.42**). The size ranges between 2 to 6 cm in diameter. The clinical characteristics are not diagnostic and the definitive diagnosis is exclusively based on histologic criteria.

Differential diagnosis

- Fibrosarcoma
- Liposarcoma
- Kaposi's sarcoma
- Other types of sarcomas
- Squamous cell carcinoma
- Peripheral giant cell granuloma
- Pyogenic granuloma

Pathology

Histologically, malignant fibrous histiocytoma consists of atypical, plump spindled fibrous cells and histiocytes with large atypical nuclei and pale cytoplasm that are arranged in bundles. There are also areas of multinucleated giant cells with different degrees of differentiation. The spindle cells and histiocytes are vimentin positive. Additionally, the spindle cells are actin and vimentin positive, while the histiocytes are α_1-antitrypsin and α_1-antichymotrypsin positive. However, there is no specific immunophenotype to characterize the neoplasm.

Treatment

Radical surgical excision is the treatment of choice. Radiotherapy and chemotherapy may also be used as adjunctive therapy.

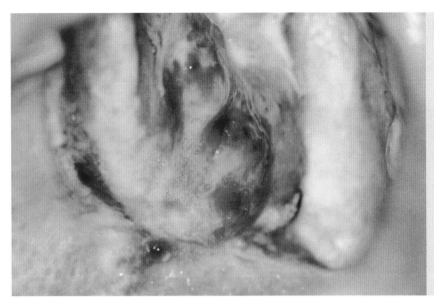

Fig. 39.40 Fibrosarcoma on the palate.

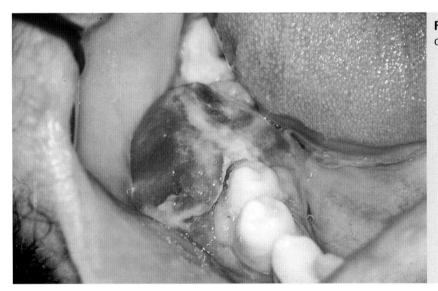

Fig. 39.41 Malignant fibrous histiocytoma on the lower gingiva.

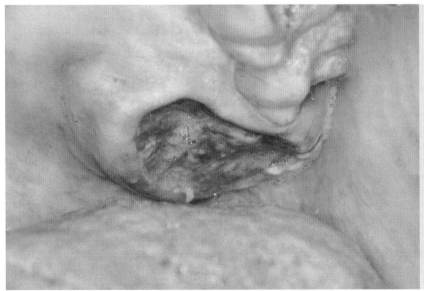

Fig. 39.42 Malignant fibrous histiocytoma on the maxillary alveolar mucosa.

3. Muscle Tissue

Leiomyosarcoma

Key points

- Leiomyosarcoma derives from the smooth muscle cells.
- More often it develops in the gastrointestinal tract, uterus, and the skin.
- It is rare in the mouth.
- The diagnosis is based exclusively on histologic criteria.

Introduction

Leiomyosarcoma is a malignant neoplasm of the smooth muscle tissue which accounts for 4 to 8% of total soft tissue sarcomas. The tumor most commonly occurs in the gastrointestinal tract, the uterus, and the skin, while it is very rare in the mouth. Primary oral leiomyosarcoma is uncommon and may derive from smooth muscle cells of the blood vessels and the circumvallate papillae of the tongue or from pluripotent remnants of embryonic mesenchyme.

Clinical features

Oral leiomyosarcoma most often affects females, usually over age 50. Clinically, the tumor presents as a slow-growing, painless or painful, raised firm mass with a smooth red surface that may or may not exhibit ulceration (**Figs. 39.43, 39.44**). The gingiva and tongue are the most common sites affected. The neoplasm can also occur intraosseously in the jaws. The clinical features are not characteristic and the diagnosis is exclusively based on histologic criteria.

Differential diagnosis

- Squamous cell carcinoma
- Rhabdomyosarcoma
- Fibrosarcoma
- Angiosarcoma
- Other soft tissue sarcomas
- Leiomyoma
- Peripheral gingival fibroma

Pathology

Histologically, leiomyosarcoma consists of atypical spindled cells with abundant eosinophilic cytoplasm and cigar-shaped nuclei. These cells have the characteristics of smooth muscle cells with variable polymorphism and cellular atypia, as well as multiple mitoses. Immunohistochemical markers are h-caldesmon, α smooth muscle actin, desmin, and myosin. However, they are not specific to smooth muscle fibers as they can also be detected in other cell types such as myofibroblasts. If they are negative, a diagnosis of leiomyosarcoma is not considered.

Treatment

The treatment of choice is radical surgical excision with or without adjunctive radiotherapy or/and chemotherapy.

Rhabdomyosarcoma

Key points

- A malignant neoplasm that originates from the striated muscles.
- The head and neck area and the genitourinary tract are the most frequent sites of involvement.
- Much more common in children and adolescents.
- It is very rare in the mouth.
- The tumor is classified into two basic types: *embryonal* and *alveolar*.
- The diagnosis is based on histologic criteria.

Introduction

Rhabdomyosarcoma is a rare malignant tumor in which the cells present with striated muscle differentiation. The tumor is common in children and adolescents and rare in young adults. The most frequent affected site is the head and neck area, followed by the genitourinary system, while it is rare in the mouth. It is classified into two basic types: *embryonal* and *alveolar*.

Clinical features

The tumor usually affects the 5- to 15-year-olds and is a little more common in males. Oral rhabdomyosarcoma presents as a rapidly growing, firm or hard mass that can gradually become painful. It can ultimately cause deformity of the affected area and of the face (**Fig. 39.45**). Trismus, facial nerve palsy, and hypoesthesia may also occur. The most commonly affected sites are the palate and the buccal mucosa. Embryonal rhabdomyosarcoma is most common during the first 10 years of life, accounting for 50 to 60% of the cases. The alveolar form develops in older children and teenagers or young adults, accounting for 20 to 30% of the cases. The diagnosis is based on the history, clinical features, and especially on the histologic findings.

Differential diagnosis

- Leiomyosarcoma
- Neuroblastoma
- Non-Hodgkin's lymphoma
- Burkitt's lymphoma
- Lymphangioma

Pathology

Histologically, rhabdomyosarcoma is characterized by cells of variable size and shape with polymorphism, hyperchromatic nuclei, and multiple mitoses. Based on histologic criteria,

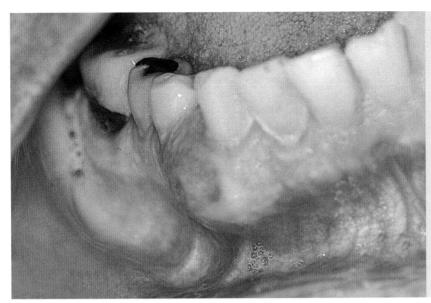

Fig. 39.43 Leiomyosarcoma on the lower gingiva, in the canine area.

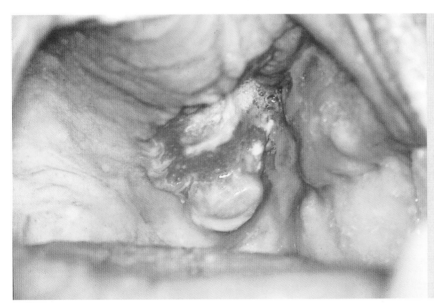

Fig. 39.44 Ulcerated leiomyosarcoma on the palate and the alveolar mucosa.

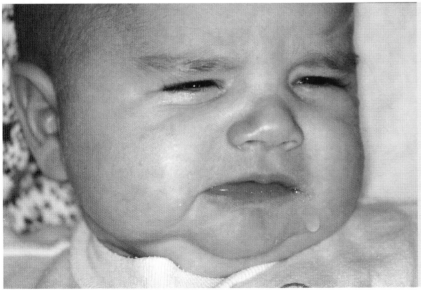

Fig. 39.45 Rhabdomyosarcoma in the right buccal mucosa.

rhabdomyosarcoma is classified into two basic types: *embryonal* and *alveolar* and three more rare types: *anaplastic*, *pleomorphic*, and *sclerosing*. There are differences in the cellular structure and morphology depending on the type of tumor. The cells are positive to vimentin, desmin, myogenin/myo-D1, and myoglobin.

Treatment

The first line of treatment is surgical excision combined with radiotherapy and chemotherapy. The prognosis is usually poor.

4. Vascular Tissue

Hemangioendothelioma

Key points
- Hemangioendothelioma is a malignant neoplasm of the vascular wall endothelial cells.
- It is probably a variety of angiosarcoma.
- Most commonly occurs in the head and neck area.
- The tumor is quite rare in the mouth.

Introduction

Hemangioendothelioma is a rare malignant neoplasm, of the angiosarcoma type, that originates from the endothelial cells of the blood or lymph vessel wall. It usually occurs on the skin of the head and neck and is very rare in the mouth.

Clinical features

Hemangioendothelioma more often affects females, usually over age 50. Clinically, it presents as an elevated firm mass with a characteristic deep red or brown-red color, with or without ulceration that bleeds easily (**Figs. 39.46, 39.47**). The tumor most commonly occurs in the tongue, buccal mucosa, palate, gingiva, and the lips. The clinical diagnosis has to be confirmed by histology.

Differential diagnosis
- Kaposi's sarcoma
- Hemangiopericytoma
- Malignant fibrous histiocytoma
- Hemangioma
- Leiomyoma
- Pyogenic granuloma
- Peripheral giant cell granuloma

Pathology

Histologically, hemangioendothelioma is characterized by multiple vascular spaces that are lined by atypical endothelial cells with hyperchromatic nuclei and several mitoses. The neoplastic cells are positive to CD31 and factor VIII.

Treatment

The treatment of choice is surgical excision usually combined with radiotherapy.

Hemangiopericytoma

Key points
- A rare neoplasm of the vascular tissue.
- Originates from the vascular wall pericytes.
- The tumor is classified into two types: *benign* and *malignant*.
- Very rare in the mouth.

Introduction

Hemangiopericytoma is a neoplasm that arises from the pericytes of the vascular wall. It is classified into *benign* and *malignant* type. It is difficult to distinguish between the two.

Clinical features

Hemangiopericytoma equally affects both sexes, usually under age 50. It is rare on the oral mucosa. The most commonly affected sites are the buccal mucosa, tongue, and the palate. Clinically, the tumor usually presents as a well-circumscribed painless, elevated mass of normal or red color and firm consistency (**Fig. 39.48**). The malignancy usually progresses quickly and may become ulcerated. The clinical feature is not diagnostic and the final diagnosis has to be confirmed by histology.

Differential diagnosis
- Hemangioendothelioma
- Kaposi's sarcoma
- Malignant fibrous histiocytoma
- Leiomyoma
- Hemangioma
- Glomus tumor

Pathology

Histologically, hemangiopericytoma is characterized by multiple vascular spaces that are intersecting irregularly giving it a

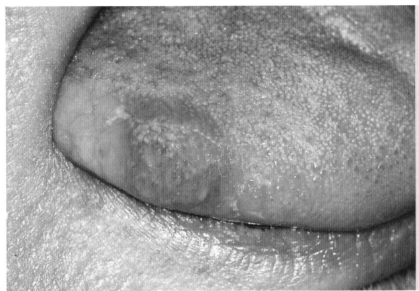

Fig. 39.46 Hemangioendothelioma on the lateral border of the tongue.

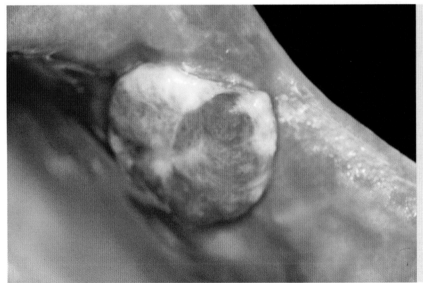

Fig. 39.47 Hemangioendothelioma on the buccal mucosa.

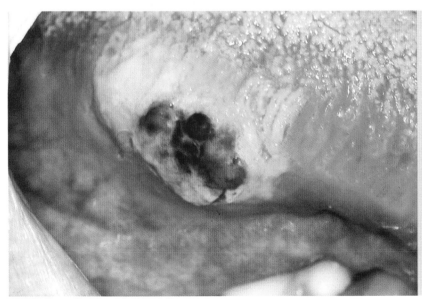

Fig. 39.48 Hemangiopericytoma on the lateral border of the tongue.

shape that has been compared with a deer antler. These spaces are lined by endothelial cells and are surrounded by crowded pericytes. The latter have almost round or ovoid nuclei, indistinct cytoplasmic borders, and sometimes spindle morphology. Reticulin stain highlights the dense network of fibers that surround the vessels and the isolated cells. Indications of possible malignant behavior are the detection of four or more mitoses per 10 high-power fields and the presence of necrosis.

Treatment

The first-line treatment is surgical excision. The extent of the excision depends on the degree of differentiation observed that is an indicator of the tumor's degree of malignancy.

Kaposi's Sarcoma

Key points

- Kaposi's sarcoma is classified into four groups: *classic*, *African-endemic*, *iatrogenic* (immunosuppression–related), and *epidemic* (acquired immunodeficiency syndrome [AIDS]-related).
- The main etiologic factor is human herpes virus, type 8 (HHV-8).
- In the last four decades, the epidemic type has been widespread.
- It predominantly affects the skin.
- The oral mucosa can commonly be affected in the epidemic type and rarely in the three other types.
- The first line of treatment is chemotherapy with or without radiotherapy.

Introduction

Kaposi's sarcoma was first described in 1872 by the Hungarian dermatologist Moritz Kaposi, on elderly individuals. It was observed to have good biological behavior, slow development, and unknown cause. With HIV infection and AIDS, Kaposi's sarcoma was found in the epicenter of scientific interest since its incidence multiplied. Following that, the tumor was studied and the progress in the findings was impressive on molecular, histologic, clinical, etiologic, and therapeutic level. Since the introduction of highly active antiretroviral therapy (HAART), the prevalence of AIDS-related Kaposi's sarcoma has dramatically been reduced.

Kaposi's sarcoma is classified into four groups: *classic*, *African-endemic*, *iatrogenic immunosuppression–related*, and *epidemic AIDS-related*. HHV-8 has been isolated from both the tumor and the patients' peripheral blood and is the cause of this lesion. However, it still remains unclear whether Kaposi's sarcoma is a true neoplasm or a hyperplastic reaction resulting from great proliferation of the endothelial cells following cytokine and growth factors' action. Immunohistochemical and electron microscope studies have confirmed that Kaposi's sarcoma originates from endothelial cells without making clear whether these are of the blood or lymph vessels.

Clinical features

The classic Kaposi's sarcoma more commonly affects males (ratio between 3:1 and 8:1), between the age of 50 and 70 years, and has a slow development. It is more common in the Balkans, the Mediterranean countries, and Jewish and Greek populations. It mainly affects the skin and rarely the oral and other mucosae, gastrointestinal tract, and viscera. Clinically, the lesions present as solitary or multiple macules, plaques, nodules, or tumors with a deep red, or brown-red color (**Figs. 39.49– 39.51**). The most commonly affected sites are the feet, hands, nose, and the ears. The oral mucosa is affected relatively rarely and usually after spread of the disease, while it is very uncommon to be the only affected site. Clinically, the oral lesions appear as single or multiple macules, plaques, or tumors that might ulcerate and are of

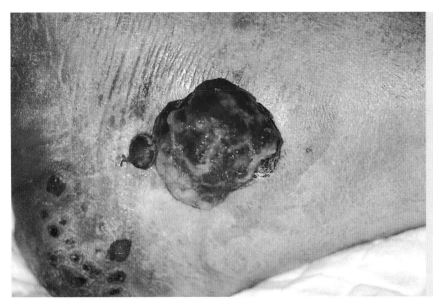

Fig. 39.49 Classic Kaposi's sarcoma, multiple tumors on the skin of the foot.

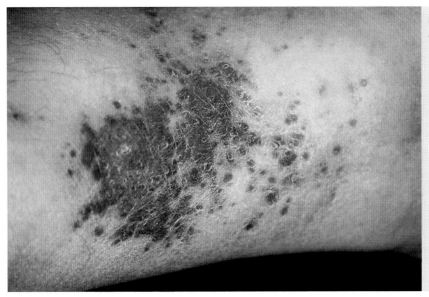

Fig. 39.50 Classic Kaposi's sarcoma on the skin.

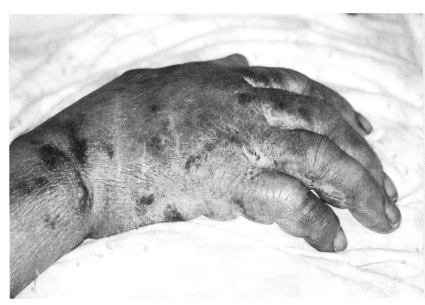

Fig. 39.51 Classic Kaposi's sarcoma, generalized lesions on the hand.

bright red or brown-red color (**Figs. 39.52–39.54**). The most commonly affected sites are the palate and gingiva, followed by lips, tongue, and the buccal mucosa. The clinical diagnosis has to be confirmed by histopathologic examination. African (endemic) Kaposi's sarcoma is common in Uganda and other African countries, primarily involves the skin and lymph nodes but rarely the oral mucosa, and usually has an indolent course. Kaposi's sarcoma is observed in patients with kidney transplantation as well as those having received immunosuppressive drugs for a variety of diseases. The clinical course of this form is indolent, but sometimes can be very aggressive, involving the viscera, but rarely the oral mucosa. AIDS-related (epidemic) Kaposi's sarcoma, without race predilection and of high incidence among AIDS patients, involves primarily the skin, lymph nodes, viscera, and frequently the oral mucosa. It has a rapid, usually fatal course.

Differential diagnosis

- Bacillary angiomatosis
- Angiosarcoma
- Hemangioendothelioma
- Hemangiopericytoma
- Leiomyosarcoma
- Hemangioma
- Peripheral giant cell granuloma
- Pyogenic granuloma
- Non-Hodgkin's lymphoma
- Malignant melanoma

Pathology

There are no histologic differences between the four types of Kaposi's sarcoma. The main histologic findings are the presence of multiple vascular spaces lined by flat and/or occasionally atypical, endothelial cells with hyaline droplets, extravasated erythrocytes, and hemosiderin deposits. There are also more solid areas with spindled cells that are usually arranged in bundles. A characteristic immunologic finding is the expression of HHV-8 antinuclear antigens (LNA-1). HHV-8 genome can also be detected with polymerase chain reaction (PCR). Moreover, immunohistochemically the endothelial cells are FLI-1, CD31, CD34, and D2–40 positive.

Treatment

Because of the multifocal nature of Kaposi's sarcoma, the first line of treatment is chemotherapy with or without radiotherapy. The chemotherapeutic agents that have been used are vincristine, doxorubicin, bleomycin, and interferon α, in various combinations. In localized lesions, surgical excision, cryotherapy, laser, and photodynamic therapy (PDT) have been applied.

5. Osseous and Chondroid Tissue

Osteosarcoma

Key points

- The most common primary malignancy of the bones.
- Common between age 10 and 20, but when located in the jaws, usually affects patients of 30 to 40.
- Jaw osteosarcoma represents 6 to 7% of the tumor's total cases.
- Enlargement and pain are the principal signs and symptoms.

Introduction

Osteosarcoma is the most common primary malignancy of mesenchymal cells that have the capability to create bone. The etiology remains unknown. However, occasionally, the neoplasm seems to develop after bone trauma or in patients irradiated for other oral lesions or in patients with Paget's disease. It is more common in males, usually between age 10 and 20. Osteosarcoma of the jaws represents 6 to 7% of the total cases and usually occurs 10 to 15 years later at other skeletal sites. The mandible and maxilla are equally affected.

Clinical features

Clinically, oral osteosarcoma presents as a hard enlargement on the jaw bone that develops relatively rapidly. It can cause teeth movement and displacement and facial deformity

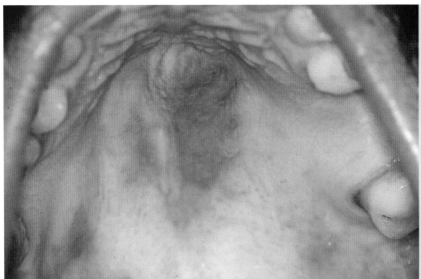

Fig. 39.52 Kaposi's sarcoma on the hard palate.

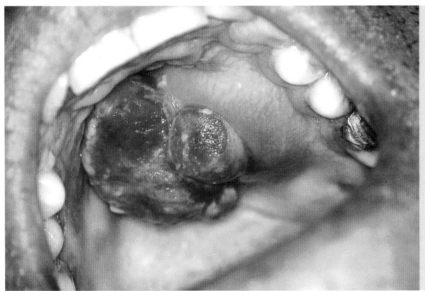

Fig. 39.53 Ulcerated Kaposi's sarcoma on the palate.

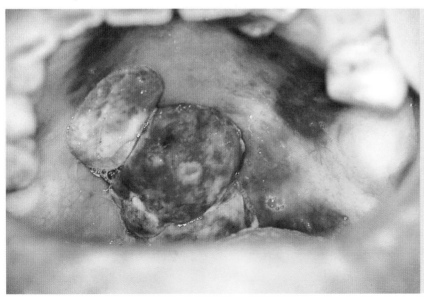

Fig. 39.54 Kaposi's sarcoma, multiple tumors on the palate and the gingiva.

(**Fig. 39.55**). Following the osseous destruction, the tumor may occasionally present as a soft exophytic mass with an irregular ulcerated surface (**Fig. 39.56**). Characteristic symptoms include pain, bleeding, paresthesia, and nasal obstruction. It can equally affect the maxilla and the mandible and has a poor prognosis. The oral lesions usually develop 10 years after the primary tumor elsewhere in the skeleton. The diagnosis is based on clinical, radiological, and mainly histologic criteria.

Differential diagnosis
- Chondrosarcoma
- Ewing's sarcoma
- Odontogenic tumors of the jaws
- Paget's disease of bone
- Fibrous dysplasia
- Cherubism
- Osteoblastoma

Pathology

Histologic examination of the tumor is required for the diagnosis. Microscopically, osteosarcoma shows significant cytologic diversity with consistent characteristic in the formation of osteoid, osseous tissue, occasionally chondroid or even fibrous connective tissue by the neoplastic mesenchymal cells. The latter are spindled or round with high polymorphism and irregular hyperchromatic nuclei. Depending on the dominant histologic feature, osteosarcoma is classified into *osteoblastic*, *chondroblastic*, and *fibroblastic*. However, this classification is not indicative of the prognosis. Radiographically (computed tomography [CT] scan, panoramic and occlusal radiographs), radiopacity is observed together with radiolucent areas, while in 20 to 30% of the cases a characteristic appearance that is described as *sunray* or *sunburst* is observed. Additionally, there is often symmetrical enlargement of the periodontal space that is caused by periodontal membrane infiltration by neoplastic cells. Prior to surgery, CT scan can also be useful.

Treatment

Preoperative or postoperative chemotherapy together with radical surgical excision of the tumor are the first line of treatment.

Ewing's Sarcoma

Key points
- A primary malignant neoplasm of undifferentiated mesenchymal cells of bone.
- Represents 6 to 7% of the total of primary bone neoplasias.
- Commonly affects the long bones, the pelvis, and the ribs.
- Uncommon in the jaws.

Introduction

Ewing's sarcoma was first described as an independent entity by James Ewing (1866–1942). It is a distinctive primary malignant neoplasm of the bones and third in frequency after osteosarcoma and chondrosarcoma. It consists 6 to 7% of the total primary malignancies of the bones. It has an unclear histogenesis, however, the neuroectodermal origin of the tumor is the most supported. Over 90% of the tumor cells demonstrate translocation between chromosomes 11 and 22, t(11;22) and development of a new chimeric gene.

Clinical features

Ewing's sarcoma mainly affects children and young adults, particularly males with more than 80% of patients being under 20 years at the time of diagnosis. In the head and neck area, the average patient's age is 11. Ewing's sarcoma most commonly presents in the long bones, the pelvis and the ribs, while the head and neck area represents approximately 4 to 6% of the total cases. Jaw involvement is under 1% with predilection to the angle and the ascending ramus of the mandible. Clinically, jaw expanding associated with pain are the most common signs and symptoms. It progresses to osseous destruction and teeth mobility while there is often an ulcerated soft mass originating from the affected area of the bone (**Fig. 39.57**). Facial disfigurement, paresthesia, and fever may occur. The clinical diagnosis has to be confirmed by histology and imaging.

Differential diagnosis
- Osteosarcoma
- Chondrosarcoma
- Neuroblastoma
- Osteomyelitis
- Giant cell tumor
- Odontogenic tumors

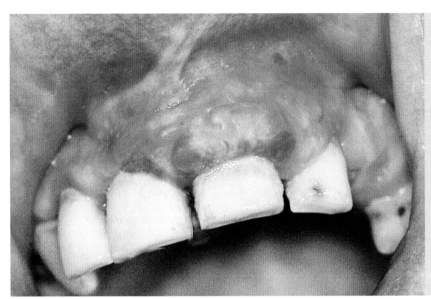

Fig. 39.55 Osteosarcoma on the anterior part of the maxilla.

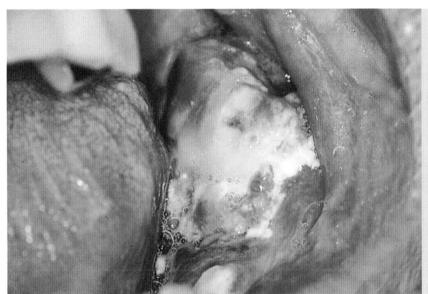

Fig. 39.56 Osteosarcoma on the mandible.

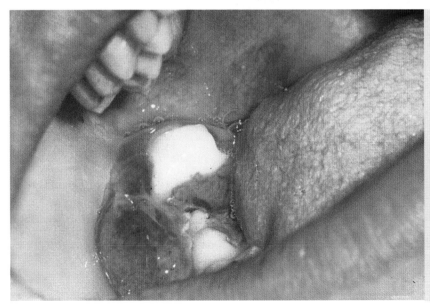

Fig. 39.57 Ewing's sarcoma, enlargement on the mandible.

Pathology

Histologic examination is required for the definitive diagnosis of Ewing's sarcoma. Microscopically, a uniform cellular population, arranged in large sheets, is observed, with small round cells that have an ovoid, small, well-defined nucleus and indistinct cell membrane. The cytoplasm is periodic acid–Schiff (PAS) positive due to the presence of glycogen. Areas of hemorrhage and necrosis are common findings. Reverse transcription polymerase chain reaction (RT-PCR) and in situ hybridization for the identification of the 11.22 gene translocation can be used as specific diagnostic techniques.

Radiographic examination and CT are also of great diagnostic help, exhibiting either a *sunray* or an *onion-peel* pattern due to new bone deposition in layers.

Treatment

First-line treatment is the combination of radical surgical excision with radiotherapy and chemotherapy. These therapeutic regimens have greatly improved the 5-year survival rate (50–80%).

Chondrosarcoma

Key points

- Chondrosarcoma is a malignant neoplasm characterized by the formation of aberrant cartilage tissue.
- It consists 8–10% of all the primary malignancies of the skeleton.
- The limbs and pelvis are more commonly affected and less frequently the head and neck area.
- Jaw involvement is rare.
- The diagnosis is based on histology.

Introduction

Chondrosarcoma is a malignant neoplasm that is characterized by cartilage formation by the tumor cells. It represents 8 to 10% of all the primary tumors of the skeleton. It is relatively rare in the head and neck area (1–3%) and very rare in the jaws (0.5–1%). It is classified into *primary*, when it develops de novo and *secondary*, when it develops from a preexisting benign cartilage tumor. *Mesenchymal* chondrosarcoma is an uncommon histologically distinct variant of chondrosarcoma that may also occur in the jaws.

Clinical features

Chondrosarcoma more commonly affects males, usually between age 30 and 50. Clinically, the tumor presents as a painless, hard swelling that develops rapidly, causing extensive osseous destruction with pain and loosening and displacement of the teeth. Occasionally, a large, erythematous, lobulated, and ulcerated exophytic, soft mass may present in the oral cavity (**Figs. 39.58, 39.59**). The maxilla is more commonly affected than the mandible (ratio 4:1) and when present, it can cause epistaxis, nasal obstruction, photophobia, and visual disturbances.

Differential diagnosis

- Osteosarcoma
- Ewing's sarcoma
- Malignant fibrous histiocytoma
- Squamous cell carcinoma
- Giant cell granuloma
- Odontogenic tumors

Pathology

Histologic examination is required for the diagnosis of chondrosarcoma. Microscopically, the tumor is characterized by cartilage formation with increased cellularity consisting of atypical chondrocytes. Depending on the degree of differentiation of the neoplastic cells and the stroma, it is classified into three histologic grades that have prognostic significance (I, II, and III). Radiographs and CT scans are useful toward the diagnosis.

Treatment

First-line treatment is radical surgical excision of the tumor. Radiotherapy and chemotherapy can be used as adjuncts in selected cases.

6. Pigmented Tissue

Malignant Melanoma

Key points

- Melanoma is a malignant neoplasm deriving from melanocytes.
- It affects mainly the skin and less often the mucosae and other areas.
- In recent decades, the incidence of melanoma has increased.
- Primary melanoma of the oral mucosa is rare, accounting for 0.5 to 1% of all melanomas.
- Primary cutaneous melanoma is classified into four basic types: *superficial spreading melanoma*, *nodular melanoma*, *lentigo maligna melanoma*, and *acral lentiginous* melanoma.
- Early detection is an important goal in melanoma management and prognosis.
- The prognosis of oral melanoma is usually poor due to late diagnosis.

Introduction

Malignant melanoma arises from melanocytes, is of poor prognosis, and occurs mainly on the skin, but can also occur in any area of the body where pigmented tissue exists (**Fig. 39.60**). The incidence and mortality rates of skin

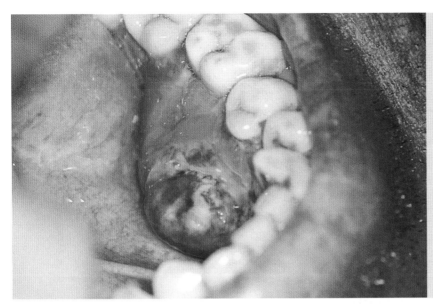

Fig. 39.58 Chondrosarcoma on the lingual aspect of the mandible.

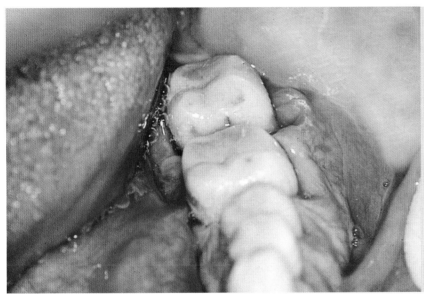

Fig. 39.59 Chondrosarcoma, lingual and buccal enlargement of the mandible.

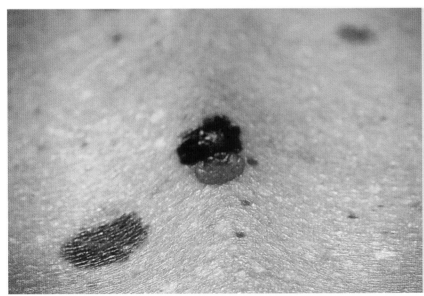

Fig. 39.60 Malignant melanoma, multiple lesions on the skin of the trunk.

melanoma has increased greatly worldwide during the last four decades. In Australia, where the highest percentage of melanoma cases occur, there are 50 new cases per 100,000 individuals, in the United States 15 new cases per 100,000, and in the United Kingdom 10 to 12 new cases per 100,000. The great increase is attributed to prolonged sunlight exposure. Risk factors are classified into three groups: genetic factors, environmental factors, and phenotypic factors reflecting gene/environmental interaction such as melanocytic nevi, dysplastic nevi, and ephelides. Primary melanoma of the oral mucosa accounts for 0.5 to 1% of total melanomas. The tumor can also affect other mucosae (larynx, rhinopharynx, conjunctivae, vagina, and anus). It develops either de novo or on a preexisting benign pigmented lesion from skin or mucosal melanocytes. The tumor cells present with two growth phases, the *horizontal* or *radial* and *vertical* with deeper extension. These are indicative of the type of extension and the prognosis of the neoplasm.

The prognosis of the melanoma of the skin depends on the clinical type of melanoma and the depth of invasion histologically (Breslow's depth). There is an 11-grade scale that places great importance on the invasion thickness that is based on the *Breslow's* method (measuring in millimeters from the top of the granular cell layer of the epidermis and the deepest point of tumor penetration, using an ocular micrometer). However, the above criteria are not of practical help with oral melanoma.

Clinical features

Malignant melanoma of the oral mucosa equally affects both sexes usually between age 50 and 60 . Melanoma is classified by clinical and histologic criteria into four basic types. *Nodular melanoma* presents as exophytic black or black-brown nodule or tumor that grows very rapidly, bleeds easily, and is frequently ulcerated (**Figs. 39.61–39.63**). It occurs quite often in the mouth and has the worst prognosis because it grows vertically. The *superficial spreading melanoma* presents as a circumscribed flat or slightly raised black plaque that grows peripherally (**Fig. 39.64**). It is relatively rare in the mouth and has better prognosis compared with the nodular type, as it spreads horizontally. *Lentigo maligna melanoma* is extremely rare intraorally and has the best prognosis, because it has the lowest spread on a horizontal plane (**Fig. 39.65**). *Acral lentiginous* melanoma is a rare type (5–10%) that characteristically occurs on the palms and soles and around or beneath the nail apparatus. *Amelanotic melanoma* is rare variant of melanoma without pigmented element that can histologically be classified under one of the four basic types.

In the mouth, over 80% of the melanomas present in the hard palate, maxillary gingiva, and alveolar mucosa. The remaining 20% is distributed in the mandibular gingiva, buccal mucosa, tongue, floor of the mouth, and the lips. The diagnosis of melanoma is based on clinical criteria, but mainly on the histopathologic findings. On the skin, the ABCDE system* is the most common sensitive clinical signs for melanoma. The prognosis of oral melanoma is worst of that of the skin due to delay in detection and rapid metastases.

Differential diagnosis

- Lentigo maligna
- Pigmented nevi
- Ephelides
- Lentigo simplex
- Melanoacanthoma
- Kaposi's sarcoma
- Bacterial angiomatosis
- Pyogenic granuloma
- Amalgam tattoo
- Cavernous hemangioma
- Other black foreign materials
- Physiologic pigmentation

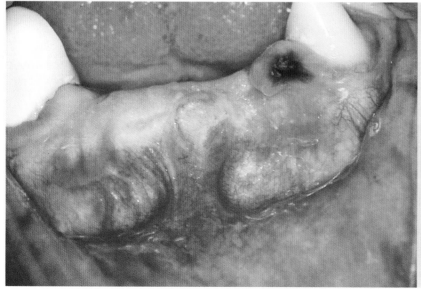

Fig. 39.61 Malignant melanoma, nodular type, primary on the alveolar mucosa.

*****ABCDE** system: **A**symmetry, **B**order irregularity, **C**olor variegation, **D**iameter (> 5 mm), and **E**volving.

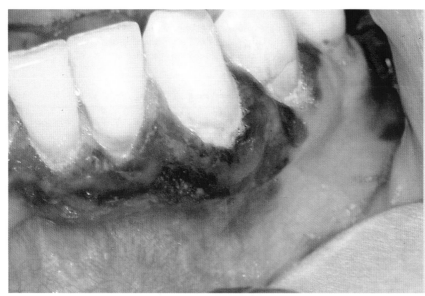

Fig. 39.62 Malignant melanoma, nodular type, multiple lesions on the gingiva.

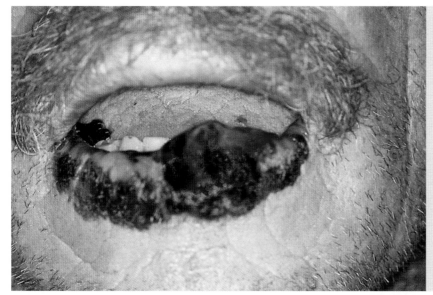

Fig. 39.63 Malignant melanoma, nodular type, on the lower lip.

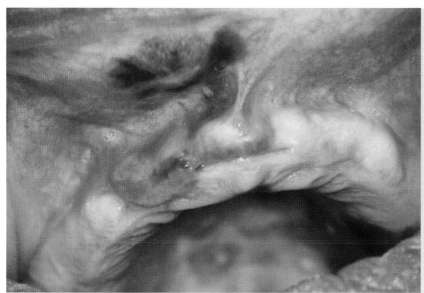

Fig. 39.64 Malignant melanoma, early, superficial spreading.

Pathology

Histopathologic examination is the most reliable criterion toward diagnosis. Indicators with strong prognostic value are the architecture of the tumor, the cellular morphology, Clark's scale of infiltration, and mainly the Breslow's scale that examines the depth of invasion from the top of the granular layer down to the lowest part of tumor invasion. Histologically, atypical melanocytes with large nuclei, multiple mitoses, and cellular polymorphism are observed. They form nests in the epidermis, the dermal–epidermal junction, and the underlying connective tissue. S100 protein is positive. Other immunohistochemical markers that help the histologic differential diagnosis are HMB45, Melan-A/MART-1, and tyrosinase.

Treatment

The first-line treatment is radical surgical excision of the tumor. Regional lymph node dissection is undertaken in cases of positive sentinel lymph node biopsy. Adjuvant therapy after surgical excision includes chemotherapy in combination with immunotherapy or hormonal therapy or molecularly targeted therapy. The management of malignant melanoma includes prevention, early diagnosis, treatment, and close follow-up.

Lentigo Maligna

Key points

- A precancerous lesion of melanocytes.
- It mainly occurs on the face with a preference for the cheek and nose.
- It is uncommon in the oral mucosa.
- Histologically, it is an in situ melanoma which progresses in approximately 5% to invasive melanoma.

Introduction

Lentigo maligna, also known as Hutchinson's melanotic freckle, is a precancerous lesion of the pigmented tissue.

Lentigo maligna is usually an in situ melanoma that in over 5% progresses to invasive melanoma with better prognosis than the other types of melanomas. It usually occurs on sun-damaged skin, frequently on the face.

Clinical features

Lentigo maligna equally affects both sexes, usually over age 60. The most commonly affected sites are the cheeks and the nose (**Fig. 39.66**). It is uncommon in the oral mucosa. Clinically, oral lentigo maligna presents as a black or black-brown plaque of variable size with irregular or smooth surface. It has slow progression and can occur on the buccal mucosa, palate, floor of the mouth, and the lower lip (**Fig. 39.67**). The clinical diagnosis has to be confirmed by histologic examination.

Differential diagnosis

- Actinic melanosis
- Lentigo simplex
- Ephelides
- Pigmented nevi
- Melanoacanthoma
- Malignant melanoma
- Amalgam tattoo
- Physiologic pigmentation
- Smoker's melanosis

Pathology

Histologically, lentigo maligna is an in situ melanoma characterized by an increased number of atypical neoplastic melanocytes that are commonly present within the epithelium.

Treatment

Conservative surgical excision or radiotherapy are recommended. Cryosurgery is also useful as an alternative modality for lentigo maligna. If it has evolved into malignant melanoma, the treatment options for melanoma are followed.

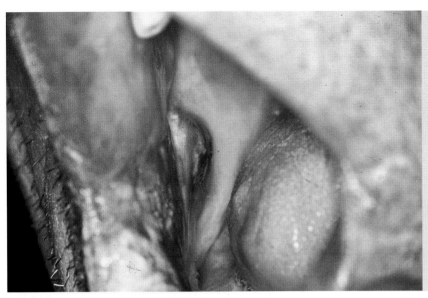

Fig. 39.65 Malignant melanoma, (buccal tumor) on a lentigo maligna.

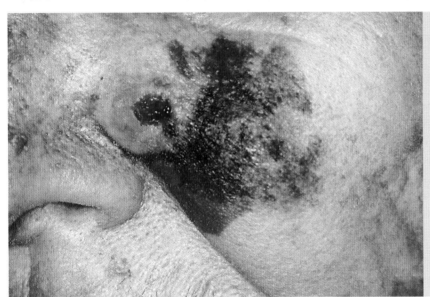

Fig. 39.66 Lentigo maligna on the skin of the face.

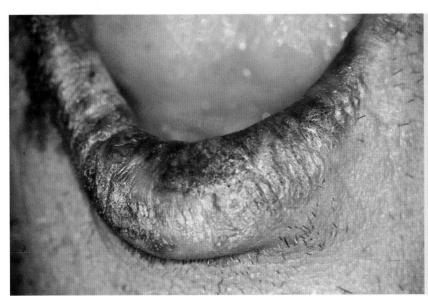

Fig. 39.67 Lentigo maligna on the lower lip.

7. Metastatic Neoplasms

Key points
- Metastases in the oral cavity are uncommon.
- They can occur both in the soft tissues and the jaws.
- The clinical features do not have special characteristics.
- Any malignancy is capable of metastasis in the oral cavity.

Introduction

Metastatic tumors in the oral cavity are rare, representing approximately 1 to 2% of all oral cancers. They usually occur in the jaws and less frequently in the soft tissues. The significance of metastatic tumors is great as it can be the first presentation of a malignancy with an unknown primary or may be the first metastasis of an already diagnosed primary.

Clinical features

Oral metastases can usually occur from gastrointestinal tract carcinomas (**Fig. 39.68**), lungs (**Fig. 39.69**), prostate, renal, breast, and melanoma. Theoretically, any malignancy may be metastasized to the mouth (**Fig. 39.70**). Most commonly, the metastatic tumors affect the gingiva, followed by the tongue and the palate. Clinically, it presents as an asymptomatic tumor with or without ulceration, without any special clinical characteristics. It may mimic benign oral lesions or primary oral carcinoma. The diagnosis is exclusively based on histology and the finding of the primary tumor. Usually, at the time of the diagnosis of the oral lesion, the primary tumor already is known. The final diagnosis is based on the histopathologic features.

Differential diagnosis
- Squamous cell carcinoma
- Pyogenic granuloma
- Peripheral giant cell granuloma
- Peripheral odontogenic tumors
- Minor salivary gland tumors
- Non-Hodgkin's lymphoma

Pathology

Histopathologic and occasionally detailed immunohistochemical examination is required for accurate diagnosis and determination of the primary malignancy.

Treatment

The management of the oral lesion is palliative and the main treatment follows the recommended protocol of the primary tumor.

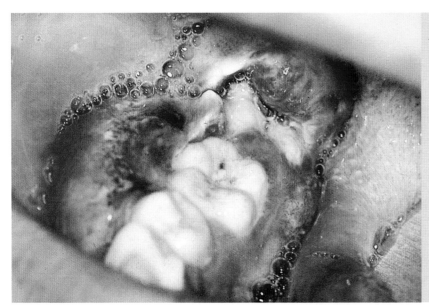

Fig. 39.68 Metastatic carcinoma on the gingiva from a primary carcinoma in the rectum.

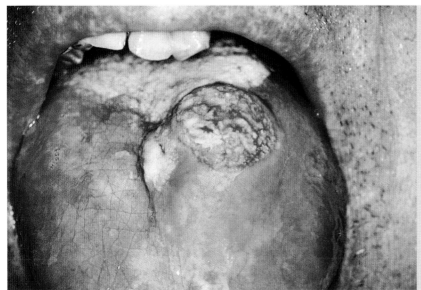

Fig. 39.69 Metastatic carcinoma on the tongue from a primary carcinoma in the lungs.

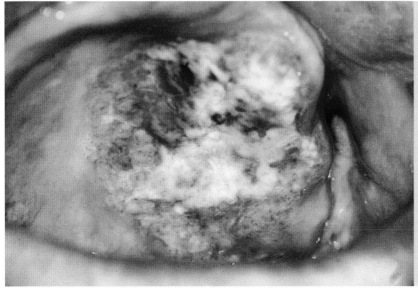

Fig. 39.70 Metastatic carcinoma on the palate from breast adenocarcinoma.

40 Malignancies of the Hematopoietic and Lymphatic Tissues

Leukemias

Key points

- A group of neoplastic disorders of the hematopoietic system.
- Many types of leukemia exist each of which has its own epidemiologic characteristics.
- Certain types of leukemia are linked to specific chromosomal abnormalities (Philadelphia chromosome of chronic myelogenous leukemia).
- Leukemias are classified into *acute* and *chronic*, depending on the clinical course, and into *myelogenous* or *myeloid* and *lymphocytic* or *lymphoblastic*, depending on the histogenesis.
- All forms of leukemias cause oral lesions to a different degree.

Introduction

Leukemias belong to a heterogeneous group of malignant neoplasias of the blood-forming tissues. They present an abnormal stem cell proliferation and maturation of bone marrow and the peripheral blood. Both genetic and environmental factors (i.e., ionizing radiation, viruses, chemicals, etc.) play a great role in the etiology of leukemias. Some types of leukemias are caused by specific chromosomal abnormalities, such as chronic myelogenous leukemia that represents a translocation between chromosomes 9 and 22. Chromosomal analysis can be very useful toward better understanding of the pathogenesis, prognosis, and more effective targeted therapies.

Depending on the clinical course and the degree of maturation of the neoplastic cells, leukemias are classified into *acute* and *chronic*. Depending on the affected cell line that dominates and also its origin, they are subclassified into *myelogenous* or *myeloid*, *lymphocytic* or *lymphoblastic*, *hairy cell*, *monocytic*, *eosinophilic*, *basophilic*, *megacaryoblastic*, and *erythroleukemia*. The incidence of all types is approximately 10 to 15 new cases per 100,000 people per year. The systemic clinical manifestations of acute and chronic leukemias are almost similar. All types may cause oral manifestations and symptoms to a different degree, during their course.

Acute Leukemia

Of all acute leukemias, the lymphocytic mainly affects children. Acute myelogenous leukemia and chronic myelogenous occur primarily in adults while chronic lymphocytic leukemia and hairy cell leukemia occur most frequent in elderly patients.

Clinical features

This group of leukemias is of acute onset and is clinically characterized by generalized lymphadenopathy, chills, fever, headaches, fatigue, weight loss, liver and spleen enlargement, petechiae, ecchymoses, mucosal and skin pallor, hemorrhage, and symptoms of anemia (**Fig. 40.1**). The oral mucosa is commonly affected (70–80%) and often these manifestations may proceed the development of the disease in the peripheral smear. The lesions are more common in monocytic leukemia, followed by the myelogenous and more rarely the lymphocytic leukemia. Petechiae, ecchymoses, gingival enlargement, spontaneous gingival bleeding, delayed wound healing, ulceration, necrosis, and submandibular and cervical lymph node enlargement are included in the spectrum of the clinical features of acute leukemias in the oral cavity (**Fig. 40.2**). The ulceration is the result of small vessel thrombosis by the leukemic cells and infection by the oral microflora. Ulceration may also reflect a side effect treatment with chemotherapeutic agents or minor trauma. A characteristic early and common finding, mainly in the monocytic and myelomonocytic types, is localized or generalized gingival enlargement caused by gingival infiltration by leukemic cells (**Figs. 40.3, 40.4**). The gingivae bleed spontaneously and are enlarged, edematous, erythematous, and inflamed to the extent of even covering the crowns of the teeth. Other common oral complications are infectious such as candidiasis, herpetic infections, aspergillosis, and infections from bacteria and cocci. Acute leukemias may cause nonspecific reactive skin lesions or specific infiltrate of leukemia cutis and several other inflammatory skin disorders. The clinical diagnosis has to be confirmed by hematologic investigations and bone marrow biopsy.

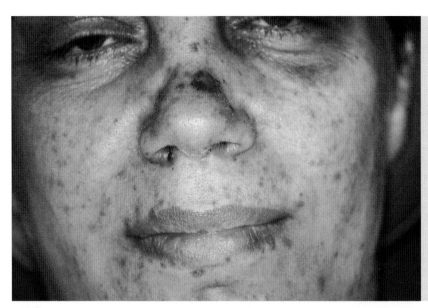

Fig. 40.1 Acute marrow leukemia, pallor, and petechiae in the skin.

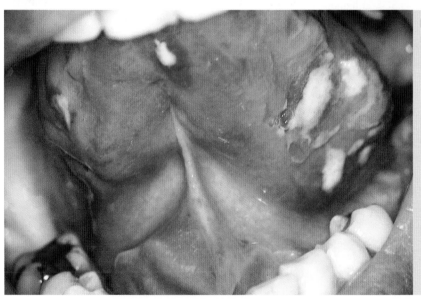

Fig. 40.2 Acute myelogenous leukemia ulcerations on the tongue.

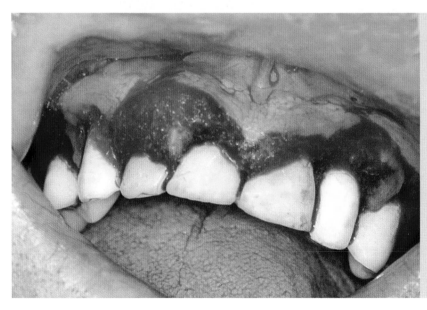

Fig. 40.3 Acute myelomonocytic leukemia, hemorrhagic swelling in the gums.

Chronic Leukemias

Chronic leukemias are more common in the middle age and elderly people. Males are affected almost twice as often than females.

Clinical features

A chronic leukemia begins usually in a mild fashion and may continue asymptomatic for months or even years before being detected by routine hematologic investigations. The most common signs are pallor, weight loss, night sweats, enlargement of the lymph nodes, liver, spleen, salivary glands, and tonsils. Petechiae, ecchymoses, small vessel vasculitis, papules, nodules (chloromas), pigmentation, pruritus, and herpes zoster may be observed on the skin, while more rarely bullous pemphigoid or pemphigus may occur (paraneoplastic diseases).

The oral mucosa is less commonly affected than in acute leukemias. Clinical manifestations may include mucosal pallor, petechiae, superficial ulceration (**Fig. 40.5**), and hemorrhage following tooth extraction or subgingival cleaning. Gingival enlargement may occur in lymphocytic leukemia and less frequently in myelogenous type (**Fig. 40.6**). Candidiasis and herpetic infections may also occur intraorally.

Differential diagnosis

- Neutropenias
- Cyclic neutropenia
- Agranulocytosis
- Aplastic anemia
- Thrombocytopenic purpura
- Traumatic lesions
- Drugs-induced gingival enlargement
- Acute necrotizing ulcerative gingivitis
- Scurvy
- Hereditary gingival fibromatosis

Pathology

Hematologic examination of the peripheral blood and myelogram are required for the diagnosis of leukemia. Histopathologic examination of oral lesion can only be indicative of the disease.

Treatment

Treatment of leukemia involves management of both the disease and the complications. The treatment of leukemias lies upon the hematologist. Multiagent chemotherapy, peripheral blood stem cell or bone marrow transplantation, radiotherapy, and cytostatic medication are used in various combinations toward treatment.

Erythroleukemia

Key points

- A rare variant of acute, nonlymphocytic leukemia.
- It is characterized by proliferation of erythroblasts in the bone marrow.
- Oral lesions are rare and nonspecific.

Introduction

Erythroleukemia or Di Guglielmo's syndrome is a rare variant of acute nonlymphocytic leukemia that is characterized by atypical proliferation of the erythroblasts in the bone marrow.

Clinical features

Clinically, anemia, fever, enlargement of the liver and spleen as well as hemorrhage may be observed. The clinical course is similar to that of acute myeloblastic leukemia with the exception of absence of lymph node enlargement. The oral mucosa is rarely affected by hemorrhage and gingival enlargement (**Fig. 40.7**).

Differential diagnosis

- Acute leukemias
- Chronic leukemias
- Aplastic anemia
- Myelodysplastic syndrome

Pathology

Myelogram and examination of the peripheral blood are required.

Treatment

Chemotherapy.

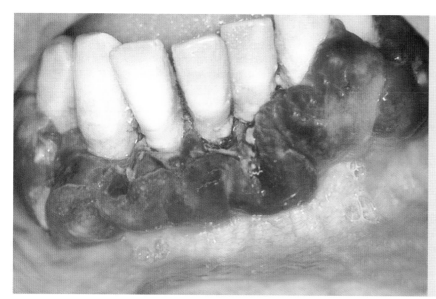

Fig. 40.4 Acute monocytic leukemia, pronounced swelling of the gums.

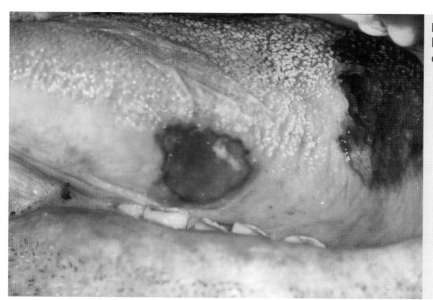

Fig. 40.5 Chronic myelogenous leukemia, ulcerations and ecchymoses of the tongue.

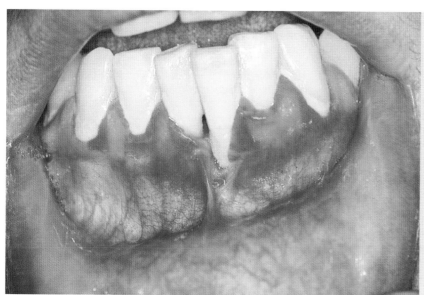

Fig. 40.6 Chronic lymphocytic leukemia, erythema and mild enlargement of the lower gingiva.

Hodgkin's Disease

Key points

- A malignant lymphoproliferative disorder.
- Histologically, it is characterized by the presence of Reed-Sternberg cells.
- Predominantly affects lymph nodes, mainly cervical and supraclavicular.
- Intraoral manifestations are rare.

Introduction

Hodgkin's disease or Hodgkin's lymphoma is a malignant lymphoproliferative disorder. It is characterized by the presence of the Reed-Sternberg cells and their variants that have relatively recently been found to derive from B lymphocytes. The exact etiology remains unknown. However, there are recognized factors that play part in its appearance, such as genetic and environmental factors and mainly infection by the Epstein-Barr virus. There is also an increased risk of developing the disease among patients with autoimmune disorders, AIDS, and other immunodeficiencies. It affects most commonly males, presenting with two age peaks, one around 15 to 35 years and a second one after age of 50 years. Hodgkin's disease is classified into four stages depending on the lymph nodes affected and any other organs involved: I, II, III, and IV (Ann Arbor classification system). Additionally, it is classified into stage A, where there are no systemic manifestations and stage B, when systemic manifestations are present (fever, night sweats, weight loss over 10% within 6 months). The incidence is approximately 3–4 cases per 100,000 population per year.

Clinical features

A characteristic clinical sign of Hodgkin's disease is persistent enlargement of lymph node groups, particularly the cervical and supraclavicular (80%) and less frequently the mediastinal, axillary, inguinal, and others (**Fig. 40.8**). At an early stage the enlarged lymph nodes are firm, mobile, and asymptomatic while at a later stage these are sensitive and fixed into the surrounding tissues. If the disease remains untreated, it spreads to more lymph node groups, the spleen, and other organs (lungs, liver, bones). As the disease progresses, other signs and symptoms include loss of appetite, fever, night sweats, weight loss, and pruritus (30–40%). Cutaneous manifestations include one or several ulcerated nodules, erythema nodosum, and exfoliative dermatitis, while association with dermatomyositis and pemphigus may occur. The mouth is rarely affected by soft mass swelling that may ulcerate (**Fig. 40.9**). The prognosis is relatively good and depends on the stage of the disease and the histopathologic findings.

Differential diagnosis

- Non-Hodgkin's lymphoma
- Leukemias
- Wegener's granulomatosis
- Infectious mononucleosis

Pathology

Histologically, Hodgkin's disease is characterized by the presence of the Reed-Sternberg cells and some other variants. These are large cells with a characteristic bipolar nucleus resembling an "*owl's eye*" appearance. Applying histopathologic criteria, Hodgkin's lymphoma is classified into two large groups: *nodular, lymphocyte predominant* and *classical* which is then further divided into four subtypes: *lymphocyte-rich, nodular sclerosing, mixed cellularity, and lymphocyte depleted*. In the classical type, using immunohistochemical and molecular techniques, the neoplastic cells are found to be B lymphocytes, positive for CD30 and CD15, while they do not express the leukocyte common antigen (LCA). In the nodular, lymphocyte-predominant type, the neoplastic cells with a popcorn-like appearance are B lymphocytes; they express LCA, are positive for EMA, and are negative for CD30 and CD15.

Treatment

The treatment of Hodgkin's disease lies with the hematologist and the oncologist. The treatment regimens are selected and adapted depending on the stage of the disease at the time of diagnosis, the histologic type, the resistance to treatment, relapse, etc.

Non-Hodgkin's Lymphoma

Key points

- A heterogeneous group of lymphoid tissue malignancies with varied clinical presentation.
- Mainly affects lymph nodes, but in contrast to Hodgkin's disease, extranodal manifestations are common.
- Intraorally, it is the third most frequent malignancy.
- Over 90% of non-Hodgkin's lymphomas derive from B lymphocytes, while 10% from T lymphocytes.
- The diagnosis is based on histologic and molecular criteria.

Introduction

Non-Hodgkin's lymphomas comprise a heterogeneous group of lymphoid tissue malignancies which account for 70 to 80% of all lymphomas. Over 90% of the cases derive from B lymphocytes, 10% derive from T lymphocytes, and very rarely from histiocytes. The exact etiology remains unknown. Genetic and environmental factors seem to play a significant role in its causation (viruses—mainly Epstein-Barr and human T-cell lymphotropic virus 1 [HTLV-1], medication, radiation, etc.). Additionally, non-Hodgkin's lymphomas occur in patients with AIDS, hereditary and acquired immunodeficiencies, autoimmune conditions (Sjögren's syndrome, rheumatoid arthritis), and patients who had a transplant. *Helicobacter pylori* has been implicated in mucosa-associated lymphoid tissue (MALT) lymphoma etiology.

Based on the disease progression and the degree of cellular aggression, non-Hodgkin's lymphomas are classified into three categories: *low grade, intermediate*, and *high grade*. This depends on the histopathologic, immunologic, molecular, and cytogenetic findings. The classification has been reviewed and modified many times in the past. The most recent

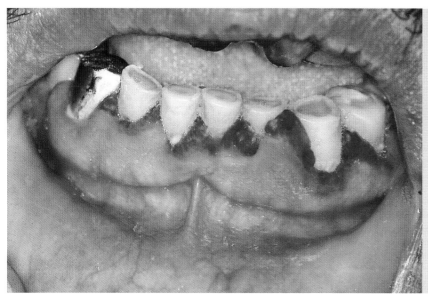

Fig. 40.7 Erythroleukemia, hemorrhagic enlargement of the lower gingiva.

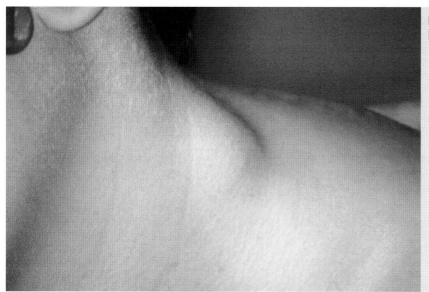

Fig. 40.8 Hodgkin's disease, cervical lymph node enlargement.

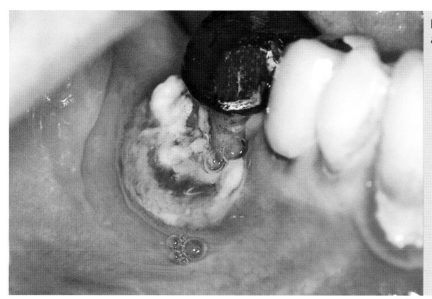

Fig. 40.9 Hodgkin's disease, ulceration of the lower gingiva.

system of classification is that by the WHO (2008) that divides lymphomas into two major groups: (1) *B-cell* derived and (2) *T-cell* derived. There are many subtypes (over 30 types of non-Hodgkin's lymphomas have been described).

Clinical features

Clinically, the disease is characterized by persistent peripheral lymphadenopathy, lymphoid organ involvement, and up to 40% extranodal manifestations including the oral cavity. The head and neck are the most commonly affected sites. The incidence is approximately 6 to 8 new cases per 100,000 of population. Non-Hodgkin's lymphomas may affect individuals of any age and sex. The clinical presentation may be acute, or take a more gradual course. The clinical manifestations include lymphadenopathy, symptoms from the lungs and the gastrointestinal tract, and less often weight loss, night sweats, etc. The mouth is rarely the first and only manifestation of the disease. More often it is involved in the systemic disease process. A soft enlargement may appear that rapidly evolves and might ulcerate (**Figs. 40.10–40.12**). The ulcer surface appears irregular with surrounding inflammation and firm on palpation, together with the adjacent tissues. The most commonly affected oral site is the soft palate, followed by posterior gingiva, base of the tongue, and floor of the mouth. Skin lesions may also occur (**Fig. 40.13**).

The clinical diagnosis has to be confirmed by histology and immunophenotyping using molecular techniques. Non-Hodgkin's lymphomas' staging is based on the modified Ann Arbor system as well as other systems for more specified sites. For the staging is important, the history and clinical presentation of the disease, chest radiograph, computed tomography (CT) scan of head, neck, chest, and abdomen, bone marrow biopsy, and biopsy of other organs as required. The staging results determine the type of treatment.

Differential diagnosis

- Hodgkin's disease
- Different types of non-Hodgkin's lymphomas
- Wegener's granulomatosis
- Eosinophilic ulcer
- Necrotizing sialadenometaplasia
- Squamous cell carcinoma
- Systemic mycoses

Pathology

Histologically, non-Hodgkin's lymphoma is characterized by a great and uniform proliferation of lymphocytes that demonstrate different degree of atypia and differentiation depending on the type of the lymphoma. Further analysis of the different histologic characteristics of each type of non-Hodgkin's lymphoma is outside the remit of this book, but can be sought in more specific hematopathology manuals.

Treatment

The treatment of non-Hodgkin's lymphomas is the responsibility of the specialized hemato-oncologist. The therapeutic regimen may include different types of chemotherapy depending on the type and the cellular differentiation. More recently, good results have been achieved with the use of monoclonal antibodies against the CD20 antigen of the B-lymphocyte membrane, in combination with CHOP.

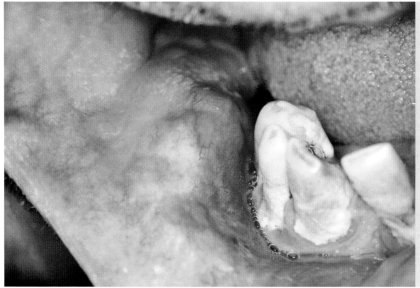

Fig. 40.10 Non-Hodgkin's lymphoma, multiple enlargements on the buccal mucosa.

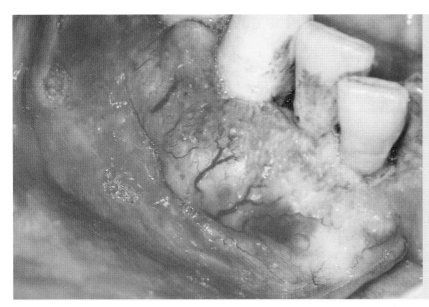

Fig. 40.11 Non-Hodgkin's lymphoma, localized enlargement on the lower gingiva.

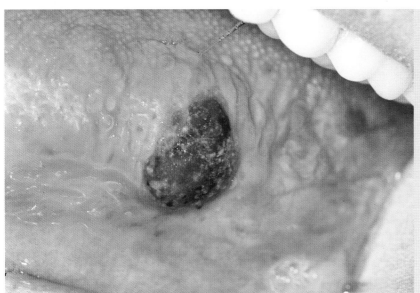

Fig. 40.12 Non-Hodgkin's lymphoma, vegetative enlargement on the lateral border of the tongue.

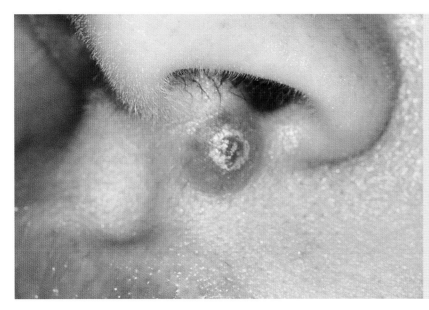

Fig. 40.13 Non-Hodgkin's lymphoma, ulcerated nodule on the skin.

Burkitt's Lymphoma

- A high-grade, non-Hodgkin's B-cell lymphoma.
- Endemic in Africa and usually affects children.
- Epstein-Barr virus is implicated in the pathogenesis.
- It affects immunocompromised and AIDS patients more frequently.
- It occurs mostly in the jaws (60–70%).

Introduction

Burkitt's lymphoma was first described by the English surgeon Dennis Burkitt in 1956 in central Africa. It is classified under high-grade non-Hodgkin's lymphomas and is derived from B lymphocytes. There is a strong indication that Epstein-Barr virus (EBV) is responsible for the disease, since over 90% of the neoplastic cells present with antigen expression against the virus and the patients have high titers of anti-EBV antibodies. Recently, translocation has been observed between chromosomes 8 and 14.

Burkitt's lymphoma is classified using epidemiologic and histologic criteria into two basic types: (1) *classic African* or *endemic* and (2) *non-African* or *sporadic*. The latter presents outside Africa and affects specific patient groups such as patients with AIDS, immunocompromised patients, and patients that had undergone transplantation.

Clinical features

The classic African Burkitt's lymphoma affects mostly children between 2 and 14 years. It occurs most commonly in the jaws (70–80%) and less frequently in other organs. Clinically, enlargement of the jaw is observed that is very rapidly advancing, causing osseous destruction, teeth displacement, mobility, and eventually loss, pain, paresthesia, and facial disfiguration (**Fig. 40.14**). The maxilla is more commonly affected compared with the mandible (ratio 2:1). Rarely, large ulcerating or nonulcerating masses may be seen, mainly on the gingiva and other oral soft tissues (**Fig. 40.15**).

In the non-African, sporadic type the most common early symptom is enlargement of the abdomen that has started from the intestine. Moreover, other organs may be affected such as the lymph nodes, kidneys, adrenals, ovaries, breasts, thyroid gland, tonsils, mouth and eyes, causing relevant symptoms. The oral lesions are identical to those seen in the classic African type. Night sweats and unjustified fever are also common. The prognosis is usually poor, but has improved over the last few years. The clinical diagnosis has to be confirmed by histology.

Differential diagnosis

- Other forms of non-Hodgkin's lymphomas
- Neuroblastoma
- Cherubism
- Melanotic neuroectodermal tumor of infancy
- Ewing's sarcoma
- Osteosarcoma
- Multiple myeloma
- Chondrosarcoma
- Odontogenic tumors

Pathology

Microscopically, the tumor consists of small, undifferentiated B lymphocytes with small hyperchromatic nuclei and little cytoplasm. Among the neoplastic B lymphocytes are many macrophages that give the characteristic "*starry-sky*" appearance.

Treatment

The treatment of choice is chemotherapy in various combinations. The CHOP regimen (cyclophosphamide, doxorubicin, vincristine, and prednisone) is one of the most successful treatments against Burkitt's lymphoma, alone or in combination with radiotherapy and surgery. Radiotherapy is a second-line treatment, alone or combined with chemotherapy. Finally, surgical excision has a place in more early, localized lesions.

Mycosis Fungoides

Key points

- The most common type of cutaneous non-Hodgkin's lymphoma from T lymphocytes.
- Genetic, immunologic, and environmental factors play part in the histogenesis.
- The cutaneous lesions are classified into three stages: *patch* (atrophic or nonatrophic), *plaque*, and *tumor*.
- The oral mucosa is rarely affected usually during the last two stages of the disease.

Introduction

Mycosis fungoides derives from T lymphocytes and is the most common type of cutaneous non-Hodgkin's lymphoma. It primarily affects the skin and is of unknown etiology. Genetic, immunologic, and environmental factors seem to play a role in the pathogenesis. The cutaneous lesions persist for years until the disease spreads to the lymph nodes and internal organs. It usually affects older individuals (mean age of diagnosis being 55–60 years). It is more common in males. The incidence is 0.3 to 0.5 new cases per 100,000 individuals per year.

Clinical features

The skin lesions may persist for years, but the disease eventually involves the lymph nodes and other organs, commonly resulting in death. The clinical course progresses in three stages: (1) the *premycotic* or *patch stage*, which begins with an intensely pruritic eruption and may resemble psoriasis, parapsoriasis en plaque, or eczema; (2) the *plaque stage*, which is characterized by the presence of irregularly shaped, well-demarcated and slightly elevated and indurated plaques; (3) the *tumor stage*, in which most of the plaques develop into raised tumors that often ulcerate, or tumors that may arise de novo (**Fig. 40.16**). Erythroderma and poikiloderma are also among the clinical presentations. The disease is chronic and before diagnosis the patients may present with psoriasis or eczematous skin lesions for some years. The average time between the first symptoms and the final diagnosis is approximately 4 and 8 years. Involvement of the oral mucosa is rare and

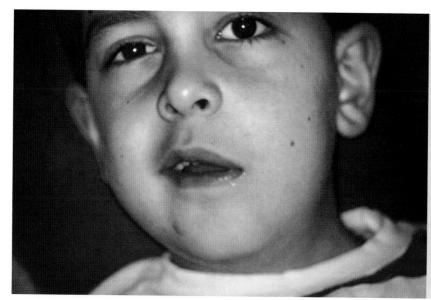

Fig. 40.14 Burkitt's lymphoma, jaw enlargement with mild facial palsy.

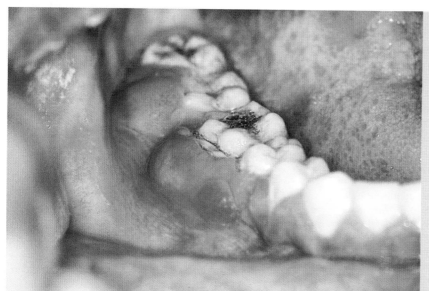

Fig. 40.15 Burkitt's lymphoma, enlargement on the lower gingiva.

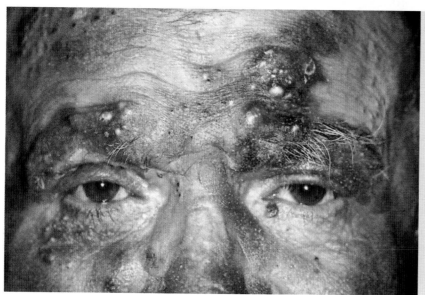

Fig. 40.16 Mycosis fungoides, tumor stage on the face.

usually occurs during the plaque and tumor stages of the disease. Clinically, the oral mucosa shows an extensive erythema, which later progresses to indurated plaques or ulcerated tumors (**Fig. 40.17**). The most commonly affected sites are the vermilion border of the lips, buccal mucosa, palate, gingiva, and tongue. Other sites of extracutaneous involvements are the regional lymph nodes and rarely other organs. The staging systems used are the tumor node metastasis (TNM) staging system as well as the clinical four-stage system I, II, III, IV for mycosis fungoides and Sezary's syndrome.

Sezary's syndrome is an aggressive form of mycosis fungoides characterized by the presence of the triad of erythroderma, generalized lymphadenopathy, and the presence of characteristic neoplastic T cells (Sezary's cells) in the skin, lymph nodes, and peripheral blood. The lungs, kidneys, and central nervous system may also be affected. There is no oral manifestation. The disease is slowly progressing and the prognosis is poor. The diagnosis has to be confirmed by histology.

Differential diagnosis

- Other types of non-Hodgkin's lymphoma
- Leukemia
- Sezary's syndrome
- Psoriasis
- Eczema
- Drug reactions

Pathology

Histologically, mycosis fungoides is characterized by small, atypical lymphocytes with hyperchromatic, cerebriform nuclei and clear cytoplasm. Initially, they are found in the basal layer and along the basement membrane. In the later stages, there is a proliferation of these neoplastic cells that can form little nests in the epidermis (*Pautrier microabscesses*) and also infiltrate the underlying connective tissue. Finally, in the tumor stage, there is infiltration by large neoplastic T lymphocytes with great polymorphism, that extends beyond the epidermis, throughout the underlying connective tissue and the subcutaneous tissues. The neoplastic cells are typically CD2+, CD3+, TCRb+, CD5+, CD4+, CD8−, and CD7− T lymphocytes. A CD8+ and CD4− phenotype can be rarely seen. This immunologic profile appears at the plaque and tumor stage and rarely in early patch stage. It is therefore of little diagnostic help in early diagnosis.

Treatment

The choice of an initial treatment in mycosis fungoides depends on the stage of the disease and the general condition and age of the patient. It can include topical corticosteroids, topical chemotherapy, topical radiation, phototherapy (psoralen and ultraviolet A [PUVA], UVA), chemotherapy (CHOP, purine analogues-gemcitabine-liposomal doxorubicin), and biological response modifiers (cytokines, retinoids, interferon-α). All treatment regimens are used in various combinations that are decided by the hematologist, oncologist, and dermatologist. The prognosis of patients is dependent on the stage, the type, and extent of skin lesions as well as the presence of extracutaneous involvements.

Extranodal NK/T-Cell Lymphoma, Nasal Type

Key points

- A specific type of non-Hodgkin's lymphoma from highly aggressive NK/T malignant cells.
- Predominantly affects the nasal cavity, nasopharynx, mouth and skin.
- Progresses rapidly causing destruction mainly around the facial midline.
- EBV is observed in over 95% of the cases.
- First-line treatment is CHOP chemotherapy combined with radiation.

Introduction

Extranodal natural killer (NK)-/T-cell lymphoma—nasal type (angiocentric T-cell lymphoma or midline lethal granuloma) is a very aggressive type of non-Hodgkin's lymphoma that derives from NK/T cells. WHO classifies the tumor as a specific type of non-Hodgkin's lymphoma from NK/T cells—nasal type. The disease most commonly affects the nasopharynx, palate, skin, and more rarely the gastrointestinal tract and testes. The lymph nodes can be secondarily affected in some of the cases. When the tumor is observed outside the nasal cavity, it is CD56+ and the EBV is detected. The nasal type represents 1.5 to 8% of all non-Hodgkin's lymphomas. It affects more often male (ratio 3:1) of 55 to 65 years. The prognosis is poor with mean survival rate of 1 year. Lately, there has been staging of the disease (four stages) that is based on clinical factors and determines the treatment and prognosis.

Clinical features

Clinically, the disease is characterized by prodromal signs and symptoms such as fever, weight loss, weakness, nocturnal sweating, epistaxis, nasal stuffiness, foul-smelling nasal discharge and obstruction, edema and erythema of the palate, trismus, and visual disturbances. As the disease progresses, there are deep necrotic ulcers that spread both peripherally and in depth (**Figs. 40.18–40.21**). The lesions deteriorate causing major midfacial destruction of the palate, the nasal septum, the eyes, the base of the skull, and the face resulting in severe disfiguration. Bleeding and secondary infection are common complications. The prognosis is unfavorable, with an extremely high fatality rate. The clinical diagnosis has to be confirmed by histology and immunohistochemistry.

Differential diagnosis

- Other types of non-Hodgkin's lymphoma
- Wegener's granulomatosis
- Necrotizing sialadenometaplasia
- Adenocarcinomas of the minor salivary glands
- Squamous cell carcinoma
- Rhabdomyosarcoma
- Mucormycosis
- Aspergillosis
- Tuberculosis
- Gumma

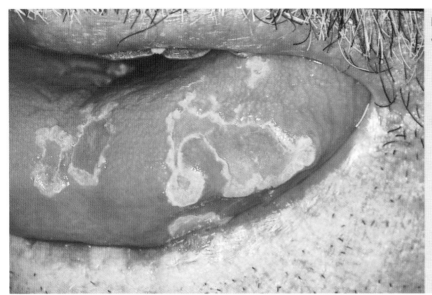

Fig. 40.17 Mycosis fungoides, ulcerations on the tongue.

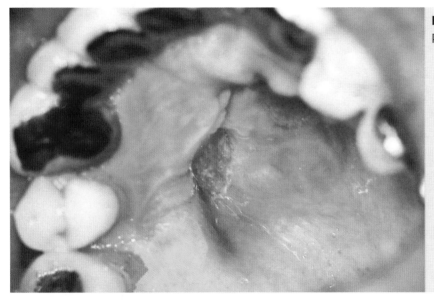

Fig. 40.18 Extranodal NK/T-cell lymphoma, early ulceration on the palate.

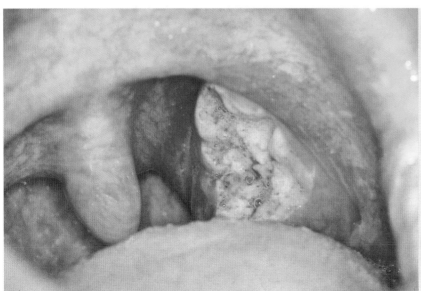

Fig. 40.19 Extranodal NK/T-cell lymphoma, necrotic ulceration on the tonsil and the soft palate.

Pathology

Histologically, extranodal NK/T-cell lymphoma—nasal type is characterized by atypical neoplastic cells of various size that have irregular nucleus, granular chromatin, small nucleoli, and clear cytoplasm. There is an inflammatory infiltrate with lymphocytes, plasma cells, eosinophils, and histiocytes. Necrosis and vascular infiltration is observed as well as pseudoepitheliomatous hyperplasia of the epithelium. Immunohistochemically, the tumor is CD2+ (membrane marker) and CD43+ and CD56+ (cytoplasmic markers). Finally, using molecular techniques, Epstein-Barr genome is often detected in the neoplastic cells.

Treatment

The treatment regimen is dependent on the stage of the disease and decided by the hemato-oncologist. First-line treatment is usually systemic CHOP chemotherapy combined with radiation. Surgical intervention is not recommended.

Multiple Myeloma

Key points

- A malignant proliferation of plasma cells.
- Mainly affects the spine, ribs, and skull.
- The jaws are involved in approximately 25 to 30% of the cases.
- The signs and symptoms include osseous pain, kidney failure, anemia, neurologic disturbances, and infections.
- Monoclonal serum paraprotein or urine protein electrophoresis or immunofixation.
- Primary systemic amyloidosis coexists in approximately 10 to 20% of the patients with multiple myeloma.

Introduction

Multiple myeloma is a generalized malignant plasma cell disorder of unknown cause. The neoplastic cells replace the bone marrow, produce osseous destruction, and paraproteinemia (monoclonal immunoglobulin/M protein). The incidence is approximately 2 to 4 new cases per year per 100,000 individuals. It constitutes the second–in–frequency hematologic malignancy (10–15%) and represents 1% of all malignancies. The pathogenesis is not entirely clear. However, chromosomal translocations have been observed in approximately 50% of the cases (involving chromosome 14—locus 14q32—and several other chromosomes). Additionally, environmental chemical factors may also be implicated.

Clinical features

Multiple myeloma more often occurs in males over 60 years of age. The main signs and symptoms include painful osseous lesions, kidney failure, anemia, neurologic disturbances, and infections (pneumonia, pyelonephritis). The most common affected sites are the skull, spine, ribs, pelvis, and clavicles. The jaws can also be affected in approximately 25 to 30% of the cases and even constitute the only site. Signs and symptoms can be osseous pain, paresthesia, fractures, osseous enlargement, and teeth movements (**Fig. 40.22**). Less often petechiae, bleeding, and painless soft tissue enlargement that occur in the gingiva, alveolar mucosa, and palate can be observed (**Fig. 40.23**).

Osseous destruction leads to calcium release in the peripheral blood which results in pronounced hypercalcemia, a characteristic feature of the disease. In approximately 10 to 20% of the cases, multiple myeloma coexists with primary systemic amyloidosis.

Diagnostic criteria have been set by the International Myeloma Working Group and classify the spectrum of plasma cell dyscrasias where multiple myeloma belongs to (1) *symptomatic myeloma*, (2) *asymptomatic myeloma*, (3) *monoclonal gammopathy of undetermined significance* (*MGUS*). Regarding

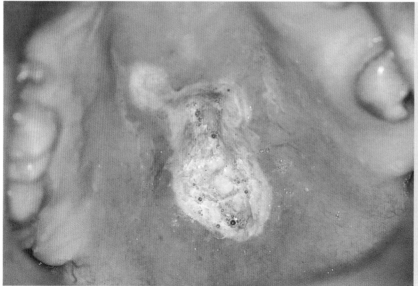

Fig. 40.20 Extranodal NK/T-cell lymphoma, ulceration with inflammatory reaction on the center of the palate.

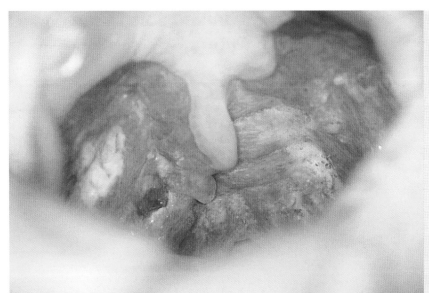

Fig. 40.21 Extranodal NK/T-cell lymphoma, great ulceration, and destruction of the palate.

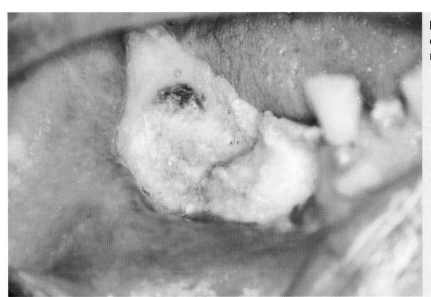

Fig. 40.22 Multiple myeloma, osseous destruction, and necrosis on the mandible.

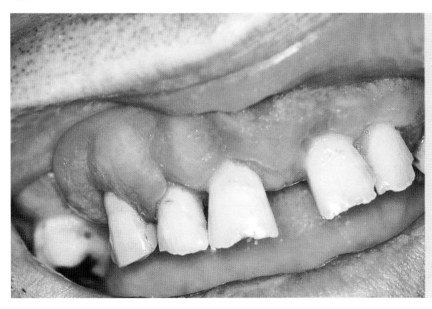

Fig. 40.23 Multiple myeloma, localized gingival enlargement.

the disease staging, the same group has published the International Staging System (ISS) that is based on serum β_2-microglobulin and albumin levels. The older Durie-Salmon Staging System is still in use but has been largely replaced by the simpler ISS. The prognosis is generally poor with survival rates of 2 to 5 years, depending on the disease stage at the beginning of the treatment. However, there has been significant progress within the past 10 years.

The diagnosis is based on clinical and laboratory findings.

Differential diagnosis

- MGUS
- Waldenstrom's macroglobulinemia
- Non-Hodgkin's lymphomas
- Burkitt's lymphoma
- Plasmacytoma
- Osteosarcoma
- Squamous cell carcinoma
- Odontogenic tumors

Pathology

Histologically, the bone marrow is replaced by abnormal plasma cells. Radiographically, skeletal osseous destruction with a characteristic image of round radiolucent areas on the skull known as *punched-out lesions* is present. Magnetic resonance imaging (MRI), CT, and positron emission tomography (PET) are diagnostically very helpful. Immunochemically, the neoplastic cells have monotypic cytoplasmic immunoglobulin (Ig) and they are CD56+, CD38+ CD138+, CD19−, and CD45−. Protein electrophoresis of blood and urine reveals paraproteins (monoclonal protein) with or without reduction of the normal proteins. The paraprotein Bence Jones is detected in urine.

Treatment

The therapeutic regimen depends on the disease stage during diagnosis. It is a decision of the hemato-oncology team. It includes chemotherapy in various combinations (dexamethasone, thalidomide, lenalidomide, bortezomib) and also autologous stem cell transplant.

Extramedullary Soft Tissue Plasmacytoma

Key points

- A monoclonal neoplasia of either the bone marrow or the soft tissues.
- It is classified into *solitary* and *multiple*. The solitary can then be subclassified into *skeletal* and *extramedullary*.
- In the mouth, the extramedullary soft tissue plasmacytoma originates from the mucosal plasma cells.

Introduction

Extramedullary soft tissue plasmacytoma is a monoclonal neoplastic disorder of the mucosal plasma cells rather than the bone marrow. However, both subtypes of solitary plasmacytoma (of the bones and the soft tissues) have the same biological characteristics. The extramedullary type represents approximately 3% of all plasma cell neoplasias and in 10 to 30% of the cases it progresses into multiple myeloma within 10 years. It is more common in males than females (ratio 3:1) of 50 to 60 years. In 80 to 90% of the cases, it occurs in the head and neck area and particularly the initial parts of the respiratory and digestive systems. The ipsilateral lymph nodes are often affected. The disease is rare in the mouth.

Clinical features

Oral extramedullary soft tissue plasmacytoma appears as painless, soft enlargement with a smooth surface and diameter that varies from 1 to many centimeters that can eventually ulcerate (**Figs. 40.24, 40.25**). The most commonly affected oral sites are the palate and gingiva, followed by buccal mucosa, tongue, lips, and floor of the mouth. It may also occur in the tonsils, nasal cavity and paranasal sinuses, pharynx, and parotid. It is recommended that patients should be followed upon the completion of treatment due to risk of multiple myeloma development. The diagnosis is mainly based on histologic and other laboratory findings.

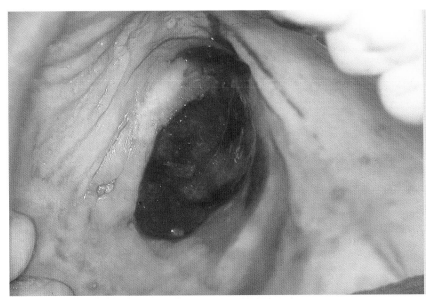

Fig. 40.24 Soft tissue plasmacytoma, hemorrhagic enlargement on the palate.

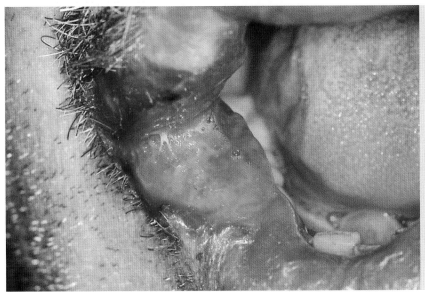

Fig. 40.25 Soft tissue plasmacytoma, ulceration on the commissure.

Differential diagnosis

- Non-Hodgkin's lymphoma
- Pleomorphic adenoma
- Minor salivary gland adenocarcinomas
- Necrotizing sialadenometaplasia
- Plasma cell gingivitis

Pathology

Histologically, extramedullary soft tissue plasmacytoma is characterized by monoclonal plasma cells of different degree of differentiation, as in multiple myeloma. However, in contrast with multiple myeloma, the bone marrow does not present significant plasma cell infiltration (< 5% of all the enucleated cells). There are no osteodestructive lesions or kidney failure. Finally, serum hypercalcemia and hyperproteinemia are not observed.

Treatment

In small lesions, surgical excision is the first line of treatment with very good results. Radiotherapy and chemotherapy are considered in extensive lesions.

Waldenstrom's Macroglobulinemia

Key points

- A malignancy of the hematopoietic blast cells that differentiate into precursor hybrid of plasma cells and B lymphocytes.
- Monoclonal IgM paraprotein production is a characteristic of these cells.
- Infiltrations of bone marrow by plasmacytic lymphocytes.
- In the mouth, bleeding from the gingiva and other areas is a characteristic of the disease.

Introduction

Waldenstrom's macroglobulinemia is a rare malignancy of the hematopoietic stem cells differentiated as preplasma B cells that morphologically are hybrid of lymphocytes and plasma cells. These cells characteristically secrete an IgM paraprotein. The disease affects usually males between 60 and 70 years and is of poor prognosis.

Clinical features

Clinically, Waldenstrom's macroglobulinemia is characterized by pallor, loss of appetite and weight, weakness, nausea, vertigo, lymphadenopathy, liver and spleen enlargement, and neurologic and visual disturbances. Mucosal and gastrointestinal bleeding is caused by vessel dilation and platent dysfunction. Intraorally, persistent bleeding is observed as well as petechiae and ecchymoses, while ulcerations have also been described (**Figs. 40.26, 40.27**).

Differential diagnosis

- MGUS
- Leukemias, mainly chronic lymphoblastic
- Thrombocytopenic purpura
- Thrombocytopenias

Pathology

Anemia is a common finding. The bone marrow analysis demonstrates great infiltration by plasma cells and lymphocytes. The most characteristic finding, however, remains the monoclonal paraprotein IgM in the serum electrophoresis in the β-globulin region. Osseous lesions and kidney failure are not observed.

Treatment

The hemato-oncologist decides on the course of treatment. Plasmapheresis can be used in acute cases. In more chronic cases, first line of treatments are fludarabine and the monoclonal antibody rituximab as well as bortezomib which is a selective proteasome inhibitor. Periodic plasmapheresis can also be used.

Langerhans Cell Histiocytosis

Key points

- A clonal group of proliferative disorders characterized by Langerhans cell dysfunction.
- Langerhans cells are S100, SD1a, and CD207 positive.
- Four clinical variants have been recognized.
- Oral lesions are common in the three basic variants.

Introduction

Langerhans cell histiocytosis is a heterogeneous group of clonal proliferative disorder of Langerhans cells that express a positive immunophenotype for S100, CD1a, and CD207 (Langerin) which contain cytoplasmic *Birbeck granules*.

The pathogenesis of the disease remains unclear. Recent findings suggest that there is a genetic link between the two cell lines. The presence of clonal CD1a histiocytes within the lesions is an indication that Langerhans cell histiocytosis may be a clonal neoplastic disorder of varied biological behavior. WHO classifies Langerhans cell histiocytosis under dendritic and histiocytic cell neoplasms of the lymphatic tissue. The annual incidence varies between 0.5 and 5.5 new cases per 1,000,000 children while the adult incidence is significantly less. It is more common in males than females (ratio 2:1) and usually affects groups of early life (1–3 years) to any age. Familiar cases have also been described. The spectrum of the disease includes four prominent clinical types: *Letterer-Siwe* disease, *Hand-Schüller-Christian* disease, *Eosinophilic granuloma*, and *Hashimoto-Pritzker* disease or congenital self-healing reticulohistiocytosis.

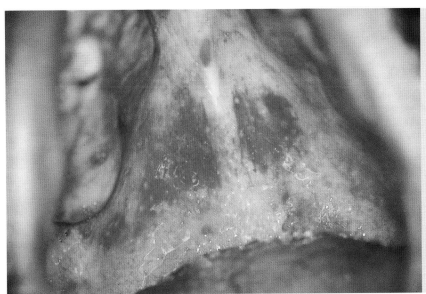

Fig. 40.26 Waldenstrom's macro-globulinemia, palatal ecchymoses.

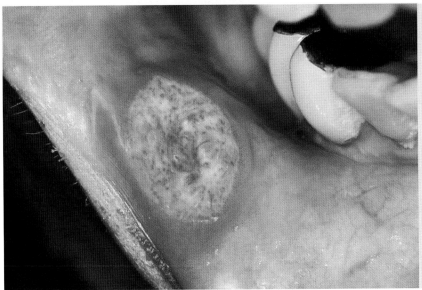

Fig. 40.27 Waldenstrom's macro-globulinemia, ulceration of the mucosa of the lower lip.

Clinical features

The disease manifestations vary from asymptomatic, mild, single-organ affecting to severe multisystemic disease. Oral manifestations are common in the first three basic clinical variants.

Letterer-Siwe disease is the acute multisystemic form that manifests prior to second year of life and has poor prognosis. Clinically, it is characterized by fever, chills, weakness, generalized skin manifestations (erythema, scaly, papules, vesicles, pustules, petechiae, ecchymoses, ulceration, particularly on the scalp, trunk, and flexural area of the neck), onycholysis (**Fig. 40.28**), lymphadenopathy, liver and spleen enlargement, anemia, thrombocytopenia, lung involvement, and osteolytic bone lesions. The oral lesions appear as ecchymoses, ulceration, gingivitis, periodontitis, and loose tooth (**Fig. 40.29**).

Hand-Schüller-Christian disease is the chronic, multifocal form with a milder course and generally of better prognosis. It occurs between ages 2 and 6. Clinically, the classic triad is *osteolytic lesions* (particularly of the scull), *exophthalmos*, and *diabetes insipidus* (**Fig. 40.30**). The triad is present in only 25% of the patients. Additionally, chronic otitis media, otitis externa, and skin rash may occur. Involvement of liver, spleen, lungs and lymph nodes is less common. The mouth is commonly affected in the early stages of the disease. Ulceration, edema, enlargement and necrosis of the gingiva, halitosis, and taste disturbance are the prominent features (**Fig. 40.31**). When the jaw bones are affected, there is tooth mobility and loss, resembling advanced periodontal disease, and delayed healing of tooth sockets after extraction may be seen.

Eosinophilic granuloma is the localized form of the disease that does not affect the viscera and is of good prognosis. It most frequently affects children between 7 and 15 years of age. Clinically, it is characterized primarily by solitary or multiple osseous lesions. The cranium is most frequently affected followed by ribs, vertebrae, pelvis, and long bones. The jaw bones may be affected and result in osseous destruction and tooth mobility and loss. Ulcerations may be observed usually on the gingiva and palate (**Figs. 40.32, 40.33**). The salivary glands are rarely affected, while skin lesions are rare.

Hashimoto-Pritzker disease or congenital self-healing reticulohistiocytosis is a benign, self-healing clinical variant which is limited to the skin and occurs at birth or soon after. Painless red-brown papules and nodules or vesicles might be observed on the skin that can be localized or widespread and may ultimately ulcerate. The oral mucosa is not involved. An association between Langerhans cell histiocytosis and malignancies (leukemia and solid tumors) has been described.

The diagnosis of all variants of the disorder is based on the history, the clinical features, and should be confirmed by the histologic examination and radiographic findings.

Differential diagnosis

- Acrodermatitis enteropathica
- Incontinentia pigmenti
- Neonatal acropustulosis
- Mastocytosis
- Leukemia
- Multiple myeloma
- Non-Hodgkin's lymphomas
- Mycosis fungoides
- Agranulocytosis
- Aplastic anemia
- Aggressive periodontal disease
- Acatalasemia
- Hypophosphatemia
- Metastatic neoplasms

Pathology

Histologically, Langerhans cell histiocytosis is characterized by the presence of large mononuclear cells with a kidney-shaped nucleus. Special stains demonstrate that these are Langerhans cells without the dendrites. On electron microscopy, these cells demonstrate *Birbeck granules* which are rod or racquet-shaped cytoplasmic structures characteristic for Langerhans cells. Additionally, special enzyme histochemical techniques and electron microscope studies can help toward the identification of the cells. These cells are found among multinucleated giant cells, eosinophils, plasma cells, lymphocytes, and mastocytes. Radiographic examination as well as CT and MRI scans are necessary for the identification of osseous and other lesions. Full blood and liver workout are also recommended.

Treatment

As a rule, all patients with Langerhans cell histiocytosis should undergo evaluation of the hematologic, pulmonary, hepatic, splenic, renal, and skeletal systems to determine the activity and extent of the disease. Surgical curettage with or without radiotherapy is the treatment of choice for eosinophilic granuloma. Corticosteroids may also be used. For the systemic forms of the disease, corticosteroids and chemotherapy in various combinations and dosages are used. These are decided in special centers by pediatricians and pediatric oncologists.

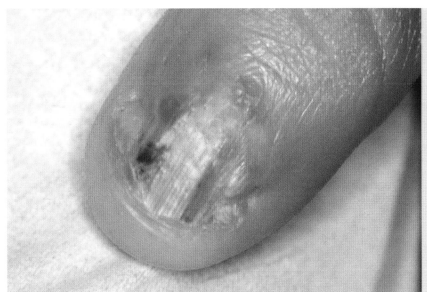

Fig. 40.28 Letterer-Siwe disease, onycholysis.

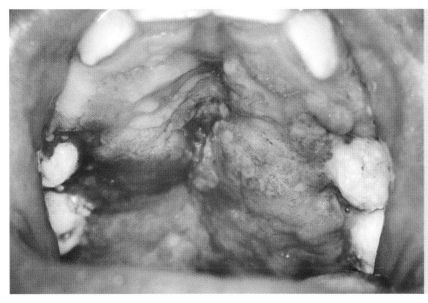

Fig. 40.29 Letterer-Siwe disease, palatal ulcerations, and periodontal disease with tooth displacement.

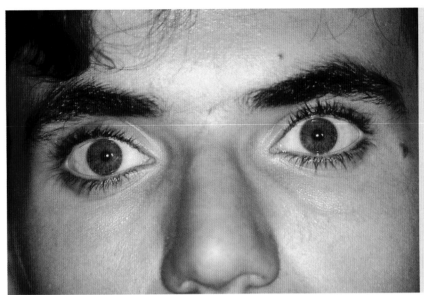

Fig. 40.30 Hand-Schüller-Christian disease, exophthalmos.

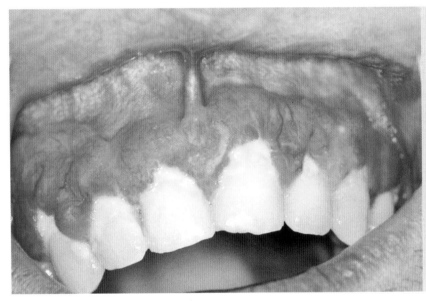

Fig. 40.31 Hand-Schüller-Christian disease, enlargement and ulcerations on the gingiva.

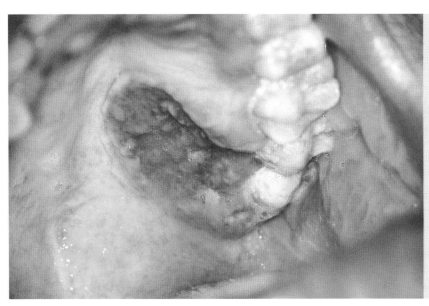

Fig. 40.32 Eosinophilic granuloma, palatal ulceration, and osseous destruction of the maxilla.

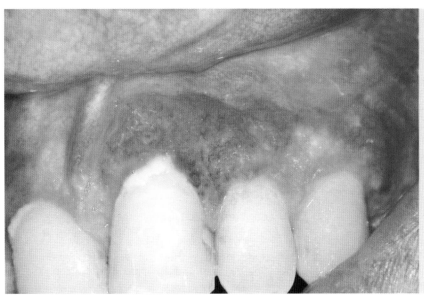

Fig. 40.33 Eosinophilic granuloma, localized gingival enlargement with periodontal osseous destruction.

41 Paraneoplastic Mucocutaneous Diseases

It is a group of disorders that present with cutaneous, oral, and other mucosal manifestations. These lesions are not malignant themselves, but directly are linked with visceral and hematologic malignancies. The criteria used to associate a mucocutaneous disease and malignancy (Curth's postulates) are (1) concurrent onset, (2) parallel course, (3) uniform site or type of malignancy, (4) statistical association, (5) genetic linkage.

In **Table 41.1,** mucocutaneous diseases of paraneoplastic nature are summarized. Some of them are separately described in the relevant chapters. In **Table 41.2,** there are some genetic syndromes with strong genetic base that may predispose or coexist with the presence of malignancies and may present with oral lesions.

Malignancy-Associated Acanthosis Nigricans

Key points
- The most common paraneoplastic diseases that can affect the skin and mucosae.
- Most frequently associated with stomach adenocarcinoma (60–70% of the cases) and less often with other malignancies.
- The oral mucosa and lips are often involved (40–60% of the cases).
- The oral and cutaneous lesions are benign.
- The disease course is parallel to the malignancy.

Introduction

Malignancy-associated acanthosis nigricans is a type of acanthosis nigricans that affects adults and is always accompanied by a malignancy, usually adenocarcinoma of the stomach, or other viscera and less commonly by Hodgkin's disease, squamous cell carcinoma, etc. It is believed that the development is driven by factors secreted by the neoplasia (growth factor α, insulin) that stimulate the mucosal and epidermal cells causing hyperplasia. Usually, the neoplasia and

mucocutaneous lesions appear simultaneously whereas less frequently the diagnosis of neoplasia precedes (22%) or follows (20–30%) the skin and mucosal lesions. The oral mucosa is affected in 40 to 60% of the cases.

Clinical features

Clinically, the oral lesions appear as multiple asymptomatic verrucous or papillomatous lesions of normal color, which rapidly grow and may occupy large areas. The lips and tongue are the most frequently affected sites followed by the palate, gingiva, and buccal mucosa (**Figs. 41.1, 41.2**). Similar lesions may develop in other mucosae (conjunctiva, anus, pharynx, vagina, esophagus, intestine, etc.) (**Fig. 41.3**). The skin is rough with pigmentation while multiple papillomatous lesions or tags occur on the axillae, inguinal area, neck, and rarely on the palms and soles (**Figs. 41.4, 41.5**). The diagnosis is based on clinical criteria.

Differential diagnosis
- Benign acanthosis nigricans
- Lipoid proteinosis
- Goltz's syndrome
- Pemphigus vegetans
- Cowden's disease
- Multiple papillomas

Pathology

The investigations undertaken are the ones required for the detection of malignancy. Histologically, the cutaneous lesions are characterized by hyperkeratosis, acanthosis, and papillomatosis of stratum spinosum, as well as increased melanin production. The latter is not observed in the oral lesions.

Treatment

The treatment of oral and skin lesions is symptomatic. Usually, the mucocutaneous lesions may regress with the successful treatment of the underlying malignancy.

Table 41.1 Paraneoplastic mucocutaneous diseases

Disease	Clinical Features			Malignancy
	Skin	Oral mucosa	Other	
I. Strong correlation				
Malignant acanthosis nigricans	Papillomatous lesions, pigmentation mainly on the axillae, inguinal areas, neck, palms, and soles	Papillomatous lesions on the lips, palate, gingiva, tongue. Normal color	Conjunctiva, pharynx, esophagus, anus	Stomach adenocarcinoma (70%), other sites of the gastrointestinal and other internal malignancies
Paraneoplastic pemphigus	Erythema multiforme-like exanthems	Extensive erosions in the mouth and lips	Conjunctiva, pharynx, larynx, esophagus	Chronic lymphocytic leukemia, non-Hodgkin's lymphoma, Castleman's disease
II. Mild correlation				
Bullous pemphigoid	Bullae	Bullae, superficial ulceration	Mucosae of the nose, eye, pharynx, larynx, esophagus, and genitalia	Gastrointestinal, urogenital, lungs neoplasias, leukemias, non-Hodgkin's lymphoma
Antiepiligrin mucous membrane pemphigoid	Bullae	Bullae, superficial ulceration, desquamative gingivitis, mucosal atrophy	Mucusae of the nose, pharynx, larynx, esophagus, and genitalia	Adenocarcinoma
Dermatitis herpetiformis	Papules, plaques, vesicles, pruritus	Papules, vesicles, erosions	Gluten enteropathy	Non-Hodgkin's lymphoma
Dermatomyositis	Poikiloderma, macules, plaques, heliotrope rash, alopecia	Erythema, erosions	Myositis	Ovarian, lungs, intestinal, pancreas, non-Hodgkin's lymphoma
Sweet's syndrome	Erythematous papules and plaques, bullae, necrotic lesions	Ulceration mimicking major aphthous ulcer	Ocular lesions, arthritis, myalgia, fever, gastrointestinal disorders	Acute myelogenic leukemia, urogenital carcinoma, plasma cell dyscrasia (IgA)
Primary systemic amyloidosis	Papules, plaques, bullae	Erythematous plaques and nodules, bullae, macroglossia	Internal organ involvement (heart, kidneys, etc.)	Multiple myeloma, plasma cell dyscrasia (monoclonal gammopathy)

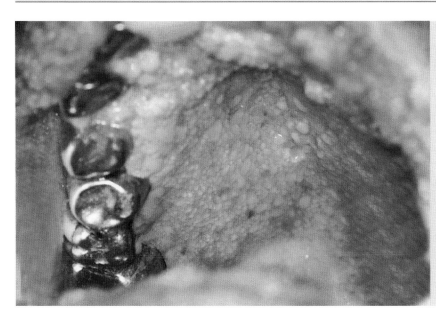

Fig. 41.1 Malignancy-associated acanthosis nigricans, papillomatous lesions on the palate.

Table 41.2 Genetic syndromes (genodermatoses) with oral lesions associated with malignancies

	Clinical Features			
Syndrome	**Oral**	**Skin**	**Other**	**Malignancy**
Howel-Evans syndrome (palmoplantar hyperkeratosis and esophageal carcinoma)	Leukoplakia	Hyperkeratosis of palms and soles	–	Esophageal carcinoma
Gorlin's syndrome or nevoid basal cell carcinoma syndrome	Odontogenic keratocysts, interdental spacing, occlusal abnormalities	Epidermal cysts, multiple basal cell carcinomas, broad nasal root, small depressions (pits) in the skin of the palms and soles	Skeletal abnormalities, skeletal and CNS involvement	Basal cell carcinoma, fibrosarcoma, medulloblastoma
Cowden's syndrome	Multiple small nodules	Papules, small nodules, hair follicles hamartomas, lipomas, xanthomas, hemangiomas	Hamartomas, gastrointestinal polyps	Breast, thyroid carcinomas
Multiple endocrine neoplasia syndrome, type 2B	Multiple neuromas, high-arched palate, big lips	Pigmentation, neuromas	Multiple neuromas on the mucosae of eyes, larynx, nose	Thyroid, adrenals, parathyroid carcinomas
Neurofibromatosis, type I	Multiple neurofibromas	Multiple neurofibromas	Skeletal and endocrine abnormalities	Rhabdomyosarcoma, pheochromocytoma, neurosarcoma
Dyskeratosis congenital	Leukoplakia	Poikiloderma, hyperhidrosis of palms and soles, bullae	Blepharitis, ectropion, gastrointestinal and hepatic disorders	Verrucous and squamous cell carcinoma of the mouth, leukemia, non-Hodgkin's lymphoma
Gardner's syndrome	Osteomas of the jaws, fibromas, cysts, odontomas, supernumerary and impacted or unerupted teeth	Epidermoid cysts, fibromas, lipomas, hair cortex cell tumors	Intestinal polyps	Gastrointestinal adenocarcinoma
Peutz-Jeghers syndrome	Round pigmented macules on the lips and intraorally	Pigmented macules on the face	Intestinal polyps	Gastrointestinal adenocarcinoma, other solid tumors

Abbreviation: CNS, central nervous system.

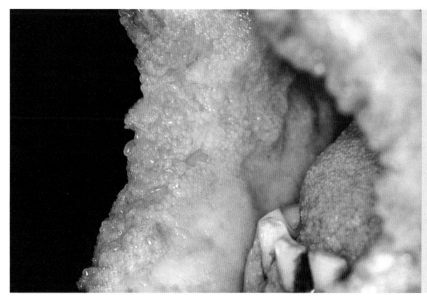

Fig. 41.2 Malignancy-associated acanthosis nigricans, papillomatous lesions on the commissure and the buccal mucosa.

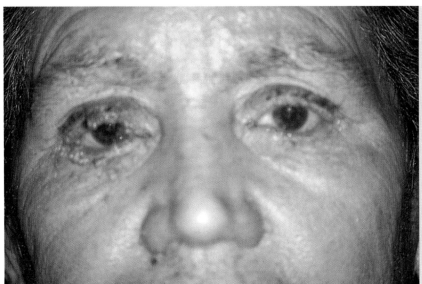

Fig. 41.3 Malignancy-associated acanthosis nigricans, papillomatous lesions on the conjunctiva and the eyelids.

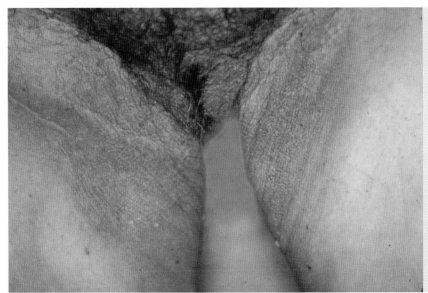

Fig. 41.4 Malignancy-associated acanthosis nigricans, black-brown papillomatous lesions on the skin of the inguinal area and the thigh.

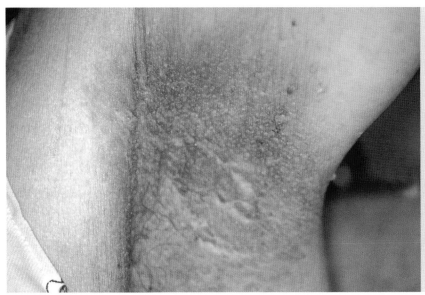

Fig. 41.5 Malignancy-associated acanthosis nigricans, black-brown papillomatous lesions on the axilla.

42 Nonneoplastic Diseases of the Jaws

Fibrous Dysplasia

Key points

- A nonneoplastic tumor-like developmental process caused by *GNAS1* gene mutation.
- Classified into *monostotic* and *polyostotic*.
- The jaws are the most commonly affected sites mainly in the monostotic type.

Introduction

Fibrous dysplasia is a benign developmental disorder of unknown etiology. It is characterized by the replacement of normal bone by immature, cellular fibrous tissue containing irregular trabeculae of woven bone. It is a sporadic disorder caused by *GNAS1* gene mutation, which is the gene responsible for the proliferation and differentiation of osteoblasts and osteoclasts. Two forms of fibrous dysplasia are recognized: the *monostotic*, which is limited to a single bone and accounts for 80 to 90% of all cases and the *polyostotic* or *McCune-Albright syndrome*, which affects more than two bones and is rare. The latter in approximately 2 to 4% of the cases and may evolve into osteosarcoma or chondrosarcoma.

Clinical features

Monostotic fibrous dysplasia equally affects males and females, usually during the first three decades of life. The jaws are frequently involved with the maxilla been affected more often that the mandible. Clinically, jaw lesions usually present as a painless, slow-growing bone swelling. The swelling may be firm, elastic, or hard on palpation, and may cause intraoral bone deformity and tooth displacement and/or facial asymmetry (**Figs. 42.1–42.3**). The lesions are usually unilateral and rarely bilateral. The ribs, femur, and shin are most frequently affected.

The polyostotic form is characterized by multiple bone involvement, skin pigmentation or *café au lait* macules (**Fig. 42.4**), and endocrine disorders of the pituitary, the parathyroids, the thyroid gland, and sexual precocity. The long bones are more frequently affected while jaw involvement is relatively rare. The clinical features of jaw lesions are similar to those seen in the monostotic form. Chronic osteomyelitis and osteosarcoma of the jaws are rare complications. The clinical diagnosis should be confirmed by laboratory tests.

Differential diagnosis

- Cherubism
- Odontogenic tumors
- Ossifying fibroma
- Chronic osteomyelitis
- Central giant cell granuloma
- Paget's disease
- Hyperparathyroidism
- Ewing's sarcoma
- Osteosarcoma
- Chondrosarcoma
- Exostoses

Pathology

Histologically, fibrous dysplasia is characterized by immature, cellular fibrous stroma containing islands of immature woven bone and irregular trabeculae, also known as "*Chinese characters*." In places, the bone presents more mature. Radiography can be useful as it reveals not well-demarcated radiopacities and radioluscencies with unclear borders that are characterized as "*ground-glass*" opacification. Computed tomography (CT) scan can also be useful in determining the extent of the disease.

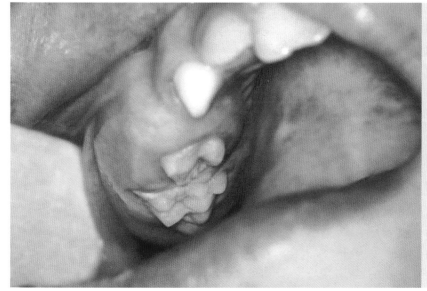

Fig. 42.1 Fibrous dysplasia, enlargement of the maxilla with teeth displacement.

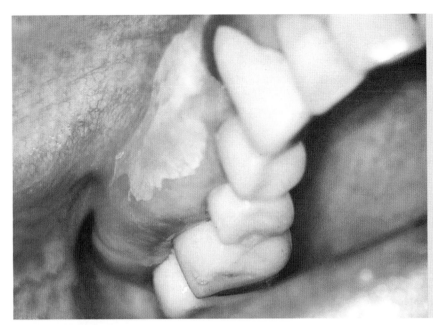

Fig. 42.2 Fibrous dysplasia, osseous enlargement of the maxilla.

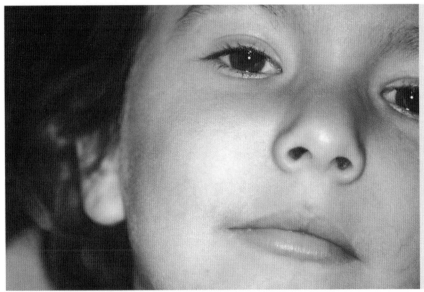

Fig. 42.3 Fibrous dysplasia, enlargement of the face to the right.

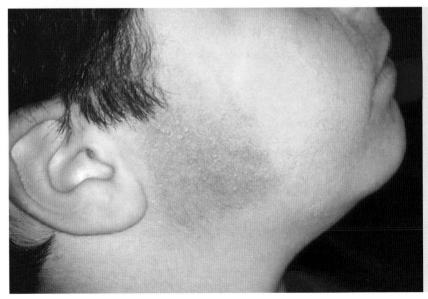

Fig. 42.4 Fibrous dysplasia, *café au lait* macules on the skin of the cheek.

Treatment

Small asymptomatic and inactive jaw bone lesions do not usually require treatment, or can be treated with conservative surgery. More extensive lesions require surgery for cosmetic reasons wherever necessary. Finally, more recently the systemic use of bisphosphonates has considerably helped, especially in the polyostotic type.

Cherubism

Key points

- An autosomal dominant genetic disorder with high penetrance and variable expressivity.
- It is caused by *SH3BP2* gene mutation.
- Exclusively affects the jaws, usually in a symmetric pattern.
- Facial deformity, premature exfoliation of deciduous teeth, and delayed eruption of permanent teeth are common.

Introduction

Cherubism is a rare benign genetic fibro-osseous disorder transmitted as an autosomal dominant trait with high penetrance and variable expressivity. Sporadic cases may also develop which represents spontaneous mutations. In over 80% of the cases, the *SH3BP2* genetic mutation is observed of chromosomes 4p16.3. The disease is characterized by bone loss, replaced by fibrous connective tissue with abundant osteoclastic cells and inflammation cells, and the presence of cystic spaces. It exclusively affects the maxilla and mandible. In severe cases, extensive maxillary involvement causes stretching of the skin of the upper face, exposing the sclerae, and thus creating the "*cherubic*" appearance.

Clinical features

The first signs and symptoms of cherubism usually appear early during the first decade of life and progress until puberty, when they stabilize and many times regress. Clinically, it appears as a painless, symmetrical, bilateral expansion of the jaw bones and cheeks, producing a chubby facial appearance similar to that of the plump-cheeked angels depicted in Renaissance painting (**Figs. 42.5, 42.6**). Premature exfoliation of deciduous teeth, tooth displacement, and unerupted permanent teeth are common findings. In severe cases, extensive maxillary involvement causes stretching of the skin of the upper face, exposing the sclerae and creating the "*cherubic*" pattern. In addition, difficulties in eating, speech or even vision, and hearing impairment lead to psychological problems. The spectrum of clinical presentation varies from mild to severe. The diagnosis is based on the history, the clinical features, and the necessary laboratory tests.

Differential diagnosis

- Fibrous dysplasia
- Odontogenic tumors
- Odontogenic cysts
- Central giant cell granuloma
- Langerhans cell histiocytosis
- Ramon's syndrome
- Noonan's syndrome
- Ewing's sarcoma
- Osteosarcoma
- Rhabdomyosarcoma

Pathology

Histologically, cherubism is characterized by a vascular fibrous stroma with great cellularity containing variable number of multinucleated giant cells and hemorrhagic areas. Radiographically, multilocular radiolucent, cystic spaces are observed in the jaws.

Treatment

Spontaneous resolution of the lesions after puberty may occur in most cases, so that by the end of 30 to 40 years the facial appearance looks almost normal. Only in severe cases, conservative surgical correction can be suggested. It would then aim to reduce the size of the jaws by removing some of the fibrous tissue and cystic spaces. Orthodontic intervention may be required to aid the eruption of impacted/unerupted permanent teeth.

Central Giant Cell Granuloma

Key points

- A benign lesion of the jaws of unknown etiology.
- It affects more commonly the mandible (70–80%).
- Classified into two types: *aggressive* and *nonaggressive*.
- The first line of treatment is surgical excision.

Introduction

Central giant cell granuloma is a benign nonneoplastic lesion of unknown etiology that affects the jaws. The mandible is more commonly affected (70–80%), especially the anterior portions. It equally affects both sexes usually under age of 30 years.

Clinical features

The signs and symptoms of central giant cell granuloma depends on the course of the disease and the size and number of lesions. Using clinical and radiologic criteria, the disease is classified into two types: aggressive and nonaggressive. The *aggressive type*, which is rare and is characterized by rapid growth, pain, cortical perforation, paresthesia or hypoesthesia, root resorption, and tooth displacement. Occasionally, a great jaw expansion with bone destruction that leads to the tumor's protrusion intraorally may occur (**Fig. 42.7**).

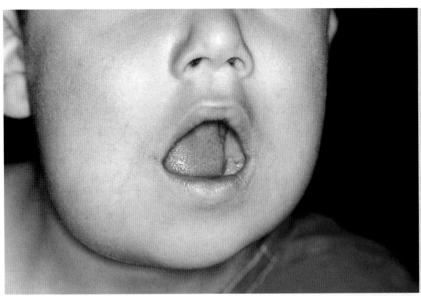

Fig. 42.5 Cherubism, bilateral facial enlargement.

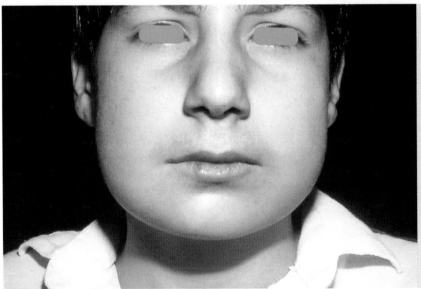

Fig. 42.6 Cherubism, symmetrical enlargement of the face.

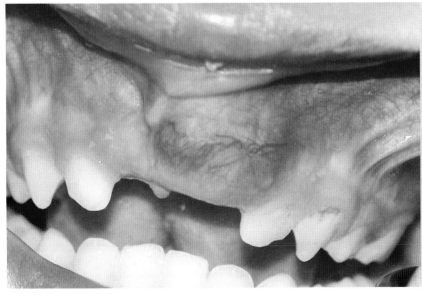

Fig. 42.7 Central giant cell granuloma, enlargement of the mandible on the upper anterior area.

The *nonaggressive type*, which is more common with slow growth and usually asymptomatic or accompanied by mild pain. It is usually detected as an incidental finding during routine radiologic examination. The diagnosis is based on clinical, but mainly radiologic and histologic findings.

Differential diagnosis

- Cherubism
- Fibrous dysplasia
- Aneurysmal bone cyst
- Odontogenic tumors
- Brown tumor of hyperparathyroidism
- Peripheral giant cell granuloma
- Neurofibromatosis, type 1
- Noonan's syndrome

Pathology

Histologically, central giant cell granuloma is characterized by a vascular stroma of spindled, large mesenchymal cells with macrophages, erythrocytes extravasation, and hemosiderin deposition. The presence of multiple multinucleated giant cells is typical of the disease. Radiographically, radioluscent areas are observed that may be multilocular or unilocular. Root and bone resorption are observed in approximately 30 to 40% of the cases.

Treatment

The first line of treatment is surgical excision. In extensive lesions intralesional injection of corticosteroids had been tried as well as systemic calcitonin and interferon α, but with unclear effectiveness.

Paget's Disease of Bone

Key points

- It is characterized by abnormal turnover of the bones resulting in weaker bone structure and osseous deformities.
- Classified into *monostotic* and *polyostotic*.
- Commonly affects the pelvis, skull, limbs, and spine.
- The jaws are affected in approximately 15 to 20% of the cases.

Introduction

Paget's disease or osteitis deformans is a chronic, relatively common, disorder. The disease is characterized by abnormal turnover of the bones resulting in defective bone architecture, deformity, and mechanical weakness. The etiology remains unknown. However, recently genetic mutations (gene *SQSTM1*), slow viral infection in early age, and hormonal disorders have been implicated. Geographically, the disease presents with different incidence with increased incidence in Europe (mainly England), Australia, and New Zealand. It is estimated that in these countries the disease reflects one new case in 100 to 200 individuals over age 50 years. Males are more frequently affected than females.

Clinical features

Paget's disease is often mild and usually asymptomatic. Only 27 to 30% of affected people are symptomatic at the time of diagnosis. The disease may involve multiple bones (*polyostotic form*) or just limited to one bone (*monostotic form*). It can also be classified depending on the presence or absence of symptoms into *symptomatic* and *asymptomatic* types. Clinically, the signs and symptoms develop gradually and become apparent over the age of 50 years. They can include bone pain, headache, joint pain, reduction in hearing, visual disorders, progressive enlargement of the skull, limbs deformities, nasal cavity narrowing, reduction in height and scoliosis, and frequent "*chalk stick*" fractures with mild trauma. Increased skin temperature around the affected bones may also be observed.

The jaws are affected in approximately 15 to 20% of the cases with the maxilla being involved more often than the mandible (ratio 3:1).

The affected bones become thickened, enlarged, and weakened. Clinically, progressive expansion of the jaw bones occurs with accompanying pain of different degree (**Figs. 42.8–42.10**). Characteristically, edentulous patients may complain that dentures do not fit, as due to alveolar enlargement they seem small. Similarly, if the patient is wearing hats, they are no longer fitting due to skull expansion. The signs and symptoms of the disease present a wide spectrum, ranging from asymptomatic to very serious ones. The patients are susceptible to pathologic bone fractures, cardiovascular disease, and rarely the development of osteosarcoma (1–3%). The diagnosis is based on both clinical and laboratory criteria.

Differential diagnosis

- Fibrous dysplasia
- Multiple exostoses
- Cemento-osseous dysplasia
- Fibrogenesis imperfecta ossium
- Osteosarcoma
- Multiple myeloma

Pathology

The investigations required for Paget's disease include (1) biochemical investigation that reveals marked elevation of serum alkaline phosphatase, elevated markers of bone breakdown, serum N-telopeptide and C-telopeptide, increased urinary hydroxyproline; (2) radiographic examination with the typical osteolytic focal radioluscencies (osteoporosis circumscribed) in the skull or advancing flame-shaped lytic lesions in long bones (during the osteoblastic phase, patchy areas of sclerotic bone are formed with "*cotton wool*" appearance); (3) CT scan; and (4) histopathologic examination. Histologically, there

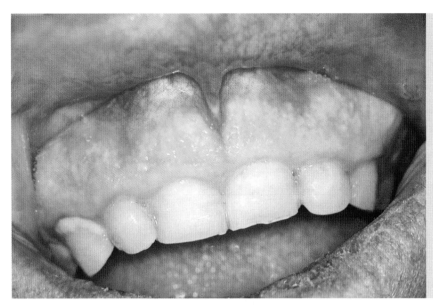

Fig. 42.8 Paget's disease, enlargement of the maxilla, and expansion into the sulcus.

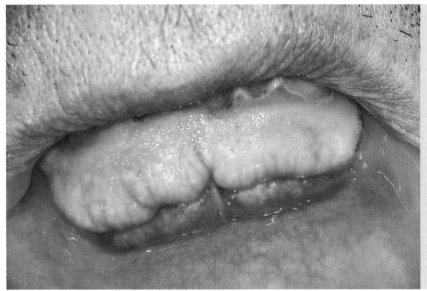

Fig. 42.9 Paget's disease, enlargement of the mandible, and expansion into the sulcus.

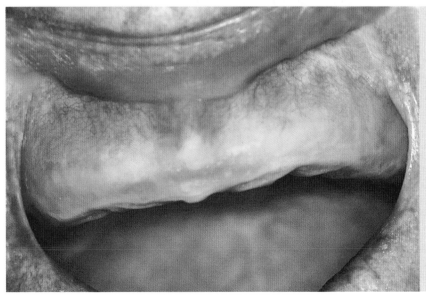

Fig. 42.10 Paget's disease, enlargement of an edentulous maxilla.

is abnormal osseous destruction and new bone formation. Depending on the disease phase, there may be numerous osteoclasts or osteoblasts with increased activity around bone trabeculae. The stroma comprises of a greatly vascular connective tissue that replaces the bone marrow. A characteristic finding is the presence of basophilic reversal lines where new bone is formed.

Treatment

Asymptomatic patients with limited involvement may require only clinical surveillance and no treatment. Treatment tends to be advised in (1) symptomatic patients, (2) patients with osseous deformities, and (3) patients with polyostotic disease and susceptibility to pathologic fractures. The first-line treatment is bisphosphonates with nasal calcitonin salmon and plicamycin as alternatives. Analgesics and nonsteroidal anti-inflammatory drugs are also used. Surgical intervention is advised in cases with great osseous deformities.

Dry Socket

Key points

- A serious postextraction complication.
- It occurs more often in the posterior area of mandible.
- Caused by a disturbance in the fibrinolytic mechanism of the clot and release of kinins and other pain mediators.
- Clinical characteristics are the absence of clot, an empty socket, intense pain, and halitosis.

Introduction

Dry socket or alveolar osteitis is a common complication following dental extraction. It most commonly occurs after the extraction of mandible molars and especially an impacted third molar. It is caused by the failure of clot formation due to a disturbance in the fibrinolytic mechanism. It results in the breakdown of fibrin and the release of kinins and other enzymes that are pain mediators. Predisposing and risk fac-

tors in the development of dry socket are a difficult extraction that may lead to damage of the surrounding tissues, preexisting infection, previous episodes of dry socket, etc. The frequency of a dry socket is 1 to 2% of all extractions and up to 10 to 20% of impacted mandibular third molars.

Clinical features

Clinically, the alveolar bone is bear with small dirty gray clot remnants (**Fig. 42.11**). The diagnosis is confirmed by probing of the socket, which reveals the exposed alveolar bone which is very sensitive. The most characteristic symptom is intense pain, halitosis, mild edema, and regional lymphadenopathy. The symptoms begin 2 to 3 days following the tooth extraction and without treatment may last up to 2 to 4 weeks. The diagnosis is based on the history and the clinical features.

Differential diagnosis

- Impacted foreign body
- Osteosarcoma
- Malignant fibrous histiocytoma
- Trigeminal neuralgia

Pathology

It is not required.

Treatment

Packing of the socket with an iodoform gauze containing eugenol and butamben, a local anesthetic, is used widely. Topical antibiotics offer only limited help, while systemic antibiotics should be avoided, as their effects are controversial. The systemic use of corticosteroids in a low dose (i.e., prednisolone 10–20 mg/d for only 4–5 days) along with local carbamide peroxide (oxygen-releasing) drops inside the socket three to four times per day for 4–5 days can stop the pain immediately.

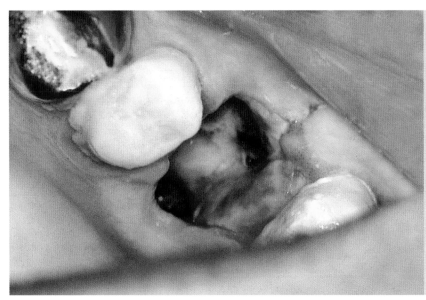

Fig. 42.11 Dry socket, empty, without a clot, postextraction alveolar socket.

43 Odontogenic Tumors

General considerations
- Odontogenic tumor is a heterogeneous group of tumors that derive from tooth germ tissues.
- They are classified into three groups based on their origin: (1) *epithelial*, that originate from the odontogenic epithelium, (2) *mesenchymal*, that originate from the odontogenic mesenchyme, and (3) *mixed*, with origin in both the odontogenic epithelium and mesenchyme (**Table 43.1**).
- Every odontogenic tumor has a different biological behavior and histologic features.
- Depending on the site, they are classified into *intraosseous* or *central* that account for 99% of all cases and *extraosseous* or *peripheral* that are very rare.
- The tumors may be generated at any period during the life of an individual.
- In this chapter, we have discussed the extraosseous odontogenic tumors and those of the intraosseous group that protrude intraorally. Both groups can cause diagnostic problems.

Ameloblastoma

Key points
- The second more frequent odontogenic tumor after odontoma.
- It derives from the odontogenic epithelium.
- The mandible (80%) is most commonly affected than the maxilla (20%).
- Using radiologic criteria, it is classified into *unicystic* (10–13%), *multicystic* or *solid* (85–90%), and *extraosseous*.
- The extraosseous or peripheral type represents 1 to 2% of all cases.

Introduction

Ameloblastoma is the most common tumor of odontogenic epithelial origin. It is benign, although occasionally it can be locally aggressive, causing osseous destruction. Extremely rarely, it can undergo malignant transformation that gives rise to metastases. It is more common between the age of 30 and 60 years and affects males and females equally. Depending on the affected site, ameloblastomas are classified into *intraosseous* or *central* and *extraosseous* or *peripheral*. The intraosseous type affects the mandible in over 80% of the cases, usually the molar–ramus region, while in the maxilla they present in the premolar area.

The extraosseous or peripheral ameloblastoma represents 1 to 2% of all cases and arises nearly always in the posterior tooth-bearing mucosa.

Clinical features

Clinically, intraosseous ameloblastoma is usually asymptomatic for a long time and is detected during a routine radiographic examination of the jaws. It develops slowly causing osseous enlargement. That can lead to destruction of the alveolar bone, cause tooth displacement, and may extend intraorally as an exophytic soft, red-brown mass (**Figs. 43.1, 43.2**). It may cause pain or paresthesia and often resorption and destruction of the roots of the teeth. In 20% of the cases, the tumor is associated with an impacted tooth or a dentigerous cyst. Using radiologic criteria, it is classified into *unicystic* and *multicystic*. The most typical radiographic pattern is a well-defined, multilocular, radiolucent area, usually with scalloped margin. Resorption of the teeth apices are common. The extraosseous or peripheral ameloblastoma is rare and may originate from dental lamina remnants or from basal cells of the surface epithelium. Clinically, it appears as a painless, slowly growing, erythematous mass with a smooth or papillary surface that rarely ulcerates (**Fig. 43.3**). Most commonly, there are no radiographic findings, as the tumor may cause mild or no osseous destruction. It can cause clinical diagnostic problems and the final diagnosis should be confirmed by histology.

Differential diagnosis
Intraosseous type
- Odontogenic myxoma
- Adenomatoid odontogenic tumor
- Aneurysmal cyst
- Dentigerous cyst
- Calcifying cystic odontogenic tumor
- Calcifying odontogenic tumor
- Other odontogenic tumors
- Gorlin's syndrome
- Cherubism
- Fibrous dysplasia
- Central giant cell granuloma

Extraosseous type
- Pyogenic granuloma
- Peripheral giant cell granuloma
- Fibroma
- Peripheral calcifying odontogenic tumor
- Non-Hodgkin's lymphoma
- Squamous cell carcinoma

Table 43.1 Histologic classification of odontogenic tumors (WHO 2005) (partly modified)

Epithelial	Mesenchymal	Mixed
I. Benign		
Ameloblastoma	Odontogenic myxoma	Ameloblastic fibroma
Adenomatoid odontogenic tumor	Odontogenic fibroma	Ameloblastic fibro-odontoma
Calcifying epithelial odontogenic tumor	Cementoblastoma	Ameloblastic fibrodentinoma
Squamous odontogenic tumor		Odontoameloblastoma
Keratocystic odontogenic tumor		Odontoma
		Calcifying cystic odontogenic tumor
II. Malignant		
Malignant ameloblastoma	Ameloblastic fibrosarcoma	
Ameloblastic carcinoma	Ameloblastic	
Primary	fibro-odontosarcoma	
Secondary—intraosseous	Ameloblastic	
—extraosseous	fibrodentinosarcoma	
Squamous cell carcinoma from odontogenic cyst		
Other types		

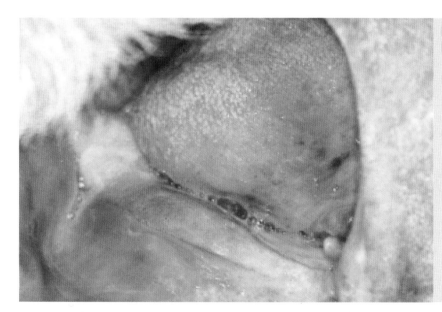

Fig. 43.1 Central ameloblastoma, enlargement that protrudes intraorally.

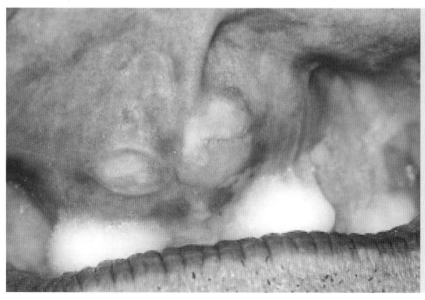

Fig. 43.2 Central ameloblastoma, enlargement of the maxilla with poor displacement.

Pathology

Using histologic criteria, ameloblastoma has been classified into six types: *follicular* and *plexiform* that are the most common and *acanthomatous, granular cell, basal cell*, and *desmoplastic* that are rare. Histopathologically, ameloblastoma can be solid or cystic. *The follicular type* consists of central stellate cells that resemble the developing enamel organ. This central formation is surrounded by a layer of cuboidal or columnar basal cells in palisading arrangement with vacuolated cytoplasm and hyperchromatic nuclei that are polarized away from the basement membrane. Often multiple small cysts or larger cystic spaces are common within the epithelial islands. The *prexiform type* is characterized by irregular masses or a network of strands. Each mass or strand is bounded by a layer of columnar cells and includes cells resembling stellate reticulum. There is minimal loose and vascular connective tissue. Other useful diagnostic adjuncts are radiographs and computed tomography (CT) and magnetic resonance imaging (MRI) scans.

Treatment

En bloc resection is the first line of treatment. More conservative surgical approach with curettage can lead to recurrence in 45 to 90% of the cases. A conservative surgical approach is the first line of treatment for the extraosseous type and gives excellent results.

Ameloblastic Carcinoma

Key points
- Very rarely ameloblastoma undergoes malignant transformation.
- This malignant behavior is described as *ameloblastic carcinoma* or *malignant ameloblastoma*.
- The metastases occur in the lungs, bones, and the lymph nodes.

Introduction

Ameloblastoma with malignant behavior and metastases represents 0.5 to 1% of all the cases of ameloblastoma. The term ameloblastic carcinoma is used when there are definite histologic elements of malignancy in the primary tumor and in the metastases. The term malignant ameloblastoma is used when metastases occur in the absence of malignant characters in both the primary tumor and the metastases.

Clinical features

Clinically, ameloblastic carcinoma presents as a rapidly progressing, usually painful, enlargement, mostly affecting the mandible. The tumor destroys the alveolar bone early, protruding intraorally as an exophytic, ulcerated mass (**Fig. 43.4**). In contrast, malignant ameloblastoma presents with the characters and biological behavior of typical ameloblastoma but it metastasizes. It is not unusual for the metastases to be diagnosed 10 to 15 years following the treatment of the primary tumor. Most commonly, metastasis occurs on the lungs, bones, and lymph nodes. The diagnosis is based mainly on the histologic features of the primary tumor and the metastasis.

Differential diagnosis
- Benign ameloblastoma
- Odontogenic myxoma
- Squamous cell carcinoma
- Osteosarcoma
- Chondrosarcoma

Pathology

Histopathologic examination of the primary lesion and the metastasis is a prerequisite for the correct and definite diagnosis. In ameloblastic carcinoma, both the typical characteristics of ameloblastoma and features of malignancy (cellular pleomorphism, hyperchromatic nuclei, mitoses etc.) are seen. In malignant ameloblastoma, there are areas retaining the typical characteristics of ameloblastoma without any features of malignancy.

Treatment

Surgery combined with chemotherapy is the first line of treatment. It is usually of poor prognosis.

Calcifying Epithelial Odontogenic Tumor

Key points
- A rare epithelial odontogenic tumor.
- The mandible is most frequently affected than the maxilla with a ratio of 2:1.
- It is classified into *intraosseous* and *extraosseous* types.
- The tumor displays a characteristic histologic pattern and presence of amyloid-like material.

Introduction

Calcifying epithelial tumor or Pindborg's tumor is a rare epithelial odontogenic tumor representing only 1% of all odontogenic tumors. The exact histogenesis remains unclear. However, the most accepted theory defines its origin from the dental lamina remnants or the stratum intermedium layer of the enamel organ. Depending on the affected site, it is classified into *intraosseous* or *central* and *extraosseous* or *peripheral*. The tumor equally affects both sexes between 20 and 60 years, with a mean age of around 40 years.

Clinical features

The intraosseous type is the most common (95–97%) and mostly affects the mandible at a ratio of 2:1 with a predilection in the premolar–molar area. Clinically, it appears as a painless, slow-growing expansile mass of the jaw (**Fig. 43.5**). This can rarely result to osseous destruction of the alveolar bone, protruding intraorally as a firm mass. Smaller lesions are asymptomatic and are usually diagnosed after a routine radiographic examination. In 60% of the cases, the tumor coexists with an impacted tooth or an odontoma.

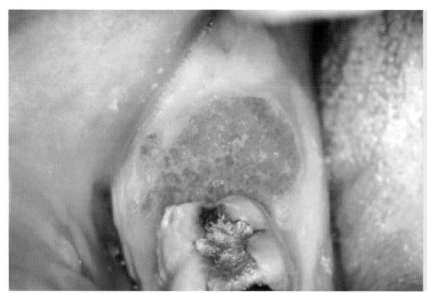

Fig. 43.3 Peripheral ameloblastoma, ulcerated erythematous mass on the retromolar area.

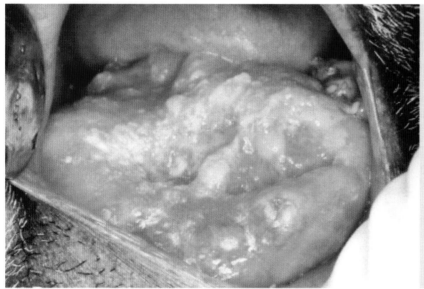

Fig. 43.4 Ameloblastic carcinoma, large, ulcerated tumor that protrudes intraorally.

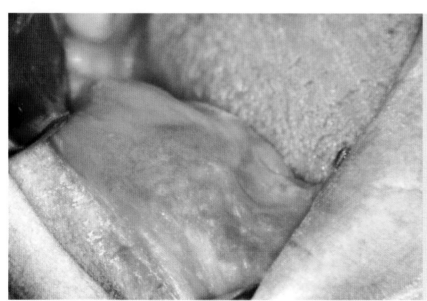

Fig. 43.5 Calcifying epithelial odontogenic tumor, central type. Enlargement of the mandible that protrudes intraorally.

The extraosseous type is rare (3–5%) and clinically presents as a painless, firm mass on the gingiva lacking in more specific characteristics (**Fig. 43.6**). The overlying mucosa might be intact or ulcerated. The diagnosis of calcifying epithelial odontogenic tumor is based mostly on histologic criteria and secondarily on radiographic findings.

Differential diagnosis

Intraosseous type
- Calcifying cystic odontogenic tumor
- Other odontogenic tumors
- Ameloblastic fibro-odontoma
- Fibrous dysplasia
- Osteosarcoma
- Intraosseous squamous cell carcinoma

Extraosseous type
- Peripheral ossifying fibroma
- Fibroma
- Peripheral giant cell granuloma
- Chondrosarcoma
- Non-Hodgkin's lymphoma
- Squamous cell carcinoma

Pathology

Histologically, calcifying epithelial odontogenic tumor is characterized by the presence of polygonal epithelial cells with abundant eosinophilic cytoplasm and prominent intercellular bridges, arranged in islands and sheets in a fibrous stroma. The nuclei are frequently pleomorphic with common giant features and no mitotic figures. A characteristic is the presence of amorphous eosinophilic, amyloid-like material that stains positive with Congo red and fluorescence with Thioflavin T while reacts metachromatically with methyl and crystal violet. There are also multiple spherical calcified areas arranged in concentric rings (*Liesegang ring calcification*). Radiographically, they can be uni- or multiloculated with scattered areas of calcification, while impacted teeth are not uncommon.

Treatment

Conservative surgical excision is the first line of treatment. Recurrence is rare.

Calcifying Cystic Odontogenic Tumor

Key points
- It is classified by the World Health Organization (WHO) under odontogenic tumors.
- The tumor is classified into *intraosseous* or *central* and *extraosseous* or *peripheral*.
- The diagnosis is based on histologic and radiographic criteria.

Introduction

Calcifying cystic odontogenic tumor or calcifying odontogenic cyst or Gorlin's cyst, is a rare odontogenic lesion characterized by an ameloblastoma-like epithelium with ghost cells that may calcify. WHO (2005) defined it as a benign cystic neoplasm of odontogenic origin. Depending on the affected site, it is classified into *intraosseous* or *central* (80–90%) and *extraosseous* or *peripheral* (10–20%). Often (20–30%) coexists with impacted teeth or odontoma and more rarely with ameloblastoma or adenomatoid odontogenic tumor. It equally affects both jaws. The age spectrum of the patients is great, ranging between 5 and 80 years with a peak around 20 to 30 years old, without gender predilection.

Clinical features

Clinically, the *intraosseous* type presents as a painless, slow-growing swelling that progresses to expansion of the jaw bone and occasionally perforates the jaw bone. At the time of diagnosis, the size ranges between 2 and 10 cm. Clinically, the *extraosseous* type presents as a painless well-circumscribed, pedunculated, or sessile pink to reddish elevated gingival mass, measuring up to 4 cm in diameter (**Fig. 43.7**). It is soft in palpation and lacks specific characteristics. The diagnosis of both types is based on the histology of the lesion.

Differential diagnosis

Intraosseous type
- Calcifying epithelial odontogenic tumor
- Other odontogenic tumors
- Dentigerous cyst
- Cherubism
- Central giant cell granuloma

Extraosseous type
- Peripheral giant cell granuloma
- Peripheral ossifying fibroma
- Gingival cyst of adult
- Peripheral calcifying epithelial odontogenic tumor
- Peripheral ameloblastoma

Pathology

Histologically, the cyst wall is lined by odontogenic epithelium. The basal cell layers resemble ameloblasts (tall cuboidal or cylindrical), while the overlying layers are formed by stellate reticulum-like cells. A specific characteristic is the presence of large eosinophilic cells, within the epithelial layers in nests or large surfaces known as "*ghost cells*," due to the lack of nuclei. These cells may be calcified. Radiographically, the intraosseous type is usually unilocular and more rarely multilocular radioluscent and well circumscribed. In about 50% of the patients, a variable amount of radiopaque material or an impacted tooth or an odontoma may be seen.

Treatment

Surgical excision is the treatment of choice. Recurrence is rare and prognosis is generally good.

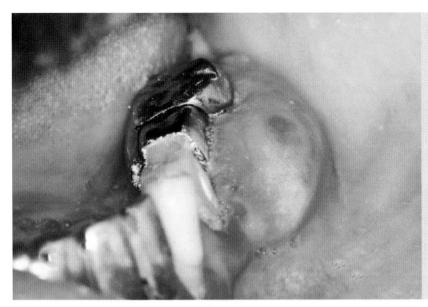

Fig. 43.6 Calcifying epithelial odontogenic tumor, peripheral type. Tumor of the lower gingivae on the buccal aspect.

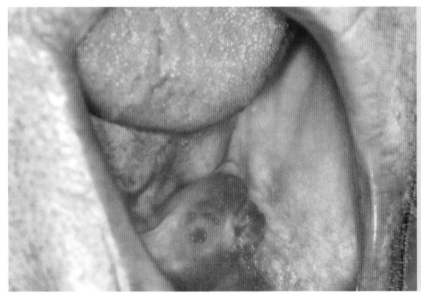

Fig. 43.7 Calcifying cystic odontogenic tumor, peripheral type. Exophytic tumor on the mandibular alveolar mucosa.

649

Odontogenic Myxoma

Key points
- A rare, benign odontogenic tumor of mesenchymal or ectomesenchymal origin.
- Most commonly affects the mandible (60–65%).
- Small lesions are asymptomatic while larger can cause bone enlargement.
- Surgical excision is the treatment of choice; recurrence rate is high (25–35%).

Introduction

Odontogenic myxoma is a rare benign odontogenic tumor that derives from the mesenchyme of the tooth germ. It represents 3 to 6% of all odontogenic tumors and affects both sexes with mean age of diagnosis between 20 and 30 years. The mandible is more often affected (60–65%) than the maxilla, usually in the molar regions.

Clinical features

Clinically, small lesions are asymptomatic and are discovered only during a routine radiographic examination of the jaws. However, as the tumor grows, it causes a painless slow-growing expansion of the involved bone. Rarely, the tumor may destroy the bone and appears intraorally as a soft mass with abnormal surface. Radiographically, the tumor appears as a multilocular or unilocular radioluscent area with irregular or scalloped margins and frequently with a "*honeycombed*" pattern similar to that seen in ameloblastoma (**Fig. 43.8**). The diagnosis is mainly based on radiographic and histologic criteria.

Differential diagnosis
- Ameloblastoma
- Chondromyxoid fibroma
- Myxosarcoma
- Intraosseous hemangioma
- Odontogenic cysts
- Fibrous dysplasia

Pathology

Histologically, odontogenic myxoma is characterized by multiple stellate, round or spindle-shaped cells into an abundant myxoid stroma with little collagen. Histochemical analysis of the stroma reveals hyaluronic acid, chondroitin sulfate, and glycosaminoglycans. Immunohistochemically, the cells react to antibodies for actin and vimentin. Rest of odontogenic epithelium are not obvious in most lesions and not required for establishing the diagnosis.

Treatment

Surgical excision is the first line of treatment. Recurrence rate of 25 to 35% has been reported.

Odontoma

Key points
- The most common odontogenic tumor.
- It is a developmental lesion than a true neoplasm.
- Classified into two types: *complex* and *compound*.
- Most commonly affects the maxilla.
- Usually asymptomatic, being discovered during routine radiographic examination.

Introduction

Odontomas are developmental malformations and not neoplasms. It derives from the odontogenic epithelium and dental mesenchyme and is characterized by dental tissue that has not grown in the normal way. It represents 40 to 50% of all odontogenic tumors. Odontomas are classified into two types: *complex* that is characterized by an irregular mass of enamel, dentine, and cementum that are not arranged in a tooth-like fashion and *compound* that consists of multiple, tooth-like structures (odontoids). Odontomas are equally frequent in males and females and the average age at the time of diagnosis is below 20 years. It occurs more frequently in the maxilla than in the mandible.

Clinical features

Most odontomas are small and asymptomatic and are usually detected accidentally in a routine radiographic examination. Clinically, large odontomas may cause osseous enlargement and, even destruction, protruding intraorally, as what would resemble "teeth" (**Fig. 43.9**). Radiographically, complex odontoma presents as a compact, amorphous, calcified, spherical, or ovoid radiopaque mass without any tooth-like structure. Compound odontoma appears as a collection of tooth-like structures, of varied shapes and sizes, surrounded by a narrow radiolucent rim. The diagnosis is mainly based on radiographic and histologic criteria.

Differential diagnosis
- Osteoma
- Gardner's syndrome
- Calcifying odontogenic tumor
- Calcifying cystic odontogenic tumor
- Fibro-odontoma
- Odontoameloblastoma

Pathology

Histologically, complex odontoma consists of mixed elements and layers of enamel, dentine, cementum, and pulpal tissues, without any tooth formation or structure. The compound type consists of all the structural elements of a tooth, in smaller and not fully formed teeth, with cords and islands of odontogenic epithelium. The distinction between complex and compound odontoma is mainly based on the presence of tooth-like structures in compound odontomas.

Treatment

Local surgical excision is the treatment of choice with very good results.

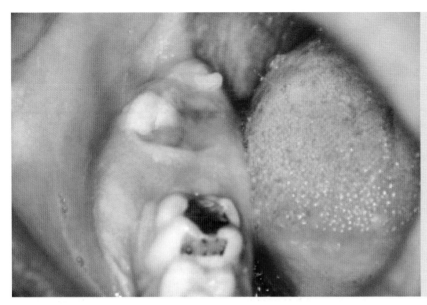

Fig. 43.8 Odontogenic myxoma, enlargement of the mandible.

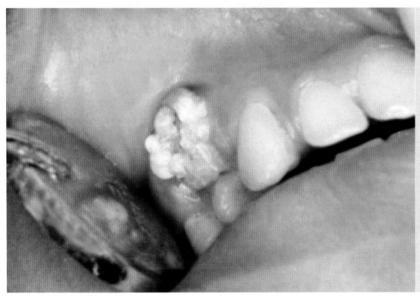

Fig. 43.9 Compound odontoma protruding intraorally.

References

1. Normal Mucosal Variants

Abidullah M, Raghunath V, Karpe T, et al. Clinicopathologic correlation of white, non scrapable oral mucosal surface lesions: a study of 100 cases. J Clin Diagn Res 2016;10(2):ZC38–ZC41

Al-Mobeeriek A, AlDosari AM. Prevalence of oral lesions among Saudi dental patients. Ann Saudi Med 2009;29(5):365–368

Amir E, Gorsky M, Buchner A, Sarnat H, Gat H. Physiologic pigmentation of the oral mucosa in Israeli children. Oral Surg Oral Med Oral Pathol 1991;71(3):396–398

Macdonald JB, Tobin CA, Hurley MY. Oral leukoedema with mucosal desquamation caused by toothpaste containing sodium lauryl sulfate. Cutis 2016;97(1):E4–E5

Madani FM, Kuperstein AS. Normal variations of oral anatomy and common oral soft tissue lesions: evaluation and management. Med Clin North Am 2014;98(6):1281–1298

Martin JL. Leukoedema: an epidemiological study in white and African Americans. J Tenn Dent Assoc 1997;77(1):18–21

Moghadam BK, Gier RE. Melanin pigmentation disorders of the skin and oral mucosa. Compendium 1991;12(1):14, 16–20

Parlak AH, Koybasi S, Yavuz T, et al. Prevalence of oral lesions in 13- to 16-year-old students in Duzce, Turkey. Oral Dis 2006;12(6):553–558

Ponti G, Meschieri A, Pollio A, et al. Fordyce granules and hyperplastic mucosal sebaceous glands as distinctive stigmata in Muir-Torre syndrome patients: characterization with reflectance confocal microscopy. J Oral Pathol Med 2015;44(7):552–557

2. Developmental Anomalies

Agha-Hosseini F, Etesam F, Rohani B. A boy with oral hair: case report. Med Oral Patol Oral Cir Bucal 2007;12(5):E357–E359

Bhattacharya V, Khanna S, Bashir SA, Kumar U, Garbyal RS. Cleft palate associated with hamartomatous bifid tongue. Report of two cases. J Plast Reconstr Aesthet Surg 2009;62(11):1442–1445

Campbell A, Costello BJ, Ruiz RL. Cleft lip and palate surgery: an update of clinical outcomes for primary repair. Oral Maxillofac Surg Clin North Am 2010;22(1):43–58

Canoglu E, Turgut MD, Tekcicek M. Healing of external inflammatory root resorptions and periapical lesions without surgical treatment in an operated oblique facial cleft case. Eur J Dent 2010;4(2):208–214

Chohayeb AA, Volpe AR. Occurrence of torus palatinus and mandibularis among women of different ethnic groups. Am J Dent 2001;14(5):278–280

Cox SE, Soderberg JM. Idiopathic hemifacial atrophy treated with serial injections of calcium hydroxylapatite. Dermatol Surg 2010;36(4):542–545

Francis DO, Krishnaswami S, McPheeters M. Treatment of ankyloglossia and breastfeeding outcomes: a systematic review. Pediatrics 2015;135(6):e1458–e1466

García-García AS, Martínez-González JM, Gómez-Font R, Soto-Rivadeneira A, Oviedo-Roldán L. Current status of the torus palatinus and torus mandibularis. Med Oral Patol Oral Cir Bucal 2010;15(2):e353–e360

Hamamci N, Özer T, Hamamci O, Tümen EC, Ağaçkiran E. Treatment of an adolescent with total ankyloglossia. World J Orthod 2010;11(3):278–283

Hiebert JC, Johnson AB, Tran HH, Yu Z, Glade RS. Congenital tongue mass with concomitant cleft palate and bifid tongue: a case report and review of the literature. Cleft Palate Craniofac J 2016;53(2):245–248

Hong P, Lago D, Seargeant J, Pellman L, Magit AE, Pransky SM. Defining ankyloglossia: a case series of anterior and posterior tongue ties. Int J Pediatr Otorhinolaryngol 2010;74(9):1003–1006

Hou M, Liu C, Wang J, Zhang L, Gao Q. Lateral or oblique facial clefts associated with accessory maxillae: Review of the literature and report of a case. J Craniomaxillofac Surg 2015;43(5):585–592

James AW, Culver K, Hall B, Golabi M. Bifid tongue: a rare feature associated with infants of diabetic mother syndrome. Am J Med Genet A 2007;143A(17):2035–2039

Jamilian A, Lucchese A, Darnahal A, Kamali Z, Perillo L. Cleft sidedness and congenitally missing teeth in patients with cleft lip and palate patients. Prog Orthod 2016;17:14

Jugessur A, Farlie PG, Kilpatrick N. The genetics of isolated orofacial clefts: from genotypes to subphenotypes. Oral Dis 2009;15(7):437–453

Kajikawa A, Ueda K, Katsuragi Y, Hirose T, Asai E. Surgical repair of transverse facial cleft: oblique vermilion-mucosa incision. J Plast Reconstr Aesthet Surg 2010;63(8):1269–1274

Kamble V, Mitra K. A rare association of bilateral and unilateral masseter hypertrophy with hypertrophy of pterygoids. J Clin Diagn Res 2016;10(2):TJ03–TJ04

Kaul B, Mahajan N, Gupta R, Kotwal B. The syndrome of pit of the lower lip and its association with cleft palate. Contemp Clin Dent 2014;5(3):383–385

Kim NH, Park RH, Park JB. Botulinum toxin type A for the treatment of hypertrophy of the masseter muscle. Plast Reconstr Surg 2010;125(6):1693–1705

Laskaris G, Hatziolou E, Vareltzidis A. A real hair on the tip of the tongue. J Eur Acad Dermatol Venereol 1994;3(3):383–385

Matsumoto K, Nozoe E, Okawachi T, Ishihata K, Nishinara K, Nakamura N. Preliminary analysis of the 3-dimensional morphology of the upper lip configuration at the completion of facial expressions in healthy Japanese young adults and patients with cleft lip. J Oral Maxillofac Surg 2016;74(9):1834–1846

Naidoo S, Bütow KW. Oblique lip-alveolar banding in patients with cleft lip and palate. Br J Oral Maxillofac Surg 2015;53(4):390–392

Rispoli DZ, Camargo PM, Pires JL Jr, Fonseca VR, Mandelli KK, Pereira MA. Benign masseter muscle hypertrophy. Rev Bras Otorrinolaringol (Engl Ed) 2008;74(5):790–793

Seah YH. Torus palatinus and torus mandibularis: a review of the literature. Aust Dent J 1995;40(5):318–321

Shobana R, Aithal S, Srikanth S. Congenital lip pits without associated anomalies. Indian J Dermatol Venereol Leprol 2014;80(5):459–460

Souto LR. Congenital bilateral lower lip pits associated with fistulae of the minor salivary glands: case report of the principal Van der Woude syndrome's trait. Aesthetic Plast Surg 2008;32(1):172–174

Suliman MT, Alhassan M. Double lip: report of five cases and review of the literature. Aesthet Surg J 2007;27(3):289–291

3. Mechanical Injuries

Al-Mobeeriek A, AlDosari AM. Prevalence of oral lesions among Saudi dental patients. Ann Saudi Med 2009;29(5):365–368

Ceyhan AM, Yildirim M, Basak PY, Akkaya VB, Ayata A. Traumatic lingual ulcer in a child: Riga-Fede disease. Clin Exp Dermatol 2009;34(2):186–188

Compilato D, Cirillo N, Termine N, et al. Long-standing oral ulcers: proposal for a new 'S-C-D classification system'. J Oral Pathol Med 2009;38(3):241–253

Damevska K, Gocev G, Nikolovska S. Eosinophilic ulcer of the oral mucosa: report of a case with multiple synchronous lesions. Am J Dermatopathol 2014;36(7):594–596

Damm DD, Fantasia JE. Bilateral white lesions of buccal mucosa. Morsicatio buccarum. Gen Dent 2006;54(6):442, 444

Elnayef B, Monje A, Lin GH, et al. Alveolar ridge split on horizontal bone augmentation: a systematic review. Int J Oral Maxillofac Implants 2015;30(3):596–606

Fonseca FP, de Andrade BA, Coletta RD, et al. Clinicopathological and immunohistochemical analysis of 19 cases of oral eosinophilic ulcers. Oral Surg Oral Med Oral Pathol Oral Radiol 2013;115(4):532–540

Hong P. Riga-Fede disease: traumatic lingual ulceration in an infant. J Pediatr 2015;167(1):204

Kovacić I, Celebić A, Zlatarić DK, et al. Decreasing of residual alveolar ridge height in complete denture wearers. A five year follow up study. Coll Antropol 2010;34(3):1051–1056

Kumar S, Gupta R, Arora R, Saxena S. Severe oropharyngeal trauma caused by toothbrush--case report and review of 13 cases. Br Dent J 2008;205(8):443–447

Kumar T, Puri G, Aravinda K, Arora N, Patil D, Gupta R. Oral sex and oral health: an enigma in itself. Indian J Sex Transm Dis 2015;36(2):129–132

Li J, Zhang YY, Wang NN, Bhandari R, Liu QQ. Riga-Fede disease in a child. Clin Exp Dermatol 2016;41(3):285–286

Macedo Firoozmand L, Dias Almeida J, Guimarães Cabral LA. Study of denture-induced fibrous hyperplasia cases diagnosed from 1979 to 2001. Quintessence Int 2005;36(10):825–829

Sciallis AP, Law ME, Inwards DJ, et al. Mucosal CD30-positive T-cell lymphoproliferations of the head and neck show a clinicopathologic spectrum similar to cutaneous CD30-positive T-cell lymphoproliferative disorders. Mod Pathol 2012;25(7):983–992

Segura S, Pujol RM. Eosinophilic ulcer of the oral mucosa: a distinct entity or a non-specific reactive pattern? Oral Dis 2008;14(4):287–295

Sklavounou A, Laskaris G. Eosinophilic ulcer of the oral mucosa. Oral Surg Oral Med Oral Pathol 1984;58(4):431–436

Taghi A, Motamedi MH. Riga-Fede disease: a histological study and case report. Indian J Dent Res 2009;20(2):227–229

Terezhalmy GT, Riley CK, Moore WS. Oral lesions secondary to fellatio. Quintessence Int 2000;31(5):361

Turker SB, Sener ID, Koçak A, Yilmaz S, Ozkan YK. Factors triggering the oral mucosal lesions by complete dentures. Arch Gerontol Geriatr 2010;51(1):100–104

4. Chemical Burns

Allen CL, Loudon J, Mascarenhas AK. Sanguinaria-related leukoplakia: epidemiologic and clinicopathologic features of a recently described entity. Gen Dent 2001;49(6):608–614

Coetzee E, Whitelaw A, Kahn D, Rode H. The use of topical, un-buffered sodium hypochlorite in the management of burn wound infection. Burns 2012;38(4):529–533

Cote V, Prager JD. Iatrogenic phenol injury: a case report and review of medication safety and labeling practices with flexible laryngoscopy. Int J Pediatr Otorhinolaryngol 2014;78(10):1769–1773

Eversole LR, Eversole GM, Kopcik J. Sanguinaria-associated oral leukoplakia: comparison with other benign and dysplastic leukoplakic lesions. Oral Surg Oral Med Oral Pathol Oral Radiol Endod 2000;89(4):455–464

Ganatra S, Cohen D. Silver nitrate burn of the lower lip: a case report. Gen Dent 2016;64(1):75–77

Gilvetti C, Porter SR, Fedele S. Traumatic chemical oral ulceration: a case report and review of the literature. Br Dent J 2010;208(7):297–300

Goswami M, Chhabra N, Kumar G, Verma M, Chhabra A. Sodium hypochlorite dental accidents. Paediatr Int Child Health 2014;34(1):66–69

Holmes RG, Chan DC, Singh BB. Chemical burn of the buccal mucosa. Am J Dent 2004;17(3):219–220

Iacomino E, Junquera LM, Vendettuoli M, González AM, Olay S, Corbacelli A. Distraction of oral scars contractures following caustic ingestion. A form of conservative treatment. Med Oral 2003;8(1):61–65

Kawashima Z, Flagg RH, Cox DE. Aspirin-induced oral lesion: report of case. J Am Dent Assoc 1975;91(1):130–131

Kozam G, Mantell GM. The effect of eugenol on oral mucous membranes. J Dent Res 1978;57(11-12):954–957

Maron FS. Mucosal burn resulting from chewable aspirin: report of case. J Am Dent Assoc 1989;119(2):279–280

Ribeiro AC, Simonato LE, Santos-Silva AR, de Moraes NP, Soubhia AM. Formalin burn. Br Dent J 2010;209(1):4

Rihani FB, Al-Bataineh MM. Iatrogenic paraformaldehyde orofacial chemical burn. BMJ Case Rep 2013;2013:2013

Rostami AM, Brooks JK. Intraoral chemical burn from use of 3% hydrogen peroxide. Gen Dent 2011;59(6):504–506

Shetty K. Hydrogen peroxide burn of the oral mucosa. Ann Pharmacother 2006;40(2):351

5. Thermal and Electricity Lesions

Hedin CA, Pindborg JJ, Axéll T. Disappearance of smoker's melanosis after reducing smoking. J Oral Pathol Med 1993;22(5):228–230

Jones KB, Jordan R. White lesions in the oral cavity: clinical presentation, diagnosis, and treatment. Semin Cutan Med Surg 2015;34(4):161–170

McMullin BT, Blumin JH, Merati AL. Thermal injury to the tongue from an operative laryngoscope. Otolaryngol Head Neck Surg 2007;137(5):798–802

Newland JR. Differential diagnosis in dentistry. Nicotinic stomatitis. J Gt Houst Dent Soc 1998;69(6):3

Samatha Y, Sankar AJ, Ganapathy KS, Srinivas K, Ankineedu D, Choudary AL. Clinicopathologic evaluation of lesions associated with tobacco usage. J Contemp Dent Pract 2014;15(4):466–472

Taybos G. Oral changes associated with tobacco use. Am J Med Sci 2003;326(4):179–182

Unsal E, Paksoy C, Soykan E, Elhan AH, Sahin M. Oral melanin pigmentation related to smoking in a Turkish population. Community Dent Oral Epidemiol 2001;29(4):272–277

Wakefield Y, Pemberton MN. Oro-facial thermal injury caused by food heated in a microwave oven. Dent Update 2009;36(1):26–27

6. Metal and Other Deposits

Gooi Z, Mydlarz WK, Tunkel DE, Eisele DW. Submandibular venous malformation phleboliths mimicking sialolithiasis in children. Laryngoscope 2014;124(12):2826–2828

Khalil A. Lead poisoning. Br Dent J 2009;206:608

Cankaya H, Unal O, Ugras S, Yuca K, Kiriş M. Hemangioma with phleboliths in the sublingual gland: as a cause of submental opacity. Tohoku J Exp Med 2003;199(3):187–191

Kissel SO, Hanratty JJ. Periodontal treatment of an amalgam tattoo. Compend Contin Educ Dent 2002;23(10):930–932, 934, 936

Mandel L, Perrino MA. Phleboliths and the vascular maxillofacial lesion. J Oral Maxillofac Surg 2010;68(8):1973–1976

Scolozzi P, Laurent F, Lombardi T, Richter M. Intraoral venous malformation presenting with multiple phleboliths. Oral Surg Oral Med Oral Pathol Oral Radiol Endod 2003;96(2):197–200

ten Bruggenkate CM, Lopes Cardozo E, Maaskant P, van der Waal I. Lead poisoning with pigmentation of the oral mucosa. Review of the literature and report of a case. Oral Surg Oral Med Oral Pathol 1975;39(5):747–753

Thumbigere-Math V, Johnson DK. Treatment of amalgam tattoo with a subepithelial connective tissue graft and acellular dermal matrix. J Int Acad Periodontol 2014;16(2):50–54

Tran HT, Anandasabapathy N, Soldano AC. Amalgam tattoo. Dermatol Online J 2008;14(5):19

Vera-Kellet C, Del Barrio-Díaz P. Images in clinical medicine. Oral amalgam tattoo mimicking melanoma. N Engl J Med 2016;374(17):e21

7. Foreign Materials

Corlianò F, Falco P, Cambi J, Brindisi L. Iron supplement tablet embedded in the oral cavity mimicking neoplasm: a case report. J Korean Assoc Oral Maxillofac Surg 2016;42(2):111–114

da Silva EJ, Deng Y, Tumushime-Buturo CG. An unusual foreign body in the tongue. Br J Oral Maxillofac Surg 2000;38(3):241–242

Odzili FA, Guimbi KC, Diembi S, et al. Oral metal foreign bodies [in French]. Odontostomatol Trop 2015;38(150):46–48

Parray T, Siddiqui MS, Abraham E, Apuya J, Shah S. A case of an unusual foreign body of the tongue. South Med J 2010;103(9):966–967

Patel KS. Foreign body in the tongue: an unusual site for a common problem. J Laryngol Otol 1991;105(10):849–850

Vieira EdeO, Fidel Junior RA, Figueredo CM, Fischer RG. Clinical evaluation of a dermic allograft in procedures to increase attached gingiva width. Braz Dent J 2009;20(3):191–194

8. Oral Complications of Radiation and Chemotherapy

Alterio D, Jereczek-Fossa BA, Fiore MR, Piperno G, Ansarin M, Orecchia R. Cancer treatment-induced oral mucositis. Anticancer Res 2007;27(2):1105–1125

Barasch A, Epstein J, Tilashalski K. Palifermin for management of treatment-induced oral mucositis in cancer patients. Biologics 2009;3:111–116

Buglione M, Cavagnini R, Di Rosario F, et al. Oral toxicity management in head and neck cancer patients treated with chemotherapy and radiation: xerostomia and trismus (Part 2). Literature review and consensus statement. Crit Rev Oncol Hematol 2016;102:47–54

Cheng SC, Wu VW, Kwong DL, Ying MT. Assessment of post-radiotherapy salivary glands. Br J Radiol 2011;84(1001):393–402

De Sanctis V, Bossi P, Sanguineti G, et al. Mucositis in head and neck cancer patients treated with radiotherapy and systemic therapies: Literature review and consensus statements. Crit Rev Oncol Hematol 2016;100:147–166

Jereczek-Fossa BA, Orecchia R. Radiotherapy-induced mandibular bone complications. Cancer Treat Rev 2002;28(1):65–74

Kwon Y. Mechanism-based management for mucositis: option for treating side effects without compromising the efficacy of cancer therapy. Onco Targets Ther 2016;9:2007–2016

Madrid C, Abarca M, Bouferrache K. Osteoradionecrosis: an update. Oral Oncol 2010;46(6):471–474

Mason H, DeRubeis MB, Burke N, et al. Symptom management during and after treatment with concurrent chemoradiotherapy for oropharyngeal cancer: a review of the literature and areas for future research. World J Clin Oncol 2016;7(2):220–226

Moslemi D, Nokhandani AM, Otaghsaraei MT, Moghadamnia Y, Kazemi S, Moghadamnia AA. Management of chemo/radiation-induced oral mucositis in patients with head and neck cancer: a review of the current literature. Radiother Oncol 2016;120(1):13–20

Nadella KR, Kodali RM, Guttikonda LK, Jonnalagadda A. Osteoradionecrosis of the jaws: Clinico-therapeutic management: a literature review and update. J Maxillofac Oral Surg 2015;14(4):891–901

Otmani N, Alami R, Hessissen L, Mokhtari A, Soulaymani A, Khattab M. Determinants of severe oral mucositis in paediatric cancer patients: a prospective study. Int J Paediatr Dent 2011;21(3):210–216

Rice N, Polyzois I, Ekanayake K, Omer O, Stassen LF. The management of osteoradionecrosis of the jaws--a review. Surgeon 2015;13(2):101–109

9. Contact Allergic Reactions

Aggarwal V, Jain A, Kabi D. Oral lichenoid reaction associated with tin component of amalgam restorations: a case report. Am J Dermatopathol 2010;32(1):46–48

Calapai G, Miroddi M, Mannucci C, Minciullo P, Gangemi S. Oral adverse reactions due to cinnamon-flavoured chewing gums consumption. Oral Dis 2014;20(7):637–643

Collet E, Jeudy G, Dalac S. Cheilitis, perioral dermatitis and contact allergy. Eur J Dermatol 2013;23(3):303–307

Georgakopoulou EA. Cinnamon contact stomatitis. J Dermatol Case Rep 2010;4(2):28–29

Hensten-Pettersen A. Skin and mucosal reactions associated with dental materials. Eur J Oral Sci 1998;106(2, Pt 2):707–712

Isaac-Renton M, Li MK, Parsons LM. Cinnamon spice and everything not nice: many features of intraoral allergy to cinnamic aldehyde. Dermatitis 2015;26(3):116–121

Koutis D, Freeman S. Allergic contact stomatitis caused by acrylic monomer in a denture. Australas J Dermatol 2001;42(3):203–206

Pemberton MN, Gibson J. Chlorhexidine and hypersensitivity reactions in dentistry. Br Dent J 2012;213(11):547–550

Pigatto PD, Bombeccari G, Spadari F, Guzzi G. Oral lichenoid reaction, dental amalgam, and tin allergy. Am J Dermatopathol 2011;33(4):414–415

Vivas AP, Migliari DA. Cinnamon-induced oral mucosal contact reaction. Open Dent J 2015;9:257–259

10. Oral Lesions Due to Drugs

Almazrooa SA, Woo SB, Mawardi H, Treister N. Characterization and management of exfoliative cheilitis: a single-center experience. Oral Surg Oral Med Oral Pathol Oral Radiol 2013;116(6):e485–e489

Amici C, La Frazia S, Brunelli C, Balsamo M, Angelini M, Santoro MG. Inhibition of viral protein translation by indomethacin in vesicular stomatitis virus infection: role of eIF2a kinase PKR. Cell Microbiol 2015;17(9):1391–1404

Beguerie JR, Gonzalez S. Angina bullosa hemorrhagica: report of 11 cases. Dermatol Rep 2014;6(1):5282

Cohen M, Nabili V, Chhetri DK. Palatal perforation from cocaine abuse. Ear Nose Throat J 2008;87(5):262

Di Cosola M, Turco M, Acero J, Navarro-Vila C, Cortelazzi R. Cocaine-related syndrome and palatal reconstruction: report of a series of cases. Int J Oral Maxillofac Surg 2007;36(8):721–727

Faiman B, Pillai AL, Benghiac AG. Bisphosphonate-related osteonecrosis of the jaw: historical, ethical, and legal issues associated with prescribing. J Adv Pract Oncol 2013;4(1):25–35

Femiano F, Lanza A, Buonaiuto C, et al. Oral manifestations of adverse drug reactions: guidelines. J Eur Acad Dermatol Venereol 2008;22(6):681–691

Gallo CB, Luiz AC, Ferrazzo KL, Migliari DA, Sugaya NN. Drug-induced pigmentation of hard palate and skin due to chronic chloroquine therapy: report of two cases. Clin Exp Dermatol 2009;34(7):e266–e267

Gupta MK, McClymont LG, El-Hakim H. Case of sublingual hematoma threatening airway obstruction. Med Sci Monit 2003;9(11):CS95–CS97

Henao MP, Kraschnewski JL, Kelbel T, Craig TJ. Diagnosis and screening of patients with hereditary angioedema in primary care. Ther Clin Risk Manag 2016;12:701–711

Kharazmi M, Sjöqvist K, Rizk M, Warfvinge G. Oral ulcer associated with alendronate: a case report. Oral Surg Oral Med Oral Pathol Oral Radiol Endod 2010;110(6):e11–e13

Kumar B, Saraswat A, Kaur I. Mucocutaneous adverse effects of hydroxyurea: a prospective study of 30 psoriasis patients. Clin Exp Dermatol 2002;27(1):8–13

Laskaris G, Satriano RA. Drug-induced blistering oral lesions. Clin Dermatol 1993;11(4):545–550

O'Sullivan EM. Nicorandil-induced severe oral ulceration. J Ir Dent Assoc 2004;50(4):157–159

Paleri V, Lindsey L. Oral ulcers caused by hydroxyurea. J Laryngol Otol 2000;114(12):976–977

Patel S, Choyee S, Uyanne J, et al. Non-exposed bisphosphonate-related osteonecrosis of the jaw: a critical assessment of current definition, staging, and treatment guidelines. Oral Dis 2012;18(7):625–632

Pierard-Franchimont C, Lesuisse M, Humbert P, Delvenne P, Pierard GE. Toxic epidermal necrolysis and antifolate drugs in cancer chemotherapy. Curr Drug Saf 2012;7(5):357–360

Radtke S, Zolk O, Renner B, et al. Germline genetic variations in methotrexate candidate genes are associated with pharmacokinetics, toxicity, and outcome in childhood acute lymphoblastic leukemia. Blood 2013;121(26):5145–5153

Silvestre FJ, Perez-Herbera A, Puente-Sandoval A, Bagán JV. Hard palate perforation in cocaine abusers: a systematic review. Clin Oral Investig 2010;14(6):621–628

Tovaru S, Parlatescu I, Dumitriu AS, Bucur A, Kaplan I. Oral complications associated with D-penicillamine treatment for Wilson disease: a clinicopathologic report. J Periodontol 2010;81(8):1231–1236

Trimarchi M, Bertazzoni G, Bussi M. Cocaine induced midline destructive lesions. Rhinology 2014;52(2):104–111

Troeltzsch M, von Blohn G, Kriegelstein S, et al. Oral mucositis in patients receiving low-dose methotrexate therapy for rheumatoid arthritis: report of 2 cases and literature review. Oral Surg Oral Med Oral Pathol Oral Radiol 2013;115(5):e28–e33

11. Gingival and Periodontal Diseases

Abu-Saleh T. Interleukin-1 composite polymorphism as a risk factor for chronic periodontitis: a review. SADJ 2010;65(4):160–162, 164–166

Al Sayed AA, Al Sulaiman MH, Mishriky A, Anil S. The role of androgen receptor gene in cyclosporine induced gingival overgrowth. J Periodontal Res 2014;49(5):609–614

Arabaci T, Köse O, Kizildağ A, Albayrak M, Ciçek Y, Kara A. Role of nuclear factor kappa-B in phenytoin-induced gingival overgrowth. Oral Dis 2014;20(3):294–300

Bhatavadekar N, Khandelwal N, Bouquot JE. Oral and maxillofacial pathology case of the month. Plasma cell gingivitis. Tex Dent J 2008;125(4):372–373, 380–383

Bushehri S. Hereditary gingival fibromatosis--review of the literature. J West Soc Periodontol Periodontal Abstr 2014;62(1):3–6

Camilotti RS, Jasper J, Ferreira TB, Antonini F, Poli VD, Pagnoncelli RM. Resection of gingival fibromatosis with high power laser. J Dent Child (Chic) 2015;82(1):47–52

Deas DE, Mealey BL. Response of chronic and aggressive periodontitis to treatment. Periodontol 2000 2010;53:154–166

Eberhard J, Jervøe-Storm PM, Needleman I, Worthington H, Jepsen S. Full-mouth treatment concepts for chronic periodontitis: a systematic review. J Clin Periodontol 2008;35(7):591–604

Eslami A, Sadeghi EM. Mouthbreather's gingivitis: a clinicopathologic review. Compendium 1987;8(1):20–22, 24

Ford PJ, Gamonal J, Seymour GJ. Immunological differences and similarities between chronic periodontitis and aggressive periodontitis. Periodontol 2000 2010;53:111–123

Gawron K, Lazarz-Bartyzel K, Lazarz M, et al. In vitro testing the potential of a novel chimeric IgG variant for inhibiting collagen fibrils formation in recurrent hereditary gingival fibromatosis: chimeric antibody in a gingival model. J Physiol Pharmacol 2014;65(4):585–591

Herrera D, Alonso B, de Arriba L, Santa Cruz I, Serrano C, Sanz M. Acute periodontal lesions. Periodontol 2000 2014;65(1):149–177

Herrera D, Roldán S, Sanz M. The periodontal abscess: a review. J Clin Periodontol 2000;27(6):377–386

Holzhausen M, Ribeiro FS, Gonçalves D, Corrêa FO, Spolidorio LC, Orrico SR. Treatment of gingival fibromatosis associated with Zimmermann-Laband syndrome. J Periodontol 2005;76(9):1559–1562

Jadwat Y, Meyerov R, Lemmer J, Raubenheimer EJ, Feller L. Plasma cell gingivitis: does it exist? Report of a case and review of the literature. SADJ 2008;63(7):394–395

Keestra JA, Grosjean I, Coucke W, Quirynen M, Teughels W. Non-surgical periodontal therapy with systemic antibiotics in patients with untreated aggressive periodontitis: a systematic review and meta-analysis. J Periodontal Res 2015;50(6):689–706

Laskaris G, Demetriou N, Angelopoulos A. Immunofluorescent studies in desquamative gingivitis. J Oral Pathol 1981;10(6):398–407

Laudenbach JM, Simon Z. Common dental and periodontal diseases: evaluation and management. Med Clin North Am 2014;98(6):1239–1260

Lo Russo L, Fedele S, Guiglia R, et al. Diagnostic pathways and clinical significance of desquamative gingivitis. J Periodontol 2008;79(1):4–24

Lo Russo L, Fierro G, Guiglia R, et al. Epidemiology of desquamative gingivitis: evaluation of 125 patients and review of the literature. Int J Dermatol 2009;48(10):1049–1052

Lourenço SV, Lobo AZ, Boggio P, Fezzi F, Sebastião A, Nico MM. Gingival manifestations of orofacial granulomatosis. Arch Dermatol 2008;144(12):1627–1630

Meng HX. Periodontal abscess. Ann Periodontol 1999;4(1):79–83

Mishra MB, Sharma S, Sharma A. Plasma cell gingivitis: an occasional case report. N Y State Dent J 2015;81(5):57–60

Ratcliff PA, Johnson PW. The relationship between oral malodor, gingivitis, and periodontitis. A review. J Periodontol 1999;70(5):485–489

Ruokonen H, Helve T, Arola J, Hietanen J, Lindqvist C, Hagstrom J. "Strawberry like" gingivitis being the first sign of Wegener's granulomatosis. Eur J Intern Med 2009;20(6):651–653

Scully C, Laskaris G. Mucocutaneous disorders. Periodontol 2000 1998;18:81–94

Shangase L, Feller L, Blignaut E. Necrotising ulcerative gingivitis/periodontitis as indicators of HIV-infection. SADJ 2004;59(3):105–108

Silva GL, Soares RV, Zenóbio EG. Periodontal abscess during supportive periodontal therapy: a review of the literature. J Contemp Dent Pract 2008;9(6):82–91

Sklavounou A, Laskaris G. Frequency of desquamative gingivitis in skin diseases. Oral Surg Oral Med Oral Pathol 1983;56(2):141–144

Straka M, Varga I, Erdelský I, Straka-Trapezanlidis M, Krňoulová J. Drug-induced gingival enlargement. Neuroendocrinol Lett 2014;35(7):567–576

Tatakis DN, Trombelli L. Modulation of clinical expression of plaque-induced gingivitis. I. Background review and rationale. J Clin Periodontol 2004;31(4):229–238

Ye X, Shi L, Yin W, Meng L, Wang QK, Bian Z. Further evidence of genetic heterogeneity segregating with hereditary gingival fibromatosis. J Clin Periodontol 2009;36(8):627–633

12. Diseases of the Tongue

Assimakopoulos D, Patrikakos G, Fotika C, Elisaf M. Benign migratory glossitis or geographic tongue: an enigmatic oral lesion. Am J Med 2002;113(9):751–755

Binmadi NO, Jham BC, Meiller TF, Scheper MA. A case of a deeply fissured tongue. Oral Surg Oral Med Oral Pathol Oral Radiol Endod 2010;109(5):659–663

Darwazeh AM, Almelaih AA. Tongue lesions in a Jordanian population. Prevalence, symptoms, subject's knowledge and treatment provided. Med Oral Patol Oral Cir Bucal 2011;16(6):e745–e749

Dreyer WP, de Waal J. Oral medicine case book 7. Migratory stomatitis and geographic tongue. SADJ 2008;63(4):246–247

Fenerli A, Papanicolaou S, Papanicolaou M, Laskaris G. Histocompatibility antigens and geographic tongue. Oral Surg Oral Med Oral Pathol 1993;76(4):476–479

Gurvits GE, Tan A. Black hairy tongue syndrome. World J Gastroenterol 2014;20(31):10845–10850

Kalifatidis A, Albanidou-Farmaki E, Daniilidis M, Markopoulos AK, Karyotis N, Antoniades DZ. HLA alleles and fissured tongue. Int J Immunogenet 2010;37(6):509–511

Klasser GD, Fischer DJ, Epstein JB. Burning mouth syndrome: recognition, understanding, and management. Oral Maxillofac Surg Clin North Am 2008;20(2):255–271, vii

Klosterman T, Tatum SA. Current surgical management of macroglossia. Curr Opin Otolaryngol Head Neck Surg 2015;23(4):302–308

Madani FM, Kuperstein AS. Normal variations of oral anatomy and common oral soft tissue lesions: evaluation and management. Med Clin North Am 2014;98(6):1281–1298

Mock D, Chugh D. Burning mouth syndrome. Int J Oral Sci 2010;2(1):1–4

Pemberton MN. Sublingual varices are not unusual. BMJ 2006;333(7560):202–210

Perkins JA. Overview of macroglossia and its treatment. Curr Opin Otolaryngol Head Neck Surg 2009;17(6):460–465

Thompson DF, Kessler TL. Drug-induced black hairy tongue. Pharmacotherapy 2010;30(6):585–593

Thorp MA, de Waal PJ, Prescott CA. Extreme microglossia. Int J Pediatr Otorhinolaryngol 2003;67(5):473–477

Yarom N, Cantony U, Gorsky M. Prevalence of fissured tongue, geographic tongue and median rhomboid glossitis among Israeli adults of different ethnic origins. Dermatology 2004;209(2):88–94

Zargari O. The prevalence and significance of fissured tongue and geographical tongue in psoriatic patients. Clin Exp Dermatol 2006;31(2):192–195

13. Diseases of the Lips

Agar N, Freeman S. Cheilitis caused by contact allergy to cocamidopropyl betaine in '2-in-1 toothpaste and mouthwash'. Australas J Dermatol 2005;46(1):15–17

Almazrooa SA, Woo SB, Mawardi H, Treister N. Characterization and management of exfoliative cheilitis: a single-center experience. Oral Surg Oral Med Oral Pathol Oral Radiol 2013;116(6):e485–e489

Andrade ES, Sobral AP, Laureano Filho JR, Santos ME, Camargo IB. Cheilitis glandularis and actinic cheilitis: differential diagnoses - report of three unusual cases. Dermatol Online J 2009;15(1):5

Baghestani S, Sadeghi N, Yavarian M, Alghasi H. Lower lip pits in a patient with van der Woude syndrome. J Craniofac Surg 2010;21(5):1380–1381

Connolly M, Kennedy C. Exfoliative cheilitis successfully treated with topical tacrolimus. Br J Dermatol 2004;151(1):241–242

Cross DL, Short LJ. Angular cheilitis occurring during orthodontic treatment: a case series. J Orthod 2008;35(4):229–233

Daniel FI, Alves SR, Vieira DS, Biz MT, Daniel IW, Modolo F. Immunohistochemical expression of DNA methyltransferases 1, 3a, and 3b in actinic cheilitis and lip squamous cell carcinomas. J Oral Pathol Med 2016;45(10):774–779

dos Santos JN, de Sousa SO, Nunes FD, Sotto MN, de Araújo VC. Altered cytokeratin expression in actinic cheilitis. J Cutan Pathol 2003;30(4):237–241

Hanami Y, Motoki Y, Yamamoto T. Successful treatment of plasma cell cheilitis with topical tacrolimus: report of two cases. Dermatol Online J 2011;17(2):6

Jin SP, Cho KH, Huh CH. Plasma cell cheilitis, successfully treated with topical 0.03% tacrolimus ointment. J Dermatolog Treat 2010;21(3):130–132

Junqueira JL, Bönecker M, Furuse C, et al. Actinic cheilitis among agricultural workers in Campinas, Brazil. Community Dent Health 2011;28(1):60–63

Kodama M, Watanabe D, Akita Y, Tamada Y, Matsumoto Y. Photodynamic therapy for the treatment of actinic cheilitis. Photodermatol Photoimmunol Photomed 2007;23(5):209–210

López-Urbano MJ, Villar MA, Ruiz Villaverde R, Avila IR. Granulomatous cheilitis: a condition that merits inclusion in the differential diagnosis of angioedema. J Investig Allergol Clin Immunol 2009;19(1):68–70

Mehta V, Nayak S, Balachandran C. Pigmented contact cheilitis to paraphenylenediamine. Indian J Dermatol 2010;55(1):119–120

Miura M, Isami M, Yagami A, Matsunaga K. Allergic contact cheilitis caused by ditrimethylolpropane triethylhexanoate in a lipstick. Contact Dermat 2011;64(5):301–302

Nico MM, Melo JN, Lourenço SV. Cheilitis glandularis: immunohistochemical expression of protein water channels (aquaporins) in minor labial salivary glands. J Eur Acad Dermatol Venereol 2014;28(3):382–387

Nico MM, Nakano de Melo J, Lourenço SV. Cheilitis glandularis: a clinicopathological study in 22 patients. J Am Acad Dermatol 2010;62(2):233–238

Noonan V, Kemp S, Gallagher G, Kabani S. Exfoliative cheilitis. J Mass Dent Soc 2007;56(2):39

O'Gorman SM, Torgerson RR. Contact allergy in cheilitis. Int J Dermatol 2016;55(7):e386–e391

Oliveira AM, Martins M, Martins A, Ramos de Deus J. Granulomatous cheilitis associated with Crohn's disease. Am J Gastroenterol 2016;111(4):456

Reichart PA, Scheifele Ch, Philipsen HP. [Glandular cheilitis. 2 case reports]. Mund Kiefer Gesichtschir 2002;6(4):266–270

Reiter S, Vered M, Yarom N, Goldsmith C, Gorsky M. Cheilitis glandularis: clinico-histopathological diagnostic criteria. Oral Dis 2011;17(3):335–339

Rocha N, Mota F, Horta M, Lima O, Massa A, Sanches M. Plasma cell cheilitis. J Eur Acad Dermatol Venereol 2004;18(1):96–98

Rosenquist BE. Median lip fissure. J Craniofac Surg 1995;6(5):390–391

Sbano P, Rubegni P, Risulo M, De Nisi MC, Fimiani M. A case of idiopathic granulomatous cheilitis and vulvitis. Int J Dermatol 2007;46(7):720–721

Shah V, Krasemann T. Symmetric lower lip pits - Van Der Woude syndrome. J Paediatr Child Health 2011;47(10):757

Sharon V, Fazel N. Oral candidiasis and angular cheilitis. Dermatol Ther (Heidelb) 2010;23(3):230–242

Skinner N, Junker JA, Flake D, Hoffman R. Clinical inquiries. What is angular cheilitis and how is it treated? J Fam Pract 2005;54(5):470–471

Veysey EC, Orton DI. Photoallergic contact cheilitis due to oxybenzone found in a lip cosmetic. Contact Dermat 2006;55(1):54

Yenidünya MO, Emsen IM, Ozdengil E. Median lower lip fissure. Plast Reconstr Surg 2001;107(3):888–889

14. Soft Tissue Cysts

Adachi P, Soubhia AM, Horikawa FK, Shinohara EH. Mucocele of the glands of Blandin-Nuhn--clinical, pathological, and therapeutical aspects. Oral Maxillofac Surg 2011;15(1):11–13

Aghaghazvini L, Mazaher H, Sharifian H, Aghaghazvini S, Assadi M. Invasive thyroglossal duct cyst papillary carcinoma: a case report. J Med Case Reports 2009;3:9308

Aikawa T, Iida S, Fukuda Y, et al. Nasolabial cyst in a patient with cleft lip and palate. Int J Oral Maxillofac Surg 2008;37(9):874–876

Asami S, Naomoto Y, Yamatsuji T, et al. Lymphoepithelial cyst of the cervical esophagus. J Gastroenterol 2006;41(1):88–89

Bonet-Coloma C, Minguez-Martinez I, Aloy-Prósper A, Galán-Gil S, Peñarrocha-Diago M, Mínguez-Sanz JM. Pediatric oral ranula: clinical follow-up study of 57 cases. Med Oral Patol Oral Cir Bucal 2011;16(2):e158–e162

Brown FH, Houston GD, Lubow RM, Sagan MA. Cyst of the incisive (palatine) papilla. Report of a case. J Periodontol 1987;58(4):274–275

Carlson ER, Ord RA. Benign pediatric salivary gland lesions. Oral Maxillofac Surg Clin North Am 2016;28(1):67–81

Derin S, Koseoglu S, Sahan L, Dere Y, Sahan M. Giant dermoid cyst causing dysphagia and dyspnea. J Craniofac Surg 2016;27(3):e260–e261

Dmytriw AA, Song JS, Gullane P, terBrugge KG, Yu E. Venous vascular malformation of the flor of mouth masquerading as a dermoid tumor. Am J Otolaryngol 2016;37(4):383–386

Fantasia JE, Damm DD. Yellow nodule of floor of mouth. Lymphoepithelial cyst. Gen Dent 2001;49(1):36, 100

Hadi U, Younes A, Ghosseini S, Tawil A. Median palatine cyst: an unusual presentation of a rare entity. Br J Oral Maxillofac Surg 2001;39(4):278–281

Harrison JD. Modern management and pathophysiology of ranula: literature review. Head Neck 2010;32(10):1310–1320

Hayes PA. Hamartomas, eruption cyst, natal tooth and Epstein pearls in a newborn. ASDC J Dent Child 2000;67(5):365–368

Holland AJ, Sparnon AL, LeQuesne GW. Thyroglossal duct cyst or ectopic thyroid gland? J Paediatr Child Health 1997;33(4):346–348

Huang LD, Gao SQ, Dai RJ, et al. Intra-thyroid thyroglossal duct cyst: a case report and review of literature. Int J Clin Exp Pathol 2015;8(6):7229–7233

Jones RS, Dillon J. Non odontogenic cysts of the jaws and treatment in the pediatric population. Oral Maxillofac Surg Clin North Am 2016;28(1):31–44

Karaçal N, Ambarcoğlu O, Kutlu N. Median palatine cyst: report of an unusual entity. Plast Reconstr Surg 2005;115(4):1213–1214

Kuczek A, Beikler T, Herbst H, Flemmig TF. Eruption cyst formation associated with cyclosporin A. J Clin Periodontol 2003;30(5):462–466

Kyriakidou E, Howe T, Veale B, Atkins S. Sublingual dermoid cysts: case report and review of the literature. J Laryngol Otol 2015;129(10):1036–1039

Lee DH, Lim SC, Lee JK. Thyroglossal duct cyst presenting with airway obstruction in an infant. Otolaryngol Head Neck Surg 2011;144(1):127–128

Lin HW, Silver AL, Cunnane ME, Sadow PM, Kieff DA. Lateral dermoid cyst of the floor of mouth: unusual radiologic and pathologic findings. Auris Nasus Larynx 2011;38(5):650–653

Mamabolo MM. General practitioner's pathology case 1. Gingival cyst. SADJ 2006;61(1):23

Mandel L. Salivary gland disorders. Med Clin North Am 2014;98(6):1407–1449

Pedron IG, Galletta VC, Azevedo LH, Corrêa L. Treatment of mucocele of the lower lip with diode laser in pediatric patients: presentation of 2 clinical cases. Pediatr Dent 2010;32(7):539–541

Pereira KM, Nonaka CF, Santos PP, Medeiros AM, Galvão HC. Unusual coexistence of oral lymphoepithelial cyst and benign migratory glossitis. Rev Bras Otorrinolaringol (Engl Ed) 2009;75(2):318

Puranik RS, Vanaki SS. Dentigerous cyst vs. eruption cyst. Aust Dent J 2007;52(4):345

Sheikh AB, Chin OY, Fang CH, Liu JK, Baredes S, Eloy JA. Nasolabial cysts: a systematic review of 311 cases. Laryngoscope 2016;126(1):60–66

Tkaczuk AT, Bhatti M, Caccamese JF Jr, Ord RA, Pereira KD. Cystic lesions of the jaw in children: a 15-year experience. JAMA Otolaryngol Head Neck Surg 2015;141(9):834–839

Wagner VP, Martins MD, Curra M, Martins MA, Munerato MC. Gingival cysts of adults: Retrospective analysis from two centers in South Brazil and a review of the literature. J Int Acad Periodontol 2015;17(1):14–19

Yigit N, Karslioglu Y, Yildizoglu U, Karakoc O. Dermoid cyst of the parotid gland: report of a rare entity with literature review. Head Neck Pathol 2015;9(2):286–292

Zhang B, Yang Z, Zhang RM, et al. Are the patients with anatomic variation of the sublingual/Wharton's duct system predisposed to ranula formation? Int J Pediatr Otorhinolaryngol 2016;83:69–73

15. Viral Infections

Afzal MA, Minor PD, Schild GC. Clinical safety issues of measles, mumps and rubella vaccines. Bull World Health Organ 2000;78(2):199–204

Badger GR. Oral signs of chickenpox (varicella): report of two cases. ASDC J Dent Child 1980;47(5):349–351

Balasubramaniam R, Kuperstein AS, Stoopler ET. Update on oral herpes virus infections. Dent Clin North Am 2014;58(2):265–280

Chen KT, Chang HL, Wang ST, Cheng YT, Yang JY. Epidemiologic features of hand-foot-mouth disease and herpangina caused by enterovirus 71 in Taiwan, 1998-2005. Pediatrics 2007;120(2):e244–e252

Chen YK, Hsue SS, Lin LM, et al. Oral verruca vulgaris. Quintessence Int 2002;33(2):162–163

Cuberos V, Perez J, Lopez CJ, et al. Molecular and serological evidence of the epidemiological association of HPV 13 with focal epithelial hyperplasia: a case-control study. J Clin Virol 2006;37(1):21–26

dos Santos-Pinto L, Giro EM, Pansani CA, Ferrari J, Massucato EM, Spolidório LC. An uncommon focal epithelial hyperplasia manifestation. J Dent Child (Chic) 2009;76(3):233–236

Dreyer WP, de Waal J. Oral medicine case book 15. Intraoral verruca vulgaris. SADJ 2009;64(2):80–81

Dunmire SK, Hogquist KA, Balfour HH. Infectious mononucleosis. Curr Top Microbiol Immunol 2015;390(Pt 1):211–240

Ebell MH, Call M, Shinholser J, Gardner J. Does this patient have infectious mononucleosis? The rational clinical examination systematic review. JAMA 2016;315(14):1502–1509

Falaki F, Amir Chaghmaghi M, Pakfetrat A, Delavarian Z, Mozaffari PM, Pazooki N. Detection of human papilloma virus DNA in seven cases of focal epithelial hyperplasia in Iran. J Oral Pathol Med 2009;38(10):773–776

Feller L, Lemmer J, Wood NH, Jadwat Y, Raubenheimer EJ. HIV-associated oral Kaposi sarcoma and HHV-8: a review. J Int Acad Periodontol 2007;9(4):129–136

Field HJ, Vere Hodge RA. Recent developments in anti-herpesvirus drugs. Br Med Bull 2013;106:213–249

Frydenberg A, Starr M. Hand, foot and mouth disease. Aust Fam Physician 2003;32(8):594–595

Hosoya M, Kawasaki Y, Sato M, et al. Genetic diversity of coxsackievirus A16 associated with hand, foot, and mouth disease epidemics in Japan from 1983 to 2003. J Clin Microbiol 2007;45(1):112–120

Inoue H, Motani-Saitoh H, Sakurada K, et al. Detection of varicella-zoster virus DNA in 414 human trigeminal ganglia from cadavers by the polymerase chain reaction: a comparison of the detection rate of varicella-zoster virus and herpes simplex virus type 1. J Med Virol 2010;82(2):345–349

Jones AC, McGuff HS, Alderson GL. Oral and maxillofacial pathology case of the month. Molluscum contagiosum. Tex Dent J 2005;122(11):1158, 1162

Johnson RW, Alvarez-Pasquin MJ, Bijl M, et al. Herpes zoster epidemiology, management, and disease and economic burden in Europe: a multidisciplinary perspective. Ther Adv Vaccines 2015;3(4):109–120

Katz J, Guelmann M, Stavropolous F, Heft M. Gingival and other oral manifestations in measles virus infection. J Clin Periodontol 2003;30(7):665–668

Kui LL, Xiu HZ, Ning LY. Condyloma acuminatum and human papilloma virus infection in the oral mucosa of children. Pediatr Dent 2003;25(2):149–153

Laskaris G, Sklavounou A. Molluscum contagiosum of the oral mucosa. Oral Surg Oral Med Oral Pathol 1984;58(6):688–691

Lefebvre N, Camuset G, Bui E, Christmann D, Hansmann Y. Koplik spots: a clinical sign with epidemiological implications for measles control. Dermatology 2010;220(3):280–281

López-Pintor RM, Hernández G, de Arriba L, Morales JM, Jiménez C, de Andrés A. Oral ulcers during the course of cytomegalovirus infection in renal transplant recipients. Transplant Proc 2009;41(6):2419–2421

Ma H, Yang H, Zhou Y, Jiang L. Molluscum contagiosum on the lip. J Craniofac Surg 2015;26(7):e681–e682

Nucci V, Torchia D, Cappugi P. Condyloma acuminatum of the tongue treated with photodynamic therapy. Clin Infect Dis 2009;48(9):1330–1332

Ramdass P, Mullick S, Farber HF. Viral skin diseases. Prim Care 2015;42(4):517–567

Ruan F, Yang T, Ma H, et al. Risk factors for hand, foot, and mouth disease and herpangina and the preventive effect of hand-washing. Pediatrics 2011;127(4):e898–e904

Sanchez-Vargas LO, Diaz-Hernandez C, Martinez-Martinez A. Detection of human papilloma virus in oral mucosa of women with cervical lesions and their relation to oral sex practices. Infect Agent Cancer 2010;5(1):25

Steichen O, Dautheville S. Koplik spots in early measles. CMAJ 2009;180(5):583

Steigman AJ, Lipton MM, Braspennickx H. Acute lymphonodular pharyngitis: a newly described condition due to Coxsackie A virus. J Pediatr 1962;61:331–336

Stoopler ET, Balasubramaniam R. Topical and systemic therapies for oral and perioral herpes simplex virus infections. J Calif Dent Assoc 2013;41(4):259–262

Suzuki Y, Taya K, Nakashima K, et al. Risk factors for severe hand foot and mouth disease. Pediatr Int 2010;52(2):203–207

Taylor GS, Long HM, Brooks JM, Rickinson AB, Hislop AD. The immunology of Epstein-Barr virus-induced disease. Annu Rev Immunol 2015;33:787–821

Triantos D, Horefti E, Paximadi E, et al. Presence of human herpes virus-8 in saliva and non-lesional oral mucosa in HIV-infected and oncologic immunocompromised patients. Oral Microbiol Immunol 2004;19(3):201–204

Tovaru S, Parlatescu I, Tovaru M, Cionca L. Primary herpetic gingivostomatitis in children and adults. Quintessence Int 2009;40(2):119–124

Zhuang ZC, Kou ZQ, Bai YJ, et al. Epidemiological research on hand, foot and mouth disease in Mainland China. Viruses 2015;7(12):6400–6411

16. Oral Manifestations of HIV Infection

Akpa OM, Oyejola BA. Modeling the transmission dynamics of HIV/AIDS epidemics: an introduction and a review. J Infect Dev Ctries 2010;4(10):597–608

Baccaglini L, Atkinson JC, Patton LL, Glick M, Ficarra G, Peterson DE. Management of oral lesions in HIV-positive patients. Oral Surg Oral Med Oral Pathol Oral Radiol Endod 2007;103(Suppl):50.e1–50.e23

Blank LJ, Rompalo AM, Erbelding EJ, Zenilman JM, Ghanem KG. Treatment of syphilis in HIV-infected subjects: a systematic review of the literature. Sex Transm Infect 2011;87(1):9–16

EC-Clearinghouse on Oral Problems Related to HIV Infection and WHO Collaborating Centre on Oral Manifestations of the Immunodeficiency Virus. Classification and diagnostic criteria for oral lesions in HIV infection. J Oral Pathol Med 1993;22(7):289–291

Economopoulou P, Laskaris G, Kittas C. Oral histoplasmosis as an indicator of HIV infection. Oral Surg Oral Med Oral Pathol Oral Radiol Endod 1998;86(2):203–206

Guidelines on the Treatment of Skin and Oral HIV-Associated Conditions in Children and Adults. Geneva: World Health Organization; 2014

Gonçalves LS, Gonçalves BM, Fontes TV. Periodontal disease in HIV-infected adults in the HAART era: Clinical, immunological, and microbiological aspects. Arch Oral Biol 2013;58(10):1385–1396

Greenspan JS, Greenspan D. The epidemiology of the oral lesions of HIV infection in the developed world. Oral Dis 2002;8(Suppl 2):34–39

Greenspan JS, Greenspan D, Webster-Cyriaque J. Hairy leukoplakia; lessons learned: 30-plus years. Oral Dis 2016;22(Suppl 1):120–127

Laskaris G, Hadjivassiliou M, Stratigos J. Oral signs and symptoms in 160 Greek HIV-infected patients. J Oral Pathol Med 1992;21(3):120–123

Laskaris G, Laskaris M, Theodoridou M. Oral hairy leukoplakia in a child with AIDS. Oral Surg Oral Med Oral Pathol Oral Radiol Endod 1995;79(5):570–571

Laskaris G, Potouridou I, Laskaris M, Stratigos J. Gingival lesions of HIV infection in 178 Greek patients. Oral Surg Oral Med Oral Pathol 1992;74(2):168–171

Laskaris G, Stergiou G, Kittas C, Scully C. Hodgkin's disease involving the gingiva in AIDS. Eur J Cancer B Oral Oncol 1992;28B(1):39–41

Laskaris G. AIDS and the dental profession in Greece. EDS Mag 1993;4:19–22

Laskaris G. Oral manifestations of HIV disease. Clin Dermatol 2000;18(4):447–455

Levy A, Johnston K, Annemans L, Tramarin A, Montaner J. The impact of disease stage on direct medical costs of HIV management: a review of the international literature. Pharmacoeconomics 2010;28(Suppl 1):35–47

Nakou M, Kamma J, Gargalianos P, Laskaris G, Mitsis F. Periodontal microflora of HIV infected patients with periodontitis. Anaerobe 1997;3(2-3):97–102

Patton LL. Current strategies for prevention of oral manifestations of human immunodeficiency virus. Oral Surg Oral Med Oral Pathol Oral Radiol 2016;121(1):29–38

Patton LL, Ranganathan K, Naidoo S, et al. Oral lesions, HIV phenotypes, and management of HIV-related disease: Workshop 4A. Adv Dent Res 2011;23(1):112–116

Scully C, Laskaris G, Pindborg J, Porter SR, Reichart P. Oral manifestations of HIV infection and their management. I. More common lesions. Oral Surg Oral Med Oral Pathol 1991;71(2):158–166

Scully C, Laskaris G, Pindborg J, Porter SR, Reichart P. Oral manifestations of HIV infection and their management. II. Less common lesions. Oral Surg Oral Med Oral Pathol 1991;71(2):167–171

Vidya KM, Rao UK, Nittayananta W, Liu H, Owotade FJ. Oral mycoses and other opportunistic infections in HIV: therapy and emerging problems - a workshop report. Oral Dis 2016; 22(Suppl 1):158–165

Wild R, Balmer MC. Have we forgotten? Oral manifestations of Kaposi's sarcoma. Sex Transm Infect 2015;91(5):345

Zhang X, Reichart PA, Song Y. Oral manifestations of HIV/AIDS in China: a review. Oral Maxillofac Surg 2009;13(2):63–68

17. Bacterial Infections

Aguiar AM, Enwonwu CO, Pires FR. Noma (cancrum oris) associated with oral myiasis in an adult. Oral Dis 2003;9(3):158–159

Al Yaghchi C, Cruise A, Kapoor K, Singh A, Harcourt J. Out-patient management of patients with a peritonsillar abscess. Clin Otolaryngol 2008;33(1):52–55

Amin AN, Cerceo EA, Deitelzweig SB, Pile JC, Rosenberg DJ, Sherman BM. Hospitalist perspective on the treatment of skin and soft tissue infections. Mayo Clin Proc 2014;89(10):1436–1451

Atzori L, Ferreli C, Zucca M, Fanni D, Aste N. Facial cellulitis associated with Pseudomonas aeruginosa complicating ophthalmic herpes zoster. Dermatol Online J 2004;10(2):20

Bloom MW, Carter EL. Bullous impetigo of the face after epilation by threading. Arch Dermatol 2005;141(9):1174–1175

Bouman MA, Marck KW, Griep JE, Marck RE, Huijing MA, Werker PM. Early outcome of noma surgery. J Plast Reconstr Aesthet Surg 2010;63(12):2052–2056

Canzi P, Occhini A, Pagella F, Marchal F, Benazzo M. Sialendoscopy in juvenile recurrent parotitis: a review of the literature. Acta Otorhinolaryngol Ital 2013;33(6):367–373

Dahlén G, Blomquist S, Carlén A. A retrospective study on the microbiology in patients with oral complaints and oral mucosal lesions. Oral Dis 2009;15(4):265–272

de Abreu MA, Alchorne MM, Michalany NS, Weckx LL, Pimentel DR, Hirata CH. The oral mucosa in paucibacillary leprosy: a clinical and histopathological study. Oral Surg Oral Med Oral Pathol Oral Radiol Endod 2007;103(5):e48–e52

de Abreu MA, Michalany NS, Weckx LL, Neto Pimentel DR, Hirata CH, de Avelar Alchorne MM. The oral mucosa in leprosy: a clinical and histopathological study. Rev Bras Otorrinolaringol (Engl Ed) 2006;72(3):312–316

Delli K, Spijkervet FK, Vissink A. Salivary gland diseases: infections, sialolithiasis and mucoceles. Monogr Oral Sci 2014;24:135–148

Duijsters CE, Halbertsma FJ, Kornelisse RF, Arents NL, Andriessen P. Recurring staphylococcal scalded skin syndrome in a very low birth weight infant: a case report. J Med Case Reports 2009;3:7313

Feller L, Altini M, Chandran R, et al. Noma (cancrum oris) in the South African context. J Oral Pathol Med 2014;43(1):1–6

Gelesko S, Blakey GH, Partrick M, et al. Comparison of periodontal inflammatory disease in young adults with and without pericoronitis involving mandibular third molars. J Oral Maxillofac Surg 2009;67(1):134–139

Götz C, Reinhart E, Wolff KD, Kolk A. Oral soft tissue infections: causes, therapeutic approaches and microbiological spectrum with focus on antibiotic treatment. J Craniomaxillofac Surg 2015;43(9):1849–1854

Handler MZ, Schwartz RA. Staphylococcal scalded skin syndrome: diagnosis and management in children and adults. J Eur Acad Dermatol Venereol 2014;28(11):1418–1423

Herrera D, Alonso B, de Arriba L, Santa Cruz I, Serrano C, Sanz M. Acute periodontal lesions. Periodontol 2000 2014;65(1):149–177

Hidaka H, Kuriyama S, Yano H, Tsuji I, Kobayashi T. Precipitating factors in the pathogenesis of peritonsillar abscess and bacteriological significance of the Streptococcus milleri group. Eur J Clin Microbiol Infect Dis 2011;30(4):527–532

Huang L, Jiang B, Cai X, et al. Multi-space infections in the head and neck: Do underlying systemic diseases have a predictive role in life-threatening complications? J Oral Maxillofac Surg 2015;73(7):1320.e1–1320.e10

Kadam S, Tagare A, Deodhar J, Tawade Y, Pandit A. Staphylococcal scalded skin syndrome in a neonate. Indian J Pediatr 2009;76(10):1074

Kato T, Fujimoto N, Nakanishi G, et al. Adult staphylococcal scalded skin syndrome successfully treated with plasma exchange. Acta Derm Venereol 2015;95(5):612–613

Klotz SA, Ianas V, Elliott SP. Cat-scratch disease. Am Fam Physician 2011;83(2):152–155

Kolokotronis A, Doumas S, Lambroudi M, Lysitsa S, Epivatianos A, Antoniades D. Facial and perioral primary impetigo: a clinical study. J Clin Pediatr Dent 2005;29(4):341–345

Laskaris G. PL10: Oral manifestations of orogenital bacterial infections. Oral Dis 2006;12(s1):2–3

Laskaris GC, Nicolis GD. Lupus vulgaris of the oral mucosa. Report of 4 cases associated with asymptomatic pulmonary tuberculosis. Dermatologica 1981;162(3):183–190

Lee YJ, Jeong YM, Lee HS, Hwang SH. The efficacy of corticosteroids in the treatment of peritonsillar abscess: a meta-analysis. Clin Exp Otorhinolaryngol 2016;9(2):89–97

Lepelletier D, Pinaud V, Le Conte P, et al; French PTA Study Group. Peritonsillar abscess (PTA): clinical characteristics, microbiology, drug exposures and outcomes of a large multicenter cohort survey of 412 patients hospitalized in 13 French university hospitals. Eur J Clin Microbiol Infect Dis 2016;35(5):867–873

López de Blanc S, Sambuelli R, Femopase F, et al. Bacillary angiomatosis affecting the oral cavity. Report of two cases and review. J Oral Pathol Med 2000;29(2):91–96

Mazur-Melewska K, Mania A, Kemnitz P, Figlerowicz M, Służewski W. Cat-scratch disease: a wide spectrum of clinical pictures. Postepy Dermatol Alergol 2015;32(3):216–220

Moghimi M, Salentijn E, Debets-Ossenkop Y, Karagozoglu KH, Forouzanfar T. Treatment of cervicofacial actinomycosis: a report of 19 cases and review of literature. Med Oral Patol Oral Cir Bucal 2013;18(4):e627–e632

Mohammed-Ali RI, Collyer J, Garg M. Osteomyelitis of the mandible secondary to pericoronitis of an impacted third molar. Dent Update 2010;37(2):106–108

Nuwwareh S. Managing a patient with pericoronitis. J Can Dent Assoc 2013;79:d169

Ochs MW, Dolwick MF. Facial erysipelas: report of a case and review of the literature. J Oral Maxillofac Surg 1991;49(10):1116–1120

Paul SP, Heaton PA. At a glance: scarlet fever in children. J Fam Health Care 2014;24(3):25–27

Prabhu K, Nair S, Chacko AG; Ramamani. Acute submandibular sialadenitis as a cause of unilateral neck swelling after posterior fossa surgery in sitting position. Neurol India 2010;58(6):963–964

Romani L, Steer AC, Whitfeld MJ, Kaldor JM. Prevalence of scabies and impetigo worldwide: a systematic review. Lancet Infect Dis 2015;15(8):960–967

Sammut S, Malden N, Lopes V. Facial cutaneous sinuses of dental origin - a diagnostic challenge. Br Dent J 2013;215(11):555–558

Smolka W, Burger H, Iizuka T, Smolka K. Primary tuberculosis of the oral cavity in an elderly nonimmunosuppressed patient: case report and review of the literature. Arch Otolaryngol Head Neck Surg 2008;134(10):1107–1109

Todescan S, Nizar R. Managing patients with necrotizing ulcerative periodontitis. J Can Dent Assoc 2013;79:d44

Uluğ M. Evaluation of cat scratch disease cases reported from Turkey between 1996 and 2013 and review of the literature. Cent Eur J Public Health 2015;23(2):146–151

Wilson KF, Meier JD, Ward PD. Salivary gland disorders. Am Fam Physician 2014;89(11):882–888

Yamalik K, Bozkaya S. The predictivity of mandibular third molar position as a risk indicator for pericoronitis. Clin Oral Investig 2008;12(1):9–14

Yemisen M, Sagit M, Karakas O. Facial bullous cellulitis caused by acute sinusitis. Int J Infect Dis 2009;13(6):e525–e526

18. Sexually Transmitted Bacterial Infections

Ahmed N, Pillay A, Lawler M, Bobat R, Archary M. Donovanosis causing lymphadenitis, mastoiditis, and meningitis in a child. Lancet 2015;385(9987):2644

Balmelli C, Günthard HF. Gonococcal tonsillar infection--a case report and literature review. Infection 2003;31(5):362–365

Compilato D, Amato S, Campisi G. Resurgence of syphilis: a diagnosis based on unusual oral mucosa lesions. Oral Surg Oral Med Oral Pathol Oral Radiol Endod 2009;108(3):e45–e49

Copeland NK, Decker CF. Other sexually transmitted diseases chancroid and donovanosis. Dis Mon 2016;62(8):306–313

Dan M, Poch F, Amitai Z, Gefen D, Shohat T. Pharyngeal Gonorrhea in female sex workers: Response to a single 2-g dose of azithromycin. Sex Transm Dis 2006;33(8):512–515

Doddridge M, Muirhead R. Donovanosis of the oral cavity. Case report. Aust Dent J 1994;39(4):203–205

Duarte EC, da Silva LM, Naves MD, do Carmo MA, de Aguiar MC. Primary syphilis of oral mucosa: case report of an unusual manifestation. Quintessence Int 2004;35(9):728–730

French P, Gomberg M, Janier M, Schmidt B, van Voorst Vader P, Young H. IUST: 2008 European guidelines on the management of syphilis. Int J STD AIDS 2009;20(5):300–309

Holmes KK, Sparling PF, Stamm WE, et al. Sexually Transmitted Diseases. 4th ed. New York, NY: McGraw-Hill; 2008

Nissanka-Jayasuriya EH, Odell EW, Phillips C. Dental stigmata of congenital syphilis: a historic review with present day relevance. Head Neck Pathol 2016;10(3):327–331

O'Farrell N, Moi H. 2016 European guideline on donovanosis. Int J STD AIDS 2016;27(8):605–607

Pires FR, da Silva PJ, Natal RF, et al. Clinicopathologic features, microvessel density, and immunohistochemical expression of ICAM-1 and VEGF in 15 cases of secondary syphilis with oral manifestations. Oral Surg Oral Med Oral Pathol Oral Radiol 2016;121(3):274–281

Ramos-E-Silva M. Facial and oral aspects of some venereal and tropical diseases. Acta Dermatovenerol Croat 2004;12(3):173–180

Veeranna S, Raghu TY. Oral donovanosis. Int J STD AIDS 2002;13(12):855–856

19. Fungal Infections

Abreu e Silva MA, Salum FG, Figueiredo MA, Cherubini K. Important aspects of oral paracoccidioidomycosis--a literature review. Mycoses 2013;56(3):189–199

Akin L, Herford AS, Cicciù M. Oral presentation of disseminated histoplasmosis: a case report and literature review. J Oral Maxillofac Surg 2011;69(2):535–541

Brazão-Silva MT, Andrade MF, Franco T, et al. Paracoccidioidomycosis: a series of 66 patients with oral lesions from an endemic area. Mycoses 2011;54(4):e189–e195

Chambers MS, Lyzak WA, Martin JW, Lyzak JS, Toth BB. Oral complications associated with aspergillosis in patients with a hematologic malignancy. Presentation and treatment. Oral Surg Oral Med Oral Pathol Oral Radiol Endod 1995;79(5):559–563

Cho H, Lee KH, Colquhoun AN, Evans SA. Invasive oral aspergillosis in a patient with acute myeloid leukaemia. Aust Dent J 2010;55(2):214–218

Dimaka K, Mallis A, Naxakis SS, et al. Chronic rhinocerebral mucormycosis: a rare case report and review of the literature. Mycoses 2014;57(11):699–702

Dogan MC, Leblebisatan G, Haytac MC, Antmen B, Surmegozler O. Oral mucormycosis in children with leukemia: report of 2 cases. Quintessence Int 2007;38(6):515–520

Economopoulou P, Laskaris G, Ferekidis E, Kanelis N. Rhinocerebral mucormycosis with severe oral lesions: a case report. J Oral Maxillofac Surg 1995;53(2):215–217

Klein IP, Martins MA, Martins MD, Carrard VC. Diagnosis of HIV infection on the basis of histoplasmosis-related oral ulceration. Spec Care Dentist 2016;36(2):99–103

Kruse AL, Zwahlen RA, Bredell MG, Gengler C, Dannemann C, Grätz KW. Primary blastomycosis of oral cavity. J Craniofac Surg 2010;21(1):121–123

Liu X, Hua H. Oral manifestation of chronic mucocutaneous candidiasis: seven case reports. J Oral Pathol Med 2007;36(9):528–532

Mignogna MD, Fortuna G, Leuci S, et al. Mucormycosis in immunocompetent patients: a case-series of patients with maxillary sinus involvement and a critical review of the literature. Int J Infect Dis 2011;15(8):e533–e540

Monteil RA, Hofman P, Michiels JF, Loubière R. Oral cryptococcosis: case report of salivary gland involvement in an AIDS patient. J Oral Pathol Med 1997;26(1):53–56

Motta-Silva AC, Aleva NA, Chavasco JK, Armond MC, França JP, Pereira LJ. Erythematous oral candidiasis in patients with controlled type II diabetes mellitus and complete dentures. Mycopathologia 2010;169(3):215–223

Muzyka BC, Epifanio RN. Update on oral fungal infections. Dent Clin North Am 2013;57(4):561–581

Nelwan EJ, Wisaksana R. Clinical manifestation of oral candidiasis in a HIV patient. Acta Med Indones 2010;42(1):43–44

Nittayananta W. Oral fungi in HIV: challenges in antifungal therapies. Oral Dis 2016;22(Suppl 1):107–113

Pedreira RdoP, Guimarães EP, de Carli ML, Magalhães EM, Pereira AA, Hanemann JA. Paracoccidioidomycosis mimicking squamous cell carcinoma on the dorsum of the tongue and review of published literature. Mycopathologia 2014;177(5-6):325–329

Rucci J, Eisinger G, Miranda-Gomez G, Nguyen J. Blastomycosis of the head and neck. Am J Otolaryngol 2014;35(3):390–395

Silva CO, Almeida AS, Pereira AA, Sallum AW, Hanemann JA, Tatakis DN. Gingival involvement in oral paracoccidioidomycosis. J Periodontol 2007;78(7):1229–1234

Vidya KM, Rao UK, Nittayananta W, Liu H, Owotade FJ. Oral mycoses and other opportunistic infections in HIV: therapy and emerging problems - a workshop report. Oral Dis 2016; 22(Suppl 1):158–165

20. Protozoal and Parasitic Infections

Cruz AF, Resende RG, Albuquerque DR, de Lacerda JC, Leite CF, Ferreira Aguiar MC. Mucosal leishmaniasis in Brazilian patients: two case reports with similar clinical presentation and different approaches. Oral Surg Oral Med Oral Pathol Oral Radiol 2016;S2212-4403(16)00088-2

Delgado-Azañero WA, Mosqueda-Taylor A, Carlos-Bregni R, Del Muro-Delgado R, Díaz-Franco MA, Contreras-Vidaurre E. Oral cysticercosis: a collaborative study of 16 cases. Oral Surg Oral Med Oral Pathol Oral Radiol Endod 2007;103(4):528–533

de Souza PE, Barreto DC, Fonseca LM, de Paula AM, Silva EC, Gomez RS. Cysticercosis of the oral cavity: report of seven cases. Oral Dis 2000;6(4):253–255

Hassona Y, Scully C, Aguida M, de Almeida OP. Flies and the mouth. J Investig Clin Dent 2014;5(2):98–103

Hosur MB, Byakodi S, Puranik RS, Vanaki SS, Puranik SR, Shivakumar MS. Oral cysticercosis: A case report and review of literature. J Maxillofac Oral Surg 2015;14(3):853–857

Kulkarni PG, Palakurthy P, Muddana K, Nandan RK. Oral cysticercosis: a diagnostic dilemma. J Clin Diagn Res 2015;9(6):ZD01–ZD02

Kumar P, Sharma PK, Jain RK, Gautam RK, Bhardwaj M, Kar HK. Oral ulcer as an unusual feature of visceral leishmaniasis in an AIDS patient. Indian J Med Sci 2007;61(2):97–101

Kumar P, Singh V. Oral myiasis: case report and review of literature. Oral Maxillofac Surg 2014;18(1):25–29

Milián MA, Bagán JV, Jiménez Y, Pérez A, Scully C. Oral leishmaniasis in a HIV-positive patient. Report of a case involving the palate. Oral Dis 2002;8(1):59–61

Sankari LS, Ramakrishnan K. Oral myiasis caused by Chrysomya bezziana. J Oral Maxillofac Pathol 2010;14(1):16–18

Sharma J, Mamatha GP, Acharya R. Primary oral myiasis: a case report. Med Oral Patol Oral Cir Bucal 2008;13(11):E714–E716

21. Orofacial Granulomatosis

Al-Hamad A, Porter S, Fedele S. Orofacial granulomatosis. Dermatol Clin 2015;33(3):433–446

Alawi F. An update on granulomatous diseases of the oral tissues. Dent Clin North Am 2013;57(4):657–671

Fukuhara K, Fukuhara A, Tsugawa J, Oma S, Tsuboi Y. Radiculopathy in patients with Heerfordt's syndrome: two case presentations and review of the literature [in Japanese]. Brain Nerve 2013;65(8):989–992

Govender P, Berman JS. The diagnosis of sarcoidosis. Clin Chest Med 2015;36(4):585–602

Hagen JW, Swoger JM, Grandinetti LM. Cutaneous manifestations of Crohn disease. Dermatol Clin 2015;33(3):417–431

Kittisupamongkol W. Heerfordt syndrome. QJM 2009;102(2):149

Lazzerini M, Bramuzzo M, Ventura A. Association between orofacial granulomatosis and Crohn's disease in children: systematic review. World J Gastroenterol 2014;20(23):7497–7504

Liu R, Yu S. Melkersson-Rosenthal syndrome: a review of seven patients. J Clin Neurosci 2013;20(7):993–995

Mandel L. Salivary gland disorders. Med Clin North Am 2014;98(6):1407–1449

Motswaledi MH, Khammissa RA, Jadwat Y, Lemmer J, Feller L. Oral sarcoidosis: a case report and review of the literature. Aust Dent J 2014;59(3):389–394

Ozgursoy OB, Karatayli Ozgursoy S, Tulunay O, Kemal O, Akyol A, Dursun G. Melkersson-Rosenthal syndrome revisited as a misdiagnosed disease. Am J Otolaryngol 2009;30(1):33–37

Petropoulos IK, Zuber JP, Guex-Crosier Y. Heerfordt syndrome with unilateral facial nerve palsy: a rare presentation of sarcoidosis. Klin Monatsbl Augenheilkd 2008;225(5):453–456

Sciubba JJ, Said-Al-Naief N. Orofacial granulomatosis: presentation, pathology and management of 13 cases. J Oral Pathol Med 2003;32(10):576–585

Sobjanek M, Michajłowski I, Zelazny I, Medrzycka-Dabrowska W, Włodarkiewicz A. What is the most effective treatment of cheilitis granulomatosa in Melkersson-Rosenthal syndrome? J Eur Acad Dermatol Venereol 2010;24(3):364–365

Thomas TK, Neelakandan RS, Bhargava D, Deshpande A. Orofacial granulomatosis: a clinicopathologic correlation. Head Neck Pathol 2011;5(2):133–136

Troiano G, Dioguardi M, Giannatempo G, et al. Orofacial granulomatosis: clinical signs of different pathologies. Med Princ Pract 2015;24(2):117–122

22. Diseases with Possible Immunopathogenesis

Alpsoy E. Behçet's disease: a comprehensive review with a focus on epidemiology, etiology and clinical features, and management of mucocutaneous lesions. J Dermatol 2016;43(6):620–632

Feder HM, Salazar JC. A clinical review of 105 patients with PFAPA (a periodic fever syndrome). Acta Paediatr 2010;99(2):178–184

Greco A, Marinelli C, Fusconi M, et al. Clinic manifestations in granulomatosis with polyangiitis. Int J Immunopathol Pharmacol 2016;29(2):151–159

Laskaris G. Advances in the classification and treatment of recurrent aphthous stomatitis. Balk J Stomatol 1999;3:83–84

Lopalco G, Rigante D, Venerito V, et al. Management of small vessel vasculitides. Curr Rheumatol Rep 2016;18(6):36

Messadi DV, Younai F. Aphthous ulcers. Dermatol Ther (Heidelb) 2010;23(3):281–290

Muñoz-Gómez S, Cunha BA. Recurrent fever of unknown origin (FUO) due to periodic fever, aphthous stomatitis, pharyngitis and adenitis (FAPA) syndrome in an adult. J Clin Med 2013;2(1):45–48

Ní Ríordáin R, Shirlaw P, Alajbeg I, et al. World Workshop on Oral Medicine VI: Patient-reported outcome measures and oral mucosal disease: current status and future direction. Oral Surg Oral Med Oral Pathol Oral Radiol 2015;120(2):152–60.e11

O'Devaney K, Ferlito A, Hunter BC, Devaney SL, Rinaldo A. Wegener's granulomatosis of the head and neck. Ann Otol Rhinol Laryngol 1998;107(5, Pt 1):439–445

Ruokonen H, Helve T, Arola J, Hietanen J, Lindqvist C, Hagstrom J. "Strawberry like" gingivitis being the first sign of Wegener's granulomatosis. Eur J Intern Med 2009;20(6):651–653

Scully C, Hodgson T. Recurrent oral ulceration: aphthous-like ulcers in periodic syndromes. Oral Surg Oral Med Oral Pathol Oral Radiol Endod 2008;106(6):845–852

Sfikakis PP, Markomichelakis N, Alpsoy E, et al. Anti-TNF therapy in the management of Behçet's disease--review and basis for recommendations. Rheumatology (Oxford) 2007;46(5):736–741

Shiva Prasad BN, Balasubramanian R. Chronic otitis media and facial paralysis as a presenting feature of Wegener's granulomatosis. Singapore Med J 2009;50(4):e155–e157

Shivhare P, Gupta A, Yadav M, Konidena A, Shankarnarayan L. Evaluation of different diagnostic criteria of diseases manifesting the oral cavity - a review. Part-1. J Oral Biol Craniofac Res 2016;6(2):135–141

Skef W, Hamilton MJ, Arayssi T. Gastrointestinal Behçet's disease: a review. World J Gastroenterol 2015;21(13):3801–3812

Stratigos AJ, Laskaris G, Stratigos JD. Behçet disease. Semin Neurol 1992;12(4):346–357

Tarakji B, Gazal G, Al-Maweri SA, Azzeghaiby SN, Alaizari N. Guideline for the diagnosis and treatment of recurrent aphthous stomatitis for dental practitioners. J Int Oral Health 2015;7(5):74–80

Wojciechowska J, Krajewski W, Krajewski P, Kręcicki T. Granulomatosis with polyangiitis in otolaryngologist practice: a review of current knowledge. Clin Exp Otorhinolaryngol 2016;9(1):8–13

Wong KK, Finlay JC, Moxham JP. Role of tonsillectomy in PFAPA syndrome. Arch Otolaryngol Head Neck Surg 2008;134(1):16–19

23. Autoimmune Diseases

Aliko A, Alushi A, Tafaj A, Lela F. Oral mucosa involvement in rheumatoid arthritis, systemic lupus erythematosus and systemic sclerosis. Int Dent J 2010;60(5):353–358

Bascones-Martínez A, García-García V, Meurman JH, Requena-Caballero L. Immune-mediated diseases: what can be found in the oral cavity? Int J Dermatol 2015;54(3):258–270

Cohen SJ, Pittelkow MR, Su WP. Cutaneous manifestations of cryoglobulinemia: clinical and histopathologic study of seventy-two patients. J Am Acad Dermatol 1991;25(1, Pt 1):21–27

Cornella SL, Stine JG, Kelly V, Caldwell SH, Shah NL. Persistence of mixed cryoglobulinemia despite cure of hepatitis C with new oral antiviral therapy including direct-acting antiviral sofosbuvir: A case series. Postgrad Med 2015;127(4):413–417

del Olmo JA, Pascual I, Bagán JV, et al. Prevalence of hepatitis C virus in patients with lichen planus of the oral cavity and chronic liver disease. Eur J Oral Sci 2000;108(5):378–382

Fauchais AL, Martel C, Gondran G, et al. Immunological profile in primary Sjögren syndrome: clinical significance, prognosis and long-term evolution to other auto-immune disease. Autoimmun Rev 2010;9(9):595–599

Fedele S, Wolff A, Strietzel F, López M, Porter SR, Konttinen YT. Neuroelectrostimulation in treatment of hyposalivation and xerostomia in Sjögren's syndrome: a salivary pacemaker. J Rheumatol 2008;35(8):1489–1494

Ferro F, Vagelli R, Bruni C, et al. One year in review 2016: Sjögren's syndrome. Clin Exp Rheumatol 2016;34(2):161–171

Fortuna G, Brennan MT. Systemic lupus erythematosus: epidemiology, pathophysiology, manifestations, and management. Dent Clin North Am 2013;57(4):631–655

Gordon JK, Domsic RT. Clinical trial design issues in systemic sclerosis: an update. Curr Rheumatol Rep 2016;18(6):38

Grossmann SdeM, Teixeira R, de Aguiar MC, de Moura MD, do Carmo MA. Oral mucosal conditions in chronic hepatitis C Brazilian patients: a cross-sectional study. J Public Health Dent 2009;69(3):168–175

Healy CM, Tobin AM, Kirby B, Flint SR. Oral lesions as an initial manifestation of dermatomyositis with occult malignancy. Oral Surg Oral Med Oral Pathol Oral Radiol Endod 2006;101(2):184–187

Helenius LM, Meurman JH, Helenius I, et al. Oral and salivary parameters in patients with rheumatic diseases. Acta Odontol Scand 2005;63(5):284–293

Imanguli MM, Pavletic SZ, Guadagnini JP, Brahim JS, Atkinson JC. Chronic graft versus host disease of oral mucosa: review of available therapies. Oral Surg Oral Med Oral Pathol Oral Radiol Endod 2006;101(2):175–183

Imanguli MM, Swaim WD, League SC, Gress RE, Pavletic SZ, Hakim FT. Increased T-bet+ cytotoxic effectors and type I interferon-mediated processes in chronic graft-versus-host disease of the oral mucosa. Blood 2009;113(15):3620–3630

Klasser GD, Balasubramaniam R, Epstein J. Topical review-connective tissue diseases: orofacial manifestations including pain. J Orofac Pain 2007;21(3):171–184

Kojima M, Nakamura N, Matsuda H, Kaba S, Itoh H, Masawa N. HIV-unrelated benign lymphoepithelial cyst of the parotid glands containing lymphoepithelial lesion--like structures: a report of 3 cases. Int J Surg Pathol 2009;17(6):421–425

Márton K, Hermann P, Dankó K, Fejérdy P, Madléna M, Nagy G. Evaluation of oral manifestations and masticatory force in patients with polymyositis and dermatomyositis. J Oral Pathol Med 2005;34(3):164–169

Margaix-Muñoz M, Bagán JV, Jiménez Y, Sarrión MG, Poveda-Roda R. Graftversus-host disease affecting oral cavity. A review. J Clin Exp Dent 2015;7(1):e138–e145

Mays JW, Fassil H, Edwards DA, Pavletic SZ, Bassim CW. Oral chronic graftversus-host disease: current pathogenesis, therapy, and research. Oral Dis 2013;19(4):327–346

Mays JW, Sarmadi M, Moutsopoulos NM. Oral manifestations of systemic autoimmune and inflammatory diseases: diagnosis and clinical management. J Evid Based Dent Pract 2012;12(3, Suppl):265–282

Mignogna MD, Fedele S, Lo Russo L, Lo Muzio L, Wolff A. Sjögren's syndrome: the diagnostic potential of early oral manifestations preceding hyposalivation/xerostomia. J Oral Pathol Med 2005;34(1):1–6

Nocturne G, Cornec D, Seror R, Mariette X. New biological therapies in Sjögren's syndrome. Best Pract Res Clin Rheumatol 2015;29(6):783–793

Ponte C, Rodrigues AF, O'Neill L, Luqmani RA. Giant cell arteritis: current treatment and management. World J Clin Cases 2015;3(6):484–494

Porter S, Scully C. Connective tissue disorders and the mouth. Dent Update 2008;35(5):294–296, 298–300, 302

Quock RL. Xerostomia: current streams of investigation. Oral Surg Oral Med Oral Pathol Oral Radiol 2016;122(1):53–60

Reiter S, Winocur E, Goldsmith C, Emodi-Perlman A, Gorsky M. Giant cell arteritis misdiagnosed as temporomandibular disorder: a case report and review of the literature. J Orofac Pain 2009;23(4):360–365

Shiboski SC, Shiboski CH, Criswell L, et al; Sjögren's International Collaborative Clinical Alliance (SICCA) Research Groups. American College of Rheumatology classification criteria for Sjögren's syndrome: a data-driven, expert consensus approach in the Sjögren's International Collaborative Clinical Alliance cohort. Arthritis Care Res (Hoboken) 2012;64(4):475–487

Steel L, Khan A, Dasgupta B. Giant cell arteritis: beyond corticosteroids. Drugs Aging 2015;32(8):591–599

Tanaka TI, Geist SM. Dermatomyositis: a contemporary review for oral health care providers. Oral Surg Oral Med Oral Pathol Oral Radiol 2012;114(5):e1–e8

Tang L, Marcell L, Kottilil S. Systemic manifestations of hepatitis C infection. Infect Agent Cancer 2016;11:29

Treister NS, Stevenson K, Kim H, Woo SB, Soiffer R, Cutler C. Oral chronic graftversus-host disease scoring using the NIH consensus criteria. Biol Blood Marrow Transplant 2010;16(1):108–114

Turner MD. Hyposalivation and xerostomia: etiology, complications and medical management. Dent Clin North Am 2016;60(2):435–443

Varga E, Field EA, Tyldesley WR. Orofacial manifestations of mixed connective tissue disease. Br Dent J 1990;168(8):330–331

Vitali C, Bombardieri S, Jonsson R, et al; European Study Group on Classification Criteria for Sjögren's Syndrome. Classification criteria for Sjögren's syndrome: a revised version of the European criteria proposed by the American-European Consensus Group. Ann Rheum Dis 2002;61(6):554–558

Vivino FB, Carsons SE, Foulks G, et al. New Treatment Guidelines for Sjogren's Disease. Rheum Dis Clin N Am 2016;42:531-551

24. Immunodeficiencies

Abinun M. Ectodermal dysplasia and immunodeficiency. Arch Dis Child 1995;73(2):185

Ariyawardana SP, Hay KD. Oral manifestations and dental management of immunocompromised patients. N Z Dent J 1999;95(421):89–97

Chinen J, Shearer WT. Secondary immunodeficiencies, including HIV infection. J Allergy Clin Immunol 2010;125(2, Suppl 2):S195–S203

Driessen G, van der Burg M. Educational paper: primary antibody deficiencies. Eur J Pediatr 2011;170(6):693–702

Fomin AB, Pastorino AC, Kim CA, Pereira CA, Carneiro-Sampaio M, Abe-Jacob CM. DiGeorge Syndrome: a not so rare disease. Clinics (Sao Paulo) 2010;65(9):865–869

Holland SM. Chronic granulomatous disease. Clin Rev Allergy Immunol 2010;38(1):3–10

Kaplan J, De Domenico I, Ward DM. Chediak-Higashi syndrome. Curr Opin Hematol 2008;15(1):22–29

Kelleher P, Misbah SA. What is Good's syndrome? Immunological abnormalities in patients with thymoma. J Clin Pathol 2003;56(1):12–16

Modell V, Gee B, Lewis DB, et al. Global study of primary immunodeficiency diseases (PI)--diagnosis, treatment, and economic impact: an updated report from the Jeffrey Modell Foundation. Immunol Res 2011;51(1):61–70

Perlman SL, Boder Deceased E, Sedgewick RP, Gatti RA. Ataxia-telangiectasia. Handb Clin Neurol 2012;103:307–332

Porter SR, Scully C. Orofacial manifestations in primary immunodeficiencies: T lymphocyte defects. J Oral Pathol Med 1993;22(7):308–309

Sponzilli I, Notarangelo LD. Severe combined immunodeficiency (SCID): from molecular basis to clinical management. Acta Biomed 2011;82(1):5–13

Szczawinska-Poplonyk A, Gerreth K, Breborowicz A, Borysewicz-Lewicka M. Oral manifestations of primary immune deficiencies in children. Oral Surg Oral Med Oral Pathol Oral Radiol Endod 2009;108(3):e9–e20

25. Genetic Diseases

Abel MD, Carrasco LR. Ehlers-Danlos syndrome: classifications, oral manifestations, and dental considerations. Oral Surg Oral Med Oral Pathol Oral Radiol Endod 2006;102(5):582–590

Adams BB. Odonto-onycho-dermal dysplasia syndrome. J Am Acad Dermatol 2007;57(4):732–733

Agarwal S, Loh YH, McLoughlin EM, et al. Telomere elongation in induced pluripotent stem cells from dyskeratosis congenita patients. Nature 2010;464(7286):292–296

Aminabadi NA, Ebrahimi A, Oskouei SG. Chondroectodermal dysplasia (Ellis-van Creveld syndrome): a case report. J Oral Sci 2010;52(2):333–336

Anchlia S, Vyas S, Bahl S, Nagavadiya V. Gorlin-Goltz syndrome in twin brothers: an unusual occurrence with review of the literature. BMJ Case Rep 2015;2015:2015

Antonoglou GN, Sándor GK, Koidou VP, Papageorgiou SN. Non-syndromic and syndromic keratocystic odontogenic tumors: systematic review and meta-analysis of recurrences. J Craniomaxillofac Surg 2014;42(7):e364–e371

Asgary S, Aminzadeh N. Unilateral gingival enlargement in patient with neurofibromatosis type I. N Y State Dent J 2012;78(6):50–53

Azeem Z, Naqvi SK, Ansar M, et al. Recurrent mutations in functionally-related EDA and EDAR genes underlie X-linked isolated hypodontia and autosomal recessive hypohidrotic ectodermal dysplasia. Arch Dermatol Res 2009;301(8):625–629

Babu NA, Rajesh E, Krupaa J, Gnananandar G. Genodermatoses. J Pharm Bioallied Sci 2015;7(Suppl 1):S203–S206

Baran I, Nalcaci R, Kocak M. Dyskeratosis congenita: clinical report and review of the literature. Int J Dent Hyg 2010;8(1):68–74

Bartholomew DW, Jabs EW, Levin LS, Ribovich R. Single maxillary central incisor and coloboma in hypomelanosis of Ito. Clin Genet 1987;31(6):370–373

Bartolucci EG, Swan RH, Hurt WC. Oral manifestations of hereditary hemorrhagic telangiectasia (Osler-Weber-Rendu disease). Review and case reports. J Periodontol 1982;53(3):163–167

Bergendal B. Orodental manifestations in ectodermal dysplasia-a review. Am J Med Genet A 2014;164A(10):2465–2471

Bhansali RS, Yeltiwar RK, Agrawal AA. Periodontal management of gingival enlargement associated with Sturge-Weber syndrome. J Periodontol 2008;79(3):549–555

Bilkay U, Erdem O, Ozek C, et al. Benign osteoma with Gardner syndrome: review of the literature and report of a case. J Craniofac Surg 2004;15(3):506–509

Bongiorno MR, Pistone G, Aricò M. Manifestations of the tongue in Neurofibromatosis type 1. Oral Dis 2006;12(2):125–129

Brauckhoff M, Gimm O, Weiss CL, et al. Multiple endocrine neoplasia 2B syndrome due to codon 918 mutation: clinical manifestation and course in early and late onset disease. World J Surg 2004;28(12):1305–1311

Cai Y, Wang R, Chen XM, Zhao YF, Sun ZJ, Zhao JH. Maffucci syndrome with the spindle cell hemangiomas in the mucosa of the lower lip: a rare case report and literature review. J Cutan Pathol 2013;40(7):661–666

Canjuga I, Mravak-Stipetić M, Kopić V, Galić J. Oral acanthosis nigricans: case report and comparison with literature reports. Acta Dermatovenerol Croat 2008;16(2):91–95

Chiaravalloti A, Payette M. Hailey-Hailey disease and review of management. J Drugs Dermatol 2014;13(10):1254–1257

Clauss F, Waltmann E, Barriere P, Hadj-Rabia S, Manière MC, Schmittbuhl M. Dento-maxillo-facial phenotype and implants-based oral rehabilitation in Ectodermal Dysplasia with WNT10A gene mutation: report of a case and literature review. J Craniomaxillofac Surg 2014;42(6):e346–e351

Cogulu O, Onay H, Aykut A, et al. Pachyonychia congenita type 2, N92S mutation of keratin 17 gene: clinical features, mutation analysis and pathological view. Eur J Pediatr 2009;168(10):1269–1272

Cross NJ, Fung DE. Tuberous sclerosis: a case report. Spec Care Dentist 2010;30(4):157–159

Cunha KS, Barboza EP, Dias EP, Oliveira FM. Neurofibromatosis type I with periodontal manifestation. A case report and literature review. Br Dent J 2004;196(8):457–460

Dar-Odeh NS, Hayajneh WA, Abu-Hammad OA, et al. Orofacial findings in chronic granulomatous disease: report of twelve patients and review of the literature. BMC Res Notes 2010;3:37

Davis T, Wyllie FS, Rokicki MJ, Bagley MC, Kipling D. The role of cellular senescence in Werner syndrome: toward therapeutic intervention in human premature aging. Ann N Y Acad Sci 2007;1100:455–469

Dessureault J, Poulin Y, Bourcier M, Gagne E. Olmsted syndrome-palmoplantar and periorificial keratodermas: association with malignant melanoma. J Cutan Med Surg 2003;7(3):236–242

Dittus C, Streiff M, Ansell J. Bleeding and clotting in hereditary hemorrhagic telangiectasia. World J Clin Cases 2015;3(4):330–337

Xuan D, Sun X, Yan Y, Xie B, Xu P, Zhang J. Effect of cleidocranial dysplasia-related novel mutation of RUNX2 on characteristics of dental pulp cells and tooth development. J Cell Biochem 2010;111(6):1473–1481

Driva T, Franklin D, Crawford PJ. Variations in expression of oral-facial-digital syndrome (type I): report of two cases. Int J Paediatr Dent 2004;14(1):61–68

Duchatelet S, Hovnanian A. Olmsted syndrome: clinical, molecular and therapeutic aspects. Orphanet J Rare Dis 2015;10:33

Engin B, Kutlubay Z, Çelik U, Serdaroğlu S, Tüzün Y. Hailey-Hailey disease: a fold (intertriginous) dermatosis. Clin Dermatol 2015;33(4):452–455

Eswar N. Chondroectodermal dysplasia: a case report. J Indian Soc Pedod Prev Dent 2001;19(3):103–106

Etöz OA, Ulu M, Kesim B. Treatment of patient with Papillon-Lefevre syndrome with short dental implants: a case report. Implant Dent 2010;19(5):394–399

Ferreira O Jr, Cardoso CL, Capelozza AL, Yaedú RY, da Costa AR. Odontogenic keratocyst and multiple supernumerary teeth in a patient with Ehlers-Danlos syndrome--a case report and review of the literature. Quintessence Int 2008;39(3):251–256

Frezzini C, Cedro M, Leao JC, Porter S. Darier disease affecting the gingival and oral mucosal surfaces. Oral Surg Oral Med Oral Pathol Oral Radiol Endod 2006;102(4):e29–e33

Goldstein E, Medina JL. Mohr syndrome or oral-facial-digital II: report of two cases. J Am Dent Assoc 1974;89(2):377–382

Haisley-Royster CA, Allingham RR, Klintworth GK, Prose NS. Hereditary benign intraepithelial dyskeratosis: report of two cases with prominent oral lesions. J Am Acad Dermatol 2001;45(4):634–636

Hanafusa T, Umegaki N, Yamaguchi Y, Katayama I. Good's syndrome (hypogammaglobulinemia with thymoma) presenting intractable opportunistic infections and hyperkeratotic lichen planus. J Dermatol 2010;37(2):171–174

Hanemann JA, de Carvalho BC, Franco EC. Oral manifestations in Ellis-van Creveld syndrome: report of a case and review of the literature. J Oral Maxillofac Surg 2010;68(2):456–460

Jain A, Chander R, Garg T, Nikita, Shetty GS. A rare multisystem disorder: Goltz syndrome - case report and brief overview. Dermatol Online J 2010;16(6):2

Javed F, Ramalingam S, Ahmed HB, et al. Oral manifestations in patients with neurofibromatosis type-1: a comprehensive literature review. Crit Rev Oncol Hematol 2014;91(2):123–129

Jerjes W, Upile T, Shah P, Abbas S, Vincent A, Hopper C. TMJ arthroscopy in patients with Ehlers Danlos syndrome: case series. Oral Surg Oral Med Oral Pathol Oral Radiol Endod 2010;110(2):e12–e20

Jham BC, Mesquita RA, Aguiar MC, Carmo MA. Hereditary benign intraepithelial dyskeratosis: a new case? J Oral Pathol Med 2007;36(1):55–57

Jones KB, Jordan R. White lesions in the oral cavity: clinical presentation, diagnosis, and treatment. Semin Cutan Med Surg 2015;34(4):161–170

Kanjanapongkul S. Chediak-Higashi syndrome: report of a case with uncommon presentation and review literature. J Med Assoc Thai 2006;89(4):541–544

Kantaputra P, Kaewgahya M, Jotikasthira D, Kantaputra W. Tricho-odonto-onycho-dermal dysplasia and WNT10A mutations. Am J Med Genet A 2014;164A(4):1041–1048

Khanna S, Kumar A, Tandon R. Good's syndrome: an unusual cause of chronic diarrhea. Indian J Gastroenterol 2004;23(4):152–153

Khocht A, Viera-Negron YE, Ameri A, Abdelsayed R. Periodontitis associated with Chediak-Higashi syndrome in a young African American male. J Int Acad Periodontol 2010;12(2):49–55

Khonsari RH, Corre P, Boukerma-Vernex Z, et al. Extreme oral manifestations in a Marfan-type syndrome. Int J Oral Maxillofac Surg 2010;39(6):622–625

Kosho T, Miyake N, Hatamochi A, et al. A new Ehlers-Danlos syndrome with craniofacial characteristics, multiple congenital contractures, progressive joint and skin laxity, and multisystem fragility-related manifestations. Am J Med Genet A 2010;152A(6):1333–1346

Laskaris G, Skouteris C. Maffucci's syndrome. Report of a case with oral hemangiomas. Oral Surg Oral Med Oral Pathol 1984;57(3):263–266

Laskaris G, Vareltzidis A, Avgerinou G. Focal palmoplantar and oral mucosa hyperkeratosis syndrome: a report concerning five members of a family. Oral Surg Oral Med Oral Pathol 1980;50(3):250–253

Lazarchick J, McRae B. Chediak-Higashi syndrome. Blood 2005;105(11):4162

Lin Z, Wang T, Sun G, Huang X. Report of a case of Zimmermann-Laband syndrome with new manifestations. Int J Oral Maxillofac Surg 2010;39(9):937–941

Longobardi G, Diana G, Poddi V, Pagano I. Follicular cyst of the jaw developing into a keratocyst in a patient with unrecognized Gorlin-Goltz syndrome. J Craniofac Surg 2010;21(3):833–836

López Jornet P. White sponge nevus: presentation of a new family. Pediatr Dermatol 2008;25(1):116–117

Lynch CD, Ziada HM, Buckley LA, O'Sullivan VR, Aherne T, Aherne S. Prosthodontic rehabilitation of hypophosphatasia using dental implants: a review of the literature and two case reports. J Oral Rehabil 2009;36(6):462–468

MacDonald DS. A systematic review of the literature of nevoid basal cell carcinoma syndrome affecting East Asians and North Europeans. Oral Surg Oral Med Oral Pathol Oral Radiol 2015;120(3):396–407

Mallineni SK, Jayaraman J, Yiu CK, King NM. Concomitant occurrence of hypohyperdontia in a patient with Marfan syndrome: a review of the literature and report of a case. J Investig Clin Dent 2012;3(4):253–257

Martelli H, Lima LS, Bonan PR, Coletta RD. Oral manifestations leading to the diagnosis of familial tuberous sclerosis. Indian J Dent Res 2010;21(1):138–140

Mevorah B, Goldberg I, Sprecher E, et al. Olmsted syndrome: mutilating palmoplantar keratoderma with periorificial keratotic plaques. J Am Acad Dermatol 2005;53(5, Suppl 1):S266–S272

Minić S, Trpinac D, Gabriel H, Gencik M, Obradović M. Dental and oral anomalies in incontinentia pigmenti: a systematic review. Clin Oral Investig 2013;17(1):1–8

Moorthy AP. Oral manifestations in Maffucci syndrome. Br Dent J 1983;155(5):160–161

Morales-Chávez MC, Rodríguez-López MV. Dental treatment of Marfan syndrome. With regard to a case. Med Oral Patol Oral Cir Bucal 2010;15(6):e859–e862

Mukamal LV, Ferreira AF, Jacques CdeM, Amorim CA, Pineiro-Maceira J, Ramos-e-Silva M. Cowden syndrome: review and report of a case of late diagnosis. Int J Dermatol 2012;51(12):1494–1499

Nico MM, Hammerschmidt M, Lourenço SV. Oral mucosal manifestations in some genodermatoses: correlation with cutaneous lesions. Eur J Dermatol 2013;23(5):581–591

Oliveira TM, Sakai VT, Candido LA, Silva SM, Machado MA. Clinical management for epidermolysis bullosa dystrophica. J Appl Oral Sci 2008;16(1):81–85

Pascual-Castroviejo I, Roche C, Martinez-Bermejo A, et al. Hypomelanosis of ITO. A study of 76 infantile cases. Brain Dev 1998;20(1):36–43

Phiske MM. An approach to acanthosis nigricans. Indian Dermatol Online J 2014;5(3):239–249

Pinto A, Haberland CM, Baker S. Pediatric soft tissue oral lesions. Dent Clin North Am 2014;58(2):437–453

Pontes FS, Conte Neto N, da Costa RM, Loureiro AM, do Nascimento LS, Pontes HA. Periodontal growth in areas of vascular malformation in patients with Sturge-Weber syndrome: a management protocol. J Craniofac Surg 2014;25(1):e1–e3

Poziomczyk CS, Recuero JK, Bringhenti L, et al. Incontinentia pigmenti. An Bras Dermatol 2014;89(1):26–36

Reibel A, Manière MC, Clauss F, et al. Orodental phenotype and genotype findings in all subtypes of hypophosphatasia. Orphanet J Rare Dis 2009;4:6

Roberts T, Stephen L, Beighton P. Cleidocranial dysplasia: a review of the dental, historical, and practical implications with an overview of the South African experience. Oral Surg Oral Med Oral Pathol Oral Radiol 2013;115(1):46–55

Scheper MA, Nikitakis NG, Sarlani E, Sauk JJ, Meiller TF. Cowden syndrome: report of a case with immunohistochemical analysis and review of the literature. Oral Surg Oral Med Oral Pathol Oral Radiol Endod 2006;101(5):625–631

Sciubba JJ, Brown AM. Oral-facial manifestations of Klippel-Trenaunay-Weber syndrome. Report of two cases. Oral Surg Oral Med Oral Pathol 1977;43(2):227–232

Scully C, Langdon J, Evans J. Marathon of eponyms: 10 Jadassohn-Lewandowsky syndrome (Pachyonychia congenita). Oral Dis 2010;16(3):310–311

Scully C, Langdon J, Evans J. Marathon of eponyms: 7 Gorlin-Goltz syndrome (Naevoid basal-cell carcinoma syndrome). Oral Dis 2010;16(1):117–118

Sharma SM, Mohan M, Baptist J. Dental considerations in hereditary epidermolysis bullosa. N Y State Dent J 2014;80(1):45–48

Shepherd V, Godbolt A, Casey T. Maffucci's syndrome with extensive gastrointestinal involvement. Australas J Dermatol 2005;46(1):33–37

Silva CA, Moraes PdeC, Furuse C, Junqueira JL, Thomaz LA, de Araújo VC. Gardner syndrome with no clinical family history. J Craniofac Surg 2009;20(4):1186–1189

Song E, Jaishankar GB, Saleh H, Jithpratuck W, Sahni R, Krishnaswamy G. Chronic granulomatous disease: a review of the infectious and inflammatory complications. Clin Mol Allergy 2011;9(1):10

Songu M, Adibelli H, Diniz G. White sponge nevus: clinical suspicion and diagnosis. Pediatr Dermatol 2012;29(4):495–497

Stuart CA, Driscoll MS, Lundquist KF, Gilkison CR, Shaheb S, Smith MM. Acanthosis nigricans. J Basic Clin Physiol Pharmacol 1998;9(2-4):407–418

Suda N, Hattori M, Kosaki K, et al. Correlation between genotype and supernumerary tooth formation in cleidocranial dysplasia. Orthod Craniofac Res 2010;13(4):197–202

Sudarsanam A, Ardern-Holmes SL. Sturge-Weber syndrome: from the past to the present. Eur J Paediatr Neurol 2014;18(3):257–266

Takagi H, Kamijo M, Ikeda S. Darier disease. J Dermatol 2016;43(3):275–279

Tsang VH, Tacon LJ, Learoyd DL, Robinson BG. Pheochromocytomas in multiple endocrine neoplasia type 2. Recent Results Cancer Res 2015;204:157–178

Vassilopoulou A, Laskaris G. Papillon-Lefevre syndrome: report of two brothers. ASDC J Dent Child 1989;56(5):388–391

Vosynioti V, Kosmadaki M, Tagka A, Katsarou A. A case of Olmsted syndrome. Eur J Dermatol 2010;20(6):837–838

Wang L, Jin X, Zhao X, et al. Focal dermal hypoplasia: updates. Oral Dis 2014;20(1):17–24

Zirbel GM, Ruttum MS, Post AC, Esterly NB. Odonto-onycho-dermal dysplasia. Br J Dermatol 1995;133(5):797–800

26. Skin Diseases

Ahmed AR, Shetty S. A comprehensive analysis of treatment outcomes in patients with pemphigus vulgaris treated with rituximab. Autoimmunity reviews 2015;14(4):323–331

Andreadis D, Gagari E, Laskaris G, Kapsokefalos P. Idiopathic Sweet's syndrome with oral manifestations. Report of a case and review of the literature. Acta Stomatol Croat 2007;41:152–158

Al-Johani KA, Fedele S, Porter SR. Erythema multiforme and related disorders. Oral Surg Oral Med Oral Pathol Oral Radiol Endod 2007;103(5):642–654

Alpsoy E, Akman-Karakas A, Uzun S. Geographic variations in epidemiology of two autoimmune bullous diseases: pemphigus and bullous pemphigoid. Arch Dermatol Res 2015;307(4):291–298

Ariyawardana A, Tilakaratne WM, Dissanayake M, et al. Oral pemphigus vulgaris in children and adolescents: a review of the literature and a case report. Int J Paediatr Dent 2005;15(4):287–293

Ayangco L, Rogers RS III. Oral manifestations of erythema multiforme. Dermatol Clin 2003;21(1):195–205

Bagan J, Lo Muzio L, Scully C. Mucosal disease series. Number III. Mucous membrane pemphigoid. Oral Dis 2005;11(4):197–218

Bain S, Ball L. Physical signs for the general dental practitioner. Case 78. Bullous pemphigoid. Dent Update 2010;37(8):569

Bascones-Martínez A, García-García V, Meurman JH, Requena-Caballero L. Immune-mediated diseases: what can be found in the oral cavity? Int J Dermatol 2015;54(3):258–270

Bermejo-Fenoll A, Sánchez-Siles M, López-Jornet P, Camacho-Alonso F, Salazar-Sánchez N. A retrospective clinicopathological study of 550 patients with oral lichen planus in south-eastern Spain. J Oral Pathol Med 2010;39(6):491–496

Beutler AM, Schumacher HR Jr. Reactive arthritis: is it a useful concept? Br J Clin Pract 1997;51(3):169–172

Black M, Mignogna M, Scully C. Mucosal diseases series number III Pemphigus Vulgaris. Oral Dis 2005;11:119–130

Bruce AJ, Rogers RS III. Oral psoriasis. Dermatol Clin 2003;21(1):99–104

Carrozzo M, Brancatello F, Dametto E, et al. Hepatitis C virus-associated oral lichen planus: is the geographical heterogeneity related to HLA-DR6? J Oral Pathol Med 2005;34(4):204–208

Chan LS, Regezi JA, Cooper KD. Oral manifestations of linear IgA disease. J Am Acad Dermatol 1990;22(2, Pt 2):362–365

Chau MN, Radden BG. Oral warty dyskeratoma. J Oral Pathol 1984;13(5):546–556

Choi Y, Lee SE, Fukuda S, Hashimoto T, Kim SC. Mucous membrane pemphigoid with immunoglobulin G autoantibodies against full-length and 120-kDa ectodomain of BP180. J Dermatol 2011;38(2):169–172

Chudomirova K, Abadjieva Ts, Yankova R. Clinical tetrad of arthritis, urethritis, conjunctivitis, and mucocutaneous lesions (HLA-B27-associated spondyloarthropathy, Reiter syndrome): report of a case. Dermatol Online J 2008;14(12):4

Cohen D, Bhattacharyya I. Case of the month. Warty dyskeratoma (isolated Darier's disease). Todays FDA 2008;20(8):17–19

Cohen PR. Sweet's syndrome—a comprehensive review of an acute febrile neutrophilic dermatosis. Orphanet J Rare Dis 2007;2:34

Cowan CG, Lamey PJ, Walsh M, Irwin ST, Allen G, McKenna KE. Linear IgA disease (LAD): immunoglobulin deposition in oral and colonic lesions. J Oral Pathol Med 1995;24(8):374–378

Craythorne E, du Viver A, Mufti GJ, Warnakulasuriya S. Rituximab for the treatment of corticosteroid-refractory pemphigus vulgaris with oral and skin manifestations. J Oral Pathol Med 2011;40(8):616–620

Economopoulou P, Laskaris G. Dermatitis herpetiformis: oral lesions as an early manifestation. Oral Surg Oral Med Oral Pathol 1986;62(1):77–80

Eguia del Valle A, Aguirre Urízar JM, Martínez Sahuquillo A. Oral manifestations caused by the linear IgA disease. Med Oral 2004;9(1):39–44

Farhi D, Dupin N. Pathophysiology, etiologic factors, and clinical management of oral lichen planus, part I: facts and controversies. Clin Dermatol 2010;28(1):100–108

Femiano F, Gombos F, Scully C. Sweet's syndrome: recurrent oral ulceration, pyrexia, thrombophlebitis, and cutaneous lesions. Oral Surg Oral Med Oral Pathol Oral Radiol Endod 2003;95(3):324–327

Femiano F. Geographic tongue (migrant glossitis) and psoriasis. Minerva Stomatol 2001;50(6):213–217

Feng S, Zhou W, Zhang J, Jin P. Analysis of 6 cases of drug-induced pemphigus. Eur J Dermatol 2011;21(5):696–699

Gagari E, Laskaris G. Pemphigoid gestationis with oral manifestations: case report and review of the literature. Bulcan J of Stomatology 2010;14(1):31–36

Haberland-Carrodeguas C, Allen CM, Lovas JG, et al. Review of linear epidermal nevus with oral mucosal involvement—series of five new cases. Oral Dis 2008;14(2):131–137

Huang A, Madan RK, Levitt J. Future therapies for pemphigus vulgaris: Rituximab and beyond. J Am Acad Dermatol 2016;74(4):746–753

Kasperkiewicz M, Sadik CD, Bieber K, et al. Epidermolysis bullosa acquisita: from pathophysiology to novel therapeutic options. J Invest Dermatol 2016;136(1):24–33

Kershenovich R, Hodak E, Mimouni D. Diagnosis and classification of pemphigus and bullous pemphigoid. Autoimmun Rev 2014;13(4-5):477–481

Knudson RM, Kalaaji AN, Bruce AJ. The management of mucous membrane pemphigoid and pemphigus. Dermatol Ther (Heidelb) 2010;23(3):268–280

Kubo Y, Urano Y, Matsuda R, et al. Ichthyosis hystrix, Curth-Macklin type: a new sporadic case with a novel mutation of keratin 1. Arch Dermatol 2011;147(8):999–1001

Lähteenoja H, Irjala K, Viander M, Vainio E, Toivanen A, Syrjänen S. Oral mucosa is frequently affected in patients with dermatitis herpetiformis. Arch Dermatol 1998;134(6):756–758

Laskaris G, Angelopoulos A. Cicatricial pemphigoid: direct and indirect immunofluorescent studies. Oral Surg Oral Med Oral Pathol 1981;51(1):48–54

Laskaris G, Nicolis G. Immunopathology of oral mucosa in bullous pemphigoid. Oral Surg Oral Med Oral Pathol 1980;50(4):340–345

Laskaris G, Papanicolaou S, Angelopoulos A. Immunofluorescent study of cytologic smears in oral pemphigus: A simple diagnostic technique. Oral Surg Oral Med Oral Pathol 1981;51(5):531–534

Laskaris G, Sklavounou A, Angelopoulos A. Direct immunofluorescence in oral lichen planus. Oral Surg Oral Med Oral Pathol 1982;53(5):483–487

Laskaris G, Sklavounou A, Bovopoulou O. Juvenile pemphigus vulgaris. Oral Surg Oral Med Oral Pathol 1981;51(4):415–420

Laskaris G, Sklavounou A, Stavrou A, Stavropoulou K. Familial pemphigus vulgaris with oral manifestations affecting two Greek families. J Oral Pathol Med 1989;18(1):49–53

Laskaris G, Sklavounou A, Stratigos J. Bullous pemphigoid, cicatricial pemphigoid, and pemphigus vulgaris. A comparative clinical survey of 278 cases. Oral Surg Oral Med Oral Pathol 1982;54(6):656–662

Laskaris G, Sklavounou A. Warty dyskeratoma of the oral mucosa. Br J Oral Maxillofac Surg 1985;23(5):371–375

Laskaris G, Stoufi E. Oral pemphigus vulgaris in a 6-year-old girl. Oral Surg Oral Med Oral Pathol 1990;69(5):609–613

Laskaris G, Satriano RA. Drug-induced blistering oral lesions. Clin Dermatol 1993;11(4):545–550

Laskaris G, Triantafyllou A, Economopoulou P. Gingival manifestations of childhood cicatricial pemphigoid. Oral Surg Oral Med Oral Pathol 1988;66(3):349–352

Laskaris G. Oral pemphigus vulgaris: an immunofluorescent study of fifty-eight cases. Oral Surg Oral Med Oral Pathol 1981;51(6):626–631

Laskaris GC, Papavasiliou SS, Bovopoulou OD, Nicolis GD. Association of oral pemphigus with chronic lymphocytic leukemia. Oral Surg Oral Med Oral Pathol 1980;50(3):244–249

Laskaris GC, Papavasiliou SS, Bovopoulou OD, Nicolis GD. Lichen planus pigmentosus of the oral mucosa: a rare clinical variety. Dermatologica 1981;162(1):61–63

Leuci S, Gürcan HM, Ahmed AR. Serological studies in bullous pemphigoid: a literature review of antibody titers at presentation and in clinical remission. Acta Derm Venereol 2010;90(2):115–121

Lewis MA, Yaqoob NA, Emanuel C, Potts AJ. Successful treatment of oral linear IgA disease using mycophenolate. Oral Surg Oral Med Oral Pathol Oral Radiol Endod 2007;103(4):483–486

Li Q, Ujiie H, Shibaki A, et al. Human IgG1 monoclonal antibody against human collagen 17 noncollagenous 16A domain induces blisters via complement activation in experimental bullous pemphigoid model. J Immunol 2010;185(12):7746–7755

Lim SW, Goh CL. Epidemiology of eczematous cheilitis at a tertiary dermatological referral centre in Singapore. Contact Dermat 2000;43(6):322–326

Lipozencic J, Ljubojevic S. Perioral dermatitis. Clin Dermatol 2011;29(2):157–161

Mattsson U, Warfvinge G, Jontell M. Oral psoriasis-a diagnostic dilemma: a report of two cases and a review of the literature. Oral Surg Oral Med Oral Pathol Oral Radiol 2015;120(4):e183–e189

McMillan R, Taylor J, Shephard M, et al. World Workshop on Oral Medicine VI: a systematic review of the treatment of mucocutaneous pemphigus vulgaris. Oral Surg Oral Med Oral Pathol Oral Radiol 2015;120(2):132–42.e61

Melato M, Gorji N, Rizzardi C, Maglione M. Associated localization of morphea and lichen planus of the lip in a patient with vitiligo. Minerva Stomatol 2000;49(11-12):549–554

Murrell DF, Marinovic B, Caux F, et al. Definitions and outcome measures for mucous membrane pemphigoid: recommendations of an international panel of experts. J Am Acad Dermatol 2015;72(1):168–174

Mutasim DF. Autoimmune bullous dermatoses in the elderly: an update on pathophysiology, diagnosis and management. Drugs Aging 2010;27(1):1–19

Nogueira PA, Carneiro S, Ramos-e-Silva M. Oral lichen planus: an update on its pathogenesis. Int J Dermatol 2015;54(9):1005–1010

Pan M, Liu X, Zheng J. The pathogenic role of autoantibodies in pemphigus vulgaris. Clin Exp Dermatol 2011;36(7):703–707

Reddy H, Shipman AR, Wojnarowska F. Epidermolysis bullosa acquisita and inflammatory bowel disease: a review of the literature. Clin Exp Dermatol 2013;38(3):225–229, quiz 229–230

Rowley AH. The complexities of the diagnosis and management of Kawasaki disease. Infect Dis Clin North Am 2015;29(3):525–537

Ruocco E, Wolf R, Ruocco V, Brunetti G, Romano F, Lo Schiavo A. Pemphigus: associations and management guidelines: facts and controversies. Clin Dermatol 2013;31(4):382–390

Scardina GA, Fucà G, Carini F, et al. Oral necrotizing microvasculitis in a patient affected by Kawasaki disease. Med Oral Patol Oral Cir Bucal 2007;12(8):E560–E564

Schifter M, Yeoh SC, Coleman H, Georgiou A. Oral mucosal diseases: the inflammatory dermatoses. Aust Dent J 2010;55(Suppl 1):23–38

Schmidt-Westhausen A, Grünewald T, Reichart PA, Pohle HD. Oral manifestations of toxic epidermal necrolysis (TEN) in patients with AIDS: report of five cases. Oral Dis 1998;4(2):90–94

Scully C, Bagan J. Oral mucosal diseases: erythema multiforme. Br J Oral Maxillofac Surg 2008;46(2):90–95

Scully C, Laskaris G. Mucocutaneous disorders. Periodontol 2000 1998;18:81–94

Seidel R, Lavi N, Chipps L. Pemphigoid gestations: a case report and review of management. J Drugs Dermatol 2015;14(8):904–907

Sedghizadeh PP, Kumar SK, Gorur A, Mastin C, Boros AL. Toxic epidermal necrolysis with a rare long-term oral complication requiring surgical intervention. Oral Surg Oral Med Oral Pathol Oral Radiol Endod 2008;105(4):e29–e33

Shimanovich I, Skrobek C, Rose C, et al. Pemphigoid gestationis with predominant involvement of oral mucous membranes and IgA autoantibodies targeting the C-terminus of BP180. J Am Acad Dermatol 2002;47(5):780–784

Shipman AR, Cooper S, Wojnarowska F. Autoreactivity to bullous pemphigoid 180: is this the link between subepidermal blistering diseases and oral lichen planus? Clin Exp Dermatol 2011;36(3):267–269

Singh S, Vignesh P, Burgner D. The epidemiology of Kawasaki disease: a global update. Arch Dis Child 2015;100(11):1084–1088

Sklavounou A, Laskaris G. Frequency of desquamative gingivitis in skin diseases. Oral Surg Oral Med Oral Pathol 1983;56(2):141–144

Sklavounou A, Laskaris G. Childhood cicatricial pemphigoid with exclusive gingival involvement. Int J Oral Maxillofac Surg 1990;19(4):197–199

Sklavounou AD, Laskaris G, Angelopoulos AP. Serum immunoglobulins and complement (C'3) in oral lichen planus. Oral Surg Oral Med Oral Pathol 1983;55(1):47–51

Sklavounou A, Laskaris G. Oral psoriasis: report of a case and review of the literature. Dermatologica 1990;180(3):157–159

Sklavounou A, Laskaris G. Paraneoplastic pemphigus: a review. Oral Oncol 1998;34(6):437–440

Speeckaert R, van Geel N. Distribution patterns in generalized vitiligo. J Eur Acad Dermatol Venereol 2014;28(6):755–762

Stratigos J, Tsambaos D. Ichthyosis hystrix and skin cancer. Clin Exp Dermatol 1995;20(1):85

Taylor J, McMillan R, Shephard M, et al. World Workshop on Oral Medicine VI: a systematic review of the treatment of mucous membrane pemphigoid. Oral Surg Oral Med Oral Pathol Oral Radiol 2015;120(2):161–71.e20

Tolat SN, Gharpuray MB. Diascopy, the lips, and vitiligo. Arch Dermatol 1995;131(2):228–229

Tomb R, Hajj H, Nehme E. [Oral lesions in psoriasis]. Ann Dermatol Venereol 2010;137(11):695–702

Tse SM, Silverman ED, McCrindle BW, Yeung RS. Early treatment with intravenous immunoglobulin in patients with Kawasaki disease. J Pediatr 2002;140(4):450–455

Vassileva S, Drenovska K, Manuelyan K. Autoimmune blistering dermatoses as systemic diseases. Clin Dermatol 2014;32(3):364–375

Woo TY, Solomon AR, Fairley JA. Pemphigus vegetans limited to the lips and oral mucosa. Arch Dermatol 1985;121(2):271–272

Wu F, Luo X, Yuan G. Sweet's syndrome representing a flare of Behçet's disease. Clin Exp Rheumatol 2009; 27(2, Suppl 53):S88–S90

Wu IB, Schwartz RA. Reiter's syndrome: the classic triad and more. J Am Acad Dermatol 2008;59(1):113–121

Yanagawa H, Nakamura Y, Yashiro M, Uehara R, Oki I, Kayaba K. Incidence of Kawasaki disease in Japan: the nationwide surveys of 1999-2002. Pediatr Int 2006;48(4):356–361

Zeppa L, Bellini V, Lisi P. Atopic dermatitis in adults. Dermatitis 2011;22(1):40–46

27. Blood Diseases

Abhinav C, Mahajan VK, Mehta KS, Chauhan PS. Angina bullosa hemorrhagica-like lesions: a rare presentation of drug-induced thrombocytopenia. Int J Dermatol 2015;54(7):819–822

Başsimitçi S, Yücel-Eroğlu E, Akalar M. Effects of thalassaemia major on components of the craniofacial complex. Br J Orthod 1996;23(2):157–162

Brennan MT, Sankar V, Baccaglini L, et al. Oral manifestations in patients with aplastic anemia. Oral Surg Oral Med Oral Pathol Oral Radiol Endod 2001;92(5):503–508

Casey C, Brooke T, Davies R, Franklin D. Case report of a family with benign familial neutropenia and the implications for the general dental practitioner. Dent Update 2011;38(2):106–108, 110

Chandra J, Ravi R, Singh V, Narayan S, Sharma S, Dutta AK. Bleeding manifestations in severely thrombocytopenic children with immune thrombocytopenic purpura. Hematology 2006;11(2):131–133

Chi AC, Prichard E, Richardson MS, Rasenberger KP, Weathers DR, Neville BW. Pseudomembranous disease (ligneous inflammation) of the female genital tract, peritoneum, gingiva, and paranasal sinuses associated with plasminogen deficiency. Ann Diagn Pathol 2009;13(2):132–139

Enomoto M, Kohmoto M, Arafa UA, et al. Plummer-Vinson syndrome successfully treated by endoscopic dilatation. J Gastroenterol Hepatol 2007;22(12):2348–2351

Flint SR, Sugerman P, Scully C, Smith JG, Smith MA. The myelodysplastic syndromes. Case report and review. Oral Surg Oral Med Oral Pathol 1990;70(5):579–583

Ganesh R, Janakiraman L, Sathiyasekaran M. Plummer-Vinson syndrome: an unusual cause of dysphagia. Ann Trop Paediatr 2008;28(2):143–147

Grein Cavalcanti L, Lyko KF, Araújo RL, Amenábar JM, Bonfim C, Torres-Pereira CC. Oral leukoplakia in patients with Fanconi anaemia without hematopoietic stem cell transplantation. Pediatr Blood Cancer 2015;62(6):1024–1026

Hou GL, Tsai CC. Oral manifestations of agranulocytosis associated with methimazole therapy. J Periodontol 1988;59(4):244–248

Jessner W, Vogelsang H, Püspök A, et al. Plummer-Vinson syndrome associated with celiac disease and complicated by postcricoid carcinoma and carcinoma of the tongue. Am J Gastroenterol 2003;98(5):1208–1209

Lele MV. Oral manifestations of polycythaemia rubra vera. J All India Dent Assoc 1965;37(11):345–348

Lu SY, Wu HC. Initial diagnosis of anemia from sore mouth and improved classification of anemias by MCV and RDW in 30 patients. Oral Surg Oral Med Oral Pathol Oral Radiol Endod 2004;98(6):679–685

Mufti G, List AF, Gore SD, Ho AY. Myelodysplastic syndrome. Hematology (Am Soc Hematol Educ Program) 2003:176–199

Pereira CM, Gasparetto PF, Coracin FL, Marquês JF, Lima CS, Corrêa ME. Severe gingival bleeding in a myelodysplastic patient: management and outcome. J Periodontol 2004;75(3):483–486

Peyvandi F, Mannucci PM. Rare coagulation disorders. Thromb Haemost 1999;82(4):1207–1214

Pontes HA, Neto NC, Ferreira KB, et al. Oral manifestations of vitamin B12 deficiency: a case report. J Can Dent Assoc 2009;75(7):533–537

Razmus TF, Fotos PG. Oral medicine in clinical dentistry: hematologic disorders. Compendium 1987;8(3):214, 216–218, 221–222

Rezaei N, Farhoudi A, Ramyar A, et al. Congenital neutropenia and primary immunodeficiency disorders: a survey of 26 Iranian patients. J Pediatr Hematol Oncol 2005;27(7):351–356

Rezaei N, Moin M, Pourpak Z, et al. The clinical, immunohematological, and molecular study of Iranian patients with severe congenital neutropenia. J Clin Immunol 2007;27(5):525–533

Rohani B. Oral manifestations and blood profile in patients with iron deficiency anemia. J Formos Med Assoc 2015;114(1):97

Samad A, Mohan N, Balaji RV, Augustine D, Patil SG. Oral manifestations of Plummer-Vinson syndrome: a classic report with literature review. J Int Oral Health 2015;7(3):68–71

Schlosser BJ, Pirigyi M, Mirowski GW. Oral manifestations of hematologic and nutritional diseases. Otolaryngol Clin North Am 2011;44(1):183–203, vii.

Scully C, Gokbuget A, Kurtulus I. Hypoplasminogenaemia, gingival swelling and ulceration. Oral Dis 2007;13(6):515–518

Scully C, MacFadyen E, Campbell A. Oral manifestations in cyclic neutropenia. Br J Oral Surg 1982;20(2):96–101

Sepúlveda E, Brethauer U, Rojas J, Le Fort P. Oral manifestations of aplastic anemia in children. J Am Dent Assoc 2006;137(4):474–478

Silva GB, Bariani C, Mendonça EF, Batista AC. Clinical manifestations due to severe plasminogen deficiency: a case report. J Dent Child (Chic) 2006;73(3):179–182

Tirali RE, Yalçınkaya Erdemci Z, Çehreli SB. Oral findings and clinical implications of patients with congenital neutropenia: a literature review. Turk J Pediatr 2013;55(3):241–245

Vinall C, Stassen LF. Dental management of the anaemic patient. J Ir Dent Assoc 2007;53(4):191–195

Vucicevic-Boras V, Topic B, Cekic-Arambasin A, Zadro R, Stavljenic-Rukavina A. Lack of association between burning mouth syndrome and hematinic deficiencies. Eur J Med Res 2001;6(9):409–412

Wang YP, Chang JY, Wu YC, Cheng SJ, Chen HM, Sun A. Oral manifestations and blood profile in patients with thalassemia trait. J Formos Med Assoc 2013;112(12):761–765

Yalçin SS, Unal S, Gümrük F, Yurdakök K. The validity of pallor as a clinical sign of anemia in cases with beta-thalassemia. Turk J Pediatr 2007;49(4):408–412

Zengin E, Sarper N, Caki Kiliç S. Clinical manifestations of infants with nutritional vitamin B deficiency due to maternal dietary deficiency. Acta Paediatr 2009;98(1):98–102

Ziv O, Ragni MV. Bleeding manifestations in males with von Willebrand disease. Haemophilia 2004;10(2):162–168

28. Gastrointestinal Diseases

Beggs AD, Latchford AR, Vasen HF, et al. Peutz-Jeghers syndrome: a systematic review and recommendations for management. Gut 2010;59(7):975–986

Bucci P, Carile F, Sangianantoni A, D'Angiò F, Santarelli A, Lo Muzio L. Oral aphthous ulcers and dental enamel defects in children with coeliac disease. Acta Paediatr 2006;95(2):203–207

da Silva PC, de Almeida PdelV, Machado MA, et al. Oral manifestations of celiac disease. A case report and review of the literature. Med Oral Patol Oral Cir Bucal 2008;13(9):E559–E562

de Carvalho FK, de Queiroz AM, Bezerra da Silva RA, et al. Oral aspects in celiac disease children: clinical and dental enamel chemical evaluation. Oral Surg Oral Med Oral Pathol Oral Radiol 2015;119(6):636–643

Fatahzadeh M, Schwartz RA, Kapila R, Rochford C. Orofacial Crohn's disease: an oral enigma. Acta Dermatovenerol Croat 2009;17(4):289–300

Fatahzadeh M. Inflammatory bowel disease. Oral Surg Oral Med Oral Pathol Oral Radiol Endod 2009;108(5):e1–e10

Iyengar S, Chambers C, Sharon VR. Bullous acrodermatitis enteropathica: case report of a unique clinical presentation and review of the literature. Dermatol Online J 2015;21(4):21

Jurge S, Hegarty AM, Hodgson T. Orofacial manifestations of gastrointestinal disorders. Br J Hosp Med (Lond) 2014;75(9):497–501

Katz J, Shenkman A, Stavropoulos F, Melzer E. Oral signs and symptoms in relation to disease activity and site of involvement in patients with inflammatory bowel disease. Oral Dis 2003;9(1):34–40

Krzywicka B, Herman K, Kowalczyk-Zając M, Pytrus T. Celiac disease and its impact on the oral health status - review of the literature. Adv Clin Exp Med 2014;23(5):675–681

Lankarani KB, Sivandzadeh GR, Hassanpour S. Oral manifestation in inflammatory bowel disease: a review. World J Gastroenterol 2013;19(46):8571–8579

Laranjeira N, Fonseca J, Meira T, Freitas J, Valido S, Leitão J. Oral mucosa lesions and oral symptoms in inflammatory bowel disease patients. Arq Gastroenterol 2015;52(2):105–110

Logan RM. Links between oral and gastrointestinal health. Curr Opin Support Palliat Care 2010;4(1):31–35

Maloney WJ, Raymond G, Hershkowitz D, Rochlen G. Oral and dental manifestations of celiac disease. N Y State Dent J 2014;80(4):45–48

Maverakis E, Fung MA, Lynch PJ, et al. Acrodermatitis enteropathica and an overview of zinc metabolism. J Am Acad Dermatol 2007;56(1):116–124

Mijandrusić-Sinčić B, Licul V, Gorup L, Brncić N, Glazar I, Lucin K. Pyostomatitis vegetans associated with inflammatory bowel disease--report of two cases. Coll Antropol 2010;34(Suppl 2):279–282

Padmavathi B, Sharma S, Astekar M, Rajan Y, Sowmya G. Oral Crohn's disease. J Oral Maxillofac Pathol 2014;18(Suppl 1):S139–S142

Pittock S, Drumm B, Fleming P, et al. The oral cavity in Crohn's disease. J Pediatr 2001;138(5):767–771

Ponti G, Tomasi A, Manfredini M, Pellacani G. Oral mucosal stigmata in hereditary-cancer syndromes: From germline mutations to distinctive clinical phenotypes and tailored therapies. Gene 2016;582(1):23–32

Rashid M, Zarkadas M, Anca A, Limeback H. Oral manifestations of celiac disease: a clinical guide for dentists. J Can Dent Assoc 2011;77:b39

Steger JW, Izuno GT. Acute zinc depletion syndrome during parenteral hyperalimentation. Int J Dermatol 1979;18(6):472–479

Tavarela Veloso F. Review article: skin complications associated with inflammatory bowel disease. Aliment Pharmacol Ther 2004;20(Suppl 4):50–53

Woo VL, Abdelsayed R. Oral manifestations of internal malignancy and paraneoplastic syndromes. Dent Clin North Am 2008;52(1):203–230, x

Xi Z, Hui Q, Zhong L. Q-switched alexandrite laser treatment of oral labial lentigines in Chinese subjects with Peutz-Jeghers syndrome. Dermatol Surg 2009;35(7):1084–1088

29. Renal Diseases

Antoniades DZ, Markopoulos AK, Andreadis D, Balaskas I, Patrikalou E, Grekas D. Ulcerative uremic stomatitis associated with untreated chronic renal failure: report of a case and review of the literature. Oral Surg Oral Med Oral Pathol Oral Radiol Endod 2006;101(5):608–613

Chuang SF, Sung JM, Kuo SC, Huang JJ, Lee SY. Oral and dental manifestations in diabetic and nondiabetic uremic patients receiving hemodialysis. Oral Surg Oral Med Oral Pathol Oral Radiol Endod 2005;99(6):689–695

Hamid MJ, Dummer CD, Pinto LS. Systemic conditions, oral findings and dental management of chronic renal failure patients: general considerations and case report. Braz Dent J 2006;17(2):166–170

Leão JC, Gueiros LA, Segundo AV, Carvalho AA, Barrett W, Porter SR. Uremic stomatitis in chronic renal failure. Clinics (Sao Paulo) 2005;60(3):259–262

McCreary CE, Flint SR, McCartan BE, Shields JA, Mabruk M, Toner ME. Uremic stomatitis mimicking oral hairy leukoplakia: report of a case. Oral Surg Oral Med Oral Pathol Oral Radiol Endod 1997;83(3):350–353

30. Metabolic Diseases

Aissi K, Rossi P, Bernard F, Granel B, Frances Y. Facial signs leading to the diagnosis of cardiac amyloidosis. Am J Med 2009;122(9):e1–e2

Angiero F, Seramondi R, Magistro S, et al. Amyloid deposition in the tongue: clinical and histopathological profile. Anticancer Res 2010;30(7):3009–3014

Behera B, Jena DK, Chhetia R, Vijayashree J. Hurler syndrome with a tuft of hair. Indian J Dermatol Venereol Leprol 2006;72(2):147–149

Chiewchanvit S, Mahanupab P, Vanittanakom P. Congenital erythropoietic porphyria: a case report. J Med Assoc Thai 1998;81(12):1023–1027

Elad S, Czerninski R, Fischman S, et al. Exceptional oral manifestations of amyloid light chain protein (AL) systemic amyloidosis. Amyloid 2010;17(1):27–31

Fayle SA, Pollard MA. Congenital erythropoietic porphyria--oral manifestations and dental treatment in childhood: a case report. Quintessence Int 1994;25(8):551–554

Juusela P, Tanskanen M, Nieminen A, et al. Xerostomia in hereditary gelsolin amyloidosis. Amyloid 2013;20(1):39–44

Kasahara M, Horikawa R, Sakamoto S, et al. Living donor liver transplantation for glycogen storage disease type Ib. Liver Transpl 2009;15(12):1867–1871

Kontos AP, Ozog D, Bichakjian C, Lim HW. Congenital erythropoietic porphyria associated with myelodysplasia presenting in a 72-year-old man: report of a case and review of the literature. Br J Dermatol 2003;148(1):160–164

Kooijman MM, Brand HS. Oral aspects of porphyria. Int Dent J 2005;55(2):61–66

Liu KL. The oral signs of Hurler-Hunter syndrome: report of four cases. ASDC J Dent Child 1980;47(2):122–127

Narang A, Maguire A, Nunn JH, Bush A. Oral health and related factors in cystic fibrosis and other chronic respiratory disorders. Arch Dis Child 2003;88(8):702–707

Nico MM, Hammerschmidt M, Lourenço SV. Oral mucosal manifestations in some genodermatoses: correlation with cutaneous lesions. Eur J Dermatol 2013;23(5):581–591

Pau M, Reinbacher KE, Feichtinger M, Kärcher H. Surgical treatment of macroglossia caused by systemic primary amyloidosis. Int J Oral Maxillofac Surg 2013;42(2):294–297

Primosch RE. Tetracycline discoloration, enamel defects, and dental caries in patients with cystic fibrosis. Oral Surg Oral Med Oral Pathol 1980;50(4):301–308

Ravi Prakash SM, Verma S, Sumalatha MN, Chattopadhyay S. Oral manifestations of lipoid proteinosis: a case report and literature review. Saudi Dent J 2013;25(2):91–94

Salapata Y, Laskaris G, Drogari E, Harokopos E, Messaritakis J. Oral manifestations in glycogen storage disease type 1b. J Oral Pathol Med 1995;24(3):136–139

Sargenti Neto S, Batista JD, Durighetto AF Jr. A case of oral recurrent ulcerative lesions in a patient with lipoid proteinosis (Urbach-Wiethe disease). Br J Oral Maxillofac Surg 2010;48(8):654–655

Schlosser BJ, Pirigyi M, Mirowski GW. Oral manifestations of hematologic and nutritional diseases. Otolaryngol Clin North Am 2011;44(1):183–203, vii.

Shaw PH, Mancini AJ, McConnell JP, Brown D, Kletzel M. Treatment of congenital erythropoietic porphyria in children by allogeneic stem cell transplantation: a case report and review of the literature. Bone Marrow Transplant 2001;27(1):101–105

Shivaswamy KN, Thappa DM, Laxmisha C, Jayanthi S. Lipoid proteinosis in two siblings: a report from south India. Dermatol Online J 2003;9(5):12

van der Waal RI, van de Scheur MR, Huijgens PC, Starink TM, van der Waal I. Amyloidosis of the tongue as a paraneoplastic marker of plasma cell dyscrasia. Oral Surg Oral Med Oral Pathol Oral Radiol Endod 2002;94(4):444–447

Van Hougenhouck-Tulleken W, Chan I, Hamada T, et al. Clinical and molecular characterization of lipoid proteinosis in Namaqualand, South Africa. Br J Dermatol 2004;151(2):413–423

Vedamurthy M. Lipoid proteinosis in siblings. Dermatol Online J 2003;9(5):13

Viggor SF, Frezzini C, Farthing PM, Freeman CO, Yeoman CM, Thornhill MH. Amyloidosis: an unusual case of persistent oral ulceration. Oral Surg Oral Med Oral Pathol Oral Radiol Endod 2009;108(5):e46–e50

31. Vitamins Deficiency

Avery KT, Shapiro S, Hamby CL. Oral manifestations of vitamin deficiencies. J Colo Dent Assoc 1985;63(6):4–7

Bacci C, Sivolella S, Pellegrini J, Favero L, Berengo M. A rare case of scurvy in an otherwise healthy child: diagnosis through oral signs. Pediatr Dent 2010;32(7):536–538

Dali-Youcef N, Andrès E. An update on cobalamin deficiency in adults. QJM 2009;102(1):17–28

Davit-Béal T, Gabay J, Antoniolli P, Masle-Farquhar J, Wolikow M. Dental complications of rickets in early childhood: case report on 2 young girls. Pediatrics 2014;133(4):e1077–e1081

Firth N, Marvan E. Oral lesions in scurvy. Aust Dent J 2001;46(4):298–300

Graells J, Ojeda RM, Muniesa C, Gonzalez J, Saavedra J. Glossitis with linear lesions: an early sign of vitamin B12 deficiency. J Am Acad Dermatol 2009;60(3):498–500

Khadim MI. Oral manifestations of malnutrition I. The effect of vitamins. J Pak Med Assoc 1981;31(2):44–48

Schlosser BJ, Pirigyi M, Mirowski GW. Oral manifestations of hematologic and nutritional diseases. Otolaryngol Clin North Am 2011;44(1):183–203, vii.

Souza AP, Kobayashi TY, Lourenço Neto N, Silva SM, Machado MA, Oliveira TM. Dental manifestations of patient with vitamin D-resistant rickets. J Appl Oral Sci 2013;21(6):601–606

32. Endocrine Diseases

Chi AC, Neville BW, Krayer JW, Gonsalves WC. Oral manifestations of systemic disease. Am Fam Physician 2010;82(11):1381–1388

Cristina de Lima D, Nakata GC, Balducci I, Almeida JD. Oral manifestations of diabetes mellitus in complete denture wearers. J Prosthet Dent 2008;99(1):60–65

Dudhia SB, Dudhia BB. Undetected hypothyroidism: a rare dental diagnosis. J Oral Maxillofac Pathol 2014;18(2):315–319

Gibson J, Lamey PJ, Lewis M, Frier B. Oral manifestations of previously undiagnosed non-insulin dependent diabetes mellitus. J Oral Pathol Med 1990;19(6):284–287

Islam NM, Bhattacharyya I, Cohen DM. Common oral manifestations of systemic disease. Otolaryngol Clin North Am 2011;44(1):161–182, vi.

Jabbour SA. Cutaneous manifestations of endocrine disorders: a guide for dermatologists. Am J Clin Dermatol 2003;4(5):315–331

Kudiyirickal MG, Pappachan JM. Diabetes mellitus and oral health. Endocrine 2015;49(1):27–34

Mancini T, Porcelli T, Giustina A. Treatment of Cushing disease: overview and recent findings. Ther Clin Risk Manag 2010;6:505–516

Quirino MR, Birman EG, Paula CR. Oral manifestations of diabetes mellitus in controlled and uncontrolled patients. Braz Dent J 1995;6(2):131–136

Venkatesh Babu NS, Patel PB. Oral health status of children suffering from thyroid disorders. J Indian Soc Pedod Prev Dent 2016;34(2):139–144

Xing H, Guan X. Necrotizing gingivostomatitis and osteonecrosis associated with antithyroid drug propylthiouracil therapy. Oral Surg Oral Med Oral Pathol Oral Radiol 2015;119(2):e65–e68

33. Peripheral Nervous System Diseases

Dziewas R, Lüdemann P. Hypoglossal nerve palsy as complication of oral intubation, bronchoscopy and use of the laryngeal mask airway. Eur Neurol 2002;47(4):239–243

Fishman JM. Corticosteroids effective in idiopathic facial nerve palsy (Bell's palsy) but not necessarily in idiopathic acute vestibular dysfunction (vestibular neuritis). Laryngoscope 2011;121(11):2494–2495

Gilden DH. Clinical practice. Bell's palsy. N Engl J Med 2004;351(13):1323–1331

Giuffrida S, Lo Bartolo ML, Nicoletti A, et al. Isolated, unilateral, reversible palsy of the hypoglossal nerve. Eur J Neurol 2000;7(3):347–349

Larsen A, Piepgras D, Chyatte D, Rizzolo D. Trigeminal neuralgia: diagnosis and medical and surgical management. JAAPA 2011;24(7):20–25

McAllister K, Walker D, Donnan PT, Swan I. Surgical interventions for the early management of Bell's palsy. Cochrane Database Syst Rev 2011;16(2):CD007468

Mathey DG, Wandler A, Rosenkranz M. Images in cardiovascular medicine. Hypoglossal-nerve palsy caused by carotid dissection. Circulation 2010;121(3):457

Sekula RF Jr, Frederickson AM, Jannetta PJ, Quigley MR, Aziz KM, Arnone GD. Microvascular decompression for elderly patients with trigeminal neuralgia: a prospective study and systematic review with meta-analysis. J Neurosurg 2011;114(1):172–179

34. Benign Tumors

A R R, Rehani S, Bishen KA, Sagari S. Warthin's tumour: a case report and review of pathogenesis and its histological subtypes. J Clin Diagn Res 2014;8(9):ZD37–ZD40

Adler BL, Krausz AE, Minuti A, Silverberg JI, Lev-Tov H. Epidemiology and treatment of angiolymphoid hyperplasia with eosinophilia (ALHE): a systematic review. J Am Acad Dermatol 2016;74(3):506–12.e11

Agarwal P, Saxena S, Kumar S, Gupta R. Melanotic neuroectodermal tumor of infancy: Presentation of a case affecting the maxilla. J Oral Maxillofac Pathol 2010;14(1):29–32

Agoumi M, Al Dhaybi R, Powell J, Brochu P, Lapointe A, Kokta V. Rapidly growing gingival mass in an infant--quiz case. Melanotic neuroectodermal tumor of infancy (MNTI). Arch Dermatol 2010;146(3):337–342

Arava-Parastatidis M, Alawi F, Stoopler ET. Multifocal pigmentation of the oral cavity. J Am Dent Assoc 2011;142(1):53–56

Arribas-García I, Alcalá-Galiano A, Gutiérrez R, Montalvo-Moreno JJ. Traumatic neuroma of the inferior alveolar nerve: a case report. Med Oral Patol Oral Cir Bucal 2008;13(3):E186–E188

Bablani D, Bansal S, Shetty SJ, et al. Pleomorphic adenoma of the cheek: a case report and review. J Oral Maxillofac Surg 2009;67(7):1539–1542

Balakrishnan K, Bauman N, Chun RH, et al. Standardized outcome and reporting measures in pediatric head and neck lymphatic malformations. Otolaryngol Head Neck Surg 2015;152(5):948–953

Barrett AW, Speight PM. Superficial arteriovenous hemangioma of the oral cavity. Oral Surg Oral Med Oral Pathol Oral Radiol Endod 2000;90(6):731–738

Baykul T, Aydın MA, Fındık Y, Yıldırım D. Huge lipoma of the right parotid gland: Case report and review of 42 cases. Ear Nose Throat J 2016;95(1):E8–E13

Belal MS, Ibricevic H, Madda JP, Al-therban W. Granular congenital cell tumor in the newborn: a case report. J Clin Pediatr Dent 2002;26(3):315–317

Bhattacharyya I. Diagnostic discussion. Melanoacanthoma. Todays FDA 2013;25(1):32–35

Bozkaya S, Uğar D, Karaca I, et al. The treatment of lymphangioma in the buccal mucosa by radiofrequency ablation: a case report. Oral Surg Oral Med Oral Pathol Oral Radiol Endod 2006;102(5):e28–e31

Brooks JK, Sindler AJ, Scheper MA. Oral melanoacanthoma in an adolescent. Pediatr Dermatol 2010;27(4):384–387

Buchner A, Merrell PW, Carpenter WM. Relative frequency of solitary melanocytic lesions of the oral mucosa. J Oral Pathol Med 2004;33(9):550–557

Bulut E, Acikgoz A, Ozan B, Gunhan O. Large peripheral osteoma of the mandible: a case report. Int J Dent 2010;2010:834761

Carlos-Bregni R, Contreras E, Netto AC, et al. Oral melanoacanthoma and oral melanotic macule: a report of 8 cases, review of the literature, and immunohistochemical analysis. Med Oral Patol Oral Cir Bucal 2007;12(5):E374–E379

Carneiro TE, Marinho SA, Verli FD, Mesquita AT, Lima NL, Miranda JL. Oral squamous papilloma: clinical, histologic and immunohistochemical analyses. J Oral Sci 2009;51(3):367–372

Carrera Grañó I, Berini Aytés L, Escoda CG. Peripheral ossifying fibroma. Report of a case and review of the literature. Med Oral 2001;6(2):135–141

Charabi B, Bretlau P, Bille M, Holmelund M. Cystic hygroma of the head and neck--a long-term follow-up of 44 cases. Acta Otolaryngol Suppl 2000;543:248–250

Chaudhary A, Wakhlu A, Mittal N, Misra S, Mehrotra D, Wakhlu AK. Melanotic neuroectodermal tumor of infancy: 2 decades of clinical experience with 18 patients. J Oral Maxillofac Surg 2009;67(1):47–51

Ciçek Y, Ertaş U. The normal and pathological pigmentation of oral mucous membrane: a review. J Contemp Dent Pract 2003;4(3):76–86

Cincik H, Gungor A, Ertugrul E, Cekin E, Dogru S. Peripheral osteoma of the mandible mimicking a parotid mass. Eur Arch Otorhinolaryngol 2007;264(4):429–431

Coelho CM, Zucoloto S, Lopes RA. Denture-induced fibrous inflammatory hyperplasia: a retrospective study in a school of dentistry. Int J Prosthodont 2000;13(2):148–151

Colella G, Tozzi U, Pagliarulo V, Bove P. Warthin tumor: a potential source of diagnostic error. J Craniofac Surg 2010;21(6):1978–1981

Corrêa PH, Nunes LC, Johann AC, Aguiar MC, Gomez RS, Mesquita RA. Prevalence of oral hemangioma, vascular malformation and varix in a Brazilian population. Braz Oral Res 2007;21(1):40–45

da Silveira EJ, Pereira AL, Fontora MC, de Souza LB, de Almeida Freitas R. Myoepithelioma of minor salivary gland--an immunohistochemical analysis of four cases. Rev Bras Otorrinolaringol (Engl Ed) 2006;72(4):528–532

de Castro LA, de Castro JG, da Cruz AD, Barbosa BH, de Spindula-Filho JV, Costa MB. Focal epithelial hyperplasia (Heck's disease) in a 57-year-old Brazilian patient: a case report and literature review. J Clin Med Res 2016;8(4):346–350

De Medts J, Dick C, Casselman J, Van Den Berghe I. Intraoral multifocal adult rhabdomyoma: a case report. B-ENT 2007;3(4):205–208

Dillenburg CS, Martins MD, Meurer L, Castilho RM, Squarize CH. Keratoacanthoma of the lip: Activation of the mTOR pathway, tumor suppressor proteins and tumor senescence. Medicine (Baltimore) 2015;94(38):e1552

Emodi O, El-Naaj IA, Gordin A, Akrish S, Peled M. Superficial parotidectomy versus retrograde superficial parotidectomy in treating benign salivary gland tumor (pleomorphic adenoma). J Oral Maxillofac Surg 2010;68(9):2092–2098

Esmeili T, Lozada-Nur F, Epstein J. Common benign oral soft tissue masses. Dent Clin North Am 2005;49(1):223–240, x

Fasanmade A, Anjum K, Hughes C, Dunnill G, Thomas S. Angiolymphoid hyperplasia with eosinophilia successfully treated with oral steroids. Quintessence Int 2010;41(1):67–69

Flaitz CM. Peripheral ossifying fibroma of the maxillary gingiva. Am J Dent 2001;14(1):56

Franco-Barrera MJ, Zavala-Cerna MG, Fernández-Tamayo R, Vivanco-Pérez I, Fernández-Tamayo NM, Torres-Bugarín O. An update on peripheral ossifying fibroma: case report and literature review. Oral Maxillofac Surg 2016;20(1):1–7

Furlong MA, Fanburg-Smith JC, Childers EL. Lipoma of the oral and maxillofacial region: Site and subclassification of 125 cases. Oral Surg Oral Med Oral Pathol Oral Radiol Endod 2004;98(4):441–450

Gabay E, Akrish S, Machtei EE. Oral focal mucinosis associated with cervical external root resorption: a case report. Oral Surg Oral Med Oral Pathol Oral Radiol Endod 2010;110(4):e75–e78

Gaitan Cepeda LA, Quezada Rivera D, Tenorio Rocha F, Leyva Huerta ER, Mendez Sánchez ER. Vascular leiomyoma of the oral cavity. Clinical, histopathological and immunohistochemical characteristics. Presentation of five cases and review of the literature. Med Oral Patol Oral Cir Bucal 2008;13(8):E483–E488

Gemigniani F, Hernández-Losa J, Ferrer B, García-Patos V. Focal epithelial hyperplasia by human papillomavirus (HPV)-32 misdiagnosed as HPV-16 and treated with combination of retinoids, imiquimod and quadrivalent HPV vaccine. J Dermatol 2015;42(12):1172–1175

Gonçalves CF, Costa NdoL, Oliveira-Neto HH, et al. Melanotic neuroectodermal tumor of infancy: report of 2 cases. J Oral Maxillofac Surg 2010;68(9):2341–2346

Grce M, Mravak-Stipetić M. Human papillomavirus-associated diseases. Clin Dermatol 2014;32(2):253–258

Gulati S, Pandiar D, Kakky S, Jiwane AY, Balan A. Keratoacanthoma of upper lip: review and report of case managed surgically. J Clin Diagn Res 2015;9(10):ZD08–ZD10

Gun BD, Ozdamar SO, Bahadir B, Uzun L. Salivary gland myoepithelioma with focal capsular invasion. Ear Nose Throat J 2009;88(7):1005–1009

Gupta AA, Nainani P, Upadhyay B, Kavle P. Oral melanoacanthoma: a rare case of diffuse oral pigmentation. J Oral Maxillofac Pathol 2012;16(3):441–443

Gupta R, Gupta R, Kumar S, Saxena S. Melanotic neuroectodermal tumor of infancy: review of literature, report of a case and follow up at 7 years. J Plast Reconstr Aesthet Surg 2015;68(3):e53–e54

Hara H, Oyama T, Saku T. Fine needle aspiration cytology of basal cell adenoma of the salivary gland. Acta Cytol 2007;51(5):685–691

Hegde U, Doddawad VG, Sreeshyla H, Patil R. Verruciform xanthoma: a view on the concepts of its etiopathogenesis. J Oral Maxillofac Pathol 2013;17(3):392–396

Heo MS, Cho HJ, Kwon KJ, Lee SS, Choi SC. Benign fibrous histiocytoma in the mandible. Oral Surg Oral Med Oral Pathol Oral Radiol Endod 2004;97(2):276–280

Hu JA, Li Y, Li S. Verruciform xanthoma of the oral cavity: clinicopathological study relating to pathogenesis. Report of three cases. APMIS 2005;113(9):629–634

Ichihara T, Kawata R, Higashino M, Terada T, Haginomori S. A more appropriate clinical classification of benign parotid tumors: investigation of 425 cases. Acta Otolaryngol 2014;134(11):1185–1191

Ishibashi N, Yanagawa T, Yamagata K, et al. Basal cell adenoma arising in a minor salivary gland of the palate. Oral Maxillofac Surg 2012;16(1):111–114

Jaju PP, Suvarna PV, Desai RS. Squamous papilloma: case report and review of literature. Int J Oral Sci 2010;2(4):222–225

Rathan JJ, Vardhan BG, Muthu MS, Venkatachalapathy, Saraswathy K, Sivakumar N. Oral lymphangioma: a case report. J Indian Soc Pedod Prev Dent 2005;23(4):185–189

Jeffcoat BT, Pitman KT, Brown AS, Baliga M. Schwannoma of the oral tongue. Laryngoscope 2010;120(Suppl 4):S154

Kaminagakura E, Andrade CR, Rangel AL, et al. Sebaceous adenoma of oral cavity: report of case and comparative proliferation study with sebaceous gland hyperplasia and Fordyce's granules. Oral Dis 2003;9(6):323–327

Karukayil D, Stephen M, Sunil A, Mukunda A. Enigma of myoepithelioma at the base of tongue: A rare case report and review of literature. J Cancer Res Ther 2015;11(4):1038

Kim Y, Moses M, Zegarelli DJ, Yoon AJ. Cartilage choristoma (soft tissue chondroma): a rare presentation in the lower lip. J Clin Pediatr Dent 2009;33(3):253–254

Kishino M, Murakami S, Toyosawa S, et al. Benign fibrous histiocytoma of the mandible. J Oral Pathol Med 2005;34(3):190–192

Kuo RC, Wang YP, Chen HM, Sun A, Liu BY, Kuo YS. Clinicopathological study of oral giant cell fibromas. J Formos Med Assoc 2009;108(9):725–729

Laskaris G, Kittas C, Triantafyllou A. Unpigmented intramucosal nevus of palate. An unusual clinical presentation. Int J Oral Maxillofac Surg 1994;23(1):39–40

Ljubojevic S, Skerlev M. HPV-associated diseases. Clin Dermatol 2014;32(2):227–234

Lipani C, Woytash JJ, Greene GW Jr. Sebaceous adenoma of the oral cavity. J Oral Maxillofac Surg 1983;41(1):56–60

López-Jornet P, Gomez-Garcia E, Camacho-Alonso F. Solitary oral neurofibroma. N Y State Dent J 2010;76(5):54–55

Luaces Rey R, Lorenzo Franco F, Gómez Oliveira G, Patiño Seijas B, Guitián D, López-Cedrún Cembranos JL. Oral leiomyoma in retromolar trigone. A case report. Med Oral Patol Oral Cir Bucal 2007;12(1):E53–E55

Macedo Firoozmand L, Dias Almeida J, Guimarães Cabral LA. Study of denture-induced fibrous hyperplasia cases diagnosed from 1979 to 2001. Quintessence Int 2005;36(10):825–829

Mahady K, Thust S, Berkeley R, et al. Vascular anomalies of the head and neck in children. Quant Imaging Med Surg 2015;5(6):886–897

Makariou E, Pikis A, Harley EH. Cystic hygroma of the neck: association with a growing venous aneurysm. AJNR Am J Neuroradiol 2003;24(10):2102–2104

Marangon Júnior H, Souza PE, Soares RV, de Andrade BA, de Almeida OP, Horta MC. Oral congenital melanocytic nevus: a rare case report and review of the literature. Head Neck Pathol 2015;9(4):481–487

Mariatos G, Gorgoulis VG, Laskaris G, Kittas C. Epithelioid hemangioma (angiolymphoid hyperplasia with eosinophilia) in the oral mucosa. A case report and review of the literature. Oral Oncol 1999;35(4):435–438

Martins MD, Anunciato de Jesus L, Fernandes KP, Bussadori SK, Taghloubi SA, Martins MA. Intra-oral schwannoma: case report and literature review. Indian J Dent Res 2009;20(1):121–125

Meleti M, Mooi WJ, Casparie MK, van der Waal I. Melanocytic nevi of the oral mucosa - no evidence of increased risk for oral malignant melanoma: an analysis of 119 cases. Oral Oncol 2007;43(10):976–981 M

Meleti M, Vescovi P, Mooi WJ, van der Waal I. Pigmented lesions of the oral mucosa and perioral tissues: a flow-chart for the diagnosis and some recommendations for the management. Oral Surg Oral Med Oral Pathol Oral Radiol Endod 2008;105(5):606–616

Minicucci EM, de Campos EB, Weber SA, Domingues MA, Ribeiro DA. Basal cell adenoma of the upper lip from minor salivary gland origin. Eur J Dent 2008;2(3):213–216

Moon WJ, Choi SY, Chung EC, Kwon KH, Chae SW. Peripheral ossifying fibroma in the oral cavity: CT and MR findings. Dentomaxillofac Radiol 2007;36(3):180–182

Narayana N, Casey J. Oral focal mucinosis: review of the literature and seven additional cases. Gen Dent 2009;57(2):e11–e13

Neto JR, Sendyk M, Uchida LM, Nunes FD, de Paiva JB. Oral focal mucinosis associated with surgically assisted rapid maxillary expansion. Am J Orthod Dentofacial Orthop 2014;145(4):534–538

Niramis R, Watanatittan S, Rattanasuwan T. Treatment of cystic hygroma by intralesional bleomycin injection: experience in 70 patients. Eur J Pediatr Surg 2010;20(3):178–182

Nishijima Sakanashi E, Sonobe J, Chin M, Bessho K. Schwannoma located in the upper gingival mucosa: case report and literature review. J Maxillofac Oral Surg 2015;14(Suppl 1):222–225

Nonaka CF, Pereira KM, Miguel MC. Oral vascular leiomyoma with extensive calcification areas. Rev Bras Otorrinolaringol (Engl Ed) 2010;76(4):539

Ogbureke KU, Nashed MN, Ayoub AF. Huge peripheral osteoma of the mandible: a case report and review of the literature. Pathol Res Pract 2007;203(3):185–188

Ojha J, Akers JL, Akers JO, et al. Intraoral cellular blue nevus: report of a unique histopathologic entity and review of the literature. Cutis 2007;80(3):189–192

Olson TS, Schmidt MA, Olson CM. Congenital granular cell tumor in the newborn. Otolaryngol Head Neck Surg 1998;118(6):907

Philipsen HPRP, Reichart PA, Takata T, Ogawa I. Verruciform xanthoma--biological profile of 282 oral lesions based on a literature survey with nine new cases from Japan. Oral Oncol 2003;39(4):325–336

Pons Vicente O, Almendros Marqués N, Berini Aytés L, Gay Escoda C. Minor salivary gland tumors: A clinicopathological study of 18 cases. Med Oral Patol Oral Cir Bucal 2008;13(9):E582–E588

Prasanna Kumar D, Umesh, Rathi T, Jain V. Benign fibrous histiocytoma: a rare case report and literature review. J Maxillofac Oral Surg 2016;15(1):116–120

Pringle GA. The role of human papillomavirus in oral disease. Dent Clin North Am 2014;58(2):385–399

Rachidi S, Sood AJ, Patel KG, et al. Melanotic neuroectodermal tumor of infancy: a systematic review. J Oral Maxillofac Surg 2015;73(10):1946–1956

Rallis G, Dais P, Kostakis G, Stathopoulos P. Osteo-cementum producing odontogenic myxomas. A literature review of a distinctive variant. J Maxillofac Oral Surg 2015;14(2):176–181

Ramos LM, Cardoso SV, Loyola AM, Rocha MA, Durighetto-Júnior AF. Keratoacanthoma of the inferior lip: review and report of case with spontaneous regression. J Appl Oral Sci 2009;17(3):262–265

Reid CO, Smith CJ. Rhabdomyoma of the floor of the mouth: a new case and review of recently reported intra-oral rhabdomyomas. Br J Oral Maxillofac Surg 1985;23(4):284–291

Sannoh S, Quezada E, Merer DM, Moscatello A, Golombek SG. Cystic hygroma and potential airway obstruction in a newborn: a case report and review of the literature. Cases J 2009;2(1):48

Santos PP, Freitas VS, Pinto LP, Freitas RdeA, de Souza LB. Clinicopathologic analysis of 7 cases of oral schwannoma and review of the literature. Ann Diagn Pathol 2010;14(4):235–239

Sayan NB, Uçok C, Karasu HA, Günhan O. Peripheral osteoma of the oral and maxillofacial region: a study of 35 new cases. J Oral Maxillofac Surg 2002;60(11):1299–1301

Scivetti M, Maiorano E, Pilolli GP, et al. Chondroma of the tongue. Clin Exp Dermatol 2008;33(4):460–462

Shekar V, Rangdhol V, Baliah WJ, Thirunavukarasu S. An unusual oral manifestation of type 1 neurofibromatosis: A case report and review of literature. J Nat Sci Biol Med 2015;6(1):261–263

Shimoyama T, Horie N, Kato T, et al. Soft tissue myxoma of the gingiva: report of a case and review of the literature of soft tissue myxoma in the oral region. J Oral Sci 2000;42(2):107–109

Silva GCVT, Vieira TC, Vieira JC, Martins CR, Silva EC. Congenital granular cell tumor (congenital epulis): a lesion of multidisciplinary interest. Med Oral Patol Oral Cir Bucal 2007;12(6):E428–E430

Sklavounou A, Laskaris G, Angelopoulos A. Verruciform xanthoma of the oral mucosa. Dermatologica 1982;164(1):41–46

Sowmya GV, Manjunatha BS, Nahar P, Aggarwal H. Oral focal mucinosis: a rare case with literature review. BMJ Case Rep 2015;2015:2015

Stănescu L, Popescu CF, Georgescu I, et al. Spitz nevus with an uncertain malignant potential. Rom J Morphol Embryol 2009;50(2):275–282

Syrjänen S, Kwong E. Human papillomavirus infections and oral tumors. Med Microbiol Immunol (Berl) 2003;192(3):123–128

Tapia JL, Quezada D, Gaitan L, Hernandez JC, Paez C, Aguirre A. Gingival melanoacanthoma: case report and discussion of its clinical relevance. Quintessence Int 2011;42(3):253–258

Tosios K, Laskaris G, Eveson J, Scully C. Benign cartilaginous tumor of the gingiva. A case report. Int J Oral Maxillofac Surg 1993;22(4):231–233

Triantafyllou AG, Laskaris GC. Papillary syringadenoma of the lower lip: report of a case. J Oral Maxillofac Surg 1987;45(10):884–887

Triantafyllou AG, Sklavounou AD, Laskaris GG. Benign fibrous histiocytoma of the oral mucosa. J Oral Med 1985;40(1):36–38

Vered M, Carpenter WM, Buchner A. Granular cell tumor of the oral cavity: updated immunohistochemical profile. J Oral Pathol Med 2009;38(1):150–159

Vesnaver A, Dovsak DA. Treatment of vascular lesions in the head and neck using Nd:YAG laser. J Craniomaxillofac Surg 2006;34(1):17–24

Wang XD, Meng LJ, Hou TT, Huang SH. Tumours of the salivary glands in northeastern China: a retrospective study of 2508 patients. Br J Oral Maxillofac Surg 2015;53(2):132–137

Werder P, Altermatt HJ, Zbären P, Bornstein MM. Canalicular adenoma of a minor salivary gland on the palate: a case presentation. Quintessence Int 2009;40(8):623–626

Woo J, Cheung WS. Bilateral oral focal mucinosis on the palate of a 2-year-old child: a case report. Int J Paediatr Dent 2011;25(1):70–72

Yuwanati M, Mhaske S, Mhaske A. Congenital granular cell tumor - a rare entity. J Neonatal Surg 2015;4(2):17

Zhou Q, Yang XJ, Zheng JW, Wang YA. Hemangioma concurrent with arteriovenous malformation in oral and maxillofacial region: report of a case and review of the literature. J Oral Maxillofac Surg 2011;69(4):1100–1102

Zwane NP, Noffke CE, Raubenheimer EJ. Solitary oral plexiform neurofibroma: review of literature and report of a case. Oral Oncol 2011;47(6):449–451

35. Reactive Tumors

Adeyemo WL, Hassan OO, Ajayi OF. Pregnancy-associated pyogenic granuloma of the lip: a case report. Niger J Med 2011;20(1):179–180

daSilva FC, Piazzetta CM, Torres-Pereira CC, Schussel JL, Amenábar JM. Gingival proliferative lesions in children and adolescents in Brazil: a 15-year-period cross-sectional study. J Indian Soc Periodontol 2016;20(1):63–66

Flaitz CM. Peripheral giant cell granuloma: a potentially aggressive lesion in children. Pediatr Dent 2000;22(3):232–233

Gbolahan O, Fatusi O, Owotade F, Akinwande J, Adebiyi K. Clinicopathology of soft tissue lesions associated with extracted teeth. J Oral Maxillofac Surg 2008;66(11):2284–2289

Gondivkar SM, Gadbail A, Chole R. Oral pregnancy tumor. Contemp Clin Dent 2010;1(3):190–192

Jafarzadeh H, Sanatkhani M, Mohtasham N. Oral pyogenic granuloma: a review. J Oral Sci 2006;48(4):167–175

Motamedi MH, Talesh KT, Jafari SM, Khalifeh S. Peripheral and central giant cell granulomas of the jaws: a retrospective study and surgical management. Gen Dent 2010;58(6):e246–e251

Omoregie FO, Ojo MA, Saheeb B, Odukoya O. Periapical granuloma associated with extracted teeth. Niger J Clin Pract 2011;14(3):293–296

Omoregie OF, Saheeb BD, Odukoya O, Ojo MA. A clinicopathologic correlation in the diagnosis of periradicular lesions of extracted teeth. J Oral Maxillofac Surg 2009;67(7):1387–1391

Perez D, Leibold D, Liddell A, Duraini M. Vascular lesions of the maxillofacial region: a case report and review of the literature. Tex Dent J 2010;127(10):1045–1057

Razek AA, Castillo M. Imaging appearance of granulomatous lesions of head and neck. Eur J Radiol 2010;76(1):52–60

Vidyanath S, Shameena PM, Johns DA, Shivashankar VY, Sudha S, Varma S. Reactive hyperplasic lesions of the oral cavity: a survey of 295 cases at a Tertiary Health Institution in Kerala. J Oral Maxillofac Pathol 2015;19(3):330–334

36. Nonneoplastic Lesions of the Salivary Glands

Aframian DJ. Anorexia/bulimia-related sialadenosis of palatal minor salivary glands. J Oral Pathol Med 2005;34(6):383

Al-Talabani N, Gataa IS, Latteef SA. Bilateral agenesis of parotid salivary glands, an extremely rare condition: report of a case and review of literature. Oral Surg Oral Med Oral Pathol Oral Radiol Endod 2008;105(3):e73–e75

Berta E, Bettega G, Jouk PS, Billy G, Nugues F, Morand B. Complete agenesis of major salivary glands. Int J Pediatr Otorhinolaryngol 2013;77(10):1782–1785

Boyce HW, Bakheet MR. Sialorrhea: a review of a vexing, often unrecognized sign of oropharyngeal and esophageal disease. J Clin Gastroenterol 2005;39(2):89–97

Carlson ER, Ord RA. Benign pediatric salivary gland lesions. Oral Maxillofac Surg Clin North Am 2016;28(1):67–81

Chou KL, Evatt M, Hinson V, Kompoliti K. Sialorrhea in Parkinson's disease: a review. Mov Disord 2007;22(16):2306–2313

Fava M, Cherubini K, Yurgel L, Salum F, Figueiredo MA. Necrotizing sialometaplasia of the palate in a cocaine-using patient. A case report. Minerva Stomatol 2008;57(4):199–202

Femopase FL, Hernández SL, Gendelman H, Criscuolo MI, López-de-Blanc SA. Necrotizing sialometaplasia: report of five cases. Med Oral 2004;9(4):304–308

Fragoulis GE, Moutsopoulos HM. IgG4 syndrome: old disease, new perspective. J Rheumatol 2010;37(7):1369–1370

Hawkey NM, Zaorsky NG, Galloway TJ. The role of radiation therapy in the management of sialorrhea: A systematic review. Laryngoscope 2016;126(1):80–85

Hernandez S, Busso C, Walvekar RR. Parotitis and sialendoscopy of the parotid gland. Otolaryngol Clin North Am 2016;49(2):381–393

Jardim EC, Ponzoni D, de Carvalho PS, Demétrio MR, Aranega AM. Sialolithiasis of the submandibular gland. J Craniofac Surg 2011;22(3):1128–1131

Jensen SB, Pedersen AM, Vissink A, et al; Salivary Gland Hypofunction/Xerostomia Section; Oral Care Study Group; Multinational Association of Supportive Care in Cancer (MASCC)/International Society of Oral Oncology (ISOO). A systematic review of salivary gland hypofunction and xerostomia induced by cancer therapies: management strategies and economic impact. Support Care Cancer 2010;18(8):1061–1079

Keogh PV, O'Regan E, Toner M, Flint S. Necrotizing sialometaplasia: an unusual bilateral presentation associated with antecedent anaesthesia and lack of response to intralesional steroids. Case report and review of the literature. Br Dent J 2004;196(2):79–81

Koch M, Bozzato A, Iro H, Zenk J. Combined endoscopic and transcutaneous approach for parotid gland sialolithiasis: indications, technique, and results. Otolaryngol Head Neck Surg 2010;142(1):98–103

Lee LT, Wong YK. Pathogenesis and diverse histologic findings of sialolithiasis in minor salivary glands. J Oral Maxillofac Surg 2010;68(2):465–470

Mandel L. An unusual pattern of dental damage with salivary gland aplasia. J Am Dent Assoc 2006;137(7):984–989

Mandic R, Teymoortash A, Kann PH, Werner JA. Sialadenosis of the major salivary glands in a patient with central diabetes insipidus--implications of aquaporin water channels in the pathomechanism of sialadenosis. Exp Clin Endocrinol Diabetes 2005;113(4):205–207

Mihas AA, Lawson PB, Dreiling BJ, Gurram VS, Heuman DM. Mikulicz syndrome associated with a malignant large cell gastric lymphoma: a case report and review of the literature. Int J Gastrointest Cancer 2003;33(2-3):123–127

Miranda-Rius J, Brunet-Llobet L, Lahor-Soler E, Farré M. Salivary secretory disorders, inducing drugs and clinical management. Int J Med Sci 2015;12(10):811–824

Mohan RP, Verma S, Chawa VR, Tyagi K. Non-syndromic non-familial agenesis of major salivary glands: a report of two cases with review of literature. J Clin Imaging Sci 2013;3(Suppl 1):2

Nanke Y, Kobashigawa T, Yago T, Kamatani N, Kotake S. A case of Mikulicz's disease, IgG4-related plasmacytic syndrome, successfully treated by corticosteroid and mizoribine, followed by mizoribine alone. Intern Med 2010;49(14):1449–1453

Orellana MF, Lagravère MO, Boychuk DG, Major PW, Flores-Mir C. Prevalence of xerostomia in population-based samples: a systematic review. J Public Health Dent 2006;66(2):152–158

Ozdemir T, Fowler EW, Hao Y, et al. Biomaterials-based strategies for salivary gland tissue regeneration. Biomater Sci 2016;4(4):592–604

Sanan A, Cognetti DM. Rare parotid gland diseases. Otolaryngol Clin North Am 2016;49(2):489–500

Sarode SC, Sarode GS. Myoepithelial cells are functionally deficient in sialadenosis: still an assumption. Oral Surg Oral Med Oral Pathol Oral Radiol Endod 2011;112(3):286, author reply 287

Shariat-Madar B, Chun RH, Sulman CG, Conley SF. Safety of ultrasound-guided botulinum toxin injections for sialorrhea as performed by pediatric otolaryngologists. Otolaryngol Head Neck Surg 2016;154(5):924–927

Stone CA, O'Leary N. Systematic review of the effectiveness of botulinum toxin or radiotherapy for sialorrhea in patients with amyotrophic lateral sclerosis. J Pain Symptom Manage 2009;37(2):246–258

Turner MD. Hyposalivation and xerostomia: etiology, complications and medical management. Dent Clin North Am 2016;60(2):435–443

Turner M, Jahangiri L, Ship JA. Hyposalivation, xerostomia and the complete denture: a systematic review. J Am Dent Assoc 2008;139(2):146–150

37. Potential Malignant Disorders—Lesions

Anderson A, Ishak N. Marked variation in malignant transformation rates of oral leukoplakia. Evid Based Dent 2015;16(4):102–103

Brennan M, Migliorati CA, Lockhart PB, et al. Management of oral epithelial dysplasia: a review. Oral Surg Oral Med Oral Pathol Oral Radiol Endod 2007;103(Suppl):19.e1–19.e12

Cabay RJ, Morton TH Jr, Epstein JB. Proliferative verrucous leukoplakia and its progression to oral carcinoma: a review of the literature. J Oral Pathol Med 2007;36(5):255–261

Hosni ES, Salum FG, Cherubini K, Yurgel LS, Figueiredo MA. Oral erythroplakia and speckled leukoplakia: retrospective analysis of 13 cases. Rev Bras Otorrinolaringol (Engl Ed) 2009;75(2):295–299

Lapthanasupkul P, Poomsawat S, Punyasingh J. A clinicopathologic study of oral leukoplakia and erythroplakia in a Thai population. Quintessence Int 2007;38(8):e448–e455

Laskaris G. How to treat oral leucoplakia. J Eur Acad Dermatol Venereol 2000;14(6):446–447

Laskaris GC, Nicolis GD. Erythroplakia of Queyrat of the oral mucosa. A report of 2 cases. Dermatologica 1981;162:395–399

Reichart PA, Philipsen HP. Oral erythroplakia–a review. Oral Oncol 2005;41:551–561

Ribeiro AS, Salles PR, da Silva TA, Mesquita RA. A review of the nonsurgical treatment of oral leukoplakia. Int J Dent 2010;2010:186018

Scully C. Challenges in predicting which oral mucosal potentially malignant disease will progress to neoplasia. Oral Dis 2014;20(1):1–5

Shiu MN, Chen TH. Intervention efficacy and malignant transformation to oral cancer among patients with leukoplakia (Review). Oncol Rep 2003;10(6):1683–1692

Shridhar K, Walia GK, Aggarwal A, et al. DNA methylation markers for oral precancer progression: A critical review. Oral Oncol 2016;53:1–9

Zhang X, Li C, Song Y, Reichart PA. Oral leukoplakia in China: a review. Oral Maxillofac Surg 2010;14(4):195–202

38. Potentially Malignant Disorders— Conditions

Anand R, Dhingra C, Prasad S, Menon I. Betel nut chewing and its deleterious effects on oral cavity. J Cancer Res Ther 2014;10(3):499–505

Angadi PV, Rekha KP. Oral submucous fibrosis: a clinicopathologic review of 205 cases in Indians. Oral Maxillofac Surg 2011;15(1):15–19

Brain JH, Paul BF, Assad DA. Periodontal plastic surgery in a dystrophic epidermolysis bullosa patient: review and case report. J Periodontol 1999;70(11):1392–1396

Butt FM, Moshi JR, Owibingire S, Chindia ML. Xeroderma pigmentosum: a review and case series. J Craniomaxillofac Surg 2010;38(7):534–537

Feller L, Wood NH, Motswaledi MH, Khammissa RA, Meyer M, Lemmer J. Xeroderma pigmentosum: a case report and review of the literature. J Prev Med Hyg 2010;51(2):87–91

Gorsky M, Epstein JB. Oral lichen planus: malignant transformation and human papilloma virus: a review of potential clinical implications. Oral Surg Oral Med Oral Pathol Oral Radiol Endod 2011;111(4):461–464

Hadzi-Mihailovic M, Raybaud H, Monteil R, Cakic S, Djuric M, Jankovic L. Bcl-2 expression and its possible influence on malignant transformation of oral lichen planus. J BUON 2010;15(2):362–368

Hoffman RM, Jaffe PE. Plummer-Vinson syndrome. A case report and literature review. Arch Intern Med 1995;155(18):2008–2011

Jiang X, Hu J. Drug treatment of oral submucous fibrosis: a review of the literature. J Oral Maxillofac Surg 2009;67(7):1510–1515

Kalavrezos N, Scully C. Mouth cancer for clinicians. Part 1: Cancer. Dent Update 2015;42(3):250–252, 255–256, 259–260

Kao SY, Mao L, Jian XC, Rajan G, Yu GY. Expert consensus on the detection and screening of oral cancer and precancer. Chin J Dent Res 2015;18(2):79–83

Kerr AR, Warnakulasuriya S, Mighell AJ, et al. A systematic review of medical interventions for oral submucous fibrosis and future research opportunities. Oral Dis 2011;17(Suppl 1):42–57

Köklü S, Bulut M, Cakal B, Bozkurt A, Yüksel O. Gastric cancer presenting with Plummer-Vinson Syndrome. J Am Geriatr Soc 2009;57(5):933–934

Laskaris G, Bovopoulou O, Nicolis G. Oral submucous fibrosis in a Greek female. Br J Oral Surg 1981;19(3):197–201

Matsumoto Y, Dogru M, Tsubota K. Ocular surface findings in Hallopeau-Siemens subtype of dystrophic epidermolysis bullosa: report of a case and literature review. Cornea 2005;24(4):474–479

Mortazavi H, Baharvand M, Mehdipour M. Oral potentially malignant disorders: an overview of more than 20 entities. J Dent Res Dent Clin Dent Prospect 2014;8(1):6–14

Rivera-Begeman A, McDaniel LD, Schultz RA, Friedberg EC. A novel XPC pathogenic variant detected in archival material from a patient diagnosed with Xeroderma Pigmentosum: a case report and review of the genetic variants reported in XPC. DNA Repair (Amst) 2007;6(1):100–114

Tadakamadla J, Kumar S, Johnson NW. Quality of life in patients with oral potentially malignant disorders: a systematic review. Oral Surg Oral Med Oral Pathol Oral Radiol 2015;119(6):644–655

39. Malignant Neoplasms

Acar GO, Cansiz H, Acioglu E, Mercan H, Dervişoglu S. Chondrosarcoma of the mandible extending to the infratemporal fossa: report of two cases. Oral Maxillofac Surg 2008;12(3):173–176

Aguas SC, Quarracino MC, Lence AN, Lanfranchi-Tizeira HE. Primary melanoma of the oral cavity: ten cases and review of 177 cases from literature. Med Oral Patol Oral Cir Bucal 2009;14(6):E265–E271

Al-Khateeb T, Bataineh AB. Rhabdomyosarcoma of the oral and maxillofacial region in Jordanians: a retrospective analysis. Oral Surg Oral Med Oral Pathol Oral Radiol Endod 2002;93(5):580–585

Andreadis D, Nomikos A, Epivatianos A, Poulopoulos A, Barbatis C. Basaloid squamous cell carcinoma versus basal cell adenocarcinoma of the oral cavity. Pathology 2005;37(6):560–563

Angiero F, Signore A, Benedicenti S. Hemangiopericytoma/Solitary fibrous tumor of the oral cavity. Anticancer Res 2011;31(2):719–723

Arduino PG, Carrozzo M, Pagano M, Broccoletti R, Scully C, Gandolfo S. Immunohistochemical expression of basement membrane proteins of verrucous carcinoma of the oral mucosa. Clin Oral Investig 2010;14(3):297–302

Arduino PG, Carrozzo M, Pagano M, Gandolfo S, Broccoletti R. Verrucous oral carcinoma: clinical findings and treatment outcomes in 74 patients in Northwest Italy. Minerva Stomatol 2008;57(7-8):335–339, 339–341

Baum BJ, Alevizos I, Chiorini JA, Cotrim AP, Zheng C. Advances in salivary gland gene therapy - oral and systemic implications. Expert Opin Biol Ther 2015;15(10):1443–1454

Bonet J, Minguez JM, Penarrocha M, Soriano I, Vera-Sempere F. Ewing´s sarcoma of the mandible. A case report. Med Oral 2000;5(4):279–282

Bouda M, Gorgoulis VG, Kastrinakis NG, et al. "High risk" HPV types are frequently detected in potentially malignant and malignant oral lesions, but not in normal oral mucosa. Mod Pathol 2000;13(6):644–653

Bouquot JE, Servos T. Oral and maxillofacial pathology case of the month. Osteosarcoma (osteogenic sarcoma), high grade. Tex Dent J 2006;123(5):456–457, 462–463

Bovopoulou O, Sklavounou A, Laskaris G. Loss of intercellular substance antigens in oral hyperkeratosis, epithelial dysplasia, and squamous cell carcinoma. Oral Surg Oral Med Oral Pathol 1985;60(6):648–654

Campo-Trapero J, Del Romero-Guerrero J, Cano-Sánchez J, Rodríguez-Martín C, Martínez-González JM, Bascones-Martínez A. Relationship between oral Kaposi 's sarcoma and HAART: contribution of two case reports. Med Oral Patol Oral Cir Bucal 2008;13(11):E709–E713

Coca-Pelaz A, Rodrigo JP, Bradley PJ, et al. Adenoid cystic carcinoma of the head and neck--An update. Oral Oncol 2015;51(7):652–661

da Silva JM, Soave DF, Moreira Dos Santos TP, et al. Significance of chemokine and chemokine receptors in head and neck squamous cell carcinoma: a critical review. Oral Oncol 2016;56:8–16

Dantas AN, Morais EF, Macedo RA, Tinôco JM, Morais MdeL. Clinicopathological characteristics and perineural invasion in adenoid cystic carcinoma: a systematic review. Rev Bras Otorrinolaringol (Engl Ed) 2015;81(3):329–335

Dehal A, Quach L, Garrett E, Jreije K, Hussain F. Soft tissue sarcoma with tongue metastasis: a case report and literature review. J Oral Maxillofac Surg 2015;73(9):1877.e1–1877.e5

Dodd RL, Slevin NJ. Salivary gland adenoid cystic carcinoma: a review of chemotherapy and molecular therapies. Oral Oncol 2006;42(7):759–769

Edwards PC, Bhuiya T, Kelsch RD. C-kit expression in the salivary gland neoplasms adenoid cystic carcinoma, polymorphous low-grade adenocarcinoma, and monomorphic adenoma. Oral Surg Oral Med Oral Pathol Oral Radiol Endod 2003;95(5):586–593

Ethunandan M, Stokes C, Higgins B, Spedding A, Way C, Brennan P. Primary oral leiomyosarcoma: a clinico-pathologic study and analysis of prognostic factors. Int J Oral Maxillofac Surg 2007;36(5):409–416

Feller L, Khammissa RA, Kramer B, Altini M, Lemmer J. Basal cell carcinoma, squamous cell carcinoma and melanoma of the head and face. Head Face Med 2016;12:11

Feller L, Lemmer J, Wood NH, Jadwat Y, Raubenheimer EJ. HIV-associated oral Kaposi sarcoma and HHV-8: a review. J Int Acad Periodontol 2007;9(4):129–136

Femiano F, Lanza A, Buonaiuto C, Gombos F, Di Spirito F, Cirillo N. Oral malignant melanoma: a review of the literature. J Oral Pathol Med 2008;37(7):383–388

Ferreras J, Junquera LM, Lopez JS, Gonzalez M, Villarreal P, Cerrato E. Spindle cell carcinoma of the oral cavity. Report o f a case. Med Oral 2000;5(1):47–53

Folk GS, Williams SB, Foss RB, Fanburg-Smith JC. Oral and maxillofacial sclerosing epithelioid fibrosarcoma: report of five cases. Head Neck Pathol 2007;1(1):13–20

Fonseca FP, Sena Filho M, Altemani A, Speight PM, Vargas PA. Molecular signature of salivary gland tumors: potential use as diagnostic and prognostic marker. J Oral Pathol Med 2016;45(2):101–110

França CM, Caran EM, Alves MT, Barreto AD, Lopes NN. Rhabdomyosarcoma of the oral tissues--two new cases and literature review. Med Oral Patol Oral Cir Bucal 2006;11(2):E136–E140

Francisco AL, Furlan MV, Peresi PM, et al. Head and neck mucosal melanoma: clinicopathological analysis of 51 cases treated in a single cancer centre and review of the literature. Int J Oral Maxillofac Surg 2016;45(2):135–140

Fujita S, Senba M, Kumatori A, Hayashi T, Ikeda T, Toriyama K. Human papillomavirus infection in oral verrucous carcinoma: genotyping analysis and inverse correlation with p53 expression. Pathobiology 2008;75(4):257–264

Galimberti D, Galimberti G, Pontón Montaño A, Jácome LR, Galimberti R. Oral verrucous carcinoma treated with carbon dioxide laser. J Eur Acad Dermatol Venereol 2010;24(8):976–977

Georgakopoulou EA, Achtari MD, Achtaris M, Foukas PG, Kotsinas A. Oral lichen planus as a preneoplastic inflammatory model. J Biomed Biotechnol 2012;2012:759626

Georgakopoulou EA, Troupis TG, Troupis G, Gorgoulis VG. Update of the cancer-associated molecular mechanisms in oral lichen planus, a disease with possible premalignant nature. J BUON 2011;16(4):613–616

Gillenwater AM, Vigneswaran N, Fatani H, Saintigny P, El-Naggar AK. Proliferative verrucous leukoplakia: recognition and differentiation from conventional leukoplakia and mimics. Head Neck 2014;36(11):1662–1668

Gómez I, Warnakulasuriya S, Varela-Centelles PI, et al. Is early diagnosis of oral cancer a feasible objective? Who is to blame for diagnostic delay? Oral Dis 2010;16(4):333–342

Gondivkar SM, Indurkar A, Degwekar S, Bhowate R. Primary oral malignant melanoma--a case report and review of the literature. Quintessence Int 2009;40(1):41–46

Gosau M, Baumhoer D, Ihrler S, Kleinheinz J, Driemel O. Ewing sarcoma of the mandible mimicking an odontogenic abscess - a case report. Head Face Med 2008;4:24

Gupta S, Gupta S. Role of human papillomavirus in oral squamous cell carcinoma and oral potentially malignant disorders: a review of the literature. Indian J Dent 2015;6(2):91–98

Hashemi Pour MS. Malignant melanoma of the oral cavity: a review of literature. Indian J Dent Res 2008;19(1):47–51

Ishikawa Y, Ishii T, Asuwa N, Ogawa T. Adenoid cystic carcinoma originated from an anterior lingual minor salivary gland: immunohistochemical and ultrastructural studies and review of the literature. J Oral Maxillofac Surg 1997;55(12):1460–1469

Kashikar S, Steinle M, Reich R, Freedman P. Epithelioid multinodular osteoblastoma of the mandible: A case report and review of the literature. Head Neck Pathol 2016;10(2):182–187

Kesse W, Violaris N, Howlett DC. An unusual cause of facial pain: malignant change in a calcified pleomorphic adenoma in the deep lobe of the parotid gland. Ear Nose Throat J 2003;82(8):623–625

Khafif A, Anavi Y, Haviv J, Fienmesser R, Calderon S, Marshak G. Adenoid cystic carcinoma of the salivary glands: a 20-year review with long-term follow-up. Ear Nose Throat J 2005;84(10):662, 664–667

Khalili M, Mahboobi N, Shams J. Metastatic breast carcinoma initially diagnosed as pulpal/periapical disease: a case report. J Endod 2010;36(5):922–925

Kim SM, Myoung H, Choung PH, Kim MJ, Lee SK, Lee JH. Metastatic leiomyosarcoma in the oral cavity: case report with protein expression profiles. J Craniomaxillofac Surg 2009;37(8):454–460

Kobayashi M, Hattori M, Miyamoto T, et al. Basement membrane-like substance in cytologic diagnosis in clear cell adenocarcinoma of the minor salivary gland of the palate. A case report. Acta Cytol 2007;51(6):916–920

Kobayashi T, Maruyama S, Cheng J, et al. Histopathological varieties of oral carcinoma in situ: Diagnosis aided by immunohistochemistry dealing with the second basal cell layer as the proliferating center of oral mucosal epithelia. Pathol Int 2010;60(3):156–166

Kolokythas A, Connor S, Kimgsoo D, Fernandes RP, Ord RA. Low-grade mucoepidermoid carcinoma of the intraoral minor salivary glands with cervical metastasis: report of 2 cases and review of the literature. J Oral Maxillofac Surg 2010;68(6):1396–1399

Kothari RK, Ghosh A, Bhattacharyya SK, Ghosh SK. Adenosquamous carcinoma of oral cavity: a case report. J Indian Med Assoc 2007;105(9):531–532

Krishna KB, Thomas V, Kattoor J, Kusumakumari P. A radiological review of Ewing's sarcoma of mandible: A case report with one year follow-up. Int J Clin Pediatr Dent 2013;6(2):109–114

Kroumpouzos G, Frank EW, Albertini JG, et al. Lentigo maligna with spread onto oral mucosa. Arch Dermatol 2002;138(9):1216–1220

Laurie SA, Ho AL, Fury MG, Sherman E, Pfister DG. Systemic therapy in the management of metastatic or locally recurrent adenoid cystic carcinoma of the salivary glands: a systematic review. Lancet Oncol 2011;12(8):815–824

Lin SK, How SW, Wang JT, Liu BY, Chiang CP. Oral post-radiation malignant fibrous histiocytoma: a clinicopathological study. J Oral Pathol Med 1994;23(7):324–329

Iino M, Yamada H, Ishikawa H, et al. Carcinoma ex pleomorphic adenoma of the submandibular gland: report of a case with an unusual malignant component of clear cell squamous cell carcinoma. Oral Surg Oral Med Oral Pathol Oral Radiol Endod 2008;106(2):e30–e34

Maahs GS, Oppermann PdeO, Maahs LG, Machado Filho G, Ronchi AD. Parotid gland tumors: a retrospective study of 154 patients. Rev Bras Otorrinolaringol (Engl Ed) 2015;81(3):301–306

Macheret M, Halazonetis TD. DNA replication stress as a hallmark of cancer. Annu Rev Pathol 2015;10:425–448

Maestre-Rodríguez O, González-García R, Mateo-Arias J, et al. Metastasis of renal clear-cell carcinoma to the oral mucosa, an atypical location. Med Oral Patol Oral Cir Bucal 2009;14(11):e601–e604

Mahomed F, Grayson W. A rare case of lymphoepithelial carcinoma of the lip. Oral Surg Oral Med Oral Pathol Oral Radiol Endod 2008;105(5):e49–e52

Manganaris A, Patakiouta F, Xirou P, Manganaris T. Lymphoepithelial carcinoma of the parotid gland: is an association with Epstein-Barr virus possible in non-endemic areas? Int J Oral Maxillofac Surg 2007;36(6):556–559

Maresi E, Tortorici S, Campione M, et al. Hemangiopericytoma of the oral cavity after a ten-year follow-up. Ann Clin Lab Sci 2007;37(3):274–279

Marques YM, Moura MdeD, Hiraki KR, Pieri SS, de Oliveira EM, Mantesso A. Chondrosarcoma of the mandible: case report and literature review. Gen Dent 2009;57(5):e47–e50

Meleti M, Leemans CR, Mooi WJ, Vescovi P, van der Waal I. Oral malignant melanoma: a review of the literature. Oral Oncol 2007;43(2):116–121

Meurman JH, Scully C. Oral cancer: comprehending the condition, causes, controversies, control and consequences. 3. Other risk factors. Dent Update 2011;38(1):66–68

Moghadam SA, Khodayari A, Mokhtari S. Primary leiomyosarcoma of the mandible. J Oral Maxillofac Pathol 2014;18(2):308–311

Mohtasham N, Kharrazi AA, Jamshidi S, Jafarzadeh H. Epithelioid hemangioendothelioma of the oral cavity: a case report. J Oral Sci 2008;50(2):219–223

Nagao T, Gaffey TA, Kay PA, Minato H, Serizawa H, Lewis JE. Polymorphous low-grade adenocarcinoma of the major salivary glands: report of three cases in an unusual location. Histopathology 2004;44(2):164–171

Nagpal DK, Prabhu PR, Shah A, Palaskar S. Leimyosarcoma of the buccal mucosa and review of literature. J Oral Maxillofac Pathol 2013;17(1):149

Oh KY, Yoon HJ, Lee JI, Hong SP, Hong SD. Chondrosarcoma of the temporomandibular joint : a case report and review of the literature. Cranio 2016;34(4):270–278

Panwar A, Kozel JA, Lydiatt WM. Cancers of major salivary glands. Surg Oncol Clin N Am 2015;24(3):615–633

Pavithran K, Doval DC, Mukherjee G, Kannan V, Kumaraswamy SV, Bapsy PP. Rhabdomyosarcoma of the oral cavity--report of eight cases. Acta Oncol 1997;36(8):819–821

Pentenero M, Meleti M, Vescovi P, Gandolfo S. Oral proliferative verrucous leucoplakia: are there particular features for such an ambiguous entity? A systematic review. Br J Dermatol 2014;170(5):1039–1047

Petridou E, Zavras AI, Lefatzis D, et al. The role of diet and specific micronutrients in the etiology of oral carcinoma. Cancer 2002;94(11):2981–2988

Qaisi M, Vorrasi J, Lubek J, Ord R. Multiple primary squamous cell carcinomas of the oral cavity. J Oral Maxillofac Surg 2014;72(8):1511–1516

Rapidis AD, Givalos N, Gakiopoulou H, et al. Mucoepidermoid carcinoma of the salivary glands. Review of the literature and clinicopathological analysis of 18 patients. Oral Oncol 2007;43(2):130–136

Rapidis AD, Gullane P, Langdon JD, Lefebvre JL, Scully C, Shah JP. Major advances in the knowledge and understanding of the epidemiology, aetiopathogenesis, diagnosis, management and prognosis of oral cancer. Oral Oncol 2009;45(4-5):299–300

Romañach MJ, Azevedo RS, Carlos R, de Almeida OP, Pires FR. Clinicopathological and immunohistochemical features of oral spindle cell carcinoma. J Oral Pathol Med 2010;39(4):335–341

Roy L, Moubayed SP, Ayad T. Lymphoepithelial carcinoma of the sublingual gland: Case report and review of the literature. J Oral Maxillofac Surg 2015;73(9):1878.e1–1878.e5

Sáenz-Santamaría J, Catalina-Fernandez I. Polymorphous low grade adenocarcinoma of the salivary gland. Diagnosis by fine needle aspiration cytology. Acta Cytol 2004;48(1):52–56

Schick U, Pusztaszeri M, Betz M, et al. Adenosquamous carcinoma of the head and neck: report of 20 cases and review of the literature. Oral Surg Oral Med Oral Pathol Oral Radiol 2013;116(3):313–320

Schultze-Mosgau S, Thorwarth M, Wehrhan F, et al. Ewing sarcoma of the mandible in a child: interdisciplinary treatment concepts and surgical reconstruction. J Craniofac Surg 2005;16(6):1140–1146

Scully C, Bagan JV, Hopper C, Epstein JB. Oral cancer: current and future diagnostic techniques. Am J Dent 2008;21(4):199–209

Scully C, Bagan J. Oral squamous cell carcinoma: overview of current understanding of aetiopathogenesis and clinical implications. Oral Dis 2009;15(6):388–399

Scully C. Oral cancer aetiopathogenesis; past, present and future aspects. Med Oral Patol Oral Cir Bucal 2011;16(3):e306–e311

Scully C, Bagan JV, Hopper C, Epstein JB. Oral healthcare in people living with cancer. Oral Oncol 2010;46(6):401

Simpson RH, Pereira EM, Ribeiro AC, Abdulkadir A, Reis-Filho JS. Polymorphous low-grade adenocarcinoma of the salivary glands with transformation to high-grade carcinoma. Histopathology 2002;41(3):250–259

Singh P, Singh A, Saxena S, Singh S. Mesenchymal chondrosarcoma of mandible: A rare case report and review. J Oral Maxillofac Pathol 2014;18(Suppl 1):S167–S170

Su HH, Chu ST, Hou YY, Chang KP, Chen CJ. Spindle cell carcinoma of the oral cavity and oropharynx: factors affecting outcome. J Chin Med Assoc 2006;69(10):478–483

Sumida T, Otawa N, Kamata YU, et al. A clinical investigation of oral sarcomas as multi-institutions over the past 30 years. Anticancer Res 2015;35(8):4551–4555

Sun ZJ, Zhang L, Zhang WF, Chen XM, Lai FM, Zhao YF. Epithelioid hemangioendothelioma of the oral cavity. Oral Dis 2007;13(2):244–250

Sur RK, Donde B, Levin V, et al. Adenoid cystic carcinoma of the salivary glands: a review of 10 years. Laryngoscope 1997;107(9):1276–1280

Tavora F, Rassaei N, Shilo K, et al. Occult primary parotid gland acinic cell adenocarcinoma presenting with extensive lung metastasis. Arch Pathol Lab Med 2007;131(6):970–973

Triantafillidou K, Dimitrakopoulos J, Iordanidis F, Koufogiannis D. Mucoepidermoid carcinoma of minor salivary glands: a clinical study of 16 cases and review of the literature. Oral Dis 2006;12(4):364–370

Tsantoulis PK, Kastrinakis NG, Tourvas AD, Laskaris G, Gorgoulis VG. Advances in the biology of oral cancer. Oral Oncol 2007;43(6):523–534

Veltrini VC, Etges A, Magalhães MH, de Araújo NS, de Araújo VC. Solitary fibrous tumor of the oral mucosa--morphological and immunohistochemical profile in the differential diagnosis with hemangiopericytoma. Oral Oncol 2003;39(4):420–426

Wadhwan V, Chaudhary MS, Gawande M. Fibrosarcoma of the oral cavity. Indian J Dent Res 2010;21(2):295–298

Walvekar RR, Chaukar DA, Deshpande MS, et al. Verrucous carcinoma of the oral cavity: A clinical and pathological study of 101 cases. Oral Oncol 2009;45(1):47–51

Widmer IC, Erb P, Grob H, et al. Human herpesvirus 8 oral shedding in HIV-infected men with and without Kaposi sarcoma. J Acquir Immune Defic Syndr 2006;42(4):420–425

Wiesmiller K, Barth TF, Gronau S. Early radiation-induced malignant fibrous histiocytoma of the oral cavity. J Laryngol Otol 2003;117(3):224–226

Wushou A, Miao XC, Shao ZM. Treatment outcome and prognostic factors of head and neck hemangiopericytoma: meta-analysis. Head Neck 2015;37(11):1685–1690

Yan B, Li Y, Pan J, Xia H, Li LJ. Primary oral leiomyosarcoma: a retrospective clinical analysis of 20 cases. Oral Dis 2010;16(2):198–203

Zavras AI, Douglass CW, Joshipura K, et al. Smoking and alcohol in the etiology of oral cancer: gender-specific risk profiles in the south of Greece. Oral Oncol 2001;37(1):28–35

Zavras AI, Laskaris C, Kittas C, Laskaris G. Leukoplakia and intraoral malignancies: female cases increase in Greece. J Eur Acad Dermatol Venereol 2003;17(1):25–27

Zavras AI, Wu T, Laskaris G, et al. Interaction between a single nucleotide polymorphism in the alcohol dehydrogenase 3 gene, alcohol consumption and oral cancer risk. Int J Cancer 2002;97(4):526–530

Zhou DN, Yang QQ, Li ZL, Pan ZY, Deng YF. Head and neck rhabdomyosarcoma: follow-up results of four cases and review of the literature. Int J Clin Exp Pathol 2015;8(5):4277–4283

Zhu W, Hu F, Zhao T, Wang C, Tao Q. Clinical characteristics of radiation-induced sarcoma of the head and neck: Review of 15 cases and 323 cases in the literature. J Oral Maxillofac Surg 2016;74(2):283–291

40. Malignancies of the Hematopoietic and Lymphatic Tissues

Angst PD, Dutra DA, Moreira CH, Kantorski KZ. Gingival inflammation and platelet count in patients with leukemia: preliminary results. Braz Oral Res 2011;25(6):544–549

Björkholm M. Treatment options in Waldenstrom's macroglobulinemia. Clin Lymphoma 2004;5(3):155–162

Bombeccari GP, Guzzi G, Ruffoni D, Gianatti A, Mariani U, Spadari F. Mucosa-associated lymphatic tissue lymphoma of the lower lip in a child. J Pediatr Surg 2011;46(12):2414–2416

Bulut E, Bekçioğlu B, Günhan O, Sener I. Diffuse large B-cell lymphoma with oral manifestations. J Craniofac Surg 2011;22(3):1144–1147

Burke VP, Startzell JM. The leukemias. Oral Maxillofac Surg Clin North Am 2008;20(4):597–608

Cisternino A, Asa'ad F, Fusco N, Ferrero S, Rasperini G. Role of multidisciplinary approach in a case of Langerhans cell histiocytosis with initial periodontal manifestations. Int J Clin Exp Pathol 2015;8(10):13539–13545

Dereure O, Guilhou JJ. Mycosis fungoides with predominant periorificial and mucous involvement [in French]. Ann Dermatol Venereol 2005;132(11, Pt 1):877–880

Gonçalves CF, Morais MO, de Cássia Gonçalves Alencar R, Batista AC, Mendonça EF. Solitary Langerhans cell histiocytosis in an adult: case report and literature review. BMC Res Notes 2016;9:19

Gonzalez-Garcia J, Ghufoor K, Sandhu G, Thorpe PA, Hadley J. Primary extramedullary plasmacytoma of the parotid gland: a case report and review of the literature. J Laryngol Otol 1998;112(2):179–181

Guimarães LF, Dias PF, Janini ME, de Souza IP. Langerhans cell histiocytosis: impact on the permanent dentition after an 8-year follow-up. J Dent Child (Chic) 2008;75(1):64–68

Guruprasad Y, Chauhan DS. Solitary eosinophilic granuloma of mandibular condyle: literature review and report of a rare case. J Maxillofac Oral Surg 2015;14(Suppl 1):209–214

Hata T, Aikoh T, Hirokawa M, Hosoda M. Mycosis fungoides with involvement of the oral mucosa. Int J Oral Maxillofac Surg 1998;27(2):127–128

Klokkevold PR, Miller DA, Friedlander AH. Mental nerve neuropathy: a symptom of Waldenström's macroglobulinemia. Oral Surg Oral Med Oral Pathol 1989;67(6):689–693

Laskaris GC, Nicolis GD, Capetanakis JP. Mycosis fungoides with oral manifestations. Oral Surg Oral Med Oral Pathol 1978;46(1):40–42

Madrigal-Martínez-Pereda C, Guerrero-Rodríguez V, Guisado-Moya B, Meniz-García C. Langerhans cell histiocytosis: literature review and descriptive analysis of oral manifestations. Med Oral Patol Oral Cir Bucal 2009;14(5):E222–E228

Meng W, Zhou Y, Zhang H, et al. Nasal-type NK/T-cell lymphoma with palatal ulcer as the earliest clinical manifestation: a case report with literature review. Pathol Oncol Res 2010;16(1):133–137

Ponce-Torres E, Ruíz-Rodríguez MdelS, Alejo-González F, Hernández-Sierra JF, Pozos-Guillén AdeJ. Oral manifestations in pediatric patients receiving chemotherapy for acute lymphoblastic leukemia. J Clin Pediatr Dent 2010;34(3):275–279

Quiñones-Avila MdelP, Gonzalez-Longoria AA, Admirand JH, Medeiros LJ. Hodgkin lymphoma involving Waldeyer ring: a clinicopathologic study of 22 cases. Am J Clin Pathol 2005;123(5):651–656

Scully C, Epstein J, Porter S, Cox M. Viruses and chronic disorders involving the human oral mucosa. Oral Surg Oral Med Oral Pathol 1991;72(5):537–544

Stoopler ET, Vogl DT, Alawi F, et al. The presence of amyloid in abdominal and oral mucosal tissues in patients initially diagnosed with multiple myeloma: a pilot study. Oral Surg Oral Med Oral Pathol Oral Radiol Endod 2011;111(3):326–332

Subramaniam P, Babu KL, Nagarathna J. Oral manifestations in acute lymphoblastic leukemic children under chemotherapy. J Clin Pediatr Dent 2008;32(4):319–324

Susarla SM, Sharaf BA, Faquin W, Hasserjian RP, McDermott N, Lahey E. Extranodal natural killer T-cell lymphoma, nasal type, with minimal osseous involvement: report of a case and literature review. J Oral Maxillofac Surg 2010;68(3):674–681

Tanaka T, Kitabatake K, Iino M, Goto K. Immunohistochemical comparison of CD5, lambda, and kappa expression in primary and recurrent buccal mucosa-associated lymphoid tissue (MALT) lymphomas. Diagn Pathol 2011;6:82

Thomas DA, O'Brien S, Faderl S, et al. Burkitt lymphoma and atypical Burkitt or Burkitt-like lymphoma: should these be treated as different diseases? Curr Hematol Malig Rep 2011;6(1):58–66

Ustün MO, Ekinci N, Payzin B. Extramedullary plasmacytoma of the parotid gland. Report of a case with extensive amyloid deposition masking the cytologic and histopathologic picture. Acta Cytol 2001;45(3):449–453

Wain EM, Setterfield J, Judge MR, Harper JI, Pemberton MN, Russell-Jones R. Mycosis fungoides involving the oral mucosa in a child. Clin Exp Dermatol 2003;28(5):499–501

Whitt JC, Dunlap CL, Martin KF. Oral Hodgkin lymphoma: a wolf in wolf's clothing. Oral Surg Oral Med Oral Pathol Oral Radiol Endod 2007;104(5):e45–e51

Witt C, Borges AC, Klein K, Neumann HJ. Radiographic manifestations of multiple myeloma in the mandible: a retrospective study of 77 patients. J Oral Maxillofac Surg 1997;55(5):450–453, discussion 454–455

41. Paraneoplastic Mucocutaneous Diseases

Abbas O, Kibbi AG, Rubeiz N. Sweet's syndrome: retrospective study of clinical and histologic features of 44 cases from a tertiary care center. Int J Dermatol 2010;49(11):1244–1249

Allen CM, Camisa C. Paraneoplastic pemphigus: a review of the literature. Oral Dis 2000;6(4):208–214

Baran I, Nalcaci R, Kocak M. Dyskeratosis congenita: clinical report and review of the literature. Int J Dent Hyg 2010;8(1):68–74

Brucoli M, Giarda M, Benech A. Gardner syndrome: presurgical planning and surgical management of craniomaxillofacial osteomas. J Craniofac Surg 2011;22(3):946–948

Cohen PR, Kurzrock R. Mucocutaneous paraneoplastic syndromes. Semin Oncol 1997;24(3):334–359

Laskaris GC, Papavasiliou SS, Bovopoulou OD, Nicolis GD. Association of oral pemphigus with chronic lymphocytic leukemia. Oral Surg Oral Med Oral Pathol 1980;50(3):244–249

Ng PP, Rencic A, Nousari HC. Paraneoplastic pemphigus: a refractory autoimmune mucocutaneous disease. J Cutan Med Surg 2002;6(5):434–437

Nomura J, Tagawa T. Acanthosis nigricans with oral lesions and a malignant visceral tumor: a case report. J Oral Maxillofac Surg 1992;50(2):169–172

Pentenero M, Carrozzo M, Pagano M, Gandolfo S. Oral acanthosis nigricans, tripe palms and sign of leser-trélat in a patient with gastric adenocarcinoma. Int J Dermatol 2004;43(7):530–532

Ramírez-Amador V, Esquivel-Pedraza L, Caballero-Mendoza E, Berumen-Campos J, Orozco-Topete R, Angeles-Angeles A. Oral manifestations as a hallmark of malignant acanthosis nigricans. J Oral Pathol Med 1999;28(6):278–281

Scheper MA, Nikitakis NG, Sarlani E, Sauk JJ, Meiller TF. Cowden syndrome: report of a case with immunohistochemical analysis and review of the literature. Oral Surg Oral Med Oral Pathol Oral Radiol Endod 2006;101(5):625–631

Silvestris N, Chetta G, Sasso N, Lucarelli A, Berardi T. Mucocutaneous paraneoplastic syndromes (MCPS). A clinical-pathologic review. J Exp Clin Cancer Res 1998;17(4):453–464

Sklavounou A, Laskaris G. Paraneoplastic pemphigus: a review. Oral Oncol 1998;34(6):437–440

Snoeckx A, Vanhoenacker FM, Verhaert K, Chappelle K, Parizel PM. Gorlin-Goltz syndrome in a child: case report and clinical review. JBR-BTR 2008;91(6):235–239

Steele HA, George BJ. Mucocutaneous paraneoplastic syndromes associated with hematologic malignancies. Oncology (Williston Park) 2011;25(11):1076–1083

Troletti GD, Bertario L, Sala P, Pallotti F, Pigatto PD, Guzzi G. Peutz-Jeghers syndrome after oral surgery. Am J Dermatopathol 2009;31(6):614

Xi Z, Hui Q, Zhong L. Q-switched alexandrite laser treatment of oral labial lentigines in Chinese subjects with Peutz-Jeghers syndrome. Dermatol Surg 2009;35(7):1084–1088

Yan Z, Hua H, Gao Y. Paraneoplastic pemphigus characterized by polymorphic oral mucosal manifestations--report of two cases. Quintessence Int 2010;41(8):689–694

Zappasodi P, Forno C, Corso A, Lazzarino M. Mucocutaneous paraneoplastic syndromes in hematologic malignancies. Int J Dermatol 2006;45(1):14–22

42. Nonneoplastic Diseases of the Jaws

Abramovitch K, Rice DD. Benign fibro-osseous lesions of the jaws. Dent Clin North Am 2016;60(1):167–193

Blum IR. Contemporary views on dry socket (alveolar osteitis): a clinical appraisal of standardization, aetiopathogenesis and management: a critical review. Int J Oral Maxillofac Surg 2002;31(3):309–317

Cardoso CL, Rodrigues MT, Ferreira Júnior O, Garlet GP, de Carvalho PS. Clinical concepts of dry socket. J Oral Maxillofac Surg 2010;68(8):1922–1932

Daryani D, Gopakumar R. Central giant cell granuloma mimicking an adenomatoid odontogenic tumor. Contemp Clin Dent 2011;2(3):249–252

Gadodia A, Seith A. Fibrous dysplasia of the maxilla. J Pediatr Surg 2010;45(4):848, author reply 848

Godse AS, Shrotriya SP, Vaid NS. Fibrous dysplasia of the maxilla. J Pediatr Surg 2009;44(4):849–851

Gomes MF, de Souza Setúbal Destro MF, de Freitas Banzi EC, dos Santos SH, Claro FA, de Oliveira Nogueira T. Aggressive behaviour of cherubism in a teenager: 4-years of clinical follow-up associated with radiographic and histological features. Dentomaxillofac Radiol 2005;34(5):313–318

Maricic M. The use of zoledronic acid for Paget's disease of bone. Curr Osteoporos Rep 2006;4(1):40–44

Mirmohammadsadeghi A, Eshraghi B, Shahsanaei A, Assari R. Cherubism: report of three cases and literature review. Orbit 2015;34(1):33–37

Peñarrocha M, Bonet J, Mínguez JM, Bagán JV, Vera F, Mínguez I. Cherubism: a clinical, radiographic, and histopathologic comparison of 7 cases. J Oral Maxillofac Surg 2006;64(6):924–930

Seehra J, Sloan P, Oliver RJ. Paget's disease of bone and osteonecrosis. Dent Update 2009;36(3):166–168, 171–172

Segal A. Rehabilitation of a maxillary defect secondary to recurrent giant cell granuloma. J Prosthodont 2011;20(Suppl 2):S32–S37

Tarakji B, Saleh LA, Umair A, Azzeghaiby SN, Hanouneh S. Systemic review of dry socket: aetiology, treatment, and prevention. J Clin Diagn Res 2015;9(4):ZE10–ZE13

Torres-Lagares D, Serrera-Figallo MA, Romero-Ruíz MM, Infante-Cossío P, García-Calderón M, Gutiérrez-Pérez JL. Update on dry socket: a review of the literature. Med Oral Patol Oral Cir Bucal 2005;10(1):81–85, 77–81

Tsodoulos S, Ilia A, Antoniades K, Angelopoulos C. Cherubism: a case report of a three-generation inheritance and literature review. J Oral Maxillofac Surg 2014;72(2):405.e1–405.e9

43. Odontogenic Tumors

Almeida RdeA, Andrade ES, Barbalho JC, Vajgel A, Vasconcelos BC. Recurrence rate following treatment for primary multicystic ameloblastoma: systematic review and meta-analysis. Int J Oral Maxillofac Surg 2016;45(3):359–367

Amado Cuesta S, Gargallo Albiol J, Berini Aytés L, Gay Escoda C. Review of 61 cases of odontoma. Presentation of an erupted complex odontoma. Med Oral 2003;8(5):366–373

Ayoub MS, Baghdadi HM, El-Kholy M. Immunohistochemical detection of laminin-1 and Ki-67 in radicular cysts and keratocystic odontogenic tumors. BMC Clin Pathol 2011;11:4

Bridle C, Visram K, Piper K, Ali N. Maxillary calcifying epithelial odontogenic (Pindborg) tumor presenting with abnormal eye signs: case report and literature review. Oral Surg Oral Med Oral Pathol Oral Radiol Endod 2006;102(4):e12–e15

Brown NA, Betz BL. Ameloblastoma: A review of recent molecular pathogenetic discoveries. Biomark Cancer 2015;7(Suppl 2):19–24

Fernandes AM, Duarte EC, Pimenta FJ, et al. Odontogenic tumors: a study of 340 cases in a Brazilian population. J Oral Pathol Med 2005;34(10):583–587

Gallana-Alvarez S, Mayorga-Jimenez F, Torres-Gómez FJ, Avellá-Vecino FJ, Salazar-Fernandez C. Calcifying odontogenic cyst associated with complex odontoma: case report and review of the literature. Med Oral Patol Oral Cir Bucal 2005;10(3):243–247

Gomes CC, Duarte AP, Diniz MG, Gomez RS. Review article: Current concepts of ameloblastoma pathogenesis. J Oral Pathol Med 2010;39(8):585–591

Guerrisi M, Piloni MJ, Keszler A. Odontogenic tumors in children and adolescents. A 15-year retrospective study in Argentina. Med Oral Patol Oral Cir Bucal 2007;12(3):E180–E185

Ide F, Kikuchi K, Miyazaki Y, Kusama K, Saito I, Muramatsu T. The early history of odontogenic ghost cell lesions: from Thoma to Gorlin. Head Neck Pathol 2015;9(1):74–78

Krishnapillai R, Angadi PV. A clinical, radiographic, and histologic review of 73 cases of ameloblastoma in an Indian population. Quintessence Int 2010;41(5):e90–e100

Litonjua LA, Suresh L, Valderrama LS, Neiders ME. Erupted complex odontoma: a case report and literature review. Gen Dent 2004;52(3):248–251

Zanetti LS, de Carvalho BM, Garcia IR Jr, de Barros LA, Dos Santos PL, de Moraes Ferreira AC. Conservative treatment of odontogenic myxoma. J Craniofac Surg 2011;22(5):1939–1941

Patiño B, Fernández-Alba J, Garcia-Rozado A, Martin R, López-Cedrún JL, Sanromán B. Calcifying epithelial odontogenic (pindborg) tumor: a series of 4 distinctive cases and a review of the literature. J Oral Maxillofac Surg 2005;63(9):1361–1368

Pippi R. Odontomas and supernumerary teeth: is there a common origin? Int J Med Sci 2014;11(12):1282–1297

Qaisi M, Eid I. Pediatric head and neck malignancies. Oral Maxillofac Surg Clin North Am 2016;28(1):11–19

Rallis G, Dais P, Kostakis G, Stathopoulos P. Osteo-cementum producing odontogenic myxomas. A literature review of distinctive variant. J Maxillofac Oral Surg 2015;14(2):176–181

Ruhin-Poncet B, Picard A, Martin-Duverneuil N, Albertini AF, Goudot P. [Keratocysts (or keratocystic epithelial odontogenic tumors)]. Rev Stomatol Chir Maxillofac 2011;112(2):87–92

Sekerci AE, Nazlim S, Etoz M, Deniz K, Yasa Y. Odontogenic tumors: a collaborative study of 218 cases diagnosed over 12 years and comprehensive review of the literature. Med Oral Patol Oral Cir Bucal 2015;20(1):e34–e44

Sham E, Leong J, Maher R, Schenberg M, Leung M, Mansour AK. Mandibular ameloblastoma: clinical experience and literature review. ANZ J Surg 2009;79(10):739–744

Tarakji B, Ashok N, Alzoghaibi I, et al. Malignant transformation of calcifying cystic odontogenic tumour - a review of literature. Contemp Oncol (Pozn) 2015;19(3):184–186

Toida M. So-called calcifying odontogenic cyst: review and discussion on the terminology and classification. J Oral Pathol Med 1998;27(2):49–52

Van Dam SD, Unni KK, Keller EE. Metastasizing (malignant) ameloblastoma: review of a unique histopathologic entity and report of Mayo Clinic experience. J Oral Maxillofac Surg 2010;68(12):2962–2974

WHO. Who histological classification of tumours of odontogenic tumours IARC 2005. Available at: http://screening.iarc.fr/atlasoralclassifwho2.php

Appendix: Classification of Oral Lesions and Diseases According to Morphology and Color, Biopsy

Morphology and Color

In the Appendix, the reader will find grouped the diseases that are included in the book according to two main criteria: (1) *The morphology (elementary lesion)* in such a way that at first glance to be able to isolate the smaller group of diseases that are characterized from similar clinical characteristics and (2) *the color of the lesions*, so that the oral physician can eliminate further the group of diseases included in the differential diagnosis. Concurrent evaluation leads to a smaller spectrum of diseases that in addition to the medical history and the clinical features (signs and symptoms) approaches the final goal that is the accurate diagnosis which is prerequisite for a correct and successful treatment.

The diagnosis of each disease is based on three fundamental rules:
1. Patient's medical history
2. Clinical assessment of signs and symptoms
3. Laboratory tests if necessary

The later has to follow and must be relevant to the clinical examination. Furthermore, the results of the tests must be evaluated in relation to the clinical findings.

Terminology of the Lesions

Macule. Flat, nonpalpable lesion smaller than 1 cm in diameter. It is due to color or fine texture change.

Papule. Small, elevated palpable lesion less than 1 cm in diameter.

Plaque. Palpable elevated lesion, greater than or equal to 1 cm in diameter.

Tumor. Indurated, elevated lesion greater than 1 cm in diameter due to epithelium or to mesenchyma or both changes.

Vesicle. Elevated, oval lesion that contains clear fluid, less than 1 cm in diameter.

Bulla. Elevated lesion that contains clear or bloody fluid, greater than 1 cm in diameter.

Pustule. Elevated lesion that contains pus (yellowish fluid), less than 1 cm in diameter.

Ulcer. Loss at least of all epithelial layers, with variable size.

Erosion. Superficial loss of epithelium with variable size.

Papillary lesion. Exophytic growth with a verrucous of cauliflower surface.

Cyst. A soft or fluctuant swelling, usually filled with fluid.

I. Morphology

1. Vesicles
- Primary herpetic gingivostomatitis
- Secondary herpetic lesions
- Herpes zoster
- Chickenpox
- Herpangina
- Hand–foot–and–mouth disease
- Erythema multiforme
- Drug-allergic reaction

2. Bullae
- Pemphigus
- Mucous membrane pemphigoid
- Bullous pemphigoid
- Linear IgA disease
- Pemphigoid gestationis
- Dermatitis herpetiformis
- Epidermolysis bullosa acquisita
- Genetic epidermolysis bullosa
- Chronic ulcerative stomatitis
- Erythema multiforme
- Stevens-Johnson syndrome
- Toxic epidermal necrolysis (Lyell syndrome)
- Lupus erythematosus, systemic
- Bullous lichen planus
- Traumatic bulla
- Angina bullosa hemorrhagica
- Primary systemic amyloidosis
- Thrombocytopenia

3. Pustules
- Dermatitis herpetiformis
- Pyostomatitis vegetans
- Impetigo

4. Erosions—Ulcerations
- **Primary**
  - Traumatic ulcer
  - Cunnilingus
  - Aphthous ulceration
  - Eosinophilic ulcer
  - Ulcerative gingivitis
  - Ulcerative stomatitis
  - Noma
  - Necrotizing sialadenometaplasia
  - Chronic ulcerative stomatitis
  - Riga-Fede ulcer
  - Mucosal necrosis due to injection
  - Chemical burns
  - Fever, adenitis, pharyngitis, aphthous (FAPA) syndrome
  - Adamantiades-Behçet disease
  - Sweet's syndrome
  - Syphilis (stages I, II, III)
  - Tuberculosis

- ◦ Staphylococcal ulceration
- ◦ Streptococcal ulceration
- ◦ Cytomegalovirus infection
- ◦ Epstein-Barr infection
- ◦ Wegener's granulomatosis
- ◦ Histoplasmosis
- ◦ Mucormycosis
- ◦ Aspergillosis
- ◦ Cryptococcosis
- ◦ Blastomycosis
- ◦ Paracoccidioidomycosis
- ◦ Chancroid
- ◦ Donovanosis
- ◦ Squamous cell carcinoma
- ◦ Adenoid cystic carcinoma
- ◦ Mucoepidermoid carcinoma
- ◦ Polymorphous low-grade adenocarcinoma
- ◦ Other types of adenocarcinomas
- ◦ Sarcomas
- ◦ Non-Hodgkin's lymphomas
- ◦ Extranodal natural killer (NK)/T-cell lymphoma, nasal type
- ◦ Mycosis fungoides
- ◦ Benign lymphoepithelial lesion
- ◦ Langerhans' cell histiocytosis
- ◦ Leukemias
- ◦ Myelodysplastic syndrome
- ◦ Lymphoproliferative lesions
- ◦ Multiple myeloma
- ◦ Waldenström's macroglobulinemia
- ◦ Cyclic neutropenia
- ◦ Other forms of neutropenias
- ◦ Aplastic anemia
- ◦ Agranulocytosis
- ◦ Glycogen storage disease, type Ib
- ◦ Graft-versus-host disease
- ◦ Crohn's disease
- ◦ Ulcerative colitis
- ◦ Erosive lichen planus
- ◦ Lupus erythematosus
- ◦ Temporal arteritis
- ◦ Odontogenic tumors, peripheral

- **Secondary, after blisters rupture**
  - ◦ Pyostomatitis vegetans
  - ◦ Primary herpetic gingivostomatitis
  - ◦ Herpes zoster
  - ◦ Herpangina
  - ◦ Hand–foot–and–mouth disease
  - ◦ Pemphigus
  - ◦ Mucous membrane pemphigoid
  - ◦ Bullous pemphigoid

- ◦ Linear IgA disease
- ◦ Pemphigoid gestationis
- ◦ Dermatitis herpetiformis
- ◦ Epidermolysis bullosa
- ◦ Erythema multiforme
- ◦ Stevens-Johnson syndrome
- ◦ Toxic epidermal necrolysis

5. **Papillary lesions**
   - Papilloma
   - Condyloma acuminatum
   - Verruca vulgaris
   - Verrucous carcinoma
   - Verruciform xanthoma
   - Verrucous leukoplakia
   - Hairy leukoplakia
   - Cinnamon contact stomatitis
   - Squamous cell carcinoma
   - Papillary palatal hyperplasia
   - Hyperplasia due to negative pressure
   - Denture fibrous hyperplasia
   - Focal epithelial hyperplasia
   - Goltz's syndrome
   - Malignant acanthosis nigricans
   - Benign acanthosis nigricans
   - Darier's disease
   - Verrucous dyskeratoma
   - Uremic stomatitis
   - Wegener's granulomatosis
   - Crohn's disease
   - Oral myiasis

6. **Soft tissue tumors**
   - Fibroma
   - Peripheral ossifying fibroma
   - Lipoma
   - Myxoma
   - Osteoma
   - Chondroma
   - Oral focal mucinosis
   - Neurofibroma
   - Schwannoma
   - Traumatic neuroma
   - Hemangioma
   - Lymphangioma
   - Leiomyoma
   - Rhabdomyoma
   - Benign fibrous histiocytoma
   - Granular cell tumor
   - Granular cell tumor of infancy
   - Melanotic neuroectodermal tumor of infancy
   - Melanocytic nevus
   - Pyogenic granuloma

- Other forms of pyogenic granulomas
- Peripheral giant cell granuloma
- Papilloma
- Condyloma acuminatum
- Verruca vulgaris
- Keratoacanthoma
- Focal epithelial hyperplasia
- Squamous cell carcinoma
- Pleomorphic adenoma
- Monomorphic adenomas
- Adenoid cystic carcinoma
- Mucoepidermoid carcinoma
- Polymorphous low-grade adenocarcinoma
- Other forms of minor salivary glands' carcinomas
- Malignant fibrous histiocytoma
- Chondrosarcoma
- Osteosarcoma
- Ewing's sarcoma
- Fibrosarcoma
- Leiomyosarcoma
- Kaposi's sarcoma
- Hemangioendothelioma
- Hemangiopericytoma
- Malignant melanoma
- Non-Hodgkin's lymphoma
- Burkitt's lymphoma
- Soft tissue plasmacytoma
- Langerhans' cell histiocytosis
- Multiple myeloma
- Metastatic neoplasms
- Actinomycosis
- Bacillary angiomatosis
- Salivary duct inflammation
- Soft tissue abscess
- Oral tooth sinus
- Peritonsillar abscess
- Leishmaniasis
- Peripheral odontogenic tumors
- Amyloidosis
- Multiple endocrine neoplasia, type 2B
- Goltz's syndrome
- Cowden's syndrome
- Other genetic syndromes
- Oral cysticercosis

7. **Soft tissue lumps—normal**
   - Foliate papillae
   - Circumvallate papillae
   - Fungiform papillae
   - Lymphoid hyperplasia
   - Fordyce's granules
   - Stensen's duct papilla

- Hypoglossal tubercle
- Incisive papilla

8. **Soft tissue cysts**
   - Mucocele
   - Ranula
   - Lymphoepithelial cyst
   - Cervical lymphoepithelial cyst
   - Dermoid cyst
   - Epidermoid cyst
   - Eruption cyst
   - Gingival cyst of adult
   - Gingival cyst of newborn
   - Incisive papilla cyst
   - Nasolabial cyst
   - Thyroglossal duct cyst
   - Cysticercosis

9. **Gingival swellings**
   - **Localized**
     - Pyogenic granuloma
     - Fibroma
     - Peripheral ossifying fibroma
     - Peripheral giant cell granuloma
     - Granular cell tumor of the newborn
     - Melanotic neuroectodermal tumor of infancy
     - Peripheral odontogenic tumors
     - Odontogenic cysts
     - Exostoses
     - Dental abscess
     - Periodontal abscess
     - Periodontal and dental fistula
     - Gingival cyst of the adults
     - Gingival cyst of the newborns
     - Eruption cyst
     - Solitary soft tissue plasmacytoma
     - Granulomatous gingivitis
     - Denture fibrous hyperplasia
     - Various benign tumors
     - Squamous cell carcinoma
     - Other types of malignant tumors
     - Kaposi's sarcoma
     - Non-Hodgkin's lymphoma
     - Multiple myeloma
     - Metastatic neoplasms
     - Donovanosis
     - Cowden's syndrome
     - Tuberous sclerosis
   - **Generalized**
     - Hyperplastic gingivitis
     - Mouth-breathing gingivitis
     - Gingival enlargement during pregnancy

- ◦ Granulomatous gingivitis
- ◦ Scurvy
- ◦ Crohn's disease
- ◦ Plasmacytoma
- ◦ Leukemias
- ◦ Wegener's granulomatosis
- ◦ Acanthosis nigricans
- ◦ Hereditary gingival fibromatosis
- ◦ Hurler's syndrome
- ◦ Zimmermann-Laband syndrome
- ◦ Lipoid proteinosis
- ◦ Drug-induced overgrowth
  - - Phenytoin
  - - Calcium channel blockers
  - - Cyclosporine
  - - Monoclonal antibodies

10. Bone swellings
- • Torus mandibularis
- • Torus palatinus
- • Multiple exostoses
- • Osteoma
- • Fibrous dysplasia
- • Central giant cell granuloma
- • Cherubism
- • Paget's disease
- • Gardner's syndrome
- • Melanotic neuroectodermal tumor of infancy
- • Langerhans' cell histiocytosis
- • Intraosseous hemangioma
- • Odontogenic cysts
- • Odontogenic tumors
- • Osteosarcoma
- • Chondrosarcoma
- • Multiple myeloma
- • Burkitt's sarcoma
- • Ewing's sarcoma
- • Metastatic neoplasms on the jaws

II. Color Changes

1. White lesions
- • **Attached to the oral mucosa**
  - ◦ Leukoplakia
  - ◦ Hairy leukoplakia
  - ◦ Cinnamon contact stomatitis
  - ◦ Uremic stomatitis
  - ◦ Chronic mechanical irritation
  - ◦ Chronic biting
  - ◦ Linea alba
  - ◦ Chemical burns
  - ◦ Leukoedema
  - ◦ Fordyce's granules

- ◦ Nicotine stomatitis
- ◦ Cigarette smoker's lip lesions
- ◦ Tobacco pouch keratosis
- ◦ Chronic hyperplastic candidiasis
- ◦ Lichen planus
- ◦ Lichenoid reactions
- ◦ Submucous fibrosis
- ◦ White-coated tongue
- ◦ Geographic tongue and stomatitis
- ◦ Discoid lupus erythematosus
- ◦ Oral psoriasis
- ◦ Ichthyosis hystrix
- ◦ Atrophic glossitis in late syphilis
- ◦ Skin and mucosal grafts
- ◦ Mucosal horn
- ◦ Fibrous histiocytoma
- ◦ Papilloma
- ◦ Verrucous hyperplasia
- ◦ Verrucous carcinoma
- ◦ Squamous cell carcinoma
- ◦ White sponge nevus
- ◦ Dyskeratosis congenita
- ◦ Pachyonychia congenita
- ◦ Focal palmoplantar and oral mucosa hyperkeratosis syndrome
- ◦ Hereditary benign intraepithelial dyskeratosis
- ◦ Darier's disease
- ◦ Myelodysplastic syndromes

- • **Scraped off from the oral mucosa**
  - ◦ Material alba
  - ◦ White-coated tongue
  - ◦ Candidiasis, pseudomembranous
  - ◦ Thermal burns
  - ◦ Epithelial peeling
  - ◦ Cotton roll stomatitis
  - ◦ Chancre of primary syphilis
  - ◦ Mucous patches of secondary syphilis
  - ◦ Secondary pseudomembranes after erosions or ulcerations

2. Red lesions
- • Traumatic erythema
- • Fellatio
- • Cunnilingus
- • Thermal burn
- • Denture stomatitis
- • Radiation-induced mucositis
- • Chemotherapy-induced mucositis
- • Candidiasis, erythematous
- • Linear gingival erythema
- • Gonococcal stomatitis
- • Secondary syphilis

- Streptococcal stomatitis
- Herpetic gingivostomatitis
- Infectious mononucleosis
- Angular cheilitis
- Licking cheilitis and dermatitis
- Geographic stomatitis
- Median rhomboid glossitis
- Desquamative gingivitis
- Plasma cell gingivitis and stomatitis
- Granulomatous gingivitis
- Allergic contact stomatitis
- Cinnamon contact stomatitis
- Erythroplakia
- Squamous cell carcinoma
- Soft tissue plasmacytoma
- Reiter's syndrome
- Peripheral ameloblastoma
- Hemangioma
- Vascular malformations
- Angiolymphoid hyperplasia with eosinophilia
- Leiomyoma
- Granular cell tumor
- Hereditary hemorrhagic telangiectasia
- Sturge-Weber syndrome
- Klippel-Trenaunay-Weber syndrome
- Maffucci's syndrome
- Thrombocytopenic purpura
- Leukemias
- Aplastic anemia
- Cyclic neutropenia
- Thrombocytopenia
- Plasminogen deficiency
- von Willebrand's disease
- Myelodysplastic syndrome
- Lupus erythematosus
- CREST syndrome
- Anemias
- Porphyrias
- Vitamin B deficiency

3. **White and red lesions**
   - Speckled leukoplakia
   - Nicotine stomatitis
   - Chemical burns
   - Candidiasis
   - Geographic tongue
   - Cinnamon contact stomatitis
   - Lichen planus
   - Lupus erythematosus
   - Oral psoriasis
   - Reiter's syndrome
   - Scarlet fever

- Syphilis
- Actinic cheilitis
- Verruciform xanthoma
- Myelodysplastic syndromes

4. **Black and Brown lesions**
   - Racial pigmentation
   - Drug-induced pigmentation
   - Smoker's melanosis
   - Black and brown hairy tongue
   - Lentigo simplex
   - Freckles
   - Melanocytic nevus
   - Nevus of Ota
   - Nevus of Spitz
   - Oral melanoacanthoma
   - Lentigo maligna
   - Malignant melanoma
   - Addison's disease
   - Peutz-Jeghers syndrome
   - Albright's syndrome
   - Neurofibromatosis, type I
   - Amalgam tattoo
   - Graphite deposition
   - Heavy metal deposition
     - Bismuth
     - Lead
     - Silver
   - Black or brown foreign material
   - Acanthosis nigricans
   - Varicoses
   - Ecchymoses
   - Hemochromatosis
   - Kaposi's sarcoma
   - Eruption cyst

5. **Yellow lesions**
   - Fordyce's granules
   - Superficial abscess
   - Xanthomas
   - Verruciform xanthoma
   - Lipoma
   - Lymphoid aggregate
   - Lymphoepithelial cyst
   - Dermoid cyst
   - Epidermoid cyst
   - Gingival cyst of the newborn
   - Hypercarotenemia
   - Jaundice
   - Pyostomatitis vegetans
   - Molluscum contagiosum
   - Hairy tongue

Biopsy

Biopsy is the minor surgical procedure of obtaining tissue from a lesion for microscopic observation and recording of cellular and tissue abnormalities. Histopathologic examination of a lesion is an effective laboratory aid in diagnosis and appropriate treatment of the underlying disease.

Clinical practitioners are required to possess the knowledge and clinical expertise to make a clinical diagnosis based on grouping and differential diagnosis. Histopathology will confirm or reject the working clinical diagnostic hypothesis.

In conclusion, biopsy and histopathologic examination of tissue samples, are not "magic diagnostic bullets" but useful tools in the hands of an experienced clinician. A clinicopathologic correlation is the hallmark in order to arrive at the most likely diagnosis.

Indications for Biopsy

The main indications for performing a biopsy of oral lesions are as follows:

- Precancerous lesions to determine the risk of progression to malignancy.
- Lesions clinically suspicious for malignancy.
- Ulcers persisting for more than 10 days, after removal possible of trauma.
- Blistering and bullous lesions, persisting for more than a week.
- Any tumorous persistent lesion without a firm clinical diagnosis.
- Any lesion that persists in spite of appropriate therapy.
- Any clinically undiagnosed lesion.

Contradiction to Biopsy

- Patients on anticoagulant therapy.
- Patients with hematologic disorders such as neutropenias, thrombocytopenias, leukemia etc.
- Patients on severe immunosuppression.
- Lesions suspicious for melanoma.
- Hemangiomas and other vascular dysplasias.

In all of the above cases, biopsy should be performed by experts with considerable clinical and surgical experience, preferably in an inpatient basis.

Biopsy is a small scale surgical procedure. The dentist or doctor who performs this procedure must be familiar with basic surgical techniques. Mild manipulations during the procedure constitute a fundamental principle to minimize the risk of dispersion and seeding of malignant cells. It goes without saying that good knowledge of oral medicine is a must, so that the dentist or doctor performing the biopsy knows the underlying substrate of the lesion. *A good clinician is she/he whose clinical diagnosis is confirmed by biopsy.*

Common Errors in Performing a Biopsy

- The disease is at a phase that is unlikely to yield diagnostic material.
- Erroneous choice of the location for tissue sampling, particularly in extensive or multiple lesions.
- Alteration or destruction of the biopsy material due to vigorous or awkward manipulations during the procedure.
- Insufficient or nonrepresentative tissue sample.
- Obtaining a sample using cautery or electrodissection or laser.
- Inappropriate fixation.
- Providing insufficient clinical information in the accompanying document to the histopathology laboratory.

Choosing the Site of Biopsy

The choice of the site to biopsy is of vital importance and requires good knowledge of oral medicine. **Table A.1** summarizes the optimal sites to biopsy in relation to the type of lesion.

Table A.1 Choice of the site to biopsy

Type of lesion	Optimal site
Tumor	Thickest, hardest part
Ulcer	Peripheral edge of the ulcer
Vesicle or bulla	Periphery of the lesion, including neighboring healthy tissue
Plaque	One or multiple suspicious sites
Small lesions < 1 mm in diameter	Total excision including healthy tissue (2–4 mm)

Basic Equipment

- Local anesthetic
- Syringe with attached needle
- Needle holder
- Forceps and lancet
- Needle forceps
- Thin surgical forceps
- Hemostatic clamp
- Vessel clamps
- Suture scissors
- Atraumatic sutures
- Gauzes
- Hemostatic sponge
- Suction tip
- Cautery

Types of Biopsies

a. Incisional biopsy

Incisional biopsy is the most common type of biopsy. It is indicated whenever the lesion is greater than 1 cm in diameter.

It is the procedure of choice whenever the clinical suspects a malignancy.

If the lesion is greater than 2 cm in diameter, two or more samples are obtained to ensure good representation of the lesion.

Usually a wedge-shaped or oval incision 4 × 6 mm is performed making sure that neighboring, clinically healthy tissue is included in the sample (**Figs. A.1–A.5**).

Special care is required when sampling bullous lesions. The size of biopsy should be at the edge of the lesion and should measure approximately 6 mm (**Figs. A.6–A.8**).

On completion of the incisional biopsy the wound is closed with atraumatic sutures.

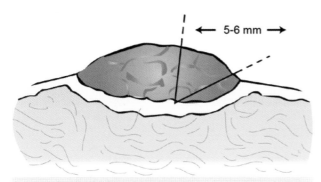

Fig. A.1 Schematic incisional biopsy from single location.

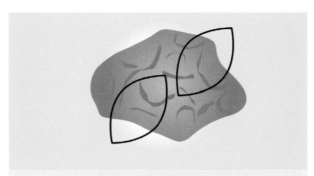

Fig. A.2 Schematic incisional biopsy from two locations.

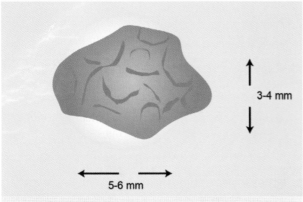

Fig. A.3 Schematic incisional biopsy, sample dimensions.

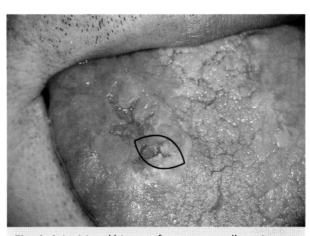

Fig. A.4 Incisional biopsy of squamous cell carcinoma.

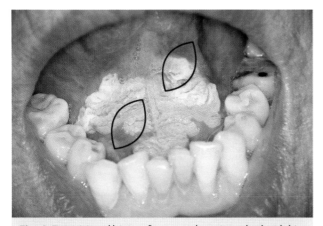

Fig. A.5 Incisional biopsy from two locations, leukoplakia.

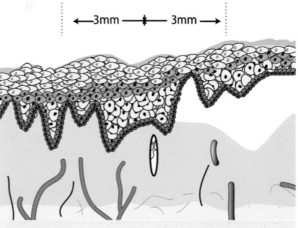

Fig. A.6 Schematic incisional biopsy, pemphigoid.

677

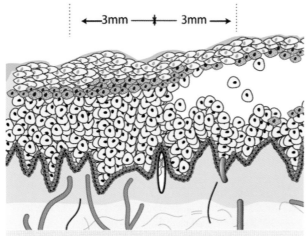

Fig. A.7 Schematic incisional biopsy, pemphigus.

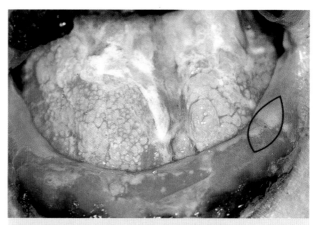

Fig. A.8 Incisional biopsy, pemphigus.

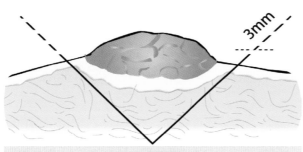

Fig. A.9 Schematic excisional biopsy, vertical incision of the lesion.

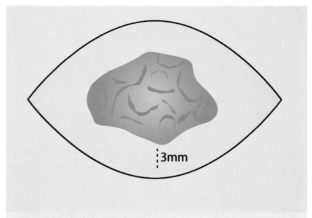

Fig. A.10 Schematic excisional biopsy, border of excision.

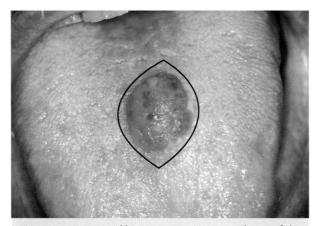

Fig. A.11 Excisional biopsy, pyogenic granuloma of the dorsum of the tongue.

b. Excisional biopsy

Excisional biopsy is the second common type of biopsy. It is indicated whenever the lesion is less than 1 cm in diameter.

Local anesthesia should be used at a distance of approximately 5 mm away from the lesion and never in the lesion. The entire lesion including a rim of adjacent normal tissue (3–4 mm) should be removed (**Figs. A.9–A.11**).

Oftentimes, when dealing with benign lesions, excisional biopsy is therapeutic.

c. Other types of biopsies

Specialized types of biopsies include **punch biopsy** (indicated in skin lesions), **scissors biopsy** (mainly skin diseases), and **fine-needle aspiration biopsy** (indicated in salivary gland lesions and enlarged lymph nodes).

Because of the specialized character of these types of biopsies, they should be performed by specialists and will not be described in this volume.

On conclusion of the excision, the specimens are placed in vials containing buffered formalin 10%. The mount of the fixing solution should be 10 times the volume of the specimen. The name and age of the patient are recorded on the vial label.

The clinician, then fills out the accompanying form that will be sent to the pathology laboratory.

The form includes the following information:

- The patient's last and first name
- Age and sex
- Site of the biopsy
- Type of biopsy

- Duration of the lesion
- Number of lesions
- Presence of lesions in other organS
- Working clinical diagnosis

The last item is the most important in the list.

The pathology report should be back within 4–6 days. The pathology laboratory should be led by a competent pathologist having excellent grasp of the pathology of the mouth and not by nonspecialists possessing only general empirical knowledge of histopathology.

The pathology report is then evaluated by the clinician in relation to the clinical picture, bearing in mind that the findings reflect the site of biopsy taken and a moment in the natural course of the disease and are not permanent.

The bottom line is that the clinician bears the ultimate responsibility for interpreting the whole body of evidence not just the pathology report and taking appropriate action.

The two pillars of medical practice are (1) diagnosis and (2) therapy. Both require a skilled physician with sound scientific background, experience, and the ability to make timely decisions and take decisive action.

In **Tables A.2–A.4** the reader may find a few more useful facts and instructions concerning biopsies.

Table A.2 Types of fixation media for different kinds of examination of biopsy specimens

Type of examination	Fixation medium
Histopathology	10% formalin
Direct immunofluorescence	Fresh tissue on gauze soaked in normal saline, fresh tissue on Michel's medium
Immunoperoxidase method	Formalin-fixed or fresh tissue
Molecular studies	Formalin-fixed tissue or specialized handling depending on the study
Electron microscopy	Glutaraldehyde

Table A.3 Important aspects of the patient's history before carrying out a biopsy

- Allergic reactions (known reactions to local anesthetics)
- Medications
- History of endocarditis, diseases affecting the cardiac valves
- History of orthopedic operations and replacement of joints
- Hypertension or hypotension
- Uncontrolled diabetes mellitus
- Primary and secondary immune deficiencies
- Hematologic malignancies
- Possible pregnancy in women of reproductive age
- History of adrenal insufficiency

Table A.4 Considerations for chemoprophylaxis before biopsy

- Patients with a history of endocarditis
- Patients with valvulopathies or artificial heart valves
- Patients with a history of major orthopedic operations
- Patients on intense immunosuppression
- Patients with uncontrolled hematologic malignancies

Index

Page numbers in *italics* refer to illustrations; those in **bold** refer to tables

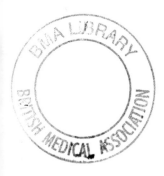